The Final FFICM Structured Oral Examination Study Guide

This book is the definitive guide to the Final Fellowship of the Faculty of Intensive Care Medicine (FFICM) Structured Oral Examination. With a broad coverage of the clinical curriculum, it equips candidates to tackle this challenging examination. Each chapter contains sample questions with concise answers, focusing on key concepts to facilitate deeper understanding. The content is organised by subject, enabling more structured revision in an easy-to-use format. This text provides references to guidance that will remain relevant in the ever-changing landscape of intensive care medicine. Not only is this book an essential resource for studying intensivists but it also forms a useful reference for any professional encountering the world of critical care in their practice.

Eryl Davies is a dual trainee in Intensive Care Medicine and Anaesthesia. She is based in the North West of England and holds a postgraduate qualification in medical education. Her experiences with the FFICM, FRCA, and MRCP examinations have allowed her to tailor this study guide to the FFICM candidate.

The Final FFICM Structured Oral Examination Study Guide

Edited by
Eryl Davies BSc (Hons) MBChB PGCert FRCA FFICM
Manchester, UK

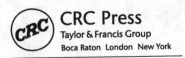

CRC Press
Taylor & Francis Group
Boca Raton London New York

CRC Press is an imprint of the
Taylor & Francis Group, an **informa** business

First edition published 2023
by CRC Press
6000 Broken Sound Parkway NW, Suite 300, Boca Raton, FL 33487-2742

and by CRC Press
4 Park Square, Milton Park, Abingdon, Oxon, OX14 4RN

CRC Press is an imprint of Taylor & Francis Group, LLC

© 2023 Taylor & Francis Group, LLC

ISBN: 9781032153421 (hbk)
ISBN: 9781032114590 (pbk)
ISBN: 9781003243694 (ebk)

DOI: 10.1201/9781003243694

Typeset in Minion Pro
by KnowledgeWorks Global Ltd.

To Aleksandr, who told me to dedicate this to myself.

To Alys, Hee Yen and Elgan. Blood is thicker than Hartmann's.

CONTENTS

SECTION 3: On the ICU

SECTION 4: Toxicology

SECTION 5: Airway

SECTION 6: Resuscitation

SECTION 7: Surgery

SECTION 8: Cardiothoracics

SECTION 9: Neurosciences

SECTION 10: Obstetrics

SECTION 11: Paediatrics

SECTION 12: Microbiology

SECTION 13: Medicine

SECTION 14: Palliative Care

FOREWORD

Postgraduate exams ensure the consultants of the future are trained and assessed to a very high standard. Specialty trainees devote a lot of time and energy in preparation for their exams, on top of their clinical commitments and shift work. Passing the Fellowship of the Faculty of Intensive Care Medicine is a major career high and should be celebrated when achieved.

The curriculum is wide, and the examinations test the whole curriculum. A resource such as this book assists candidates to pass the exams – it draws from experts in many fields and covers the entire curriculum. The author and team have spent a lot of time bringing new resources together and have ended up with, in my opinion, a first-class textbook filling a gap in the market.

As it is common for Intensive Care Medicine trainees to dual train, they often have more than one set of postgraduate examinations to pass. It is therefore especially worthwhile to have high-quality revision texts to help with these exams.

I hope you all enjoy reading this book – I certainly have and I wish you good luck for your careers.

Dr Liz Thomas

Consultant in Anaesthesia and Intensive Care Medicine
Stockport NHS Foundation Trust
Joint Medical Lead, Greater Manchester Critical Care Network

Intensive Care Medicine is a dynamic and exciting specialty, undergoing constant change. The Final Fellowship of the Faculty of Intensive Care Medicine examinations may seem daunting in this context.

This book was written through the lens of dual training in Anaesthesia alongside Intensive Care Medicine. My own preparation inspired me to create a resource that would facilitate focused study in key areas of the curriculum, whilst promoting an awareness of landmark research and best practice within the specialty.

The authors have drawn upon valuable clinical experience and knowledge of the curriculum to anticipate potential topics for discussion. We hope that the breadth of the subject matter will enable candidates to feel confident in their examinations.

The Final FFICM Structured Oral Examination Study Guide provides coverage of the Intensive Care Medicine curriculum whilst aiming to promote a deeper conceptual understanding. Appendices containing over 200 key trials and clinical guidelines should remain useful resources for years to come. I hope this text appeals to all clinicians working in critical care environments, including allied professionals and partner specialties.

Many complementary resources exist for this examination including not only books but also online pages, with a substantial contribution in the form of FOAMed. I would like to thank their creators for furthering my understanding of the specialty.

Writing this book would not have been possible without my co-authors and reviewers and the people I've spoken to along the way. I am lucky to have such wise friends, family, and colleagues. Learning from you all has been a joy. Once again, thank you.

Finally, good luck! I hope that reading *The Final FFICM Structured Oral Examination Study Guide* proves useful, and even enjoyable, and helps you to understand your critical care practice for the better.

Eryl Davies

Ozerah Choudhry MBChB MRCP (UK) FFICM PGCert
Consultant in Intensive Care Medicine
Northern Care Alliance NHS Foundation Trust, Salford, UK

Jessica Davis BSc MBChB FRCA FFICM
Consultant in Intensive Care Medicine and Anaesthesia
Bolton NHS Foundation Trust, Bolton, UK

Samuel Ford MBChB (Dist) MRCEM FFICM
Specialty Trainee in Intensive Care Medicine
Health Education England North West, Manchester, UK

Nina Hjelde BSc (Hons) MBChB (Hons) FRCA EDIC FFICM
Specialty Trainee in Intensive Care Medicine and Anaesthesia
Health Education England North West, Manchester, UK

Claire Knapp BSc (Hons) MBChB FRCA
Specialty Trainee in Anaesthesia
Health Education England North West, Manchester, UK

Katherine Phillips MBChB (Dist) FRCA FFICM
Specialty Trainee in Intensive Care Medicine and Anaesthesia
Health Education England North West, Manchester, UK

ACKNOWLEDGEMENTS

Mohammed Al-Hayali MBChB MRCP (UK)
Specialty Trainee in Endocrinology and Diabetes, Health Education England North West, Manchester, UK

Andrea Au BM BSc MRCP
Clinical Fellow in Gastroenterology, Manchester University Hospitals NHS Foundation Trust, Manchester, UK

Anandh Balu BSc MBChB FRCA FFICM
Specialty Trainee in Intensive Care Medicine and Anaesthesia, Health Education England West Midlands, Birmingham, UK

Kailash Bhatia FRCA EDRA DNB DA
Consultant in Anaesthesia, Manchester University NHS Foundation Trust, University of Manchester, Manchester, UK

Miguel Garcia MBChB MSc Internal Medicine FRCA FFICM EDIC
Consultant in Cardiothoracic Anaesthesia and ECMO, ECMO lead, Manchester University NHS Foundation Trust, Manchester, UK

James Hanison BSc MBChB FRCA FFICM
Consultant in Anaesthesia and Intensive Care Medicine; Clinical Director for Adult Critical Care (Oxford Road Campus), Manchester University NHS Foundation Trust, Manchester, UK

Gan Hanumanthu MBChB FRCA FFICM
Consultant in Intensive Care Medicine and Anaesthesia, St Helens and Knowsley Teaching Hospitals NHS Trust, Whiston, UK

Daniel Horner BA MBBS MD PGCert MRCP (UK) FRCEM FFICM
Consultant in Emergency Medicine and Intensive Care, Northern Care Alliance NHS Foundation Trust, Salford, UK; Thrombosis/Anticoagulation Committee Chair, VTE Exemplar Centre, Greater Manchester, UK; Specialty Research Lead for Trauma and Emergency Care NIHR CRN, Greater Manchester, UK

Elfateh Ibrahim MBBS
Specialty Trainee in Intensive Care Medicine, Health Education England North West, Manchester, UK

Brendan A McGrath MBChB FRCP FRCA EDIC DICM FFICM MAcadMEd AHEA HonFRCSLT PhD
Consultant in Anaesthesia and Intensive Care Medicine, Wythenshawe Hospital, Wythenshawe, UK; Honorary Senior Lecturer, University of Manchester, Manchester, UK; Difficult Airway Society Professor of Anaesthesia and Airway Management, London, UK

Sayyid M Ammar Raza MBChB MRCP PhD
Renal Academic Clinical Lecturer, University of Manchester, Manchester, UK

Reuben Roy MBChB MRes (Dis) MRCP
Research Fellow in Intensive Care and Renal Medicine, University of Manchester, Manchester, UK

Sarah Stirling MBChB MRCP FRCA FFICM
Consultant in Cardiothoracic Intensive Care Medicine and Anaesthesia, Wythenshawe Hospital, Manchester, UK

Richard Templeton BSc MBBS FRCA FFICM
Consultant in Cardiothoracic Critical Care, Anaesthesia and ECMO, Wythenshawe Hospital, Manchester, UK

Stephanie Thomas BSc (Hons) MBChB MSc DTM&H FRCPath PGCert (Med Ed)
Consultant in Medical Microbiology, Manchester University NHS Foundation Trust, Manchester, UK

Ann Tivey MBBS MRCP

Academic Clinical Fellow in Medical Oncology, Health Education England North West, Manchester, UK

Tammy Towers MBChB MPH MRCP (UK)

Specialty Trainee in Intensive Care Medicine and Respiratory Medicine, Health Education and Improvement Wales, Cardiff, UK

Robert WM Walker MBChB FRCA

Consultant in Paediatric Anaesthesia and Intensive Care, Royal Manchester Children's Hospital, Manchester, UK

5-ASA	5-Aminosalicylic acid	AIS	Abbreviated Injury Scale
5-HT	5-Hydroxytryptamine	AKD	Acute kidney disease
6MWT	6-min walk test	AKI	Acute kidney injury
βhCG	Beta human chorionic gonadotrophin	ALA	Aminolaevulinic acid
		ALF	Acute liver failure
AAA	Abdominal aortic aneurysm	ALL	Acute lymphoblastic leukaemia
AAV	ANCA-associated vasculitidies	ALP	Alkaline phosphatase
ABG	Arterial blood gas	ALS	Advanced Life Support
ABSCM	Anterior border of sternocleidomastoid	ALT	Alanine transaminase
		AMAN	Acute motor axonal neuropathy
AC	Alternating current	AML	Acute myeloid leukaemia
ACC	American College of Cardiology	AMSAN	Acute motor sensory axonal neuropathy
ACCP	Advanced critical care practitioner	ANA	Antinuclear antibodies
		ANC	Acute necrotic collection
ACE2	Angiotensin-converting enzyme 2	ANCA	Anti-neutrophil cytoplasm antibodies
ACE-I	Angiotensin-converting enzyme inhibitor	ANP	Atrial natriuretic peptide
		ANTT	Aseptic non-touch technique
ACh	Acetylcholine	ANZROD	Australia and New Zealand Risk of Death
ACHD	Adult congenital heart disease		
AChR	Acetylcholine receptor	AoA	Association of Anaesthetists
ACLF	Acute-on-chronic liver failure	AoMRC	Academy of Medical Royal Colleges
ACLS	Advanced Cardiac Life Support		
ACR	Albumin-to-creatinine ratio	APACHE	Acute Physiology and Chronic Health Evaluation
ACS	Acute coronary syndrome		
ACTH	Adrenocorticotropic hormone	APH	Antepartum haemorrhage
ADEM	Acute disseminated encephalomyelitis	APLS	Advanced Paediatric Life Support
ADH	Antidiuretic hormone	APML	Acute promyelocytic leukaemia
ADL	Activities of daily living	APRV	Airway pressure release ventilation
ADMA	Asymmetric dimethyl arginine		
ADR	Alpha-delta ratio	APTT	Activated partial thromboplastin time
AED	Anti-epileptic drugs		
AF	Atrial fibrillation	ARB	Angiotensin receptor blocker
AFB	Acid-fast bacilli	ARDS	Acute respiratory distress syndrome
AFE	Amniotic fluid embolism		
AFLP	Acute fatty liver of pregnancy	ARNI	Angiotensin receptor neurolysin inhibitor
AGEP	Acute generalised exanthematous pustulosis		
		ARVC	Arrhythmogenic right ventricular cardiomyopathy
AGP	Aerosol-generating procedure		
AHA	American Heart Association	AST	Aspartate aminotransferase
AHI	Apnoea/Hypopnoea Index	ASIA	American Spinal Injury Association
AIDP	Acute inflammatory demyelinating polyneuropathy		
		ASOT	Anti-streptolysin titre
AIDS	Acquired immunodeficiency syndrome	ASV	Adaptive support ventilation
		ATP	Adenosine triphosphate
AIHA	Autoimmune haemolytic anaemia	ATS	American Thoracic Society
		AUC	Area under curve
AIP	Acute interstitial pneumonia		

AUROC	Area under the receiver operating characteristic curve
AV	Atrioventricular
AV-ECMO	Arterio-venous ECMO
BAL	Bronchoalveolar lavage
BBB	Bundle branch block
BCNIE	Blood culture-negative infective endocarditis
BHB	Beta-hydroxybutyrate
BHIVA	British HIV Association
BiPAP	Bilevel positive airway pressure
BISAP	Bedside Index of Severity of Acute Pancreatitis
BiVAD	Biventricular assist device
BLS	Basic Life Support
BM	Boehringer Mannheim (blood glucose measurement)
BMA	British Medical Associations
BMI	Body mass index
BMR	Basal metabolic rate
BNP	Brain natriuretic peptide
BP	Blood pressure
BSA	Body surface area
BSG	British Society of Gastroenterology
BSH	British Society for Haematology
BSI	Blood stream infection
BTF	Brain Trauma Foundation
BTS	British Thoracic Society
CABG	Coronary artery bypass graft(s)
CAM-ICU	Confusion Assessment Method for ICU
cAMP	Cyclic adenosine monophosphate
CANH	Clinically assisted nutrition and hydration
CAP	Community-acquired pneumonia
CAPA	COVID-19-associated pulmonary aspergillosis
CAR-T	Chimeric antigen receptor T-cell
CAT	COPD Assessment Test
CAUTI	Catheter-associated UTI
CBF	Cerebral blood flow
CBRNE	Chemical, biological, radiological, nuclear, and explosives
CCC	Citrate-calcium complexes
CCF	Congestive cardiac failure
CDC	Centers for Disease Control
CDI	*Clostridium difficile* infection
CDT	*Clostridium difficile* toxin B
cEEG	Continuous EEG
CFS	Clinical Frailty Scale
CFTR	Cystic fibrosis transmembrane conductance regulator
CICO	Can't intubate, can't oxygenate
CIDP	Chronic inflammatory demyelinating polyneuropathy

CIM	Critical illness myopathy
CIP	Critical illness polyneuropathy
CIPNM	Critical illness polyneuromyopathy
CIRCI	Critical illness-related corticosteroid insufficiency
CJD	Creutzfeldt-Jakob disease
CK	Creatine kinase
CKD	Chronic kidney disease
CLABSI	Central line-associated blood stream infection
CLL	Chronic lymphocytic leukaemia
CMAP	Compound muscle action potential
CMD	Cerebral microdialysis
CMR	Cerebral metabolic rate
$CMRO_2$	Cerebral metabolic rate of oxygen
CMV	Cytomegalovirus
CNS	Central nervous system
COMT	Catechol-O-methyltransferase
COP	Cryptogenic organising pneumonia
COPD	Chronic obstructive pulmonary disease
COVID	COronaVIrus Disease
CPAP	Continuous positive airway pressure
CPB	Cardiopulmonary bypass
CPC	Cerebral Performance Category
CPIS	Clinical Pulmonary Infection Score
CPR	Cardiopulmonary resuscitation
CPP	Cerebral perfusion pressure
CR	Capillary refill
CRBSI	Catheter-related blood stream infection
CRH	Corticotropin-releasing hormone
CRMP5	Collapsing response mediator protein 5
CRP	C-reactive protein
CRRT	Continuous RRT
CRS	Cytokine release syndrome
CRS-R	Coma Recovery Scale – Revised
CRT	Cardiac resynchronisation therapy
CRT-D	Cardiac resynchronisation therapy with defibrillator
CRT-P	Cardiac resynchronisation therapy with pacemaker
CS	Cardiogenic shock
CSA	Central sleep apnoea
CSF	Cerebrospinal fluid
CSWS	Cerebral salt-wasting syndrome
CPE	Carbapenemase-producing *Enterobacteriaceae*
CT	Computed tomography
CTG	Cardiotocography
CTEPH	Chronic thromboembolic pulmonary hypertension

CTPA	CT pulmonary angiography	ECCO$_2$R	Extracorporeal carbon dioxide removal
CVA	Cerebrovascular accident	ECG	Electrocardiogram
CVC	Central venous catheter	Echo	Echocardiography
CVP	Central venous pressure	ECLS	Extracorporeal life support
CVST	Cerebral venous sinus thrombosis	ECMO	Extracorporeal membrane oxygenation
CVVH	Continuous veno-venous haemofiltration	ECOG	Eastern Cooperative Oncology Group
CVVHD	Continuous veno-venous haemodialysis	EDH	Extradural haematoma
CVVHDF	Continuous veno-venous haemodiafiltration	EDTA	Ethylenediaminetetraacetic acid
		EE	Energy expenditure
CXR	Chest X-ray	EEG	Electroencephalogram
DAMP	Damage-associated molecular pattern	EGDT	Early goal-directed therapy
DAPT	Dual antiplatelet therapy	eGFR	Estimated glomerular filtration rate
DAS	Difficult Airway Society	EGPA	Eosinophilic granulomatosis with polyangiitis
DBC	Detriment-Based Classification of acute pancreatitis severity	EGRIS	Erasmus GBS Respiratory Insufficiency Score
DBD	Donation after brain stem death	ELISA	Enzyme-linked immunosorbent assay
DC	Direct current		
DCCV	DC cardioversion	EMG	Electromyography
DCD	Donation after circulatory death	EN	Enteral nutrition
DCI	Delayed cerebral ischaemia	ENT	Ear, nose, and throat
DCM	Dilated cardiomyopathy	EPAP	Expiratory positive airway pressure
DDAVP	1-Desamino-8-d-arginine vasopressin	ERAS	Enhanced Recovery After Surgery
DIC	Disseminated intravascular coagulation	ERC	European Resuscitation Council
DIEP	Deep inferior epigastric perforator	ERCP	Endoscopic retrograde cholangiopancreatography
DIP	Desquamative interstitial pneumonia	ERS	European Respiratory Society
DKA	Diabetic ketoacidosis	ESBL	Extended-spectrum beta-lactamase-producing organism
DLBCL	Diffuse large B-cell lymphoma		
DMARDs	Disease-modifying anti-rheumatic drugs	ESC	European Society of Cardiology
DMSA	Dimercaptosuccinic acid	ESH	European Society of Hypertension
DNA	Deoxyribonucleic acid		
DOAC	Direct oral anticoagulant	ESICM	European Society of Intensive Care Medicine
DOLS	Deprivation of liberty safeguards		
DOPA	Dihydroxyphenylalanine	ESMO	European Society for Medical Oncology
DPP	Direct procurement and machine perfusion	ESPEN	European Society for Clinical Nutrition and Metabolism
DRESS	Drug reaction with eosinophilia and systemic symptoms	ESR	Erythrocyte sedimentation rate
		ESRF	End-stage renal failure
DSA	Digital subtraction angiography	E$_t$CO$_2$	End-tidal carbon dioxide
E-CPR	Extracorporeal cardiopulmonary resuscitation	EVAR	Endovascular aneurysm repair
		EVD	External ventricular drain
EAA	Extrinsic allergic alveolitis	f	Frequency
EASL	European Association for the Study of the Liver	FAST	Focused assessment with sonography for trauma
EAST	European Association for the Surgery of Trauma	FBC	Full blood count
		FEES	Fiberoptic endoscopic evaluation of swallowing
EBV	Epstein-Barr virus		
ECC	Excitation-contraction coupling	FES	Fat embolism syndrome
ECCO	European Crohn's and Colitis Organisation	FeNO	Fractional exhaled nitric oxide

FEV$_1$	Forced expiratory volume in 1 second	HCM	Hypertrophic cardiomyopathy
FFP	Fresh frozen plasma	Hct	Haematocrit
fHLH	Familial haemophagocytic lymphohistiocytosis	HCV	Hepatitis C virus
		HDU	High-dependency unit
F$_{ET}$O$_2$	Fraction of end-tidal oxygen	HELICS	Hospital in Europe Link for Infection Control through Surveillance
F$_I$O$_2$	Fraction of inspired oxygen		
FICM	Faculty of Intensive Care Medicine	HELLP	Haemolysis, elevated liver enzymes, and low platelets
FLAIR	Fluid attenuated inversion recovery		
FONA	Front of neck airway	HEPA	High-efficiency particulate absorbing
FRC	Functional residual capacity		
FRII	Fixed-rate insulin infusion	HES	Hydroxyethyl starch
FSH	Follicle-stimulating hormone	HF	Heart failure
fullPIERS	Pre-eclampsia Integrated Estimate of RiSk	HFmrEF	Heart failure with mildly reduced ejection fraction
FVC	Forced vital capacity	HFNO	High-flow nasal oxygen
GA	General anaesthesia	HFOV	High-frequency oscillatory ventilation
GABA	Gamma-aminobutyric acid		
GAD	Glutamic acid decarboxylase	HFpEF	Heart failure with preserved ejection fraction
GBL	Gamma butyrolactone		
GBM	Glomerular basement membrane	HFrEF	Heart failure with reduced ejection fraction
GBS	Guillain-Barré syndrome		
G-CSF	Granulocyte colony-stimulating factor	HHS	Hyperosmolar hyperglycaemic state
GCS	Glasgow Coma Scale	HHV	Human herpesvirus
GFR	Glomerular filtration rate	HIET	Hyperinsulinaemic euglycaemia therapy
GH	Growth hormone		
GHB	Gamma-hydroxybutyric acid	HIPA	Heparin-induced platelet activation assay
GHRH	Growth hormone-releasing hormone		
		HIPEC	Hyperthermic intraperitoneal chemotherapy
GI	Gastrointestinal		
GMC	General Medical Council	HIT	Heparin-induced thrombocytopaenia
GnRH	Gonadotropin-releasing hormone		
GOLD	Global Initiative for Chronic Obstructive Lung Disease	HITT	Heparin-induced thrombocytopaenia thrombosis
GOS	Glasgow Outcome Scale	HIV	Human immunodeficiency virus
GOSE	Extended GOS	HLA	Human leukocyte antigen
GP	General practitioner	HLH	Haemophagocytic lymphohistiocytosis
GPA	Granulomatosis with polyangiitis		
		HME	Heat and moisture exchanger
GPICS	Guidelines for the Provision of Intensive Care Services	HMIMMS	Hospital Major Incident Medical Management and Support
GRACE	Global Registry of Acute Coronary Events	HMOD	Hypertension-mediated organ damage
GTN	Glyceryl trinitrate	HOCM	Hypertrophic obstructive cardiomyopathy
GU	Genitourinary		
GvHD	Graft-versus-host disease	HONK	Hyperosmotic non-ketotic coma
HAGMA	High anion gap metabolic acidosis	HR	Heart rate
HAP	Hospital-acquired pneumonia	HRS	Hepatorenal syndrome
HAS	Human albumin solution	HSCT	Haematopoietic stem cell transplantation
HASU	Hyperacute stroke unit		
HAV	Hepatitis A virus	HSP	Henoch-Schönlein purpura
Hb	Haemoglobin	HSV	Herpes simplex virus
HbCO	Carboxyhaemoglobin	HTIg	Human tetanus immunoglobulin
HBV	Hepatitis B virus	HTLV	Human T-lymphotropic virus
HCID	High-consequence infectious disease	HTN	Hypertension
		HTX	Haemothorax

HUS	Haemolytic uraemic syndrome	JAK	Janus kinase
HVPG	Hepatic venous pressure gradient	JBDS-IP	Joint British Diabetes Society for Inpatient Care
IABP	Intra-aortic balloon pump		
IAH	Intra-abdominal hypertension	JPAC	Joint UK Blood Transfusion and Tissue Transplantation Services Professional Advisory Committee
IAP	Intra-abdominal pressure		
IBD	Inflammatory bowel disease		
IBW	Ideal body weight		
ICA	Internal carotid artery	JVP	Jugular venous pulse
ICANS	Immune effector cell-associated neurotoxicity syndrome	KDIGO	Kidney Disease Improving Global Outcomes
ICD	Implantable cardiac defibrillator	LA	Left atrial/atrium
ICH	Intracerebral haemorrhage	LABA	Long-acting beta agonist
ICI	Immune checkpoint inhibitors	LACS	Lacunar syndrome
ICM	Intensive care medicine	LAM	Lymphangioleiomyomatosis
ICNARC	Intensive Care National Audit and Research Centre Model	LAMA	Long-acting muscarinic antagonist
ICP	Intracranial pressure	LBBB	Left bundle branch block
ICS	Intensive Care Society	LDH	Lactate dehydrogenase
ICU	Intensive care unit	LDL	Low density lipoprotein
ICUAW	ICU-acquired weakness	LEMS	Lambert-Eaton myaesthenic syndrome
IE	Infective endocarditis		
I:E	Inspiratory:expiratory ratio	LFT	Liver function tests
IgG	Immunoglobulin G	LGR	Lower good recovery
IHCA	In-hospital cardiac arrest	LH	Luteinising hormone
IHD	Ischaemic heart disease	LMD	Lower moderate disability
IJV	Internal jugular vein	LMWH	Low-molecular-weight heparin
IL	Interleukin	LOC	Loss of consciousness
ILD	Interstitial lung disease	LocSSIP	Local Safety Standards for Invasive Procedures
IM	Intramuscular		
IMCA	Independent mental capacity advocate	LOS	Length of stay
		LP	Lumbar puncture
IMPDH	Inosine-5-monophosphate dehydrogenase	LPR	Lactate to pyruvate ratio
		LPV	Lung-protective ventilation
iNO	Inhaled nitric oxide	LR	Lindegaard ratio
INR	International normalised ratio	LRINEC	Laboratory Risk Indicator for Necrotising Fasciitis
INTERMACS	Interagency Registry for Mechanical Assisted Circulatory Support	LSD	Lower severe disability
		LTOT	Long-term oxygen therapy
IO	Intraosseous	LTRA	Leukotriene receptor antagonist
IOP	Intraocular pressure	LV	Left ventricle/ventricular
IPAP	Inspiratory positive airway pressure	LVAD	Left ventricular assist device
		LVEF	Left ventricular ejection fraction
IPF	Idiopathic pulmonary fibrosis		
IR	Interventional radiology	LVOTO	LV outflow tract obstruction
IRIS	Immune reconstitution inflammatory syndrome	MAC	Minimum alveolar concentration
		MAHA	Microangiopathic haemolytic anaemia
ISFC	International Society and Federation of Cardiology	MAHAT	Microangiopathic haemolytic anaemia and thrombocytopaenia
ISS	Injury Severity Score		
ITP	Immune thrombocytopaenic purpura	MAKE	Major adverse kidney events
		MAO	Monoamine oxidase
IU	International units	MAOI	Monoamine oxidase inhibitor
IV	Intravenous	MAP	Mean arterial pressure
IVAC	Infection-related ventilator-associated condition	MARS	Molecular adsorbent recirculation system
IVC	Inferior vena cava	MAS	Macrophage activation syndrome
IVIg	Intravenous immunoglobulin		

MBRRACE-UK	Mothers and Babies: Reducing Risk through Audits and Confidential Enquiries across the UK
MCS	Minimally conscious state
MC+S	Microscopy, culture, and sensitivities
MCA	Middle cerebral artery
MDMA	3,4-methylenedioxymethamphetamine
MDT	Multidisciplinary team
MDS	Myelodysplastic syndromes
MELAS	Mitochondrial encephalopathy, lactic acidosis, and stroke-like episodes
MELD	Model for End-Stage Liver Disease
MEOWS	Modified Early Obstetric Warning System
MERS	Middle East respiratory syndrome
MH	Malignant hyperthermia
MHRA	Medicines and Healthcare products Regulatory Agency
MI	Myocardial infarction
MIC	Minimum inhibitory concentration
MILS	Manual in-line stabilisation
MINOCA	MI with non-obstructive coronary arteries
MMR	Measles, mumps, and rubella
MND	Motor neurone disease
MODS	Multi-organ dysfunction syndrome
MOH	Major obstetric haemorrhage
MPA	Microscopic polyangiitis
mPaw	Mean airway pressure
MPM	Mortality Prediction Model
MR	Magnetic resonance
MRC	Medical Research Council
MRCP	Magnetic resonance cholangiopancreatography
mRS	Modified Rankin Scale
MRSA	Methicillin-resistant *Staphylococcus aureus*
MS	Multiple sclerosis
MSH	Melanocyte-stimulating hormone
MTC	Major trauma centre
MuSK	Muscle-specific kinase
MUST	Malnutrition Universal Screening Tool
MV	Minute ventilation
NA	Noradrenaline
NAC	N-acetylcysteine
NAP	National Audit Project of the Royal College of Anaesthetists
NAPQI	N-acetyl-p-benzoquinone imine
NAPS	National Acute Porphyria Service
NASH	Non-alcoholic steatohepatitis
NatSSIP	National Safety Standards for Invasive Procedures
NAVA	Neurally assisted ventilatory assist
NBL	Non-directed bronchial lavage
NCEPOD	National Confidential Enquiry into Patient Outcome and Death
NELA	National Emergency Laparotomy Audit
NEWS	National Early Warning Score
NG	Nasogastric
NHL	Non-Hodgkin lymphoma
NHS	National Health Service
NIBP	Non-invasive blood pressure
NICE	National Institute for Health and Care Excellence
NIHSS	National Institutes of Health Stroke Scale
NINDS	National Institute of Neurological Disorders and Stroke
NIRS	Near-infrared spectroscopy
NIV	Non-invasive ventilation
NJ	Nasojejunal
nMAB	Neutralising monoclonal antibody
NMB	Neuromuscular blockade/blocker
NMDA	N-methyl-D-aspartate
NMS	Neuroleptic malignant syndrome
NNRTI	Non-nucleoside/nucleotide reverse transcriptase inhibitor
NNT	Number needed to treat
NPi	Neurologic Pupil index
NPIS	National Poisons Information Service
NPSA	National Patient Safety Agency
NRS	Nutrition Risk Screening
NRTI	Nucleoside/nucleotide reverse transcriptase inhibitor
NSAIDs	Non-steroidal anti-inflammatory drugs
NSE	Neuron-specific enolase
NSIP	Non-specific interstitial pneumonia
NSTE-ACS	Non-ST segment elevation ACS
NSTEMI	Non-ST segment elevation MI
NTIS	Non-thyroidal illness syndrome
NTSP	National Tracheostomy Safety Project
NUTRIC	Nutrition Risk in Critically Ill
NYHA	New York Heart Association
OAA	Obstetric Anaesthetists' Association

OGD	Oesophago-gastro-duodenoscopy	PI	Pulsatility Index
OHCA	Out-of-hospital cardiac arrest	PICC	Peripherally inserted central catheter
OHS	Obesity hypoventilation syndrome	PICS	Post-intensive care syndrome
OI	Opportunistic illness	PICUPS	Post-ICU Presentation Screen
ONSD	Optic nerve sheath diameter	PIM	Paediatric Index of Mortality
OPSI	Overwhelming post-splenectomy infection	PImax	Maximum inspiratory pressure
OSA	Obstructive sleep apnoea	PIMS-TS	Paediatric multisystem inflammatory syndrome temporally associated with SARS-CoV-2
OSAHS	Obstructive sleep apnoea/ hypopnoea syndrome		
OSAS	Obstructive sleep apnoea syndrome	P_{insp}	Inspiratory pressure
		PIP	Peak inspiratory pressure
OT	Occupational Therapy	P_IO_2	Inspired oxygen tension
PA	Pulmonary artery/arterial	PJP	*Pneumocystis jirovecii* pneumonia
PAC	Pulmonary artery catheter		
PACS	Partial anterior circulation syndrome	PlGF	Placental growth factor
		PML	Progressive multifocal leukoencephalopathy
P_aCO_2	Partial pressure of carbon dioxide in arterial blood	PMMC	Pectoralis major myocutaneous
P_aO_2	Partial pressure of oxygen in arterial blood	PN	Parenteral nutrition
		PO	Per os (by mouth)
PADIS	Pain, Agitation/Sedation, Delirium, Immobility, and Sleep disruption	POCS	Posterior circulation syndrome
		PPCI	Primary PCI
		PPCM	Peripartum cardiomyopathy
PAH	Pulmonary arterial hypertension	PPE	Personal protective equipment
PAMP	Pathogen-associated molecular pattern	PPH	Post-partum haemorrhage
		PR	Per rectum
PAWP	Pulmonary artery wedge pressure	PREP-S	Prediction of complications in early-onset pre-eclampsia
PAP	Pulmonary artery pressure	PRES	Posterior reversible encephalopathy syndrome
P_{btO2}	Brain parenchymal oxygen tension		
		PSP	Primary spontaneous pneumothorax
PCA	Patient-controlled analgesia		
PCC	Prothrombin complex concentrate	PT	Prothrombin time
		PTSD	Post-traumatic stress disorder
PCI	Percutaneous coronary intervention	PTX	Pneumothorax
		PVC	Peripheral venous cannula
PCR	Polymerase chain reaction	PVL	Panton-Valentine leukocidin-producing
PCT	Procalcitonin		
PCV	Pressure control ventilation	pVO_2	Mixed venous oxygen tension
PCWP	Pulmonary capillary wedge pressure	PVR	Pulmonary vascular resistance
		qSOFA	Quick Sequential Organ Failure Assessment
PD	Peritoneal dialysis		
PDOC	Prolonged disorder of consciousness	RA	Right atrial/atrium
		RAC	Revised Atlanta Classification
PE	Pulmonary embolism	RAPD	Relative afferent pupillary defect
PEA	Pulseless electrical activity	RAS	Renin-angiotensin system
PEEP	Positive end-expiratory pressure	RASS	Richmond Agitation-Sedation Scale
PEFR	Peak expiratory flow rate		
PERC	PE rule-out criteria	RBBB	Right bundle branch block
PESI	PE Severity Index	RB-ILD	Respiratory bronchiolitis-ILD
P/F	P_aO_2/F_IO_2 ratio	RCA	Right coronary artery
PF4	Platelet factor 4	RCEM	Royal College of Emergency Medicine
PFT	Pulmonary function tests		
PGD	Primary graft dysfunction	RCM	Restrictive cardiomyopathy
PH	Pulmonary hypertension	RCoA	Royal College of Anaesthetists

RCOG	Royal College of Obstetricians and Gynaecologists	SD	Standard deviation
RCP	Royal College of Physicians	SDD	Selective decontamination of the digestive tract
RCPCH	Royal College of Paediatrics and Child Health	SDH	Subdural haematoma
RCT	Randomised controlled trial	sEng	Soluble endoglin
RCVGE	Retrograde cerebral venous gas embolism	sFlt1	Soluble FMS-like tyrosine kinase 1
		SGLT2	Sodium-glucose co-transporter-2
REBOA	Retrograde endovascular balloon occlusion of the aorta	sHLH	Secondary/acquired HLH
		SIADH	Syndrome of inappropriate ADH secretion
RESP	Respiratory ECMO Survival Prediction	SIBICC	Seattle International Brain Injury Consensus Conference
RNA	Ribonucleic acid	SIGN	Scottish Intercollegiate Guidelines Network
ROLE	Recognition of life extinct		
ROS	Reactive oxygen species	SIMV	Synchronised intermittent mandatory ventilation
ROSC	Return of spontaneous circulation		
		SIRS	Systemic inflammatory response syndrome
ROSIER	Recognition Of Stroke In the Emergency Room	SJS	Stevens-Johnson syndrome
ROTEM	Rotational thromboelastometry	SjvO$_2$	Jugular bulb venous oxygen saturation
RPGN	Rapidly progressive glomerulonephritis		
		SLE	Systemic lupus erythematosus
RR	Respiratory rate	SLEDD	Slow low-efficiency daily dialysis
RRT	Renal replacement therapy	SLT	Speech and language therapy
RSBI	Rapid Shallow Breathing Index	SMR	Standardised mortality ratio
RSI	Rapid sequence induction	SNAP	Sensory nerve action potential
RSV	Respiratory syncytial virus	SNARE	Soluble N-ethylmaleimide attachment protein receptor
RUL	Right upper lobe		
RV	Right ventricle/ventricular	SNRI	Selective noradrenaline reuptake inhibitor
RVAD	Right ventricular assist device		
S-PESI	Simplified PESI	SNS	Sympathetic nervous system
SAAG	Serum-ascites albumin gradient	SOFA	Sequential Organ Failure Assessment
SABA	Short-acting beta-2 agonist		
SAH	Subarachnoid haemorrhage	SOL	Space-occupying lesion
S$_a$O$_2$	Arterial oxygen saturation	SOB	Shortness of breath
SAP	Severe acute pancreatitis	SOS	Sinusoidal obstruction syndrome
SARC	Sexual assault referral centre	S$_p$O$_2$	Peripheral oxygen saturation
SAPS	Simplified Acute Physiology Score	SRA	Serotonin release assay
		SSC	Surviving Sepsis Campaign
SARS	Severe acute respiratory syndrome	SSEP	Somatosensory evoked potential
		SSI	Surgical site infection
SARS-CoV-2	Severe acute respiratory syndrome coronavirus 2	SSRI	Selective serotonin receptor antagonists
SBAR	Situation, Background, Assessment, Recommendation	SSP	Secondary spontaneous pneumothorax
SBP	Spontaneous bacterial peritonitis	STE-ACS	ST-segment elevation ACS
SBT	Spontaneous breathing trial	STEMI	ST-segment elevation myocardial infarction
SCA	Subclavian artery		
SCAR	Severe cutaneous adverse reaction	SV	Stroke volume
		ScvO$_2$	Central venous oxygen saturation
SCCM	Society of Critical Care Medicine		
SCORTEN	SCORe of TEN	SvO$_2$	Venous oxygen saturation
SCUF	Slow continuous ultrafiltration	SVR	Systemic vascular resistance
SCV	Subclavian vein	SVT	Supraventricular tachycardia
ScvO$_2$	Central venous oxygen saturation	T2	Transverse relaxation time
		T-RTS	Triage Revised Trauma Score

TA-GvHD	Transfusion-associated graft-versus-host disease	UA	Unstable angina
TACO	Transfusion-associated circulatory overload	UC	Ulcerative colitis
TACS	Total anterior circulation syndrome	UFH	Unfractionated heparin
TAH	Total artificial heart	UGIB	Upper GI bleeding
TA-NRP	Thoraco-abdominal normothermic regional perfusion	UGR	Upper good recovery

TA-GvHD — Transfusion-associated graft-versus-host disease
TACO — Transfusion-associated circulatory overload
TACS — Total anterior circulation syndrome
TAH — Total artificial heart
TA-NRP — Thoraco-abdominal normothermic regional perfusion
TAPVD — Total anomalous pulmonary venous drainage
TARN — Trauma Audit and Research Network
TAVI — Transcatheter aortic valve implantation
TB — Tuberculosis
TBI — Traumatic brain injury
TCA — Tricyclic antidepressants
TCCDS — Transcranial colour-coded duplex sonography
TCD — Transcranial doppler
TEG — Thromboelastography
TEN — Toxic epidermal necrolysis
TEP — Tracheo-oesophageal puncture
TFT — Thyroid function tests
THC — Tetrahydrocannabinol
t_i — Inspiratory time
t-PA — Tissue plasminogen activator
TIA — Transient ischaemic attack
TIPS — Transjugular intrahepatic portosystemic shunt
TIVA — Total intravenous anaesthesia
TLCO — Transfer factor for carbon monoxide
TLS — Tumour lysis syndrome
TMA — Thrombotic microangiopathy
TNF — Tumour necrosis factor
TOE — Transoesophageal echocardiography
TRALI — Transfusion-related acute lung injury
TRAM — Transverse rectus abdominis myocutaneous
TRH — Thyrotropin-releasing hormone
TSH — Thyroid-stimulating hormone
TSS — Toxic shock syndrome
TTE — Transthoracic echocardiography
TTM — Targeted temperature management
TTP — Thrombotic thrombocytopaenic purpura
TURP — Transurethral resection of the prostate
TXA — Tranexamic acid
U&E — Urea and electrolytes

UA — Unstable angina
UC — Ulcerative colitis
UFH — Unfractionated heparin
UGIB — Upper GI bleeding
UGR — Upper good recovery
UK — United Kingdom
UKELD — UK model for End-Stage Liver Disease
UKOSS — UK Obstetric Surveillance System
UK WPAP — UK Working Party on Acute Pancreatitis
UMD — Upper moderate disability
UO — Urine output
US — Ultrasound
USD — Upper severe disability
UTI — Urinary tract infection
VA-ECMO — Veno-arterial ECMO
VAC — Ventilator-associated condition
VAD — Ventricular assist device
VAE — Ventilator-associated event
VAP — Ventilator-associated pneumonia
VBG — Venous blood gas
VBO — Vertebrobasilar occlusion
VC+ — Volume control plus
VCO_2 — Carbon dioxide production
VDRL — Venereal disease research laboratory
VEGF — Vascular endothelial growth factor
VF — Ventricular fibrillation
VGE — Vascular gas embolism
VGKC — Voltage-gated potassium channel
VHA — Viscoelastic haemostatic assay
VITT — Vaccine-induced immune-thrombocytopaenia and thrombosis
VLE — Verification of life extinct
VO_2 — Oxygen consumption
VOC — Variants of concern
VOD — Veno-occlusive disease
VOI — Variants of interest
VRE — Vancomycin-resistant *Enterococcus*
VS — Vegetative state
VSQIP — Vascular Surgery Quality Improvement Project
V/Q — Ventilation/perfusion
VT — Ventricular tachycardia
V_T — Tidal volume
VTE — Venous thromboembolism
VUM — Variants under monitoring
VV-ECMO — Veno-venous ECMO
vWF — von Willebrand factor
VZIg — Varicella zoster immunoglobulin
VZV — Varicella zoster virus
WAO — World Allergy Organization

WBC   White blood cell
WCC   White cell count
WFNS   World Federation of
            Neurosurgical Societies
WHO   World Health Organization
WNV   West Nile virus

WON   Walled-off necrosis
WSACS   World Society of the Abdominal
            Compartment Syndrome
WSES   World Society of Emergency
            Surgery

Welcome to *The Final FFICM Structured Oral Examination Study Guide*.

The SOE is composed of four stations, each including two 7-minute questions. Questions involve a structured analysis of candidates' knowledge in clinical science applied to the practice of Intensive Care Medicine. Scores are allocated by two examiners, ranging through 0 (fail), 1 (borderline), and 2 (pass). The maximum total mark is 32, with the pass mark usually set in the range of 80–85%.

Here you will find a comprehensive bank of practice questions. The curriculum has been reflected in sections arranged by subject area. A broad spectrum of topics has been covered, including management dilemmas, organ support, significant critical care pathologies, emergency care, airway issues, surgery, sub-specialty critical care, medicine, and palliative care. The perspective is one of a critical care clinician rather than looking from the expert approach of our allied specialties.

Focused sections should facilitate deeper learning of clinical concepts whilst highlighting the main similarities and differences between similar or related subjects. To avoid duplication, references to other questions have been incorporated throughout.

Essential subjects have been expanded, requiring the selection of an appropriate number of questions for practical examination practice. The section on 'Organ Support' risks straying into OSCE territory but aims to target understanding primarily. Subject coverage is not exhaustive, and bullet points have been used to suggest memorable structures to some answers rather than verbatim responses. Further reading may be prompted, with some resources suggested below. Material tested in primary examinations is not covered extensively. This does not mean that it won't appear in the Final FFICM SOE. These areas are likely to have been covered extensively elsewhere; their exclusion allows a greater focus on the more advanced clinical issues here.

Key studies and clinical guidelines have been included in boxes. Only basic detail is given, such as important primary and secondary outcomes, and readers are encouraged to read and analyse the original papers critically. References are listed in the appendices, separate to the other resources concluding individual chapters. These appendices may prove useful resources in their own rights and act as a starting point as evidence changes in due course.

The ideal approach to the SOE is very much individual. This book can be read through in continuum, used as a reference for individual queries, or applied during mock testing. Balancing studying with other aspects of life and adequate relaxation is worth consideration. I was taught the value of 'brain rest' a few years ago and have benefitted from incorporating this in my own strategies. Ultimately, hard work is likely to be required and time is arguably the most precious resource. Use it well!

Additional Resources

- Life in the Fast Lane (https://litfl.com)
- The Internet Book of Critical Care (https://emcrit.org/ibcc/toc/)
- The Bottom Line (https://www.thebottomline.org.uk)
- Deranged Physiology (https://derangedphysiology.com)
- Bersten A, Handy JM. Oh's Intensive Care Manual, 8th ed. Amsterdam: Elsevier Limited; 2009.
- Flavin K, Morkane C, Marsh S. Questions for the Final FFICM Structured Oral Examination. Cambridge: Cambridge University Press; 2018.
- Jeyanathan J, Johnson C, Haslam J. Viva and Structured Oral Examinations in Intensive Care Medicine. Shrewsbury: TFM Publishing Ltd; 2018.

ORGANISATIONAL ISSUES

1. PROVISION OF SERVICES

What systems and tools can be adopted to ensure the early recognition and review of a deteriorating patient?

Early detection of deteriorating patients has the potential to improve outcomes. There are many models that may be used to do this. The most common is a rapid response nurse-led team with medical support. All hospitals in the UK must have a standardised approach to detection of deteriorating patients and must use a validated track and trigger early warning score system. The National Early Warning Score 2 (NEWS 2) is recommended.

What is critical care outreach?

Comprehensive critical care outreach is defined as a multidisciplinary organisational approach to ensure safe, equitable, and quality care for all acutely unwell, critically ill, and recovering patients, irrespective of location or pathway. Several core components address National Institute for Health and Care Excellence (NICE) and National Confidential Enquiry into Patient Outcome and Death (NCEPOD) recommendations:

Prepare
- Patient track and trigger
- Rapid response
- Education, training, and support
- Patient safety and clinical governance
- Audit, evaluation, and monitoring of patient outcome and continuing quality care
- Rehabilitation after critical illness
- Enhancing service delivery

What are the different levels of care?

Levels of care are described according to clinical needs, regardless of patient location. These levels should not be used alone to decide staffing requirements. Examples of patient care levels are as follows:

Level 0
- Needs met through normal ward care in an acute hospital

Level 1
- Increased levels of observation/intervention:
  - Basic support of single organ system
  - Recent 'step down'
- Requiring intervention to prevent deterioration
- Needs met with additional advice and support from critical care
- Rehabilitation needs that cannot be met on a standard ward

Level 2

- Increased observation/intervention beyond level 1
- Advanced organ support of 1 system
- Monitoring and support of ≥2 organ systems
- Extended post-op care
- Level 1 support + enhanced nursing for other reason (e.g. severe agitation)

Level 3

- Advanced respiratory monitoring and support
- Advanced support of 2 organ systems
- Level 2 support + delirium and agitation
- Chronic impairment of ≥1 organ system sufficient to restrict activities + support for acute reversible failure of another system

What do you know about the recommended ratios of medical and nursing staff?

Minimum requirements are indicated in national guidelines. This may be higher depending on the complexity of patients on the unit. A key document in UK practice is 'Guidelines for the Provision of Intensive Care Services (GPICS)', from the Faculty of Intensive Care Medicine (FICM) and Intensive Care Society (ICS), with recommendations as follows:

Medical

- Daytime consultant:patient ratio 1:8–1:12
- Daytime resident:patient ratio ≥1:8, higher if providing emergency care outside the unit
- Night-time resident:patient ratio ≥1:8
- All staff on resident rota should have basic airway skills
- 24/7 access to a doctor/advanced critical care practitioner (ACCP) with advanced airway skills
- FICM-associated ACCP with consultant supervision falls within definition of intensive care resident

Nursing

- *Level 3*: registered nurse:patient ratio ≥1:1 for direct care
- *Level 2*: registered nurse:patient ratio ≥1:2 for direct care
- Supernumerary senior registered nurse (units <6 beds may have supernumerary at peak times only)
- *Per additional 10 beds*: additional supernumerary senior registered nurse
- ≤20% temporary staff per shift from outwith the unit

GUIDELINE FICM ICS 2022 GPICS 2.1

Can you describe the key standards surrounding admission to critical care?

- Decision to admit and management plan must be discussed with the duty ICM consultant.
- Time of decision to admit must be documented.
- Unplanned admissions must occur within 4 h of decision.
- Patients must have a clear and documented treatment escalation plan.
- ICM consultant in-person review should occur within 12 h of admission or sooner if clinical state dictates.
- Transfer to other units for non-clinical reasons must be avoided where possible.

Who should attend an ICU ward round?

- There should be a consultant-led ward round twice a day.
- The nurse in charge should be present in person.

How often should allied professionals be involved in patient care?

- Daily input from nursing, microbiology, pharmacy, and physiotherapy teams
- Regular input from dietetics, speech and language therapy (SLT), occupational therapy (OT), and clinical psychology

Can you describe any standards surrounding discharge and ongoing care?

- Patients must have access to a follow-up programme
- Outpatient clinic appointment 2–3 months post-hospital discharge for specific patients
- Discharge to a general ward must occur within 4 h of decision
- Discharge must occur between 07:00 and 21:59
- Standardised handover procedure
- Formalised transfer process
- Structured rehabilitation programme
- Monitor and review causes for unplanned readmissions
- Repatriation must occur within 48 h of decision

2. SCORING SYSTEMS

Can you name some examples of commonly used critical care illness severity scores?

- *APACHE I–IV*: Acute Physiology and Chronic Health Evaluation
- *SAPS I–III*: Simplified Acute Physiology Score
- *MPM I–III*: Mortality Prediction Model
- *SOFA*: Sequential Organ Failure Assessment
- *PIM 1–3*: Paediatric Index of Mortality
- *ICNARC*: Intensive Care National Audit and Research Centre Model
- *ANZROD*: Australia and New Zealand Risk of Death

When are scoring systems used in critical care?

There are 3 main types of scoring systems used for critically ill patients:

- **Illness severity scores** (e.g. SOFA)
- **Outcome prediction models** (e.g. APACHE II–IV)
- **Decision-support tools** (e.g. NEWS)

Physiological scoring systems are designed to assess and monitor outcomes and treatments for service evaluation and research. Of note, the trauma Injury Severity Score (ISS) is anatomical rather than physiological.

Decision-support tools assist professionals to define risk, communicate it, and provide safe effective bedside care.

Describe a disease-specific illness severity score that you have used.

One example is the **Model for End-Stage Liver Disease (MELD)**, which predicts 3-month mortality in patients ≥12 years of age with liver cirrhosis. It utilises the following criteria from serum laboratory values:

- Creatinine
- Bilirubin
- INR
- Sodium

These are entered into a formula to give a score ranging from 6 to 40. Mortality is predicted as below:

- ≤9: 1.9%
- 10–19: 6.0%
- 20–29: 19.6%
- 30–39: 52.6%
- 40: 71.3%

The original version was created to estimate survival in patients undergoing elective transjugular intrahepatic portosystemic shunt (TIPS). It has since been validated to predict short-term mortality in patients with cirrhosis with variceal bleeding, acute alcoholic hepatitis, or undergoing non-transplant surgeries.

What are the limitations of scoring systems?

- *Data accuracy*: errors may generate false scores, significant on individual level
- *Applicability of cohort*: limited use at the bedside for individuals (also due to delayed/serial assessment)
- *Changing predictive ability*: through use in treatment decisions (e.g. withdrawal of life-sustaining treatment in patients with >95% mortality will result in 100% mortality in that group)
- *Score performance*

How would you evaluate a scoring system?

There are 3 relevant core characteristics: discrimination, calibration, and validity. When applied to mortality prediction models:

Discrimination describes how well the model distinguishes between patients who will die and those who will survive. It can be represented by the area under the receiver operating characteristic curve (AUROC) of observed vs predicted mortality. Reasonable discrimination is seen with AUROC >0.7 and excellent >0.9.

Calibration describes how close predicted values are to observed values (i.e. actual mortality rate).

Validity describes how well a model reflects reality. This is important both internally and in external populations. Reducing heterogeneity of populations studied limits generalisability.

Examples are as follows:

- *Discrimination*: APACHE II had a published AUROC of 0.85 and APACHE III 0.90.
- *Calibration*: Baux score (burns mortality) has strong discrimination but poor calibration.
- *Validity*: Quick SOFA (qSOFA) is valid for screening outwith the ICU but has limited validity within critical care.

Can you describe the qSOFA score in more detail?

The qSOFA score was developed to screen patients outwith critical care for greater risk of death from infection. It shows better discrimination than systemic inflammatory response syndrome (SIRS) criteria or SOFA in this context (AUROC 0.81 vs 0.76 and 0.79). It should not be used for diagnosis of sepsis. Serial assessment might be useful. A score ≥2 is deemed high risk (× 3–14 in-hospital mortality). (See Chapter 26 Sepsis)

> **KEY POINT**
>
> In qSOFA, 1 point is given for each of the 3 criteria:
>
> - *Altered mental status*: GCS <15
> - RR ≥22 min^{-1}
> - Systolic BP ≤100 mmHg

How would you use scoring systems in your decisions surrounding admission to critical care?

Caution should be exercised when interpreting scores in the context of a decision to admit to critical care. Critical care scoring systems are often not designed to support these decisions and they are likely to be inaccurate when used on an individual level. Most are calculated with significant time lag from admission, after which critical care interventions will have been instituted, resulting in bias. Disease-specific scores may grade the severity of comorbidities.

The decision should be individualised and incorporate factors other than disease severity and mortality prediction. Factors might include the following: the patient's perception of acceptable quality of life, specific circumstances, ICU-related harm, and the availability and capability of alternative clinical environments (i.e. the potential benefits versus burdens of the proposal).

The ethics surrounding application of predicted values are debatable. No clear mortality cut-off has yet to be deemed acceptable or unacceptable for admission to critical care (and this is unlikely to happen). Caution should be exercised in allowing patients to interpret such information in the context of their own disease.

Mortality prediction tools describe risk or **probabilities for whole populations** but are of limited utility in describing the best course of action for an individual. They provide additional information to a patient-centred decision-making process.

(See Chapter 60 Emergency Laparotomy)

Can you describe a score that is used to monitor service quality?

In the UK, the **standardised mortality ratio (SMR)** is an outcome-based score that is used to compare observed to predicted number of deaths in an ICU. Prediction is based on scoring systems such as APACHE II. SMR >1 implies worse performance than predicted and <1 implies better than predicted.

KEY POINT

SMR = Observed/predicted number of deaths

Limitations of the SMR

- Dependent on coding/data quality, case mix, and clinical factors
- *Does not reflect ICU care alone*: may also be dependent on care prior to admission
- Excludes readmissions ± transfers in/to other critical care units, organ donation, and palliative admission
- Only measures in-hospital deaths

How else might the quality of a critical care service be measured?

Measurement of a structure, process, or outcome can be used to ensure maintenance and improvement of standards of care. These can be described as minimum standards or quality indicators (Table 2.1).

Minimum standards assure a level of care and are linked directly to measurable effects. Quality indicators often have interdependent relationships and are more difficult to change but can help in understanding a system. They may serve as flags or pointers.

Table 2.1   Measures of critical care service quality

	Minimum standards	Quality indicators
Structure	• Participation in national comparative audit • Daily review and written management plan by consultant • Twice-daily ward rounds • Healthcare-associated infection surveillance system	• Nurse staffing and skill levels • Pharmacist in critical care • Physiotherapist in critical care
Process	• Night-time discharges • Care bundles – VAP, CVC, PVC	• Tracheostomy needs assessment • Delirium screening • Rehabilitation assessment • End-of-life care policy
Outcome	• SMR • Early discharges • Morbidity and mortality meetings	• Patient relative/experience surveys

Resources

- Barlow CJ, Pilcher D. Severity scoring and outcome prediction. In: Bersten AD, Handy JM, eds. Oh's Intensive Care Manual, 8th ed. Amsterdam: Elsevier; 2019:19–33.
- Desai N, Gross J. Scoring systems in the critically ill: uses, cautions, and future directions. BJA Educ. 2019;19(7):212–218.
- Kamath PS, Weisner RH, Malinchoc M, et al. A model to predict survival in patients with end-stage liver disease. Hepatology. 2001;33(2):464–470.
- The Scottish Intensive Care Society Quality Improvement Group. Minimum Standards and Quality Indicators for critical care in Scotland, version 3.0. December 2015. Available from: https://www.scottishintensivecare.org.uk/uploads/2015-12-29-14-19-25-QualityIndicatorsBookletW-70202.pdf. (Accessed 20 April 2022.)

3. TRANSPORT OF THE CRITICALLY ILL PATIENT

Why is safe transport of critical care patients important?

Transport of critically ill patients is becoming increasingly common and may be required to access specialist treatment (e.g. tertiary neurosurgery), to repatriate a patient closer to home or to manage capacity during times with significant bed pressures.

Transfers come with risks to patients and staff. Therefore, appropriate training and experience are essential. A number of guidelines exist regarding transfer of critically unwell adults, including those from the ICS and AAGBI (now Association of Anaesthetists [AoA]).

GUIDELINE ICS FICM 2019 Transfer

What are the hazards of patient transport?

Patient
- *Haemodynamic instability*: hypotension, effects of acceleration and deceleration
- *Clinical deterioration*: pneumothorax (PTX), aspiration
- *Dislodged equipment*: airway, drains, lines
- *Equipment failures*: drug delivery, ventilator, power supply, gas supply
- *Non-routine setting*: isolated location, limited space and personnel, travel at speed
- Patient/relative dissatisfaction
- Loss of information at handover of care

Staff
- Motion sickness
- Significant time between breaks (e.g. lengthy 'back transfer' for repatriation)
- Disruption of shift work
- Injury

Organisational
- Disruption of staffing ratios and on-call cover

What types of transfer are there?

Transfers can be classified in many different ways (Table 3.1).

Which indications might require more urgent transportation?

- Aortic surgery for dissection or ruptured aneurysm
- Primary percutaneous coronary intervention (primary PCI [PPCI]) for ST-segment elevation myocardial infarction (STEMI) or out-of-hospital cardiac arrest (OHCA)

Table 3.1 Classification of patient transfers

Classification	Details
Location	Primary, secondary, tertiary
Indication	Clinical, non-clinical, capacity, repatriation
Urgency	Time-critical, urgent, routine
Level of care	Levels 1, 2, 3
Distance	Within the unit, intra-hospital, inter-hospital, long distance
Mode of transport	Foot, road, air (helicopter or fixed wing)

- Decompressive neurosurgery (e.g. for extradural haematoma [EDH], subdural haematoma [SDH], or hydrocephalus)
- Paediatric emergency surgery

How do you carry out a transfer?

Safe transfer requires clear decision-making and communication as well as careful selection and set-up of personnel, equipment, and the patient. Checklists are recommended to support the process both before, during, and after transfer.

Decision-making

- Patient
  - Clinically assessed and physiologically stable for transfer
  - Indication for transfer identified
  - Benefit of transfer will outweigh risks to the patient
  - Patient and relatives informed of decision
- Sending and receiving hospitals aware and consultants accepting patient for transfer (both parent team and critical care)
- Decision made regarding timing and urgency of transfer
  - If time-critical, delays must be avoided
  - *Less urgent*: ideally within daytime hours to assist staffing and reduce risks

Personnel

- *Doctor*: trained in transfer and appropriate skills for patient requirements
- *Nurse/ODP*: trained in transfer and familiar with equipment
- Paramedic crew
- *Additional team members as required*: specialist support/skills (e.g. perfusionist for ECMO)

Equipment

- Transfer trolley
- *Battery-operated equipment*: adequate charge and power cables, mounted and attached to trolley where possible
- *Monitoring*: ECG, S_pO_2, NIBP, invasive BP, E_tCO_2, and temperature – lit display with visual and audible alarms
- *Infusion pumps*: cannot rely on gravity delivery (unreliable delivery and risk of air embolus)
- Airway equipment
- Portable suction
- *Drugs*: emergency, infusions, and replacements sufficient for duration of travel and potential delays
- *Oxygen*: sufficient quantity for requirement and appropriate cylinders
- *Ventilator*: variable PEEP, range of V_T, variable F_IO_2, efficient gas use, known output, and visible lit display with visual and auditory alarms
- *Mobile phone*: contact numbers for sending and receiving units

Patient

- Appropriate resuscitation and stabilisation (extent balanced with urgency)
- Consideration of likelihood of deterioration and requirement for intervention on transfer (pre-empt if possible)
- *A*: secured if required, documentation including laryngoscopy, equipment available
- *B*: stablished on transfer ventilator, tolerating settings, ABG
- *C*: fluid resuscitated and attached as required, 2 × IV access
- *D*: specific indications for intubation prior to transfer (e.g. GCS < 8), pre-intubation GCS breakdown, BM, other neurological examination as able, appropriate analgesia, sedation, and muscle relaxation
- *E*: infusions attached and being delivered, alarms set appropriately, 5-point harness secured, lines secured, warming as required (e.g. blankets, hat)

Why is handover important in this setting and which aspects of information transfer are particularly significant?

Robust and clear handover is vital for safe patient transfer. Appropriate handover should not rely on the transfer of all information by one person at a single point in time (e.g. on arrival at receiving unit).

Multilevel handover often occurs with different perspectives and priorities as follows:

- Medical handover to accepting parent team
- Critical care consultant-to-consultant handover
- Technical handover to paramedics at transferring hospital
- Medical and nursing handovers to transferring team
- Medical and nursing handovers to receiving team

Other important features are as follows:

- Clear documentation of decision-making prior to transfer
- Use of checklists in preparation for transfer
- Documentation including observations during transfer
- *Relevant personnel present for medical handover*: may include other teams (e.g. neurosurgery)
- *Structure of handover itself using SBAR*: Situation, Background, Assessment, Recommendation
- *Attention to detail*: lines, infusions, previous treatments, and investigations
- Documentation in the patient's notes following handover

Can you describe any additional considerations to transfer in specific scenarios?

- *Fixed-wing air transfer*: effects of altitude, reduced atmospheric pressure, acceleration/deceleration, training, requirement for transfer to/from airfield
- *Brain-injured patients*: continuing neuroprotection en route, time-critical
- *ECMO*: specialist retrieval team; most centres in UK commence ECMO prior to departure from base hospital (with handover of overall patient responsibility at full flow). Alternatively, a team may retrieve before commencing ECMO at a tertiary centre.
- *Paediatric critical care*: often done by dedicated regional teams but there are some alternative pathways (e.g. transfer for emergency surgery by duty anaesthetist).
- *Regional teams* exist in some adult critical care networks.

Discuss capacity transfer.

Guidance advises against transfer for capacity reasons alone. Risks to the patient, other patients, and each critical care unit will need to be considered. The decision to transfer for capacity pressure is complex and should be a last resort with consultant agreement.

The ethical principle applied is distributive justice: doing the greatest good for the greatest number of patients. This often supersedes the individual risks of transfer and care further away from a patient's home.

Resources

- Bourn S, Wijesingha S, Nordmann G. Transfer of the critically ill adult patient. BJA Educ. 2018;18(3):63–68.
- The Association of Anaesthetists of Great Britain and Ireland. AAGBI Safety Guideline: Interhospital Transfer. February 2009. Available from: https://anaesthetists.org/Portals/0/PDFs/Guidelines%20PDFs/Guideline_inter-hospital_transfer_2009_final.pdf?ver=2018-07-11-163754-600&ver=2018-07-11-163754-600. (Accessed 16 January 2022.)

4. CRITICAL INCIDENTS

What is an error?

An error is an act that can lead to an undesirable outcome. Medical error is a preventable adverse effect of care. Errors may be classified by process resulting in the error, intent, personnel involvement, and time of occurrence relative to identification.

- *Latent error*: lies dormant before situation arises in which it is identified.
- *Active error*: action directly causes an error in real time.

Unsafe acts can be subdivided as follows:

- **Unintended**
  - *Slip*: attentional failures in familiar skill-based tasks
  - *Lapse*: memory failures in complex tasks
- **Intended**
  - *Mistake*: rule-/knowledge-based mistakes
  - *Violation*: routine deviations and malevolent acts

What is a critical incident?

Errors might also be described in the context of 'critical incidents' and 'patient safety incidents':

- A **critical incident** is an active error with significant consequences.
- A **patient safety incident** is the potential or actual harm due to any healthcare event.

Why does critical care predispose to incidents?

Patient
- Altered capacity and ability to communicate
- Impaired defences (e.g. sedation affecting protection against pressure sores)
- Reduced reserve to mitigate consequences of errors

Disease/management
- Unstable and high-risk conditions
- Requirement for invasive procedures
- Multiple medical devices
- High load of parenteral/enteral therapies and polypharmacy

Environment
- High acuity
- High patient turnover
- Vulnerability to interruption and distraction

What is a never event?

Which never events are relevant to critical care?

National guidance lists several never events, including the following:

Medication
- Mis-selection of a strong potassium solution
- Administration of a medication by the wrong route
- Overdose of insulin due to abbreviations or incorrect device
- Overdose of methotrexate for non-cancer treatment
- Mis-selection of high-strength midazolam during conscious sedation

General
- Chest or neck entrapment in bed rails
- Transfusion of ABO-incompatible blood components
- Misplaced naso-/orogastric tubes
- Scalding of patients
- Unintentional connection of a patient requiring oxygen to an air flowmeter

GUIDELINE NHS 2021 Never Events

What steps would you take if a critical incident occurred?

- Prioritise patient safety
- Escalate to responsible consultant
- Seek alternative staff to manage patient if objectivity compromised
- Inform patient or representative as soon as possible (duty of candour)
- Complete incident report
- Document the event in the patient notes
- Ensure affected staff also supported appropriately

The department should engage in onward reporting as indicated and undertake a root cause analysis where required.

What is a root cause analysis?

A root cause analysis is a structured, thorough investigation attempting to determine underlying causes and contributing factors to errors. It then facilitates analysis and drawing out of learning points.

Stages
- Getting started
- Gathering and mapping information
- Identifying care and service delivery problems
- Analysis
- Generating recommendations and solutions

- Implementing solutions
- Writing report

Incidents will be categorised and investigated by level of harm as follows:

1 No/low/moderate harm
2 Severe harm or death
3 Severe harm, death, or public interest (includes never events)

The fishbone model can be used to help identify contributing factors as follows:

- Education and training
- Patient
- Individual
- Equipment and resources
- Task
- Working conditions
- Communication
- Team and social
- Organisational and strategic

How might the occurrence of errors be reduced?

Latent
- Automated systems
- Standardisation of equipment and drugs
- Equipment design and function (e.g. ergonomics, forced functions)

Active
- Checklists
- Briefing and debriefing
- Guidelines
- Handovers
- Read backs
- Simulation training
- Double checks

What are NatSSIPs and LocSSIPs?

- *NatSSIPs*: National Safety Standards for Invasive Procedures
- *LocSSIPs*: Local Safety Standards for Invasive Procedures

NatSSIPs and LocSSIPs have been introduced with the same theory behind the World Health Organization's (WHO) Surgical Safety Checklist in order to standardise processes and protect patients from adverse incidents during invasive procedures. NatSSIPs can be modified for local use, forming LocSSIPs.

Invasive procedures are those involving access to the inside of a patient's body (through a cut/hole or body cavity) or the use of electromagnetic radiation. Exclusions include simple procedures (e.g. peripheral IV cannulation, urethral catheterisation, and taking of plain X-rays).

Resources
- Adyanthaya SS, Patil V. Never events: an anaesthetic perspective. BJA Educ. 2014;14(5):197–201.
- Jhugursing M, Dimmock V, Muchandani H. Error and root cause analysis. BJA Educ. 2017;17(10):323–333.
- NHS England Patient Safety Domain and the National Safety Standards for Invasive Procedures Group. National Safety Standards for Invasive Procedures (NatSSIPs). September 2015. Available from: https://www.england.nhs.uk/wp-content/uploads/2015/09/natssips-safety-standards.pdf. (Accessed 24 February 2022.)

5.   MAJOR INCIDENTS

What is a major incident?

A major incident is "any occurrence that presents serious threat to the health of the community or causes such numbers or types of casualties as to require **special arrangements** to be implemented."

Major incidents are important to consider as the 'threat to health' may manifest in increased mortality and poor outcomes when, under normal circumstances, these would probably not occur. Special arrangements may mitigate and prevent this threat.

What types of major incidents are you aware of and can you name some examples?

Incident types can be described in terms of their characteristics with regard to timescale and origin of increased demand for resources:

- **Big bang**
  - *Sudden demand*: 1 incident or cluster of smaller incidents
  - For example, Manchester Arena bomb (2017)
- **Rising tide**
  - Gradual increase in demand
  - For example, Infectious disease epidemics, staffing/capacity crisis
- **Cloud on the horizon**
  - Predictable increase in demand ahead of time
  - For example, Music festival drug-related admissions, fighting during public celebration
- **Headline news**
  - Increased demand after public alarm
  - For example, Measles, mumps and rubella [MMR] scare (1998) causing increased engagement with healthcare services

How else might major incidents be described?

- **Internal/external**
  - *Internal*: origin within a system/hospital (e.g. power loss, flooding, fire)
  - *External*: origin outwith the affected system/hospital (e.g. rail crash)
- **Natural/man-made**
  - Natural (e.g. tsunami, earthquake, volcanic eruption)
  - Man-made (e.g. transport, industry, crowd >1000 people, terrorism)
    - ➢ *CBRNE*: chemical, biological, radiological, nuclear, and explosives
- **Simple/compound**
  - *Simple*: infrastructure remains intact
  - *Compound*: damage to infrastructure
- **Compensated/uncompensated**
  - *Compensated*: load < extraordinary capacity with additional resources in use
  - *Uncompensated*: load > capacity despite additional resources

Can you give an example?

In the COVID-19 pandemic (2020), a major incident occurred on an international scale. Its origins were debatable, but early characteristics in the UK were of a rising tide, simple, compensated incident affecting most healthcare trusts. This was arguably a 'cloud on the horizon' in the UK as incidents unfolded in other countries first.

Compensation was achieved through measures including escalating intensive care capacity and redeploying staff. As time progressed, there was a shortfall in other healthcare services and resultant delays in management of other conditions (e.g. cancer surgery), which could be described as a compound, uncompensated incident. Resultant attrition of staff and untreated existing disease led to further decompensation despite physical hospital capacity.

How is a major incident declared?

'**Major incident standby**' involves the announcement of a standby message in the hospital due to an external or internal source. An internal source might include the emergency department consultant (e.g. unusual activity noticed in the department and liaison with on-call hospital team). The METHANE model can be used to chart details received or that might need to be passed to other agencies.

KEY POINT

The **METHANE** model is recommended to promote shared situational awareness and it can be used by any member of the emergency services:

- **M**ajor incident declared?
- **E**xact location
- **T**ype of incident
- **H**azards present or suspected
- **A**ccess
- **N**umber, type, and severity of casualties
- **E**mergency services present and required

Actions during major incident standby

- *Emergency department*: staff call in, locate specific documents, establish triage station
- *Critical care*: identify patients to step down to ward, liaise with theatre coordinator for admissions
- *Wards*: assess patients for discharge/transfer, prepare trauma ward for admissions/ICU stepdowns
- *Theatres*: suspend operations that are not life-saving, set up theatre coordination point, establish clinical coordination meeting

'**Major incident declared**': This announcement confirms the major incident and will require the METHANE report to be updated. It may progress to '**major incident cancelled**' or '**major incident stand down**' states.

(H)MIMMS (Hospital Major Incident Medical Management and Support) checklist

- Prepare areas for clinical/administrative uses.
- Call in appropriate number of staff using a cascade contact system.
- Maintain internal and external communication.
- Provide a command and control structure.
- Staff already on duty should report to their clinical areas.
- Called-in staff should report to staff reporting area.
- Review specific guidance for mechanisms of injury if known (in NHS document).

GUIDELINE NHS 2020 Major Incidents

What are the priorities in major incident management?

Overall aims
- Save life
- Relieve suffering
- Prevent further escalation of incident
- Protection of environment
- Preservation of infrastructure and property
- Restoration of normality
- Facilitation of enquiries

The timeline might be divided into 4 stages:

1 **Initial response**
2 **Consolidation phase**

3 **Recovery phase**
4 **Restoration of normality**

Which processes are involved in the initial response?

CSCATTT
- Command and control
- *Safety*: self (rescuers), scene, and survivors
- *Communications*: may require radios and hand-delivered messages using runners
- Assessment of scene
- Triage
- Treatment
- Transport

Describe the triage processes used in the pre-hospital environment.

Primary triage/sieve
- Aims to deliver the right patient to the right place at the right time.
- Based on distributive justice at incident site.
- Usually performed by ambulance crew.
- Patients are labelled with colour-coded priority number using algorithm.
- Priorities relate to severity of injury.
- P1–P4 moved to casualty clearing station, and P3 sent directly to hospitals.
- P4–P5 moved to body holding area and temporary mortuary (forensic involvement may be required).
- Receiving hospitals used for sickest patients.
- Supporting hospitals for less injured or capacity transfers from receiving units.

Priorities
- *P1 – immediate (red)*: catastrophic haemorrhage, unconscious, RR/HR/CR deranged
- *P2 – urgent (yellow)*: less severe circulation abnormality (HR <120, CR <2s)
- *P3 – delayed (green)*: walking wounded
- *P4 – expectant (blue)*: unsurvivable or management would compromise resources
- *P5 – dead (black)*: occluded airway or not breathing (basic adjuncts permitted)

Secondary triage/sort
- Severity of disease graded at casualty clearing station
- e.g. Triage Revised Trauma Score (T-RTS): GCS, RR, and systolic BP allocated points
- P1–P4 used based on score (1–10, 11, 12, and 0, respectively), with expectant category removed

How does this differ in the Emergency Department?
In hospital, the following triage stages should be used with associated interventions as appropriate if high priority:

- *Catastrophic haemorrhage*: **high priority for intervention (C)**
- *Walking*: low priority (may deteriorate so reassess regularly)
- *Not breathing*: dead (declare when resources allow)
- *Not responding to voice, RR <12 or >23, or HR >100*: **high priority (ABCDE)**
- *Other*: medium priority (reassess regularly)

High priority (C)
- Tourniquet
- Pelvic binder
- Haemostatic agents

High priority (ABCDE)
- *A*: definitive airway
- *B*: thoracostomy, chest seal, and positive pressure ventilation
- *C*: blood, TXA, laparotomy, thoracotomy, pericardial window, vascular surgery/IR, and Advanced Life Support (ALS) for arrest/periarrest situations

- *D*: intracerebral haemorrhage (ICH) surgery, spinal nursing for C1–C3 fracture, and seizure termination
- *E*: correction of hypothermia, correction of hypoglycaemia, and chemical antidotes for CBRNE

What do you understand about the concept of 'command and control'?

The management of emergency response and recovery will occur at different levels involving some important concepts in order to achieve defined objectives:

- *Command*: vested authority associated with role or rank to give direction
- *Control*: application of authority and capability to manage resources
- *Coordination*: integration of multi-agency efforts and available capabilities

---

KEY POINT

Levels of management are defined by functions rather than rank/grade/status as follows:

- **Operational (bronze)**: management of 'hands-on' work within a specific area
- **Tactical (silver)**: coordination of operational level — planning/coordinating tasks, resource allocation, risk assessment, and ensuring safety
- **Strategic (gold)**: consideration of incident in wider context, defining and communicating overarching strategy and objectives, and establishing framework

---

Describe the recovery process of a major incident.

Major incident recovery will be an active process requiring coordination from all agencies involved. Recovery should start at the earliest opportunity and may be run in parallel with the response. Other services will need to be maintained throughout the response (e.g. obstetric care). Services may need to be redesigned temporarily or permanently (e.g. facilitating extra trauma theatre lists).

Debriefing should occur to identify lessons and provide support for staff as follows:

- *Hot debrief*: immediately after the incident or period of duty
- *Cold/structured/organisational debrief*: within 2 weeks of incident closure
- *Multi-agency debrief*: within 4 weeks
- *Post incident reports*: within 6 weeks

What specific standards apply to UK intensive care units?

All hospitals must have the following:

- Plans to support retrieval or transfer of placements
- Evacuation and shelter plan if critical care areas become unusable for any reason (including for highly dependent patients)
- Lockdown plan including all intensive care areas preventing unauthorised access
- Recovery plan to ensure rapid return to normality (including adequate rest and psychological support for staff)
- Action cards available for use on activation of plan (containing information and communication routes to be used)

Receiving hospitals
- Prepared to **double** normal level 3 ventilated capacity
- Maintain this for up to 96 h

Supporting hospitals
- Prepared to **double** normal capacity for level 3 beds for general use and support decanting of patients from other receiving hospitals
- Provide suitably skilled transfer teams

What other planning might mitigate the negative effects of a major incident?

- Risk management
- Staff training
- *Exercising*: communications, tabletop simulation, and live play

Resources

- Lowes AJ, Cosgrove JF. Prehospital organization and management of a mass casualty incident. BJA Educ. 2016;16(10):323–328.
- NHS England National Emergency Preparedness, Resilience and Response Unit. NHS England Emergency Preparedness, Resilience and Response Framework. November 2015. Available from: https://www.england.nhs.uk/wp-content/uploads/2015/11/eprr-framework.pdf. (Accessed 14 November 2021.)

6. FIRE

Why is fire safety a priority in the critical care unit?

Fire in the critical care unit is not unheard of, with 3 incidents occurring in the last decade requiring full-scale emergency evacuation of patients, relatives, and staff. Sources have included arson, electrical fault, and oxygen cylinders catching fire when turned on.

The potential for morbidity or loss of life from such an incident is huge. Staff may also be affected, and incidents may escalate significantly.

Why might there be greater risk of fire in the critical care environment?

The fire triangle consists of oxygen, heat, and fuel. Critical care may exacerbate risk factors in all of these categories:

- **Oxygen**
  - Requirement of high concentrations in organ failure
  - Oxygen enrichment of atmosphere and patient bedding/clothing by open circuits (e.g. high-flow nasal oxygen [HFNO], CPAP)
- **Heat**
  - Dependence on electrical equipment (e.g. ventilator and monitoring)
  - More frequent defibrillator use in theory
  - Electrosurgery (e.g. diathermy for hybrid tracheostomy)
- **Fuel**
  - Emollients including lip cream
  - Bedding and patient gowns
  - Bin contents
  - Alcohol-based skin preparations (e.g. CVC antisepsis)

What measures can be taken to reduce the risk of fire?

Pipeline oxygen

- Staff member on shift with knowledge of the unit's oxygen shut-off valves including location and how to use them

Safe use of oxygen cylinders

- Set-up
  - Upright position, facing away from patient and operator
  - Slow opening of cylinder valve
  - Appropriate flow rate using cylinder flowmeter
  - Placement in cylinder bracket, not on top of patient bed
  - Set up prior to administering (i.e. attach to patient when continuously flowing)

- Turning off
  - Close oxygen shut-off valve first
  - Then turn flow rate selector to 0
- Storage
  - Signed storage away from combustible materials
  - Tamper evident seals on cylinders
  - Shut-off valve turned off and flowmeter set to zero
  - Sufficient cylinder stock for emergencies
- Post-fire
  - Do not go back to oxygen storage area if affected by fire
  - Inform fire and rescue services of exact location of cylinders
  - Arrange collection of incident cylinders
  - Appropriate reporting

Avoiding oxygen enrichment
- Minimum F_1O_2 required should be delivered to patients
- Ventilation >10 air changes per hour in high-risk areas
- Consideration of plastic barriers to prevent enrichment of bedding and clothing

Fire training
- Mandatory fire training for all staff
- Fire extinguisher training for selected individuals

Other
- Unit design
  - Division into clinical vs non-clinical areas
  - Appropriate location within hospital
  - Small bays rather than open areas
  - Pendants for electrical equipment
- Compliance with regulations for use of fire-retardant items
- Careful maintenance of electrical equipment
- Minimised use of emollients and oil-/alcohol-based products

What resources might facilitate an emergency evacuation of patients?

- Presence of accessible evacuation policy
- *Action cards*: specific instructions for staff to follow
- *Evacuation case at bedside*: sedation, NMBs, analgesia, fluid, vasopressors, torch, and paper charts
- *Evacuation aids*: slide sheets, chairs, and mats
- *Smoke hoods*: to extend time available to safely evacuate patients
- *Power supply*: backup batteries in case of simultaneous power failure
- *Unit design*: clear evacuation routes
- *Training*: simulation of evacuation and major incident

How might an ICU be evacuated?

Evacuation of critical care areas will depend on local hospital infrastructure. Evacuation may require the temporary cessation of some treatments (e.g. ECMO, renal replacement therapy [RRT]).

Staff may also be injured and strategies should be in place to support them and counteract any absences. Risk of personal harm should be balanced against duty of care using swift risk/benefit analysis. Staff and team safety should be prioritised first.

Immediate measures
- Raise alarm
- Escalate to senior staff
- Stop open-circuit delivery to patients and seek alternatives if possible
- Trained staff to use fire extinguisher

- Provide transport oxygen cylinders for patients on the unit
- Shut off oxygen pipeline supply

Next steps
- Prepare patients for transfer
- *Evacuate to safe area*: horizontal then vertical evacuation, may require transfer to other hospital sites within a network
- Follow internal major incident policy
- Transfer notes to paper if required
- Facilitate rest for staff involved and appropriate support

Evacuation triage
- Patients closest to fire first
- Least unwell patients
- Most unwell patients
- Patients within side rooms

(See Chapter 5 Major Incidents.)

| GUIDELINE | ICS AoA 2021 Fire |

| GUIDELINE | FICM ICS 2022 GPICS 2.1 |

ORGAN SUPPORT

7. MECHANICAL VENTILATION

What are the indications for mechanical ventilation?

Airway support
- Impaired airway reflexes and risk of aspiration (e.g. trauma, impaired consciousness, secretion load)
- Patency threatened (e.g. anaphylaxis, maxillofacial trauma)

Respiratory support
- *Increased oxygen delivery*: guaranteed delivery of high F_IO_2, alveolar recruitment (e.g. pneumonia)

Ventilatory support
- Regulation of ventilation (e.g. targeted P_aCO_2 to optimise cerebral perfusion)
- Deep sedation required (e.g. to reduce oxygen demand, peri-procedural, imaging)

How can non-invasive mechanical ventilatory support be delivered?
Mechanical ventilation can be delivered by non-invasive or invasive means.

Types of NIV
- High-flow oxygen therapy
- Continuous positive airway pressure (CPAP)
- Bilevel positive airway pressure (BiPAP)

High flow oxygen therapy
- Provides heated, humidified oxygen at adjustable flows of gas and F_IO_2 (usually maximum flow 40–60 l/min, F_IO_2 1.0)
- Advantages
  - ➤ *Humidification of inspired gas*: improves secretion clearance, prevents epithelial injury, and decreases work of breathing
  - ➤ *Reduction of entrained atmospheric gas*: increases the delivered F_IO_2 when compared to variable performance devices such as nasal prongs or a reservoir mask
  - ➤ Reduction of CO_2 dead space through a 'washout' effect
  - ➤ Delivery of PEEP, particularly when closed mouth breathing

CPAP
- Continuous application of positive pressure to the upper airway throughout the respiratory cycle
- Delivered via nasal cushions, face mask, or hood interface
- Increases oxygen delivery by aiding alveolar recruitment and improving ventilation/perfusion (V/Q) matching

- Advantages
  - ➢ Cheap
  - ➢ Easily delivered
  - ➢ Usually well tolerated
  - ➢ Can be useful in LVF and associated pulmonary oedema

BiPAP
- Nomenclature varies
- Provides ventilatory support through the difference between inspiratory positive airway pressure (IPAP) and expiratory positive airway pressure (EPAP)
- Delivered via face mask from initial settings (e.g. 10/4), rapidly uptitrated according to patient status and ABG results
- Advantages
  - ➢ Clearance of CO_2 and reduced work of breathing particularly in hypercapnic respiratory failure (infective exacerbation of COPD or chest wall deformity)
  - ➢ Prevention of post-extubation respiratory failure in those with COPD

What is PEEP?

Positive end-expiratory pressure (PEEP) is the pressure present in the airway (alveolar pressure) above atmospheric pressure that exists at the end of expiration.

It is used to improve alveolar recruitment and therefore oxygenation. It also reduces the work of breathing by preventing airway collapse at the end of expiration (thereby reducing the work to reopen them during inspiration).

What are the other physiological effects of PEEP?

> **KEY POINT**
>
> Physiological effects of PEEP:
>
> - *A*: may maintain patency (e.g. preventing pharyngeal collapse in OSA)
> - *B*: alveolar recruitment; reduced shunt, overdistension, and ventilator-induced lung injury
> - *C*: initial increase then decrease in systemic venous return, increased afterload (SVR), increased pulmonary vascular resistance (PVR), raised RV pressure, and increased interventricular dependence (reducing SV)
> - *D*: raised ICP
> - *Other*: increased atrial natriuretic peptide (ANP), antidiuretic hormone (ADH), and catecholamines

Which characteristics are important to determine a mode of invasive ventilation?

Invasive ventilation can be delivered in a variety of modes which determine the interaction between ventilator and patient. PEEP and F_IO_2 can usually be manipulated independently of other characteristics:

- *Control*: pressure or volume (by controlling flow)
- *Cycling*: time, flow, or pressure
- *Trigger*: machine, patient, or operator
- *Breath type*: mandatory or spontaneous
- *Breath sequence*: mandatory, intermittent mandatory, or spontaneous
- *Synchronisation*: synchronised or independent
- *Guarantee*: V_T, MV, or pressure
- *Smart modes*: minimum pressure regulation required during volume control
  - Autoflow (Dräger)
  - Volume Control Plus (VC+) (Covidien)

Can you describe some common modes used in invasive ventilation?

Each manufacturer offers slight variations on a theme; there is no consensus taxonomy. For example, one might use a separate mode for each combination of control and support. Another might classify modes by support before control type is then set. Most modes, including hybrid variations, are based on the following concepts:

Pressure control ventilation (PCV)
- P_{insp}, PEEP, and inspiratory time (t_i) set
- V_T dependent on compliance
- Pressure rapidly delivered and held at constant level (square-wave pattern)
- Flow delivered in decelerating pattern
- Allows time for gas to equilibrate between fast and slow recruiting alveolar units
- Pressure rapidly released in expiration (elastic recoil of lungs allows expiration against PEEP)

Volume control ventilation (VCV)
- V_T, PEEP, RR, flow pattern (constant/decelerating) set
- *Constant inspiratory flow*: gradual rise in P_{insp}
- *Decelerating flow*: longer t_i may be used, improvement in alveolar time constants

Pressure support
- P_{insp}, PEEP, and expiratory flow trigger set
- ·Commonly used to aid weaning (e.g. expiratory flow trigger set at 25% or 5l for greater comfort)

How do ventilators cycle between inspiration and expiration?

Ventilator cycling can depend on the trigger to deliver a breath as well as how inspiration and expiration are defined.

The following can determine ventilator cycling:

- **Time**
  - Inspiration and expiration determined by time
  - RR = 60/f
  - Less patient interaction with the ventilator
  - Used in modes in which cycle is independent of patient effort
- **Flow**
  - Inspiration and expiration commenced after sensing change in circuit flow
  - Flow changes as patient attempts to breathe
- **Pressure**
  - Changes in pressure in ventilator circuit sensed (pressure decrease triggers inspiratory cycle)

What is adaptive support ventilation?

Adaptive support ventilation (ASV) uses a feedback loop to adjust support based on patient requirements. Support is delivered in response to RR and effort to achieve the required MV.

What is NAVA?

Neurally assisted ventilatory assist (NAVA) is a form of proportional assist ventilation. NAVA utilises electronic activity from the diaphragm. Diaphragmatic activity is monitored using a specialised NG tube. Support is based on lung dynamics and patient effort.

How would you describe SIMV?

Synchronised intermittent mandatory ventilation (SIMV) is a mode common to many manufacturers.

SIMV is a time-cycled mode involving mandatory breaths which may be machine- or patient-triggered. SIMV can be pressure- or volume-controlled, and the patient receives at least the set pressure or V_T (i.e. pressure or volume guarantee).

Spontaneous ventilation is permitted at varying parts of the cycle. If the patient effort is insufficient, a machine-triggered breath is applied.

Can you describe how airway pressure release ventilation is used?

Airway pressure release ventilation (APRV) is an open-lung mode of ventilation. It is indicated in patients who are felt to have recruitable lung disease and have shown poor response to conventional ventilatory modes.

The patient is encouraged to breathe spontaneously over time-cycling alternation in pressure. High pressure (**P-high**) is maintained for longer time (**T-high**) through an inverse ratio, allowing only a short time (**T-low**) at low pressure (**P-low**) for CO_2 clearance.

Advantages
- Promotion of alveolar recruitment
- Improvement in lung homogeneity
- Increased FRC
- Reduction in cyclical opening/closing of lung units (atelectotrauma)

Disadvantages
- Potential to aggravate lung injury if used incorrectly
  - High local transpulmonary pressures
  - Potential for RV dysfunction, cor pulmonale
  - Tachypnoea ('patient self-inflicted lung injury')
- Controversy about usefulness in patients under NMB, not spontaneously breathing

Initiating APRV
- Proposed initial settings:
  - F_IO_2 1.0 (can wean once established)
  - *P-high*: current plateau pressure (usually ≤30 cmH_2O)
  - *P-low*: 0 cmH_2O
  - *T-high*: 5 s
  - *T-low*: 0.5 s
- Reduce T-low in steps of 0.1 s until expiratory flow terminates at ≥75% peak expiratory flow (and vice versa)
- Stop NMB and titrate sedation to encourage spontaneous breathing
- Tolerate hypercapnia with pH ≥7.25 if appropriate

Weaning APRV (e.g. 'drop-and-stretch' approach)
- Reduce F_IO_2 (aim 0.4–0.5)
- Reduce P-high by 2 cmH_2O every 2–6 h (maintain F_IO_2 at 0.4–0.5)
  - If unsuccessful (i.e. hypoxaemic), increase P-high by 4 cmH_2O and wean more slowly
- Once P-high reaches 20, increase T-high by 1–2 s when P-high reduced
- This will result in weaning to CPAP < 10 cmH_2O
- Assessment of readiness for extubation
- Alternative strategy: switch to conventional pressure support once P-high reaches 12–15 cmH_2O and F_IO_2 reaches 0.4 (set PEEP to P-high with low pressure support)

What do you know about high-frequency oscillatory ventilation?

High-frequency oscillatory ventilation (HFOV) is a mode that achieves alveolar ventilation using low V_T at/below dead space volume (1–2 ml/kg) and supranormal frequencies 3–15 s^{-1}).

The inspiratory limb is connected to an electromagnetic piston that moves a flexible diaphragm to create pressure oscillation. Settings include flow, **mean airway pressure** (mPaw), '**delta P**' (power), **% t_i**, and **f**. E_tCO_2 monitoring is not possible. 'Wobble' can be described by how far oscillations propagate (e.g. to mid-thigh).

- Oxygenation α mPaw
- CO_2 removal α delta P, % t_i, and 1/f

Physiological principles
- *Bulk convection*: gas entrained when vacuum left in alveoli as oxygen absorbed into capillaries
- *Pendelluft*: gas exchanged between lung units with different time constants
- *Taylor dispersion*: gas exchanged between central column and peripheral airways
- *Coaxial flow*: bidirectional flow: central rapid inspiratory column and outer slow-expiratory sleeve
- *Augmented molecular diffusion*: force of oscillation pushes molecules to enhance Brownian motion

HFOV fell out of favour in adult critical care after the **OSCILLATE** and **OSCAR** trials and is strongly recommended against by FICM and ICS in the management of ARDS. Potential harms reported include barotrauma, hypotension, and oxygenation failure.

HFOV is still used in paediatrics when conventional ventilation fails.

GUIDELINE FICM ICS 2018 ARDS

STUDY

OSCILLATE (2013)

- New onset moderate–severe ARDS
- *Intervention*: HFOV vs conventional PCV
- *Primary*: in-hospital mortality – **significantly higher (47% vs 35%)**, trial terminated early
- *Secondary*: refractory hypoxaemia lower
- HFOV patients received more NMB, midazolam, and vasoactive drugs

STUDY

OSCAR (2013)

- ARDS
- *Intervention*: HFOV vs local practice
- *Primary*: 30-day mortality – **no difference**
- *Secondary*: oxygenation improved

Resources

- Ashraf-Kashani N, Kumar R. High-flow nasal oxygen therapy. BJA Educ. 2017;17(2):57–62.
- Swindin J, Sampson C, Howatson A. Airway pressure release ventilation. BJA Educ. 2020;20(3):80–88.
- Yartsev A. Deranged Physiology: Physiology of Gas Exchange in HFOV. 2015. Available from: https://deranged-physiology.com/required-reading/respiratory-medicine-and-ventilation/Chapter%205.1.8/physiology-gas-exchange-hfov. (Accessed 24 April 2022.)
- Webb A, Angus D, Finfer S, et al. (Eds.) Oxford Textbook of Critical Care, 2nd ed. London: Oxford University Press; 2016. Available from: https://oxfordmedicine.com/view/10.1093/med/9780199600830.001.0001/med-9780199600830. (Accessed 24 April 2022.)

8. PRONING

What are the indications for and contraindications to prone positioning?

Indications

- Critical care
  - Moderate to severe ARDS ($F_IO_2 \geq 0.6$ and P/F ratio < 150 mmHg or 20 kPa)
  - Early in disease (<48 h and after 12–24 h optimisation of mechanical ventilation)
    - ➤ Supported by **PROSEVA** trial, strongly recommended by FICM and ICS
- Surgical access (e.g. spinal and posterior fossa craniotomy)

Contraindications
- Absolute
  - Open chest (e.g. post-op cardiac surgery)
  - <24 h post-cardiac surgery
  - Central cannulation for BiVAD or ECMO
  - Spinal instability
- Relative
  - Previous poor tolerance of proning
  - Recent tracheostomy < 24 h
  - Refractory cardiovascular instability
  - High ICP/intraocular pressure
  - Frequent seizures
  - Facial fractures
  - Significant trauma (e.g. pelvic fixation device)
  - Pregnancy second to third trimester
  - Morbid obesity

STUDY

PROSEVA (2014)

- Severe ARDS
- *Intervention*: prone for ≥16 h for 28 days or until improvement vs supine
- *Primary*: 28-day all-cause mortality – **significantly lower (16% vs 33%)**

Can you describe some risks of proning?

Staff injury
Instability
- Airway displacement
- Haemodynamic instability
- Increased intra-abdominal pressure (IAP)
- CRRT, ECMO line flow issues
- Gastro-oesophageal reflux (and risk of aspiration)
- Brief period without full monitoring
- Other line or device displacement and sequelae (e.g. ECMO cannula, haemorrhage)

Patient injury
- Pressure sores (face, ears, etc.)
- Periorbital oedema, chemosis
- Ocular injury, corneal abrasion, blindness
- Brachial plexus injury
- Other nerves over bony prominences

What extra resources might you require?

Staff
- Minimum five staff: 1 airway, 2 each side
- Additional staff if required (e.g. for chest drain or ECMO cannulae)

Monitoring
- Airway trolley
- ECG electrodes
- Caps for disconnected lines

Protecting patient
- Tracheal tube tapes
- Eye ointment and patches

- NG syringe
- Absorbent pads
- Patches for nipples

Moving and handling
- Low air loss mattress
- Slide sheet
- 3–5 pillows, 2 clean bed sheets

How would you prone a ventilated patient?

Pre-procedure
- MDT decision
- Proning team introductions and brief (including emergency 'deproning' strategy) ± checklist use
- Choice of appropriate time and informing senior nurse and doctor on the unit
- Complete outstanding tasks suited to supine position (e.g. line change, wash, and stoma dressing)
- Resources ready as above
- Systems review
    - A: secure, suction mouth and tube, and note tube depth
    - B: pre-oxygenate, note compliance, ABG, ensure chest drain below patient ± clamp and ventilator close to patient
    - C: discontinue non-essential infusions, may be appropriate to cap arterial line
    - D: Richmond Agitation-Sedation Scale (RASS)-5, consider NMB
    - E: eye and nipple protection, remove other items from front (e.g. ECG stickers)
    - F: spigot urinary catheter and tape to inside leg
    - G: aspirate NG tube 1 h prior, document length, and secure to nose

Procedure
- Neutral position on slide sheet and tuck arm nearest ventilator under buttock
- Pillows over chest, iliac crests, and knees
- Wrap patient with sheet over top, keeping head and neck exposed, and roll sheet edges
- Move as directed by person managing airway
    - Horizontal move: opposite direction to ventilator and away from direction of roll
    - Lateral turn (roll): 90° on side
    - Proning completion

Post-procedure
- Immediate systems review and pressure area check
- Fine-tune positioning: swimmer's position, 30° reverse Trendelenberg
- Debrief
- Documentation
- 'Swim' patient to other side every 2–4 h
- Modifications to support (e.g. low volume feed)

GUIDELINE FICM ICS 2019 Proning

What would you do if the patient lost cardiac output on being turned into the prone position?

- Recognise situation, declare cardiac arrest, and call for help
- Commence CPR
    - Mid-thoracic level between scapulae
    - Effective if good E_tCO_2 and arterial trace
- Place defibrillator pads biaxillary or over left mid-axillary line and right scapula

- Check for equipment malfunction or disconnection
- If ineffective, turn patient supine

GUIDELINE   Resuscitation Council UK NSGBI SBNS 2014 Neurosurgery

What is 'conscious proning' and when is it used?

Conscious proning refers to utilisation of the prone position in conscious patients with respiratory failure in order to improve oxygenation. Its use increased during the COVID-19 pandemic.

The ICS recommends that patients requiring F_IO_2 ≥28% or basic respiratory support to meet their target S_aO_2 should utilise proning, provided they are able to communicate, co-operate, and adjust their position independently, and airway issues are not anticipated.

Absolute contraindications
- Respiratory distress
- Immediate requirement for intubation
- Haemodynamic instability
- Altered mental status
- Unstable spinal/thoracic injury
- Recent abdominal surgery

Reverse Trendelenburg positioning may aid comfort. Sedation should not be used to facilitate proning. If saturations are maintained for 15 min, proning should continue with position changes every 1–2 h. Proning should be discontinued if, after 15 min, the patient deteriorates, there is no improvement, proning is not tolerated, or signs of respiratory distress are present.

Position change cycle
- Fully prone
- Right lateral recumbent
- Sitting up at 30–60° (Fowler's position)
- Left lateral recumbent

GUIDELINE   ICS 2020 Conscious proning

9.   ECMO AND ECCO$_2$R

What is ECMO?

ECMO is a form of extracorporeal life support (ECLS) in which a modified heart-lung machine provides respiratory or circulatory support (or both) for refractory hypoxaemia.

Types of ECLS
- **Veno-venous ECMO (VV-ECMO)**
- **Veno-arterial ECMO (VA-ECMO)**
- **Arterio-venous ECMO (AV-ECMO)** (rarely used)
- **Extracorporeal CO$_2$ removal (ECCO$_2$R)**
- **Cardiopulmonary bypass (CPB)**
- **Ventricular assist device (VAD) with oxygenator**

ECMO was introduced in the 1970s and gained popularity during the H1N1 pandemic (2009). More recently, the COVID-19 pandemic (2020) saw a significant demand for ECMO services, and further insight has been gained about prognosis and appropriate selection criteria. It is thought that prognosis in COVID-19 is similar to that in other aetiologies. ECMO is not a benign process, and patients will require significant physiological reserve to withstand the demands and sequelae of an ECMO admission, over and above standard intensive care.

In the UK, VV-ECMO is provided by a national network of tertiary centres that have the necessary expertise and equipment to care for such patients for often several weeks. VA-ECMO is not commissioned but is used in selected cases. Extracorporeal cardiopulmonary resuscitation (E-CPR) is an emerging form of VA-ECMO that is occasionally used in cardiac arrest (Figure 9.1).

GUIDELINE   ELSO 2017 ECLS

(See Chapter 27 Out-of-Hospital Cardiac Arrest.)

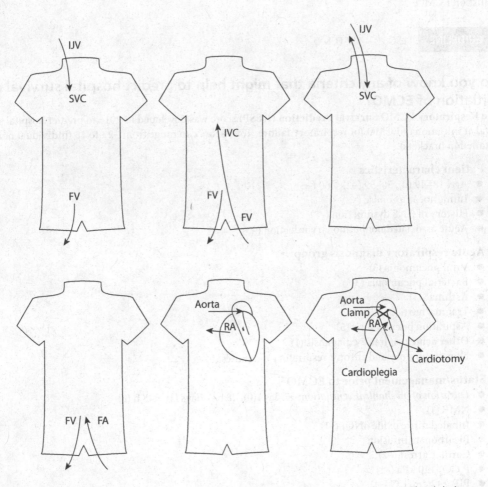

Figure 9.1   Common ECMO configurations and comparison with cardiopulmonary bypass. Blood drainage and return are indicated by bold arrows.

IJV, internal jugular vein; SVC, superior vena cava; FV, femoral vein; FA, femoral artery; RA, right atrium.

Summarise the key concepts behind how VV-ECMO works to support respiratory failure.

Gas exchange in the native circulation has failed and is replaced by exchange between the bloodstream and an extracorporeal circuit. An **oxygenator** (>1 in certain circumstances) is incorporated in the ECMO circuit, allowing diffusion of oxygen and CO_2 through a membrane along a pressure gradient.

Oxygenation is determined by the **circuit blood flow rate (l/min)** and oxygen content of post-oxygenator blood. Oxygenation can therefore be increased by increasing the circuit flow rate. It will also depend on native flow. The pump will be set to achieve a specified number of **revolutions per minute** to achieve the desired flow. Recirculation of relatively deoxygenated blood may reduce efficiency.

CO_2 also diffuses out through the oxygenator and is primarily determined by the **sweep gas flow rate (l/min)** as a substitute for ventilation. CO_2 is more soluble, so it diffuses more readily across the oxygenator membrane than oxygen. An adequate gradient is always maintained, so manipulation of CO_2 extraction involves changing the flow rate of the sweep gas rather than blood flow through the system. The sweep gas flow rate is controlled by a flowmeter and percentage of oxygen it contains – usually set to 100% unless weaning. Membrane surface area and oxygenator efficiency will also affect this process.

Whilst these processes occur, conventional **mechanical ventilation is reduced** to 'rest settings' to minimise iatrogenesis and allow lung pathology to recover. In exceptional circumstances, it may be stopped altogether (e.g. airway haemorrhage requiring tube clamp). Some patients may be suitable for extubation whilst on ECMO.

GUIDELINE ELSO 2021 VV-ECMO

Do you know of any criteria that might help to predict hospital survival on initiation of ECMO?

The **Respiratory ECMO Survival Prediction (RESP)** score was developed in 2014 to predict hospital survival at initiation of ECMO for respiratory failure. Total score can range from −22 to 15 (individual points detailed in brackets).

Patient characteristics
- *Age*: 18–49 (0), 50–59 (−2), ≥60 (−3)
- Immunocompromise (−2)
- History of CNS dysfunction (−7)
- Acute associated nonpulmonary infection (−3)

Acute respiratory diagnosis group
- Viral pneumonia (3)
- Bacterial pneumonia (3)
- Asthma (11)
- Trauma/burn (3)
- Aspiration pneumonitis (5)
- Other acute respiratory diagnosis (1)
- Non-respiratory and chronic respiratory diagnoses (0)

Status/management prior to ECMO
- *Duration of mechanical ventilation*: >7 days (0), 48 h–7 days (1), <48 h (3)
- NMB (1)
- Inhaled nitric oxide (iNO) (−1)
- Bicarbonate infusion (−2)
- Cardiac arrest (−2)
- P_aCO_2 ≥10 kPa (−1)
- PIP ≥42 cmH$_2$O (−1)

Risk class is then determined by total RESP score to give predicted in-hospital survival (in brackets):

   I ≥6 (92%)

  II 3–5 (76%)

III   −1 to 2 (57%)

IV   −5 to −2 (33%)

V   ≤−6 (18%)

When would you refer a patient for VV-ECMO?

VV-ECMO is indicated in acute, severe, potentially reversible respiratory failure. The referral criteria have evolved over time to contain:

Inclusion criteria
- Potentially reversible severe respiratory failure
- Murray Lung Injury Score ≥3
- Uncompensated hypercapnia with a pH ≤7.20 (despite RR > 35 min^{-1} or due to life-threatening airway disease)

Additional considerations
- Failed trial of ventilation in the prone position for ≥6 h unless contraindicated
- Failed optimal respiratory management with lung-protective ventilation (LPV) after discussion with a national centre

Exclusion criteria
- Refractory or established multi-organ failure
- Evidence of severe neurological injury
- Prolonged cardiac arrest (>15 min)

In the UK, at least 2 ECMO centres must agree to proceed if there is indication of low potential to recover (e.g. RESP score ≤3), or invasive mechanical ventilation has been received for >7 days.

Which criteria form the basis of the Murray score?

- Consolidation (number of quadrants on CXR)
- Compliance
- P/F ratio
- PEEP

What are the potential complications of ECMO?

Cannulation
- Haemorrhage
- *Failure* – vessels may be inadequate, end-stage vascular access
- Death
- Damage to local structures
- Lower limb ischaemia
- Stroke

General
- Bleeding (e.g. ICH, airway, GI)
- Death
- Line infection
- Circuit colonisation
- Thrombus
- Haemolysis
- Pain
- Progression of underlying disease
- Medication under-/overdosing
- Sequelae of lengthy ICU stay

Circuit failure
- Oxygenator thrombosis
- Recirculation
- Pump failure
- Gas embolism

- Unintentional decannulation
- Hypothermia

Interventions
- *Reconfiguration*: instability, cannulation related
- *Circuit change-out*: instability, gas embolism
- *Proning*: chemosis, GI reflux, decannulation
- *High-dose sedatives*: withdrawal
- *Anticoagulation*: heparin-induced thrombocytopaenia (HIT)
- Sequelae of repeated transfusion
- *Transfer (scan/theatre/IR)*: decannulation, instability, circuit failure

What is 'chatter'?

Chatter is the rapid movement of the drainage line in response to venous drainage occlusion. The pump will be unable to spin at the desired rate, and flows will decrease. Chattering also causes haemolysis. Contributing factors that may be addressed include inadequate circulating volume, patient position, cannula position, kinked tubing, and thrombosis.

What is 'recirculation'?

Recirculation refers to the portion of oxygenated blood that returns directly to the ECMO circuit without circulating to the patient first. Cannula position, intravascular volume, and pump flow affect recirculation fraction, which may be as high as 60%. It may be mitigated by higher blood flow, cannula repositioning, increased blood volume, and higher haematocrit.

Is there evidence to support the use of ECMO in severe ARDS?

Two large RCTs have examined the use of ECMO in ARDS. **CESAR** demonstrated a significant improvement in survival without severe disability. However, this was not attributable to ECMO alone, but the transfer to a tertiary centre for its consideration ± use; 75% of those transferred actually received ECMO.

More recently, **EOLIA** found no difference in mortality at 60 days. However, there was significant cross-over from conventional ventilation to ECMO.

The evidence for ECMO itself is inconclusive, but transfer to a specialist centre is advocated in the UK (CESAR criteria: Murray score > 3, and pH < 7.2 on optimum management).

STUDY

CESAR (2009)

- Severe, potentially reversible adult respiratory failure
- *Intervention*: transfer to specialist centre and consideration for ECMO vs conventional PCV
- *Primary*: survival without severe disability at 6 months – **significantly higher (63% vs 47%)**
- *Secondary*: ICU and hospital LOS – higher

STUDY

EOLIA (2018)

- Severe ARDS
- *Intervention*: VV-ECMO vs volume control ventilation (28% crossover to ECMO)
- *Primary*: 60-day mortality – **no difference**
- *Secondary*: treatment failure and RRT – lower relative risk

(See Chapter 23 ARDS.)

What do you know about ECCO$_2$R?

Extracorporeal carbon dioxide removal (ECCO$_2$R) is a low-flow technique that selectively removes CO$_2$ and is indicated in ARDS. It may be carried out through an ECMO circuit, stand-alone device, or adaptation of an existing circuit (e.g. haemofilter).

The role of specific ECCO$_2$R is under evaluation. Potential indications are as follows:

- *ARDS*: to facilitate LPV, and in refractory respiratory acidosis
- *COPD*: to prevent NIV failure, avoid invasive ventilation, and wean invasive ventilation
- Bridge to lung transplant

STUDY

SUPERNOVA (2019)

- ARDS
- Evaluation of 3 different ECCO$_2$R systems (Hemolung, Novalung, and Cardiohelp)
- *Primary*: patients achieving V$_T$ 4 ml/kg with P$_a$CO$_2$ ≤20% baseline and pH > 7.30
- *Results*: **78% at 8 h and 82% at 24 h**
- *Adverse events*: 39% overall: 14% membrane lung clot, 13% thrombocytopaenia, 12% haemolysis, 6% significant bleeding, 3% pump malfunction, 2% line displacement, and 2% infection. Six severe events: massive ICH, SVC thrombus, death, PTX, severe hypoxaemia, and haematemesis.

STUDY

REST (2021)

- Acute hypoxaemic respiratory failure
- *Intervention*: ECCO$_2$R (dual lumen catheter and heparinised) vs guideline-based mechanical ventilation
- *Primary*: 90-day all-cause mortality – **no difference**
- *Secondary*: 28-day mortality, ICU/hospital LOS – no difference; V$_T$ on day 2–3 and ventilator-free days – lower

How might you approach a rising P$_a$CO$_2$ on ECMO?

Troubleshooting on ECMO will involve complex diagnosis and may trace back to problems with the circuit, monitoring, or patient themselves.

Technical complications should be ruled out and addressed if found. Hypercarbia should prompt consideration of increased metabolic state in the patient, and it may be the first presentation of sepsis or other pathology.

The sweep gas flow rate can be increased to further remove CO$_2$.

What are the immediate priorities during an emergency involving a patient established on ECMO?

All emergencies will require appropriate delegation of complex tasks and sound leadership. Examples include the following:

Gas embolism
- Clamp return line immediately
- Clamp drainage line
- Switch off pump at console (pump head may need to be removed)
- Urgently call for help: ECMO coordinator, consultant, and perfusionist
- Identify and correct cause of air entrainment
- Remove air using syringe at oxygenator port
- May require emergency transfusion

Accidental decannulation
- Turn off pump

- Salvage if possible
- Compression of cannulation site
- Emergency recannulation
- Activation of major haemorrhage protocol

Circuit failure
- Changeout of partial/whole circuit (spare and primed circuit should be available)

Resources
- Brogan TV, Annich G, Ellis WC, et al., eds. Extracorporeal Life Support Organization: ECMO Specialist Training Manual, 4th ed. Ann Arbor: Extracorporeal Life Support Organization; 2018.
- NHS England, NHS Scotland. ECMO National Referral Pathway. Available from: https://www.signpost.health-care/ecmo-referral-pathway. (Accessed 18 January 2022.)
- Schmidt M, Bailey M, Sheldrake J, et al. Predicting survival after extracorporeal membrane oxygenation for severe acute respiratory failure. Am J Respir Crit Care Med. 2014;189(11):1374–1382.

---

10. WEANING

What is weaning?

Weaning in critical care refers to the process of liberation of the patient from organ support.

Weaning mechanical ventilation involves the reduction of ventilatory support, increase in spontaneous effort, and extubation.

What is difficult weaning?

Difficulty of weaning is described in terms of time to extubation:

- *Simple*: liberation from ventilator on first attempt (70% patients)
- *Difficult*: extubation 2–7 days after initial assessment of readiness for extubation
- *Prolonged*: >7 days after initial assessment

How is readiness to wean from mechanical ventilation assessed?

KEY POINT

Clinical assessment of readiness to wean:

- Underlying condition resolved
- Patient condition optimised
- *A*: reflexes satisfactory, secretions not problematic, and cuff leak present
- *B*: spontaneously breathing, strength adequate, F_iO_2 ≤0.4, and minimal PEEP
- *C*: cardiovascularly stable on minimal dose of vasoactive medications
- *D*: obeying commands

Objective indices
- RR < 30 min^{-1}
- V_T > 5 ml/kg or > 325 ml
- FVC > 15 ml/kg
- MV < 15 l/min
- Maximum inspiratory pressure (PI_{max}) < 30 cmH$_2$O
  - Measure of respiratory muscle strength (normally –90 to –120 cmH$_2$O)
- **Rapid Shallow Breathing Index (RSBI)** = f/V_T (litres)
  - Some evidence for progression to extubation with RSBI < 105 during spontaneous breathing trial (SBT)

- **P0.1/PImax > 0.3**
  - *P0.1*: negative airway pressure generated during the first 0.1 s of an occluded inspiration
  - Ratio correlates with central respiratory drive

Can you describe a spontaneous breathing trial?

- Screening for readiness to wean
- May be paired with sedation hold/holiday (see Chapter 14 Sedation)
- 30-min trial of T-piece or minimal CPAP ± pressure support
- Assessment of success or failure
- If well tolerated, consider extubation ± non-invasive respiratory support

---

KEY POINT

Examples of criteria for failure of SBT are as follows:

- *B*: RR > 35 min^{-1}, S_pO_2 < 90%, or high work of breathing
- *C*: HR > 140 min^{-1} or change > 20%, systolic BP > 180 or < 90 mmHg, or sweating
- *D*: agitation or anxiety

STUDY

Subirà et al. (2019)

- Adults deemed ready for weaning after ≥24 h MV
- *Intervention*: 30-min 8 cmH$_2$O pressure support vs 2-h T-piece SBT
- *Primary*: successful extubation (72 h) – **significantly higher (82.3% vs 74.0%)**
- *Secondary*: reintubation ICU/hospital LOS – no difference

What problems can be encountered in patients with weaning difficulty?

Difficult and prolonged weaning account for up to 20% of patients on the adult ICU and are associated with an increased LOS, VAP, ICU-acquired weakness (ICUAW), and mortality (though the reason for this is not clear).

As part of difficult or prolonged or difficult wean, most patients will undergo an attempt at tracheal extubation. Extubation failure may be due to either unresolved airway problems (airway obstruction, oedema, and secretion load) or ventilatory weaning problems. The process of extubation failure and subsequent reintubation is not benign. Critical care units usually have a reintubation rate of between 10 and 15%.

(See Chapter 41 Stridor)

Other causes of failure to wean
- **Increased work of breathing**
  - Inappropriate ventilator settings
  - Excessive resistance from the endotracheal tube
  - Excessive secretions
  - Pulmonary oedema
  - Decreased compliance (any cause)
  - Ongoing bronchospasm
- **Excessive cardiac work**
  - High metabolic demand
  - Unresolved cardiac failure
  - Fluid overload
  - Anaemia
  - High-dose vasopressors/inotropes
- **Poor neurological status**
  - Impaired mental state (e.g. poor central neurology, metabolic disturbance)

- Delirium
- Weakness (e.g. ICUAW, electrolyte disturbance) (see Chapter 30 ICU-Acquired Weakness)
- Pain (e.g. inadequate post-op strategy, failure of regional blockade, trauma, musculoskeletal pain)
- **Other concomitant pathology** (e.g. burns, DKA, other acidaemia, malnutrition – obesity or cachexia)

What are the indications for a tracheostomy?

- Bypass upper airway obstruction
- Allow tracheal toilet
- Decrease airway resistance
- Facilitate weaning and liberation from the ventilator
- Long-term airway support (e.g. neurological injury/disorder) .

GUIDELINE   NTSP ICS 2020 Tracheostomy

When would you perform a tracheostomy on a ventilated patient?

The optimal timing of tracheostomy is multifactorial. The **TracMan** study aimed to compare early (≤4 days) and late (≥10 days) tracheostomy insertion. There was no statistical difference in mortality at 30 days.

Patients with neurological conditions were excluded, and criticisms such as recruitment fatigue have also been applied.

STUDY

TracMan (2013)

- Mechanically ventilated adult patients with a high risk of prolonged ventilation
- *Intervention*: tracheostomy insertion ≤4 days of critical care admission vs ≥day 10 if still indicated
- *Primary*: 30-day all-cause mortality – **no difference**
- *Secondary*: survival, duration of mechanical ventilation, LOS, and antibiotics – no difference. Days of sedation in survivors at 30 days – **significantly lower (5 vs 8 days)**.

What are the advantages of tracheostomy compared to a translaryngeal tube?

- Improved patient comfort
- Reduced need for sedation
- Reduced pressure on the tongue, mouth, and oral structures
- Improved mouth care
- *Ability of the vocal cords to mobilise*: protection against aspiration and ability to phonate
- *Improved laryngeal sensation and ability to swallow*: facilitates return to oral diet and prevention of further deconditioning
- *Reduced nursing dependency*: caring for non-ventilated patients with tracheostomy

How is a tracheostomy performed?
Percutaneous, surgical, and hybrid techniques exist.

Percutaneous technique
- **Pre-procedure**
  - Ensure no contraindications, appropriate timing, and senior team members informed
  - Assent/consent

- *Prepare equipment*: airway equipment, tracheostomy tubes and insertion kit, bronchoscope, anaesthesia and analgesia (including local), sterile gown, etc.
- *Other requirements*: IV access, monitoring (including E_tCO_2 and timer), personnel
- *US neck*: identify vessels and depth of trachea
- Stop and aspirate enteral feed
- *Ventilation settings*: pre-oxygenate F_iO_2 1.0, consider volume controlled ventilation, consider 1:1 I:E ratio
- Agree sedation strategy and use of NMB
- Position patient with neck extended – shoulder bolster may be required

- **Procedure**
  - Scrub and apply antiseptic solution to skin
  - Apply local anaesthetic to skin and subcutaneous tissues (e.g. lidocaine with adrenaline)
  - Second operator visualises trachea with bronchoscope and pulls back translaryngeal tube under direct vision
  - Perform dilatational insertion of tracheostomy using Seldinger technique
  - Second operator confirms position with bronchoscopy down tracheostomy and translaryngeal tube
  - Attach breathing circuit to tracheostomy, ventilate, and confirm E_tCO_2
  - Remove translaryngeal tube
- **Post-procedure**
  - *Secure tracheostomy*: sutures not used routinely in case emergency removal required
  - Note any obvious complications (e.g. tracheal ring fracture)
  - Sign out/debrief team
  - Document procedure
  - CXR performed in some institutions

How about surgical or hybrid tracheostomy insertion?

Surgical technique involves dissecting down to the trachea before creating a window, inserting a tracheostomy tube, and confirming position. Two anaesthetists may be required: one to manipulate the translaryngeal tube and another to maintain anaesthesia, often at the opposite end of theatre.

A hybrid technique can be used, involving a combination of surgical and percutaneous techniques. This is usually carried out in theatre with skilled assistance.

'Hybrid' tracheostomy may also refer to the location, that is, performance of surgical tracheostomy on the critical care unit. This involves mobilising equipment (e.g. operating table, surgical kit, trolleys, and diathermy) and staff (e.g. scrub nurse) to the unit and associated theatre list allocation.

What are the potential complications of tracheostomy insertion?

Immediate
- Loss of airway
- Bleeding
- Subcutaneous emphysema
- Loss of PEEP and derecruitment
- Aspiration
- Bronchospasm
- *Injury to local structures*: thyroid, nerves (including recurrent laryngeal), and oesophagus
- Death

Short term
- Infection
- Bleeding
- Tracheo-innominate artery fistula (catastrophic haemorrhage)
- Accidental decannulation
- Inadequate sputum clearance
- Change in smell/taste sensation

Long term
- Tracheal stenosis
- Tracheomalacia
- Change in voice
- Scarring (see Chapter 48 Laryngeal Injury)

When can a patient with a tracheostomy be weaned and decannulated?

An improving trajectory is a prerequisite. This may be facilitated by rehabilitative interventions (e.g. physiotherapy and dietetics).

Important considerations
- Consistent approach and MDT involvement
- No single method of weaning is superior to another
- Establish the patient's ability to tolerate tracheostomy cuff deflation, ability to clear secretions, and cough:
  - Usually gradual, with increasing periods of cuff deflation time over days
  - This may cause an increased requirement for ventilatory support due to the effort of breathing around a deflated cuff.
  - Some centres wean using cuff deflation before pressure reduction or time on CPAP.
- Decannulation suitability depends on weaning method used and may be ventilator-dependent.
  - *Gradual pressure reduction*: end point of cuff down for 24 h
  - *Cuff down before pressure reduction*: 24 h without pressure support on tracheostomy mask (e.g. with Philips V60 ventilator, which is able to compensate for associated leak)

Occasionally doubt may exist as to whether the patient is able to wean with the current tracheostomy in situ due to its size (internal diameter too large, occluding the airway). If it is unclear whether the patient can breathe past a deflated cuff, the tracheostomy may be occluded with a gloved finger to see if airflow is able to pass through the upper airway. If this is not possible, downsizing of the tracheostomy may be considered.

The use of fenestrated tracheostomy tubes and speaking valves (both within/outwith ventilator breathing circuits) can be used during weaning. The ability of the patient to vocalise aids communication and their ability to engage with rehabilitation. Advanced techniques, such as above cuff vocalisation, might be used in experienced centres.

(See Chapter 48 Laryngeal Injury)

Resources
- 103. Carlucci A, Navalesi P. Weaning failure in critical illness. In: Webb A, Angus D, Finfer S, et al., eds., Oxford Textbook of Critical Care, 2nd ed. London: Oxford University Press; 2016. Available from: https://oxfordmedicine.com/view/10.1093/med/9780199600830.001.0001/med-9780199600830-chapter-103#med-9780199600830-chapter-103. (Accessed 24 April 2022.)
- Fernández R, Cabrera J, Calaf N, et al. P 0.1/PIMax: an index for assessing respiratory capacity in acute respiratory failure. Intensive Care Med. 1990;16(3):175–179.
- Lermitte J, Garfield MJ. Weaning from mechanical ventilation. CEACCP. 2005;5(4):113–117.
- National Tracheostomy Safety Project. Day-to-Day Management of Tracheostomies & Laryngectomies: Cuff Management, Vocalisation and Speaking Valves. Available from: https://www.tracheostomy.org.uk/storage/files/Cuff%20management%20Vocalisation.pdf. (Accessed 18 January 2022.)
- Nickson C. Life in the Fast Lane: Weaning from Mechanical Ventilation. Available from: https://litfl.com/weaning-from-mechanical-ventilation/. (Accessed 18 January 2022.)
- Yartsev A. Deranged Physiology: Complications of Percutaneous and Surgical Tracheostomy. 2016. Available from: https://derangedphysiology.com/main/required-reading/airway-management/Chapter%20212/complications-percutaneous-and-surgical-tracheostomy. (Accessed 18 January 2022.)

11. FLUIDS

When are intravenous fluids indicated in critical care?

The main indications for IV fluids are as follows:

- *Resuscitation*: rapidly restore circulating volume
- *Replacement*: mimic fluid that has been lost
- *Maintenance*: deliver basic electrolytes and glucose for metabolic needs

It is advocated that fluids are treated like drugs such as antibiotics and the '4 Ds' should be considered in prescription:

- *Drug*: consider indications, contraindications, and side effects
- *Dosing*: timing and rate
- *Duration*: consider 'stopping triggers'
- *De-escalation*: stop when no longer required

Fluid prescription should include the following:

- Type
- Rate
- Volume/dose
- Adaptation to current electrolyte disorders and other sources of fluid intake

What are the 4 phases of fluid therapy?

> **KEY POINT**
>
> The 4 phases of fluid therapy:
>
> - *Resuscitation*: patient rescue, early adequate fluid management, life-saving (boluses)
> - *Optimisation*: organ rescue, avoiding fluid overload and fluid creep (neutral balance)
> - *Stabilisation*: organ support (homeostasis), late conservative fluid management (2 × consecutive days in negative balance)
> - *Evacuation*: organ recovery, resolving fluid overload, active late goal directed fluid removal (negative balance)

Resuscitation aims to correct shock and achieve adequate perfusion pressure. Ongoing administration should be individualised and reassessed regularly. Ongoing losses should be replaced, and organ support should be provided. Removal of excessive fluid may be achieved by spontaneous diuresis during recovery, but ultrafiltration or diuretic prescription might be required.

What is 'fluid creep'?

'Fluid creep' is a term used to describe the discrepancy between predicted and administered fluid, with the potential for fluid overload. It may arise through the addition of fluids as drug diluents, flushes, or fluids used to maintain catheter patency.

What is the evidence for use of balanced crystalloids in critical care?

Several trials have compared balanced crystalloid solutions with saline in critically ill adults. They add weight to the argument that balanced solutions are safe. **SMART** concluded that balanced crystalloids should be favoured to reduce the composite outcome of death, new RRT, or persistent renal dysfunction at 30 days.

STUDY

SPLIT (2015)

- ICU patients requiring crystalloid fluid therapy
- *Intervention*: Plasma-Lyte 148 vs 0.9% sodium chloride (NaCl)
- *Primary*: proportion of patients with AKI within 90 days – **no difference**
- *Secondary*: AKI incidence, RRT requirement, readmission, LOS, mortality – no difference

STUDY

SMART (2018)

- Critically ill patients
- *Intervention*: balanced crystalloid vs 0.9% NaCl
- *Primary*: composite of major adverse kidney events (MAKE) at 30 days – **significantly lower**
- *Secondary*: mortality, new RRT, and persistent renal dysfunction – no difference

STUDY

BaSICS (2021)

- Adult intensive care patients
- *Interventions*: Plasma-Lyte vs 0.9% NaCl. Slow vs rapid bolus if required.
- *Primary*: 90-day mortality – **no difference**
- *Secondary*: day 7 SOFA score – **significantly lower**

STUDY

PLUS (2022)

- Adult intensive care patients
- *Interventions*: Plasma-Lyte 148 vs 0.9% NaCl
- *Primary*: 90-day mortality – **no difference**
- *Secondary*: new RRT – no difference

What are the undesirable effects of fluid administration?

Excess fluid administration can lead to 'resuscitation morbidity', including the following:

- **Fluid overload**
  - Pulmonary oedema and pleural effusions
  - Congestive cardiac failure (CCF)
  - Immobility and weakness
  - Delayed wound healing
  - Ileus
  - Limb compartment syndrome
  - Orbital compartment syndrome
  - Intra-abdominal hypertension (IAH) and abdominal compartment syndrome
  - Multi-organ failure due to the above
- **Electrolyte imbalance**
  - Water overload and hyponatraemia with dextrose solutions
  - Central pontine myelinolysis with rapid sodium shift
  - Hyperchloraemic acidosis with 0.9% sodium chloride

- **Transfusion-related effects**
- **Renal failure** with hydroxyethyl starch (HES)

What do you know about the FEAST trial?

The **FEAST** trial (2011) sought to investigate whether fluid boluses (albumin or saline), vs no fluid boluses, affected mortality in paediatric patients with severe febrile illnesses. It was carried out in a resource-limited setting in Africa.

Those receiving a fluid bolus had a statistically significant increase in mortality. However, the population had a high incidence of malaria and severe anaemia and was not managed in typical critical care facilities. It is difficult to apply these results to other populations. It would not be possible to replicate this study in non-resource limited populations from an ethical standpoint.

STUDY

FEAST (2011)

- Paediatric patients with severe febrile illness
- *Intervention*: fluid bolus (albumin vs saline) vs no fluid bolus
- *Primary*: mortality at 48 h in those without severe hypotension – **significantly higher**
- *Secondary*: mortality at 4 weeks – **significantly higher**

When is the use of human albumin solution (HAS) supported by the evidence?

Equivalence to 0.9% saline (**SAFE**)

- Volume resuscitation
- ARDS with hypoalbuminaemia
- Septic shock

Supported

- *Spontaneous bacterial peritonitis (SBP)*: lower mortality (**Sort et al.**) (see Chapter 136 Chronic Liver Disease)

Not supported

- Traumatic brain injury (TBI) (**SAFE**)

STUDY

SAFE (2004)

- ICU patients
- *Intervention*: resuscitation with 4% HAS vs 0.9% NaCl
- *Primary*: 28-day all-cause mortality – **no difference**
- *Secondary*: LOS, MV duration, and RRT duration – no difference
- Post hoc 28-day mortality in TBI – **significantly higher (24.5% vs 15.1%)**

Would you correct hypoalbuminaemia with HAS?

The **ALBIOS** study showed no difference in mortality with albumin supplementation to maintain a normal serum concentration in the context of sepsis. Most clinicians would not aim to correct hypoalbuminaemia to a target threshold in critical care.

STUDY

ALBIOS (2014)

- Adults with severe sepsis or septic shock
- *Intervention*: 20% HAS and crystalloid (target serum albumin ≥30 g/l) vs crystalloid only
- *Primary*: 28-day mortality – **no difference**
- *Secondary*: 90-day mortality – no difference

What do you know about the evidence behind the use of hydroxyethyl starches?

The use of HES has been the subject of research scandal. Numerous studies by J. Boldt on the use of HES were withdrawn after he was found guilty of research misconduct.

Subsequent RCTs examining HES have suggested that they cause significant harm including increased requirement for RRT (**CHEST, 6S**) and mortality (**6S**). There is also concern about coagulopathy. Starches are not widely used in contemporary practice as a result.

STUDY

CHEST (2012)

- Critically ill patients requiring fluid resuscitation
- *Intervention*: 6% HES vs 0.9% NaCl
- *Primary*: 90-day mortality – **no difference**
- *Secondary*: renal failure – **significantly higher**

STUDY

6S (2012)

- Critically ill adults with severe sepsis
- *Intervention*: 6% HES vs Ringer's acetate
- *Primary*: death or dialysis-dependence at 90/7 – **significantly higher (51% vs 43%)**
- *Secondary*: RRT use – **significantly higher (22% vs 16%)**

Resources

- Malbrain MLNG, Langer T, Annane D, et al. Intravenous fluid therapy in the perioperative and critical care setting: Executive summary of the International Fluid Academy (IFA). Ann Intensive Care 2020;10:64.
- Nickson C. Life in the Fast Lane: Albumin. 2020. Available from: https://litfl.com/albumin/. (Accessed 18 January 2022.)
- Wise J. Boldt: The great pretender. BMJ. 2013;346:f1738.

---

12.   MECHANICAL CIRCULATORY SUPPORT

What are ventricular assist devices?

A ventricular assist device (VAD) is a surgically implanted mechanical system that provides flow in order to maintain cardiac output whilst reducing the work of the heart.

Types
- *LVAD*: left ventricular assist device
- *RVAD*: right ventricular assist device
- *BiVAD*: biventricular assist device
- *TAH*: total artificial heart
- *Minimally invasive catheter-based assist devices* (e.g. Impella®)

Devices range from short-term large external circuits to compact wearable consoles for longer term therapy.

When might a VAD be used?

VAD use might be appropriate in acute or chronic heart failure (HF). The main indications are as follows:

- *Bridge to recovery*: cardiogenic shock (CS) (e.g. post-MI, viral cardiomyopathy, primary graft failure post-transplant)
- *Bridge to candidacy*
- *Bridge to transplantation*: limited organ availability and long waiting times
- *Destination therapy*: emerging internationally as outcomes become comparable to those of heart transplantation

Long-term therapy is usually via LVAD support as RV failure from pulmonary hypertension often improves concurrently. A minority will require a longer term BiVAD or TAH.

What are the key components of a VAD?

- Inflow cannula (to pump)
- Outflow cannula
- Pump
- Electrical controller/console
- Driveline (cable connecting device to controller – internal and external components)
- Power supply (e.g. battery pack)

How do VADs work?

Generations

1 *Pneumatic, hydraulic, or mechanical pusher plate*: energy ejects blood in a pulsatile manner
2 *Continuous non-pulsatile flow*: rotor suspended by contact bearings spins within a pipe and generates flow within the bloodstream
3 *Non-contact bearings*: centrifugal blood flow through magnetic or hydrodynamic levitation of an internal impeller

Mechanism

- **Pulsatile flow**
  - Electric pusher plate (LVAD)
  - Pneumatic sac-type (BiVAD/RVAD/LVAD/TAH)
- **Continuous flow**
  - Axial-flow pump with blood-immersed/magnetic bearings (LVAD)
  - Centrifugal pump ± magnetic levitation/hydrodynamic bearings (LVAD)

What are the main contraindications to VAD insertion?

- *General*: age > 65 years with biventricular failure
- *B*: severe dysfunction, fixed pulmonary hypertension
- *C*: severe valve lesions
- *D*: recent/evolving stroke, deficit impairing device management ability, significant psychological disease, inadequate psychosocial support
- *E*: AAA > 5 cm, metastatic cancer
- *F*: long-term RRT, high creatinine
- *G*: cirrhosis, fixed portal hypertension, BMI > 40 or < 20
- *H*: contraindication to anticoagulation, HIT
- *I*: severe sepsis, immunodeficiency

What complications might you encounter soon after device insertion?

- *Bleeding*: coagulopathy common (e.g. platelet consumption by device)
- Tamponade
- RV failure
- Fluid overload
- *Vasoplegia*: SIRS or phosphodiesterase inhibitor-induced

- *Haemodynamic instability*: septum deviation with underfilled ventricles
- GI/liver dysfunction
- Infection

Cardiac tamponade might present with decreasing device flows, high CVP, low MAP on escalating support, and metabolic acidosis.

What life-threatening complications might arise in a patient in the community with an LVAD?

Patients with VADs may be admitted to hospital with completely unrelated pathology. Some significant specific presentations in this population include the following:

- LVAD failure
- Ventricular arrhythmias
- Hypovolaemia
- Pump thrombosis
- Embolic stroke
- *Anticoagulation-related*: GI bleeding, ICH

How would you approach a patient with an LVAD who has been admitted to hospital following a collapse?

Ideally, the patient should be taken to a VAD centre, but this will depend on pre-hospital networks. Contacting a VAD centre for advice may be helpful.

Ask the patient/family if possible as they are likely to be very knowledgeable about their device. Information may also be located on an identification card/bracelet, in the controller bag, on the controller itself, or in an emergency bag carried separately by the patient.

There are several key differences in the management of these patients. Emergency resuscitation may include the following steps:

- Check for signs of life with responsiveness and breathing (pulse likely to be absent)
- If no signs of life, auscultate heart for humming sound
- If no humming sound or loud alarm from device: LVAD failure
- Ventilate but do not start chest compressions initially
- Try to restart LVAD
- Expose components and ensure connections attached
- Ensure power source working and secure
- Replace controller if unsuccessful in restarting LVAD
- *Consider cable fracture*: manipulate driveline to restore broken contact and tape it

If device has not failed or has been restored, other steps depend on pathology:

- *Ventricular arrhythmias:* defibrillation/cardioversion as indicated and consider CPR if fails
- *Other cause of inadequate circulation*: hypovolaemia likely (treat as indicated)
- Seek underlying cause of deterioration (e.g. stroke, hyperglycaemia, drug-related)

Would you perform CPR in an LVAD recipient?

This is controversial, and there is scant evidence to guide management. Risks include cannula dislodgement or anastomotic rupture, which may decrease over time (e.g. 10–30 days following implantation). Chest compressions may not be effective in the presence of an LVAD. It has been suggested that compressions should be started if attempts to restart or troubleshoot an LVAD fail (or if there is a significant delay to definitive management).

Give a brief overview of intra-aortic balloon pump (IABP) counterpulsation.

An IABP uses the inflation of a balloon in diastole and deflation in early systole to provide counterpulsation – inflation causes volume displacement of blood in each direction, increasing coronary flow (and systemic perfusion through the 'Windkessel effect'). Trials have yet to demonstrate the benefits of IABP use, but it remains a cornerstone of cardiothoracic critical care. (see Chapter 78 Heart Failure)

The balloon can be triggered using the ECG or arterial pressure waveform. Support is adjusted by programming the ratio of assisted beats. Anticoagulation is required.

Contraindications
- Aortic regurgitation
- Aortic dissection
- Aortic stents
- End-stage heart disease

Specific complications
- Limb ischaemia
- Thromboembolism
- Compartment syndrome
- Aortic dissection
- Local vascular injury
- Balloon rupture and gas embolus
- Balloon entrapment
- *Malpositioning*: renal/cerebral compromise
- Tamponade
- *Haematological*: thrombocytopaenia, haemolysis

Resources
- Bowles CT, Hards R, Wrightson N, et al. Algorithms to guide ambulance clinicians in the management of emergencies in patients with implanted rotary left ventricular assist devices. Emerg Med J. 2017;34(12):842–849.
- Harris P. Ventricular assist devices. CEACCP. 2012;12(3):145–151.
- Krishna M, Zacharowski K. Principles of intra-aortic balloon pump counterpulsation. CEACCP. 2009;9(1):24–28.

13. PACING

What are the causes of bradycardia?

Intrinsic
- Idiopathic (ageing, degenerative)
- Ischaemia
- Cardiomyopathy
- Genetic disorders
- *Infiltrative*: sarcoidosis, amyloidosis, haemochromatosis
- *Collagen/vascular*: rheumatoid, scleroderma, systemic lupus erythematosus (SLE), storage diseases, neuromuscular

- *Infectious*: perivalvular abscess, Chagas' disease, myocarditis, Lyme disease, diphtheria, toxoplasmosis
- Congenital heart disease
- *Cardiac surgery*: CABG, valve, transplant, radiotherapy, iatrogenic atrioventricular (AV) block, ablation

Extrinsic
- Physical training
- Vagal reflex
- Drug effects
- Idiopathic paroxysmal AV block
- *Electrolyte imbalance*: hypo/hyperkalaemia, hypercalcaemia, hypermagnesaemia
- *Metabolic*: hypothyroidism, anorexia, hypoxia, acidosis, hypothermia
- *Neurological*: high ICP, CNS tumour, temporal epilepsy
- OSA

Drugs of note, other than antihypertensives and antiarrhythmics:

- *Sinus node bradycardia*: opioids, muscle relaxants, propofol, steroids, proton pump inhibitors, cannabis
- *AV block*: selective serotonin receptor antagonists (SSRI), tricyclic antidepressants (TCA)
- *Either/both*: lithium, phenytoin, carbamazepine, ticagrelor, H2 antagonists, some chemotherapeutic agents

Reversible causes are as follows: ischaemia, infection, post-operative, electrolytes, and drugs.'

What are the types of pacing available?

- *Percussion*: manual technique used during resuscitation
- *Transcutaneous*: temporary resuscitative technique via external pads
- *Endocardial*: transvenous lead(s) implanted into myocardium (temporary/long term)
- *Epicardial*: implanted during thoracotomy/thoracoscopy
- *Cardiac resynchronisation therapy (CRT)*: biventricular pacing to correct dyssynchrony
- *Conduction system*: bundle pacing in high-degree AV block or bundle branch block (BBB)
- *Leadless*: miniature intracardiac leadless pacemaker

How does pacing work?
Pacing involves the delivery of an electrical impulse to the myocardium to achieve a wave of depolarisation. Successful depolarisation is termed 'electrical capture'. This should then achieve contraction of the relevant chamber(s) of the heart.

Pacing relies on intact myocardial and/or conducting tissue, and any underlying pathology may affect the ability to successfully pace a patient. Hence, it will not indefinitely achieve cardiac output in a patient with non-viable myocardium. Some conditions requiring pacing are transient. For example, the conducting system may be ineffective but recover soon after some types of cardiac surgery.

How are pacemaker modes classified?
Pacing modes are described in the Generic Pacemaker Code by a series of letters, each relating to a specific function according to their position in the series.

KEY POINT

Generic Pacemaker Code:

  I. *Chamber(s) paced*: none (O), atrium (A), ventricle (V), dual A + V (D)
 II. *Chamber(s) sensed*: none (O), atrium (A), ventricle (V), dual A + V (D)
III. *Response to sensing*: none (O), inhibited (I), triggered (T), dual T + I (D)
 IV. *Programmability*: none (O), rate modulation (R)
  V. *Multisite pacing*: none (O), atrium (A), ventricle (V), dual A + V (D)

Examples
- *VOO*: asynchronous ventricular pacing (no sensing, rate modulation, multisite pacing)
- *VVIR*: ventricular inhibitory pacing with rate modulation

- *AAI*: atrial pacing inhibited by spontaneous atrial depolarisation
- *AAT*: atrial pacing regardless of atrial sensing (diagnostic use)
- *DDD*: dual chamber pacing, inhibited by A/V sensing and ventricular pacing triggered after programmed interval
- *DDI*: dual-chamber pacing without atrial synchronous ventricular pacing

What does an 'inhibitory response' mean?

The third letter, 'I' for 'inhibited', specifically means that the pacemaker response is inhibited by spontaneous ventricular activity. The pacemaker does not inhibit ventricular activity.

Can you describe some rhythm-based indications for temporary cardiac pacing?

- **Conduction abnormality**
  - *AV delay*: post-cardiac surgery, Mobitz II, and 3° heart block
  - *Bifascicular block*: new or with 1° heart block
  - Long QT with significant bradycardia
  - PA catheter insertion in patient with LBBB
- **Tachycardia (overdrive pacing)**
  - *AV junctional tachycardia*: post-CPB
  - Re-entrant SVT or VT
  - Type I atrial flutter
- **Prophylactic**
  - Bradycardia-dependent VT
  - AF
- **Other**
  - Sinus bradycardia
  - Restoration of AV mechanical synchrony in 3° heart block, AV junctional, or ventricular rhythms
  - Hypertrophic obstructive cardiomyopathy (HOCM)
  - Post-heart transplantation (denervated heart)

What is the difference between 'cardiac resynchronisation therapy with defibrillator (CRT-D)' and 'cardiac resynchronisation therapy with pacemaker (CRT-P)'?

CRT can improve cardiac function, symptoms, well-being, morbidity, and mortality in selected patients with chronic HF. This may be combined with an implantable cardiac defibrillator (ICD).

CRT-D
- Cardiac resynchronisation therapy with defibrillator
- Used if ICD indicated in CRT-indicated patients (e.g. symptomatic with LVEF ≤35%)
- Possible survival benefit over CRT-P

CRT-P
- Cardiac resynchronisation therapy with pacemaker
- May be more suitable in non-ischaemic aetiology, short life expectancy, major comorbidities, or CKD

An ICD might be indicated alone for primary or secondary prevention, particularly in ischaemic HF, certain inherited conditions, or significant ventricular arrhythmias (e.g. post-cardiac arrest).

GUIDELINE ESC 2021 Cardiac pacing

How would you perform a pacemaker check in a patient with temporary wires?

The pacing system should be checked every day (and ideally each shift), providing the patient is not unstable due to another reason.

- **Sensitivity** is the minimum current that the pacemaker can sense, so a lower number corresponds with greater sensitivity.
- The **pacing threshold** is the sensitivity at which the sense indicator flashes during each endogenous depolarisation when tested.
- The **capture threshold** is the minimum output required to stimulate an action potential in the myocardium, confirmed with a QRS complex following each pacing spike.

Pacemaker check

1 Underlying rhythm
- Reduce rate and allow native rhythm to appear (preferable to reducing energy and risking loss of capture)

2 Sensitivity
- Reduce rate below native rate, VVI/AAI/DDD mode
- Increase sensitivity number (reducing pacemaker sensitivity) until sense indicator stops flashing
- Reduce sensitivity number until indicator flashes with each native depolarisation (pacing threshold)
- **Leave sensitivity at half the pacing threshold**
- Don't prolong test as AF/VF may develop if R-on-T phenomenon occurs

3 Capture threshold
- **Don't check** if no underlying rhythm
- Set pacemaker rate above native rate so chamber of interest consistently paced
- Reduce energy output until QRS no longer follows each pacing spike (capture threshold)
- **Leave output at twice the capture threshold** (or less if threshold > 10 mA)

4 Rate
- Optimal rate usually left at 80–90 min^{-1} after testing the above
- May 'wean' to a backup rate (e.g. 40 min^{-1}) when patient in suitable condition

What technical complications might occur during temporary epicardial pacing?

- Output failure
- Failure to capture
- Undersensing
- Oversensing
- Cross-talk
- Endless loop tachycardia

Describe your approach to the newly bradycardic patient in critical care.

- Supportive care as indicated
- Follow ALS algorithm
  - Compromising features? If so, try drugs
  - If drugs ineffective, will require transcutaneous pacing
  - Transcutaneous pacing may buy time to establish chronotropic infusion (e.g. isoprenaline)
- Treat underlying cause if reversible/known
- Involve cardiologist. Useful information when considering transvenous pacing:
  - Existing central venous access
  - Anticoagulation
  - Concurrent infection
  - Timing
  - Recording on monitor
  - 12-lead ECG
- Investigate other causes (see list above). (See Chapter 71 Cardiac Advanced Life Support)

What is overdrive pacing?

Overdrive (or antitachycardia) pacing involves the delivery of stimuli at high frequencies to convert a tachyarrhythmia to sinus rhythm. It can be used in the acute setting to disrupt a rhythm or in longer-term arrhythmias with complications (e.g. tachycardia-induced ventricular dysfunction). Risks include precipitating VT or VF.

Indications
- *Diagnostic*: VT vs SVT
- Recurrent arrhythmia
- Failure of drug therapy
- Contraindication to cardioversion (see Chapter 76 Arrhythmias)

Resources
- Bernstein AD, Daubert JC, Fletcher RD, et al. The revised NASPE/BPEG generic code for antibradycardia, adaptive-rate, and multisite pacing. Pacing Clin Electrophysiol. 2002;25(2):260–264.
- Nickson C. Life in the Fast Lane: Overdrive Pacing. 2020. Available from: https://litfl.com/overdrive-pacing/. (Accessed 01 November 2021.)
- Reade MC. Temporary epicardial pacing after cardiac surgery: a practical review. Anaesthesia. 2007;62(4):264–271.

14. SEDATION

When is sedation indicated in critical care?

Sedation is indicated in specific circumstances, and its use should be individualised. In intubated patients, the majority will require sedation to tube tolerance only. This may disappear if converted to tracheostomy. Occasionally, disease states may indicate deeper sedation. The need for analgesia should be assessed first before sedative agent requirement. Many indications for sedation go hand in hand with those for invasive ventilation.

Specific indications
- Facilitate tracheal intubation
- Obtund laryngeal reflexes and maintain tracheal intubation
- Increase tolerance of invasive procedures
- Facilitate ventilator synchrony
- Reduce oxygen demand and prevent secondary injury
  - TBI
  - Prolonged seizures
  - Serotonin syndrome
  - MH
  - Severe metabolic disturbance or instability
- Withdrawal from sedative agents
- Severe hyperactive delirium

Why is depth of sedation important?

Over- or undersedation can have significant consequences as follows:

Oversedation
- Increased ventilator days
- Increased ICU LOS
- Delirium
- Masking of significant haemodynamic responses

Undersedation
- Hypercatabolism
- Immunosuppression

Table 14.1 Richmond Agitation-Sedation Scale (RASS) and levels of stimulation required for assessment

	Criteria	Definition
+4	Combative	Overly combative, violent, immediate danger to staff
+3	Very agitated	Pulls or removes tubes or catheters; aggressive
+2	Agitated	Frequent non-purposeful movement, fights ventilator
+1	Restless	Anxious but movements not aggressively vigorous
0	Alert and calm	
−1	Drowsy	Not fully alert but has sustained awakening (eye opening/eye contact) to voice (>10 s)
−2	Light sedation	Briefly awakens with eye contact to voice (<10 s)
−3	Moderate sedation	Movement or eye opening to voice (but no eye contact)
−4	Deep sedation	No response to voice but movement or eye opening to physical stimulation
−5	Unrousable	No response to voice or physical stimulation

Note: White, no stimulation; light grey, verbal stimulation; and dark grey, physical stimulation.

- Hypercoagulability
- Increased sympathetic activity
- Risk of patient harm (e.g. self-extubation)

How do you assess depth of sedation?
Sedation may be assessed using scores such as the RASS (Table 14.1).

Can you name some examples of sedative agents used in critical care?

- *Hypnotics*: propofol, ketamine, thiopentone, etomidate
- *Opioids*: remifentanil (infusion only), alfentanil, morphine, fentanyl, oxycodone
- *Benzodiazepines*: midazolam, diazepam, lorazepam
- *Alpha agonists*: dexmedetomidine, clonidine
- *Neuroleptics*: haloperidol, olanzapine
- *Volatile anaesthetics*: sevoflurane, isoflurane
- *Other*: chlordiazepoxide (also chloral hydrate and alimemazine in paediatrics)

When might you favour or avoid specific intravenous infusion agents in critical care?
Sedative agents have different profiles of desirable and undesirable effects. Some might be used for their advantages in specific disease states, whilst others might be deleterious (Table 14.2). Most involve withdrawal syndromes if use is prolonged.

What do you know about volatile anaesthetic agent use in critical care?
Volatile anaesthetic agents may be used for patients with severe bronchospasm due to bronchodilating properties, or in patients who are difficult to sedate on multiple infusions (e.g. in paediatrics).

Sevoflurane or **isoflurane** can be administered through a dedicated anaesthetic machine on the critical care unit or through a stand-alone device incorporated into the ventilator circuit (e.g. AnaConDa® by Sedana Medical). The desired minimum alveolar concentration (MAC) is targeted and measured through a gas sampling line in both contexts. **Methoxyflurane**, through a dedicated inhaler (e.g. Penthrox®), is sometimes used for its analgesic profile in the pre-hospital trauma setting.

Difficulty might arise with limited diffusion across alveoli (e.g. excessive secretions). An understanding of the nuances of volatile agents including contraindications (e.g. MH susceptibility) and planes of anaesthesia is essential for safe use.

When might the use of muscle relaxant be indicated in critical care?

- Facilitation of airway procedures
- *Severe hypoxaemic respiratory failure*: reduces oxygen consumption (VO_2)
- *Specific ventilation modes*: high pressures and inverse ratios
- Suppression of high respiratory drive

Table 14.2 Comparison of intravenous sedative infusions in critical care

	Advantages	Disadvantages
Propofol	Relatively context insensitive Obtunds laryngeal reflexes Antiepileptic	PRIS in high doses Not used commonly in paediatrics
Midazolam	Useful to reduce propofol requirement Antiepileptic	Deliriogenic Slow elimination
Ketamine	Bronchodilation in asthma	Increased secretion load Increased myocardial oxygen demand
Thiopentone	Reliable CNS depressant	Long elimination half-life Haemodynamic instability, particularly in hypovolaemia
Alfentanil	Relatively context insensitive Analgesic	Lowers seizure threshold (as with other opioids) Physical dependence
Remifentanil	Context insensitive, quick offset Analgesic	Relatively expensive Not suitable for bolus administration (risks bradycardia and asystole)
Dexmedetomidine	Anxiolysis Analgesic Antihypertensive Bridge to extubation in agitated patients	Relatively expensive
Clonidine	Cheaper than dexmedetomidine Enteral preparation for weaning	Bradycardia and hypotension more pronounced Longer elimination half-life than dexmedetomidine

- Raised ICP unresponsive to sedation
- Abdominal compartment syndrome
- Risk of instability during some transfers

What are the caveats of common neuromuscular blocking drugs in the context of critical care?

- **Suxamethonium**
  - Hyperkalaemia risk in burns >24 h and spinal cord injury >72 h (extra-junctional ACh receptor development)
  - Muscle fasciculations may be undesirable (e.g. in rhabdomyolysis or trauma)
  - Contraindicated in MH susceptibility
  - Contraindicated in Guillain-Barré syndrome (GBS) – upregulated ACh receptors risk severe hyperkalaemia
  - Relative resistance in myasthenia gravis
- **Rocuronium**
  - Highest risk of anaphylaxis
  - Prolonged duration of action in hepatic and renal impairment
  - May be ineffective soon after sugammadex use
- **Atracurium**
  - More commonly associated with bronchospasm due to histamine release
- **Cisatracurium**
  - Most haemodynamically stable but expensive

What is a sedation hold?

A sedation hold, or sedation holiday, is the temporary cessation of sedative infusions in critical care. This allows the patient to wake and facilitates washout of drugs, preventing accumulation.

Sedation holds are thought to reduce the duration of mechanical ventilation and ICU LOS when indicated, although this was not replicated in the **SLEAP** trial, which found that light sedation protocols may increase the amount of sedative administered and nursing workload.

STUDY

ABC (2008)

- Mechanically ventilated and sedated patients
- *Intervention*: spontaneous awakening trial ± SBT vs SBT alone
- *Primary*: number of ventilator-free days – **significantly higher (14.7 vs 11.6)**
- *Secondary*: ICU LOS, hospital LOS, 1-year mortality – **significantly lower**; self-extubation – **significantly higher**

STUDY

SLEAP (2012)

- Mechanically ventilated and sedated patients (with opioids and/or benzodiazepines)
- *Intervention*: daily cessation of opioid and benzodiazepine infusions vs no planned interruption
- *Primary*: days to extubation – **no difference**
- *Secondary*: days to extubation in trauma and surgical patients – **significantly lower**

How would you manage the critical care patient with insomnia?

Sleep may be difficult to achieve in the critical care environment. Overall, non-pharmacological methods are preferred due to the risks of pharmacological agents, including delirium and disproportionate sleep architecture (deficiency of 'useful' sleep).

Anti-delirium measures should be used routinely. Environments should be adapted to prevent excessive noise (ideally < 35 dB) and lighting in keeping with the natural day-night cycle. There may be a role for targeted music therapy.

Supplementary melatonin is used by some to aid sleep-wake cycle regulation, but this has not yet been supported by improved outcomes.

(See Chapter 29 Delirium)

When would you be concerned that your patient is experiencing a withdrawal syndrome and how would you manage this?

Some patients will present with withdrawal from alcohol, benzodiazepines, or opioids soon after admission to critical care. This may be easier to anticipate, and appropriate regimes may be tailored with the assistance of pharmacy and alcohol/drug liaison colleagues. (see Chapter 33 Mental Health and Critical Care)

Iatrogenic withdrawal syndromes may occur after cessation of prolonged sedation, particularly with opioids and benzodiazepines. A third of patients in critical care for greater than 7 days have features of withdrawal from sedative or analgesic agents.

Opioid withdrawal
- Occurs with all opioids
- Characterised by adrenergic excitation and exaggerated nociception
- Prevention
  - Titrate analgesia and sedation, perform sedation holds
  - Regular paracetamol where possible
  - Alternative analgesic agents where opioids likely to be ineffective (e.g. gabapentin for neuropathic pain in GBS)
- Clonidine may be used to blunt symptoms
  - e.g. 50–100 μg 8°
  - Wean slowly with opioid
  - No evidence of superiority to slow opioid weaning

KEY POINT

Example opioid withdrawal regime:

- Calculate daily infused quantity (day 0)
- *Day 1*: reduce infusion by 20%
- *Day 2*+ reduce infusion by 10% of original dose daily

Benzodiazepine withdrawal

- Acute withdrawal lasts 1–2 weeks, followed by prolonged period of decreasing somatic/psychiatric symptoms (over months)
- *Psychiatric*: acute anxiety states, phobias, perceptual disorders, irritability, aggression
- *Somatic*: paraesthesia, tremors, myalgia, blurred vision, seizures, ataxia
- Prevention should be considered (as above)
  - Usual antidepressants and antipsychotics should be restarted early
- Withdrawal may take days to weeks and circumstances vary widely between patients
- Diazepam may be more familiar to clinicians than lorazepam, but it carries an increased risk of delirium and accumulation of active metabolites

KEY POINT

Example benzodiazepine withdrawal regime:

- Calculate daily infused dose of midazolam
- Divide by 12 to give approximate total daily dose of lorazepam
- Divide by 4 to give 6 h doses
- *After dose 2*: reduce midazolam infusion by 50%
- *After dose 3*: reduce midazolam infusion by further 50%
- *After dose 4*: discontinue midazolam infusion
- Reduce lorazepam by 500 µg to 1 mg daily until weaned completely

Resources

- Borthwick M, Bourne R, Craig M, et al. Detection, Prevention and Treatment of Delirium in Critically Ill Patients, Version 1.2. June 2006. Available from: https://www.scottishintensivecare.org.uk/uploads/2014-07-24-19-57-26-UKCPADeliriumResourcepdf-92654.pdf. (Accessed 24 April 2022.)
- Lewis SR, Pritchard MW, Schofield-Robinson OJ, et al. Melatonin for the promotion of sleep in adults in the intensive care unit. Cochrane Database Syst Rev. 2018;5(5):CD012455.
- Rowe K, Fletcher S. Sedation in the intensive care unit. CEACCP. 2008;8(2):50–55.

15.   CEREBRAL MONITORING

What is multimodal cerebral monitoring?

Multimodal monitoring refers to a variety of non-invasive and invasive techniques used to observe neurophysiological and systemic parameters. These should be used in conjunction with clinical examination and traditional haemodynamic monitoring to guide treatment before irreversible damage has occurred.

Multimodal monitoring focuses on the following domains:

- Clinical neurological examination
- ICP and cerebral perfusion pressure (CPP)

- Cerebral blood flow (CBF)
- Cerebral oxygenation
- Cerebral metabolism
- Electrophysiological activity

GUIDELINE   NCS ESICM 2014 Multimodal Monitoring

Can you describe some examples of different ICP and CPP monitoring devices?

Cranial bolt/fibre-optic device
- Transduction of sensed pressure (e.g. through piezoresistive strain gauge)
- Placed ipsilaterally to maximal pathology to optimise tissue physiology in at-risk areas and should not be placed directly within the lesion

External ventricular drain (EVD)
- Intraventricular catheter connected to an external pressure transducer via fluid-filled tubing

Optic nerve sheath diameter (ONSD)
- US used to measure the optic nerve diameter 3 mm posterior to the globe
- **ONSD > 5–6 mm** is associated with ICP > 20 mmHg

Pupillometry
- Measures pupillary reactivity and calculates the Neurologic Pupil index (NPi)
- NPi values range from 0 to 5
- **NPi < 3** is associated with ICP > 20 mmHg

How is cerebral blood flow monitored?

- **Transcranial Doppler (TCD)**
  - US of intracranial arteries to evaluate CBF velocities
  - *Blood flow velocities through cerebral arteries*: identifies emboli, stenosis, or vasospasm in subarachnoid haemorrhage (SAH)
  - *Pulsatility Index (PI)*: based on systolic and diastolic variables (**PI > 0.6** associated with ICP > 20 mmHg)
- **Parenchymal thermal diffusion flowmetry**
  - Probe placed with 2 thermistors set at different temperatures
  - Rate of temperature dissipation from applied heat is calculated
  - Increased heat dissipation indicates greater blood flow
- **Transcranial colour-coded duplex sonography (TCCDS)**
- **Laser Doppler flowmetry**

How is transcranial Doppler used in the detection of vasospasm in SAH?

Increased blood flow velocity is associated with decreased vessel diameter (vasospasm) or increased blood volume (hyperaemia). The Lindegaard ratio (LR) is used to assess discrepancy in blood flow velocities between vessels. Serial assessment is helpful.

Lindegaard ratio = Mean velocity in MCA / mean velocity in ipsilateral extracranial internal carotid artery (ICA)

Interpretation
- *Vasospasm*: **LR > 3** or MCA velocity > 120 cm/s
- *Hyperaemia*: **LR < 3**

Can you describe some examples of how cerebral oxygenation may be monitored?

Brain parenchymal oxygen tension (P_{btO2})

- P_{btO2} provides a regional measure of the balance between oxygen supply and demand via a bolt
- Normal P_{btO2} 23–35 mmHg
- **P_{btO2} < 20 mmHg** may indicate ischaemic secondary injury

Near-infrared spectroscopy (NIRS)

- Measures regional cerebral oxygen saturation
- A near-infrared light source and receiver is placed with the amount of light attenuation between the 2 measured
- Light spectra absorption between oxyhaemoglobin and deoxyhaemoglobin is compared

Jugular bulb venous oxygen saturation ($SjvO_2$)

- Fibre-optic catheter is placed in the internal jugular vein (IJV) ipsilateral to the injury and advanced superiorly to the jugular bulb
- $SjvO_2$ provides a global measure of the balance between oxygen supply and demand
- Normal $SjVO_2$ 55–75%
- **$SjvO_2$ < 55%** may indicate poor oxygen supply or increased oxygen demand and may indicate ischaemia
- **$SjvO_2$ > 75%** may indicate increased oxygen supply or poor oxygen demand and may indicate hyperaemia or cell death

How does cerebral metabolism monitoring work?

Cerebral microdialysis (CMD) is a form of cerebral metabolism monitoring. A catheter containing a semi-permeable membrane is placed into the white matter. It is constantly perfused with microdialysate. Small molecules are able to diffuse into perfusion fluid.

Measured substrates

- **Glucose**
  - Low glucose associated with poor outcome
  - Reduced in hypoxaemia/ischaemia, reduced cerebral glucose supply, and cerebral hyperglycolysis
- **Lactate and pyruvate**
  - Lactate to pyruvate ratio (LPR) > 25 associated with metabolic distress
  - Reduced in hypoxaemia/ischaemia, reduced cerebral glucose supply, and mitochondrial dysfunction
- **Glutamate**
  - Excitatory neurotransmitter associated with neuro-injury and neuro-inflammatory response cascade
  - Elevated in hypoxaemia/ischaemia and excitotoxicity
- **Glycerol**
  - Lipid-rich component of neurones and marker of neurological cell breakdown and cell death
  - Elevated in hypoxaemia/ischaemia and cell membrane degradation

Can you give examples of measuring electrophysiological activity?

- **Quantitative electroencephalogram (EEG)**
  - Continuous EEG (cEEG) via scalp electrodes
  - Raw data depicting electrical activity of the brain is collected and converted to a digital form
  - Used in coma
  - Used to monitor and target sedation (e.g. barbiturate infusion to burst suppression)
  - Delayed cerebral ischaemia (DCI) in SAH
    - ➢ *Alpha-delta ratio* (ADR): normal < 50%; > 50% may indicate ischaemia
- **Somatosensory evoked potentials (SSEPs)**
  - An electrical stimulus is applied to the median or tibial nerve
  - SSEPs are measured via scalp electrodes as evoked EEG responses

What are the advantages and disadvantages of different cerebral monitoring techniques?

There are many advantages and disadvantages of different cerebral monitoring techniques (Table 15.1).

Table 15.1 Comparison of cerebral monitoring techniques

Modality	Technique	Advantages	Disadvantages
ICP/CPP	ICP bolt	Continuous monitoring Infection < 1%	Poor positioning affects values Cannot be recalibrated (drift ≥ day 5) Local (not global) measurement Some not MR compatible
	EVD	Diagnostic and therapeutic CSF sampling Intrathecal medication administration Recalibration possible	Infection in up to 10% Intermittent ICP monitoring when system closed Difficult to place in distorted anatomy
	ONSD	Non-invasive Serially measurable at bedside	May be difficult/impossible in orbital trauma Operator-dependent Intermittent
	Pupillometry	Non-invasive Serially measurable at bedside	May be difficult/impossible in orbital trauma Operator-dependent Intermittent
CBF	TCD	Non-invasive Serially measurable at bedside	Difficult if poor acoustic windows Operator-dependent Poor assessment of posterior circulation
	Parenchymal thermal diffusion flowmetry	Continuous	Poor positioning affects values Local (not global) measurement Poor reliability in systemic hyperthermia
Cerebral oxygenation	P_{btO_2}	Early detection of cerebral hypoxia (before ICP changes)	Poor positioning affects values Local (not global) measurement Some not MR compatible
	NIRS	Non-invasive Serially measurable at bedside	Difficult if scalp oedema or thick clot present Operator-dependent
	$SjvO_2$	Continuous	Requires calibration CVC-related complications Thrombosis risk
Cerebral metabolism	CMD	Early detection of secondary injury	Poor positioning affects values Delay in results (collection over time)
Electrophysiology	Quantitative EEG	Non-invasive Continuous	Operator-dependent
	SSEPs	Non-invasive Serially measurable at bedside	Operator-dependent

Resources

- Chestnut R, Aguilera S, Buki A, et al. A management algorithm for adult patients with both brain oxygen and intracranial pressure monitoring: The Seattle International Severe Traumatic Brain Injury Consensus Conference (SIBICC). Intensive Care Med. 2020;46(5):919–929.
- Darsie ME, Moheet AM, Lau W. (Eds.) The pocket guide to neurocritical care. USA: The Neurocritical Care Society; 2020.
- Tameem A, Krovvidi H. Cerebral physiology. BJA Educ. 2013;13(4):113–118.
- Tisdall MM, Smith M. Cerebral microdialysis: research technique or clinical tool. Br J Anaesth. 2006;97(10):18–25.
- White H, Venkatesh B. Applications of transcranial Doppler in the ICU: a review. Intensive Care Med. 2006;32(7):981–994.

What is the pathophysiological rationale behind the protective effects of hypothermia?

- Decreased CMR
- Decreased cerebral oxygen demand
- Decreased production of neurotransmitters (e.g. glutamate)
- Reduced free radical exposure/oxidative stress from reperfusion injury

What is therapeutic hypothermia?

Therapeutic hypothermia is a concept involving cooling a patient to a subnormal temperature for specific indications, usually to prevent brain injury, due to its neuroprotective properties. Its use is now limited to very specific circumstances as it is not without complications.

Indications
- Neuroprotection in neonatal hypoxic ischaemic brain injury
- Deep hypothermic circulatory arrest to facilitate neuroprotection in aortic surgery

Previously, therapeutic hypothermia had been considered in the management of TBI and post-cardiac arrest syndrome.

(See Chapter 58 Hypothermia, Chapter 27 Out-of-Hospital Cardiac Arrest, and Chapter 83 Traumatic Brain Injury)

What is targeted temperature management?

Targeted temperature management (TTM) superseded therapeutic hypothermia. In TTM, a constant, targeted temperature was maintained. It has, again, been superseded by the more contemporary 'temperature control' strategy.

Previous indications for TTM in the unconscious post-cardiac arrest patient with return of spontaneous circulation (ROSC) are as follows:

- OHCA, initial shockable rhythm (previously recommended)
- OHCA, initial non-shockable rhythm (previously suggested)
- In-hospital cardiac arrest (IHCA) (previously suggested)

Contraindications to hypothermia < 33°C included severe systemic infection and pre-existing medical coagulopathy.

GUIDELINE   ERC 2021 Post-resuscitation care

Why did therapeutic hypothermia and TTM fall out of favour?

Practice has largely moved away from these concepts and towards avoidance of hyperthermia and maintenance of a low normal temperature due to a lack of supporting evidence and risk of complications.

The following variables have been examined:

- Use of TTM (vs not used)
- Duration
- Method
- Temperature
- Timing
- Rewarming

STUDY

TTM (2013)

- Unconscious patients following OHCA of presumed cardiac cause
- *Intervention*: TTM to 33°C vs 36°C
- *Primary*: all-cause mortality at end of trial – **no difference**
- *Secondary*: composite of poor neurological function or death at 180 days (CPC and Modified Rankin Scale [mRS]) – no difference

STUDY

TTM 48 (2017)

- Adults post-ROSC after OHCA of presumed cardiac cause
- *Intervention*: TTM to 33°C for 48 h vs 24 h
- *Primary*: favourable neurological outcome at 6 months (CPC) – **no difference**
- *Secondary*: 6-month mortality and time to death – no difference; adverse events – **significantly higher**

STUDY

TTM2 (2021)

- Unconscious patients following OHCA
- *Intervention*: target 33°C vs trigger 37.8°C to target 37.5°C
- *Primary*: 6-month all-cause mortality – **no difference**
- *Secondary*: poor functional outcome and quality of life – no difference
- *Adverse events*: arrhythmias with haemodynamic instability – **significantly higher (24% vs 16%)**; pneumonia, sepsis, bleeding, and skin complications – no difference

How was TTM achieved?

Previous guidance recommended TTM following ROSC in patients who had suffered a cardiac arrest. This required the following phases in management:

- **Induction**
  - Achievement of target temperature: 32–36°C (previously 32–34°C)
  - May need to warm (usually passively) to target first if unintentional excessive hypothermia
- **Maintenance**
  - Remainder of first 24 h at desired temperature
- **Rewarming**
  - Subsequent 48 h in which normothermia is achieved and maintained
  - Avoidance of hyperthermia (aim ≤37.7°C)
  - Best achieved with system using temperature feedback loop to avoid fluctuation
  - Maximum 0.5°C change per hour

Timing

- Earlier initiation associated with more favourable neurological outcomes.
- Rapid spontaneous cooling associated with worse outcome but may be a marker of more severe neurological injury.
- Possible risk of rearrest with pre-hospital IV cooling so not recommended.
- Consensus was to commence TTM early after ROSC in a suitably monitored setting in hospital.

Methods
- 'TTM devices' exist, providing a feedback loop with monitoring and delivery of targeted temperature (e.g. heat-exchange water circulating cooling pads in Arctic Sun™ 5000 [Medivance/Bard])
- Simple ice packs/wet towels
- Intravascular heat exchanger
- Air circulating blankets
- *Extracorporeal circulation*: ECMO, CBP, haemofiltration
- Transnasal evaporative cooling (under investigation)
- *Environmental*: avoidance of excess bedding, appropriate room temperature

Sedation
- Sedation with NMB was recommended to avoid shivering with lower targets such as 33°C
- Magnesium may prevent shivering by lowering the threshold temperature
- Short-acting sedative agents facilitate prognostication later (e.g. propofol, remifentanil)

Temperature
- Historical preference for 36°C over 33°C
- Avoids sequelae relating to shivering
- Potential to avoid other complications of hypothermia
- Mitigates the risk of rebound hyperthermia
- Sedation requirement may be reduced

What are the risks of rewarming?

- Rebound hyperthermia
- Hypotension (vasodilatation)
- Reperfusion injury

How would you manage a patient's temperature following cardiac arrest?

The latest guidance uses the terminology '**temperature control**', rather than TTM, and recommends **actively preventing fever (temperature > 37.7°C)** by exposing the patient, using antipyretic drugs, or using a cooling device with a target temperature of **37.5°C** if these are unsuccessful.

Actively rewarming patients with mild hypothermia following ROSC is not recommended.

GUIDELINE   ERC-ESICM 2022 Temperature management

How would you manage a patient's temperature following traumatic brain injury with raised ICP?

- Normothermia, aim central temperature 36-37°C (intracranial temperature approximately 1°C higher than tympanic temperature)
- Therapeutic hypothermia used occasionally but largely fallen out of favour (local interpretation of trial evidence, balance of risk/benefit)

Resource
- Nolan JP, Soar J, Cariou A, et al. European Resuscitation Council and European Society of Intensive Care Medicine Guidelines for Post-resuscitation Care 2015: Section 5 of the European Resuscitation Council Guidelines for Resuscitation 2015. Resuscitation 2015;95;202–222.

Why is nutritional assessment challenging in the ICU?

- *Patient factors*: varied population, age range, extremes of prior health, frailty increasing
- *Active disease*: acute gut injury, sepsis, major trauma/surgery, organ failure
- *Interventions*: ventilation, RRT, body temperature changes, sedation, rehabilitation

Which scoring systems do we use for assessment of nutritional status in hospitalised patients?

NICE recommends screening all patients with the **Malnutrition Universal Screening Tool (MUST)**:

1 Measure height and weight to calculate BMI
2 Note % unplanned weight loss
3 Establish acute disease effect and score
4 Add scores from steps 1–3 to obtain overall risk
5 Apply guidelines and/or local policy to develop care plan

A score of 0 is deemed low risk, 1 medium risk, and ≥2 high risk.

Other scores
- *Nutrition Risk in Critically Ill (NUTRIC)*: ≥6 high risk
- *Nutrition Risk Screening (NRS)*: 4 at risk and ≥5 high risk (see Chapter 140 Refeeding Syndrome)

GUIDELINE NICE 2017 CG32 Nutrition

How should we assess nutritional status in the ICU?

The European Society for Clinical Nutrition and Metabolism (ESPEN) recommend general clinical assessment rather than reliance on scoring systems due to their lack of validation or demonstrable improvement in mortality. All patients admitted to ICU > 48 h should be considered at high risk of malnutrition.

- *History*: pre-ICU weight loss, pre-ICU decline in physical performance
- *Examination*: muscle mass, body composition, strength

GUIDELINE ESPEN 2019 Nutrition

What is basal metabolic rate?

Basal metabolic rate (BMR) is the amount of energy expended per unit time during a period of rest. Normal BMR is around 40 cal/m²/h. The hypothalamus has the greatest influence on BMR as it regulates adrenal and thyroid function.

What is energy expenditure and how is it calculated?

Energy expenditure (EE) is the sum of internal heat produced and external work. The internal heat produced is composed of BMR and the thermic effect of food.

Critical illness is associated with increased catabolism and a significant energy deficit. In theory, calculating the EE is essential to minimise this deficit. The **TICACOS** trial examined its impact on hospital mortality but was limited by its design.

Indirect calorimetry is the ideal method of measuring EE but is difficult to achieve in clinical practice. It requires measurement of VO_2 and carbon dioxide production (VCO_2).

Alternatives used to estimate EE:

- Derived values
  - VCO_2 from the ventilator or VO_2 from a pulmonary artery catheter (PAC, not routinely available)
  - Resting $EE = 8.2 \times VCO_2$
- Feeding equations
  - e.g. Harris-Benedict or Schofield
  - Calculations based on gender, weight, height, age, and activity levels
  - Gives an approximation of EE (can vary by up to 60%)
- Calculations based on IBW
  - Most used as simple and easily available

What is the respiratory quotient?

The respiratory quotient is ratio of CO_2 released to O_2 absorbed during respiration. It varies depending on dietary intake:

- Carbohydrate 1.0
- Protein 0.8
- Fat 0.7

It can be applied to patients with COPD, where CO_2 can be driven down by increasing the proportion of dietary fats, reducing EE on ventilation.

Which different body weight terms are you aware of?

- *Actual/total*: measured weight during hospitalisation
- *Lean (LBW)*: excludes body fat
  - Male LBW = $9270 \times W/(6680 + 216 \times BMI)$
  - Female LBW = $9270 \times W/(8780 + 244 \times BMI)$
- *Ideal (IBW)*: related to height
  - Male IBW = $50 + 0.91$(height in cm $- 152.4$)
  - Female IBW = $45.5 + 0.91$(height in cm $- 152.4$)
- *Adjusted (ABW)*: applicable in the obese patient
  - ABW = (Actual $-$ IBW) $\times 0.33 +$ IBW

What are the daily nutritional requirements in critical illness?

KEY POINT

- **Energy: 25–35 kcal/kg**
- **Carbohydrate: 2g/kg**
- **Protein: 0.8 – 1.5 g/kg**
- *Lipid*: 1.0 – 1.5 g/kg
- *Water*: 30 ml/kg
- *Na+, Cl-, and K+*: 1 mmol/kg
- *PO4³⁻*: 0.4 mmol/kg
- *Mg²⁺ and Ca²⁺*: 0.1 mmol/kg
- *Selenium*: 100 µg
- *Zinc*: 10 mg
- *Vitamin B1*: 100 mg

ESPEN recommend that, in critically ill patients with measured low plasma levels of 25-hydroxy-vitamin D (<50 nmol/l), a single high dose of vitamin D3 should be administered within a week after admission.

When should you consider nutritional support for your patient?

Medical nutrition therapy comprises oral supplements, enteral nutrition (EN), and parenteral nutrition (PN). It may be considered in patients who have:

- Increased risk of malnutrition
- Little/no diet for 5 days, likely to continue for another 5 days
- Poor absorptive capacity
- High nutritional loss
- High nutritional demand

What are the other sources of calories delivered to critical care patients?

- Propofol (1 kcal/ml)
- Dextrose-containing infusions

When should you start feeding?

ESPEN recommend EN via NG tube to the stomach first line. This should start **within 48 h** of ICU admission once haemodynamically stable. Feed should be started at 50% of estimated target and increased to 70% of EE over 48 h, reaching 70–100% by day 3.

Early EN is recommended in the following groups of patients: ECMO, TBI, stroke, spinal cord injury, severe acute pancreatitis (SAP), GI surgery, abdominal aortic surgery, receiving NMB, prone, open abdomen, and abdominal trauma with GI tract continuity.

STUDY

CALORIES (2014)

- Critically ill patients
- *Intervention*: PN via dedicated CVC lumen vs EN via NG/NJ tube
- *Primary*: 30-day all-cause mortality – **no difference**
- *Secondary*: serious hypoglycaemia, duration of organ support, complications, and LOS – no difference; episodes of clinically significant hypoglycaemia – **significantly lower**

What are the contraindications to enteral nutrition?

Absolute

- Adequate oral intakes (>80% energy target)
- *Gut dysfunction*: anastomotic leak, ischaemia, necrosis
- Generalised peritonitis
- Uncontrolled severe shock states

Relative

- Expected period of fast ≤5 days
- Gastric aspirate volume above 500 ml for 6 h
- Localised peritonitis, intra-abdominal abscess, active upper GI tract haemorrhage
- High risk of pulmonary aspiration
- High-output intestinal fistula if reliable feeding access distal to the fistula is not achievable
- Abdominal compartment syndrome
- Dementia, agitation, confusion

What are the disadvantages unique to EN that are not applicable to PN?

- Dependent on a functional GI tract
- Recognised cause of diarrhoea
- Risk of NG tube misplacement and subsequent delivery of feed to lung (a 'never event')

- Discomfort from NG tube
- Increased VAP risk

What is post-pyloric feeding?

This refers to EN delivered distal to the pylorus of the stomach (i.e. to the jejunum). It is an alternative to NG feeding for patients at high risk of pulmonary aspiration. However, this approach is more complex and often requires input from radiology and gastroenterology teams. There is no evidence that post-pyloric feeding is superior to NG feeding.

What is the difference between trophic feeding and permissive underfeeding?

Trophic feeding is the minimal administration of nutrients via EN, typically between 10 and 20 ml/h of feed (**20%** of requirement). It is used to preserve gut integrity rather than provide nutrition.

KEY POINT

Beneficial effects of trophic feeding:

- Preserves intestinal epithelium
- Stimulates secretion of brush border enzymes
- Enhances immune function
- Preserves epithelial tight cell junctions
- Prevents bacterial translocation

Hypocaloric or permissive underfeeding is the deliberate energy administration below **70%** of the defined caloric target. It has been used to provide fewer calories deliberately. The protein, lipid, and other nutrient requirements may still meet metabolic needs.

STUDY

PermiT (2015)

- Critically ill adults
- *Intervention*: permissive underfeeding (40–60% requirement) vs standard
- *Primary*: 90-day mortality – **no difference**
- *Secondary*: other mortality time frames – no difference

What is parenteral nutrition?

PN is intravenously administered preparation of sterile nutrients. Its composition can be tailored to the patient's needs. PN should be delivered via central access (including PICC) due to risks of thrombophlebitis and infection. Initiation of PN may also carry access-related risks.

Typical composition
- Lipid triglycerides, 40% of nonprotein calories
- Carbohydrate glucose mainly, 60% of non-protein calories
- All essential amino acids
- Electrolytes

Standard PN does not contain any trace elements or vitamins due to instability. These compounds require separate prescription.

When would you supplement feeding with parenteral nutrition?

If caloric requirements are not met within 48–72 h, supplementation or replacement with PN should be considered. The ideal time frame is unclear. Late initiation of PN has been associated with improved survival, shorter duration of mechanical ventilation, and lower requirement for RRT.

STUDY

EPaNIC (2011)

- Critically ill adults
- *Intervention*: late PN (day 8) vs early PN (day 3)
- *Primary*: ICU LOS – **significantly lower**; discharge alive from ICU within 8 days – **significantly higher (75.2% vs 71.7%)**; mortality – no difference; hypoglycaemia – **significantly higher**
- *Secondary*: new infection, duration of MV, duration of RRT, hospital LOS, and health care cost – **significantly lower**; functional status on hospital discharge – no difference

Can you give some examples of clinical conditions in which protein supplementation may need to be adjusted?

- *Increased*: burns, CRRT, open abdomen, trauma, necrotising fasciitis, and BMI > 30 kg/m^2
- *Decreased*: hepatic encephalopathy (see Chapter 54 Burns)

Resource

- Critical Care Nutrition. The Nutric Score. 2015. Available from: https://www.criticalcarenutrition.com/resources/nutric-score. (Accessed 19 January 2022.)

18.   STRESS ULCER PROPHYLAXIS

Why is stress ulceration a concern in critical care?

Stress-related mucosal injury can be caused by critical illness and may increase morbidity. Its incidence has declined with effective prophylaxis.

The pathophysiology is unclear, but contributing factors may include hypoxia, hypoperfusion, and coagulopathy. Initial erosions may progress to deeper ulcers, which may cause haemorrhage or GI perforation.

How does stress ulceration compare with peptic ulcer disease?

The gastric fundus is affected most commonly, in contrast to peptic ulceration which primarily affects the gastric antrum and duodenum. Presentation is also often painless.

What are the risk factors for GI bleeding in critical care?

Highest risk (8–10%)
- Mechanical ventilation without EN
- Chronic liver disease

High risk (4–8%)
- Concerning coagulopathy
- ≥2 moderate-risk factors

Moderate risk (2–4%)
- Mechanical ventilation with EN
- AKI
- Sepsis
- Shock

Low risk (1–2%)
- Critically ill, no other risk factor
- Acute hepatic failure

- Steroids or immunosuppression
- Anticoagulants
- Cancer
- Male sex

What prophylactic measures do we take against stress ulceration?

Stress ulcer prophylaxis aims to prevent clinically significant upper GI bleeding (UGIB).

This may be achieved through:

- Optimisation of fluid status and electrolytes
- Judicious use of vasopressors
- Enteral feeding
- Pharmacological prophylaxis

Tell me more about the pharmacological prophylaxis.

Medications can be used to alkalinise gastric contents (pH > 3.5). This reduces the incidence of stress ulceration, but no mortality benefit has been demonstrated.

- Proton pump inhibitors e.g. omeprazole and lansoprazole (first line)
- H_2-receptor antagonists e.g. ranitidine (second line)
- *Sucralfate*: not widely used due to difficulty in administration of sticky compound (recommended against)
- Antacids e.g. magnesium hydroxide

Pharmacological prophylaxis is recommended if there is a high risk of GI bleeding (≥4%). This applies to patients with the 'highest risk' and 'high risk' factors in the list above, as well as those with the presence of ≥2 'moderate risk' factors.

Why is pharmacological prophylaxis avoided in patients with lower risk of bleeding?

If there is a low risk of bleeding, the risks of prophylaxis may outweigh minimal benefit. A recent meta-analysis has suggested that pharmacological prophylaxis can increase risk of bacterial overgrowth, subsequently increasing the risk of HAP.

There is less convincing evidence that these drugs lead to increased *Clostridium difficile* infection (CDI), LOS in ICU and hospital, or duration of MV.

STUDY

SUP-ICU (2018)

- ICU patients at risk of GI bleeding
- *Intervention:* pantoprazole 40mg IV daily vs placebo
- *Primary:* 90-day mortality – **no difference**
- *Secondary:* clinically important GI bleeding – **significantly lower (2.5% vs 4.2%, NNT 59)**

Resources

- Wang Y, Ye Z, Long G, et al. Efficacy and safety of gastrointestinal bleeding prophylaxis in critically ill patients: systematic review and network meta-analysis. BMJ. 2020;368:I6744.
- Ye Z, Reintam Blaser AR, Lytvyn L, et al. Gastrointestinal bleeding prophylaxis for critically ill patients: a clinical practice guideline. BMJ. 2020;368:I6722.

19. EXTRACORPOREAL LIVER SUPPORT

Can you name some endogenous toxins that accumulate in liver failure?

- Bilirubin
- Bile acids
- Prostacyclins
- Nitric oxide
- Fatty acids
- Ammonia
- Lactate

What is extracorporeal liver support?

This is the name given to systems that may be used to prevent further toxic injury in the failing liver. There are various mechanisms by which it can be provided. Use is restricted to specialist centres and in clinical trial settings. There is not much evidence available relating to their efficacy at present.

Examples
- **Cell based**
  - Bioartificial liver support systems
- **Non-cell based**
  - Haemodialysis
  - Haemofiltration with plasmapheresis
  - Plasmapheresis
  - Haemoperfusion
  - Plasma perfusion
  - Charcoal-based haemoadsorption
  - Albumin dialysis

What other considerations will be required when considering extracorporeal liver support?

- Anticoagulation
- Cannulation
- Volume shifts
- Electrolyte derangements
- Trajectory of disease and perceived benefit

What is bioartificial liver support?

Hepatocytes (human or porcine) are incorporated into plasmapheresis or other extracorporeal systems.

What is MARS?

MARS stands for 'molecular adsorbent recirculation system' and is a type of extracorporeal albumin dialysis. It involves exposing patient ultrafiltrate to albumin-rich solution across a membrane to allow albumin-bound substances to move down a concentration gradient. The ultrafiltrate then undergoes conventional dialysis (Figure 19.1).

When might MARS therapy be indicated?

- Acute liver failure (ALF)
  - Severe alcoholic steatohepatitis (Maddrey ≥32, biopsy-proven)
  - Primary graft dysfunction (PGD) following liver transplantation
  - Posthepatectomy liver failure
  - Intrahepatic cholestasis with intractable pruritus
  - Overdose/intoxication with protein-bound substance
  - Progressive intrahepatic cholestasis associated with HF, graft-versus-host disease (GvHD), etc.

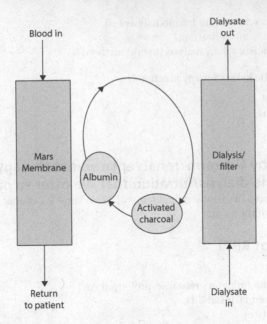

Figure 19.1 MARS.

- Acute-on-chronic liver failure (ACLF)
  - Progressive jaundice
  - Hepatic encephalopathy (grades 3–4)
  - Renal dysfunction
  - Combination of above (see Chapter 135 Acute Liver Failure and Chapter 136 Chronic Liver Disease)

Resources
- van de Kerkhove MP, Hoekstra R, Chamuleau RAFM, et al. Clinical application of bioartificial liver support systems. Ann Surg. 2004;240(2):216–230.
- Laleman W, Wilmer A, Evenepoel P, et al. Review article: non-biological liver support in liver failure. Aliment Pharmacol Ther. 2006;23(3):351–363.

---

20. RENAL REPLACEMENT THERAPY

What types of renal replacement therapy (RRT) are you aware of?
RRT can be used to substitute kidney function in acute and chronic disease. It may be classified in different ways as follows:

- Short term/long term
- Continuous/intermittent
- Vascular/peritoneal

Modalities
- *PD*: peritoneal dialysis
- *Intermittent haemodialysis*
- *CVVH*: continuous veno-venous haemofiltration
- *CVVHDF*: continuous veno-venous haemodiafiltration (hybrid method)

- *CVVHD*: continuous veno-venous haemodialysis
- *SCUF*: slow continuous ultrafiltration
- *SLEDD*: slow low-efficiency daily dialysis (hybrid method)

RRT can provide some of the kidney's many functions:

- Solute/water removal
- Electrolyte correction
- Acid-base correction

Can you suggest why the term 'renal replacement therapy' might be inappropriate for the dialysis/filtration that we offer to patients?

We can support failing kidneys in solute and fluid removal. However, RRT cannot replace the cardiovascular or endocrine functions of the kidney.

What are the risks of RRT?

- Cannula-related
- Bioincompatibility: inflammatory response, prolonged AKI
- *Fluid shifts*: hypovolaemia, instability
- Altered drug metabolism
- *Anticoagulation-related*: HIT, lactic acidosis
- Loss of circulating blood volume, anaemia (circuit clotting and wastage)
- Failure to meet RRT goal (filter downtime)
- Increased nursing workload

What are the main differences between haemofiltration and haemodialysis?

Both haemofiltration and haemodialysis involve blood passing through an extracorporeal circuit via a wide-bore cannula. The circuit will contain a blood pump and inflow/outflow of another substance depending on the modality used (Figure 20.1).

KEY POINT

Haemofiltration

- *Convection*: hydrostatic pressure gradient across a membrane
- *Ultrafiltration*: 'solute drag' pulls molecules along with mass movement of solvent.
- Transport is determined by transmembrane pressure gradient and direction.
- On the other side of the membrane, dialysate enters and effluent leaves the filter.
- Volume is lost by this process, so replacement fluid can be added after the filter.

Haemodialysis

- *Diffusion*: solutes equilibrate down concentration gradients across the membrane.
- Counter-current flow of dialysate against blood.

The choice between modes of RRT may depend on stability of the patient, resources available, and vascular access. Continuous techniques are thought to involve more haemodynamic stability, better fluid balance manipulation, enhanced inflammatory mediator clearance, and better preservation of cerebral perfusion. Kidney Disease Improving Global Outcomes (KDIGO) guidance advocates CRRT in haemodynamically unstable patients or TBI with raised ICP. (see Chapter 130 Acute Kidney Injury)

Intermittent haemodialysis may be the preferred option when faster removal of small, non-protein-bound agents (e.g. methanol and ethylene glycol) is needed. Lithium clearance is faster with intermittent haemodialysis but risks rebound toxicity.

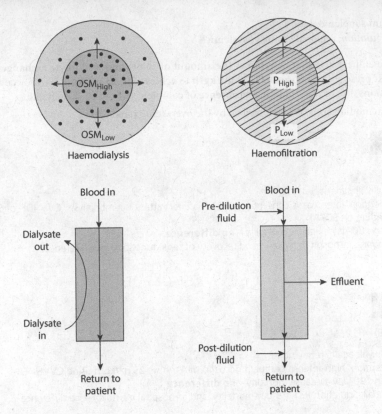

Figure 20.1 Haemodialysis and haemofiltration.

Osm, osmolality; P, pressure.

What is CVVHDF?

CVVHDF is a hybrid method of CRRT. It takes advantage of the ability of dialysis to effectively remove small molecules and the ability of ultrafiltration to remove medium/larger molecules.

How does SLEDD work?

SLEDD employs features of intermittent haemodialysis and CRRT. It utilises slow dialysis to remove solutes and ultrafiltration to remove fluid.

The key advantage is that SLEDD is relatively cheap. It takes 6–12 h daily (as opposed to continuous methods) and is most often performed overnight, allowing the patient to be active and mobile during the day. It requires no anticoagulation or frequent handling of biohazardous effluent bags. The slower solute removal avoids solute disequilibrium that is sometimes seen in intermittent haemodialysis.

Why is SLEDD not used in place of CRRT?

There has been no demonstrable survival benefit from SLEDD. CRRT is familiar, with well-established training and equipment. Since CRRT is continuous, it will allow for more stable fluid removal. CRRT also results in more continuous drug removal in comparison to SLEDD, which facilitates drug clearance at night but none during the day – this complicates daily drug dosing.

How would you prescribe RRT?

Continuous methods require prescription of the following:

- RRT dose
- Fluid removal (e.g. –100 ml/h)
- Target 24-h fluid balance (e.g. neutral)
- Replacement fluid (e.g. Hemosol® and Prismasol®)

- Potassium supplementation
- *Anticoagulation*: regional citrate vs systemic

The dose is the effluent rate that determines the amount of solute and electrolyte exchange during RRT. KDIGO suggest prescribing a dose of **25–30 ml/kg/h** to achieve **20–25 ml/kg/hr**. This accounts for treatment interruptions, use of pre-dilution, and absence of complete saturation of dialysate.

Intermittent haemodialysis is often prescribed by the overseeing renal team.

STUDY

ATN (2008)

- Critically ill patients with ATN
- *Intervention*: intensive vs conventional RRT (via intermittent haemodialysis, CVVHDF, or SLED depending on SOFA)
- *Primary*: 60-day all-cause mortality – **no difference**
- *Secondary*: in-hospital mortality and recovery of renal function – no difference

STUDY

RENAL (2009)

- Critically ill adults requiring RRT
- *Intervention*: high-intensity effluent dose (40 ml/kg/h) vs 25 ml/kg/h using CVVHDF
- *Primary*: 90-day all-cause mortality – **no difference**
- *Secondary*: duration RRT, 28-day mortality, and in-hospital mortality – no difference

STUDY

IVOIRE (2013)

- Septic shock
- *Intervention*: high-volume haemofiltration (70 ml/kg/h) vs conventional (35 ml/kg/h)
- *Primary*: 28-day mortality – **no difference** (stopped early)

What would you do if acidaemia does not improve despite RRT?

First, exclude common patient causes (e.g. sepsis). Then, address the equipment to optimise renal support:

- Increase blood flow
- Reduce pre-dilution
- Improve vascular access
- Increase effluent dose
- Minimise interruptions

What effect does RRT have on drug dosing in critical care?

Drug dosing is complex and will depend on the AKI and RRT modality.

Key principles

- *Low protein binding*: more readily removed by RRT
- *High volume of distribution*: lower clearance by RRT

Examples of adaptations

- *Vancomycin*: continuous infusion due to the narrow therapeutic index
- *Antifungals*: greater clearance so increased dosing
- *Beta-lactams*: more frequently/normal dosing

What vascular access would you use for RRT?

Vascular access may involve an acute central venous RRT line (vascath) or long-standing access. Patients known to renal services may have existing fistulae that trained staff can access for dialysis or medium-term tunnelled lines. Occasionally, these patients may have what is termed 'end-stage vascular access' and require acute lines to be inserted with assistance from IR (e.g. directly to IVC).

Successful RRT will require adequate flow, so location and position of cannulae are important. The patient's non-dominant arm is a likely site for future AV fistula if required and should be avoided if possible. SCV stenosis is a significant concern.

KEY POINT

KDIGO recommend the following order of site preference (and line length) for acute access:

1. Right IJV (15 cm)
2. Femoral vein (25 cm)
3. Left IJV (20 cm)
4. Patient dominant-hand SCV (right 15–20 cm, left 20 cm)
5. Patient non-dominant-hand SCV (as above)

What are the options for anticoagulation?

Anticoagulation is usually used unless contraindicated.

- Citrate (first line)
- Heparin (second line)
- Prostacyclin
- Argatroban
- Danaparoid

What are the strategies you can use to reduce anticoagulation needs?

General
- Minimising time on RRT
- Haemodialysis requires less anticoagulation than filtration
- Trial of no anticoagulation

Optimisation of circuit lifespan
- *Access*: optimise for good flow
- *Choice of anticoagulation*: longer lifespan with citrate
- Equipment
  - Prompt response to the filter alarms
  - Reduce blood-air contact in bubble trap
  - Minimise interruptions
  - Built in safety devices in machine (e.g. will reduce blood flow if pressures suddenly increase)
- Viscosity
  - Maintain filtration fraction < 25% (using pre-dilution and high blood flow rate)
  - Diffusion better than filtration
  - Regular 'rinsing' of membrane with saline flushes

What are the problems associated with filter clotting?

- Anaemia
- Thrombocytopaenia
- Lose blood in filter
- Interruptions
- Increased LOS
- Disrupts the pharmacokinetics and pharmacodynamics of RRT drug dosing

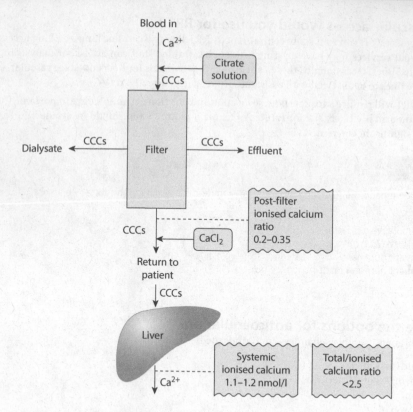

Figure 20.2 Citrate regional anticoagulation. CCC, citrated calcium complexes.

What do you know about citrate regional anticoagulation?

Systemic heparin anticoagulation risks systemic side effects including haemorrhage and HIT. Other systemic anticoagulants are available. An alternative method to systemic infusion is regional anticoagulation of the extracorporeal circuit using citrate.

Citrate is added to the bloodstream after leaving the patient. It binds ionised (free) calcium, creating citrate-calcium complexes (CCC). The plasma-ionised calcium concentration in the filter is reduced: <0.35 mmol/l results in anticoagulation. CCC cross the membrane into effluent. Calcium chloride infusion is given to compensate for the deficit and monitored using blood gases (Figure 20.2).

Residual CCC are returned to the body. Citrate is metabolised predominantly in the liver and muscles. This is less effective in liver dysfunction and muscle hypoperfusion, and its use in these settings may cause it to accumulate, resulting in citrate toxicity. Therefore, citrate regional anticoagulation is not recommended in patients with severe liver failure or shock.

Citrate metabolism produces bicarbonate, resulting in a mild metabolic alkalosis.

How is citrate monitored?

- *Efficacy of anticoagulation*: **post-filter (circuit) ionised calcium** – aim **0.2–0.35 mmol/l**
- *Adequacy of calcium replacement*: **systemic (patient) ionised calcium** – aim **1.1–1.2 mmol/l**
- *Avoidance of citrate accumulation*: **total/(patient) ionised calcium ratio** – aim **< 2.5**

What are the advantages and disadvantages of using citrate?

Advantages
- Avoidance of systemic anticoagulation
- Safe in HIT
- Prolongs circuit lifespan

- Well-established practice
- Clear safety protocols

Disadvantages
- Risk of citrate overload and toxicity
- Electrolyte imbalance (low Ca^{2+}, low Mg^{2+}, and high Na^+)

STUDY

Zarbock et al. (2020)

- Critically ill patients with AKI
- *Intervention*: regional citrate vs systemic heparin anticoagulation
- *Primary*: filter lifespan – **significantly higher (47 h vs 26 h)**; 90-day mortality – **no difference**
- *Secondary*: bleeding complications – **significantly lower (5.1% vs 16.9%)**; new infections – **significantly higher (68.0% vs 55.4%)**

What is citrate overload vs citrate toxicity?

Citrate overload occurs when the quantity of systemic citrate exceeds the body's alkalotic requirements, resulting in a metabolic alkalosis (due to raised sodium availability). This is not dangerous and is easily managed.

Citrate toxicity is more concerning. It occurs when the body is unable to metabolise CCC and acidic citrate impacts on the metabolism: high anion gap metabolic acidosis (HAGMA), hypokalaemia, and hypomagnesaemia ensue. Hypocalcaemia arises from decreased systemic ionised calcium. This occurs in 1–3% of patients and should be suspected if the following develop:

- Post-filter calcium substitution requirement continues to rise
- Total:ionised calcium ratio > 2.5
- HAGMA

Citrate delivery may need to be reduced or stopped, hepatic clearance optimised (by improving cardiac output), and hypocalcaemia treated. No difference in mortality has been shown in comparison to using heparin.

(See Chapter 132 Electrolyte Disorders)

Resources
- Gemmell L, Docking R, Black E. Renal replacement therapy in critical care. BJA Educ. 2017;17(3):88–93.
- Schneider AG, Journois D, Rimmelé T. Complications of regional citrate anticoagulation: accumulation or overload? Crit Care. 2017;21(1):281.

---

21. PLASMAPHERESIS

What are plasmapheresis and plasma exchange?

- **Apheresis** is the process of removing a component of a patient's blood using an extracorporeal device. It is often used in the donation of blood components.
- **Plasmapheresis** is a type of apheresis in which blood plasma is removed.
- **Plasma exchange** involves plasmapheresis and replacement with a substitute. It is usually performed to remove a high-molecular-weight substance from plasma that is causing pathology. Plasma exchange is used in the critical care context.

Other examples of therapeutic apheresis modalities are as follows:

- *Erythrocytapheresis*: RBC removed
- *Extracorporeal photopheresis*: blood components exposed to ultraviolet
- *Leukocytapheresis*: WBC separated out
- *Lipoprotein apharesis*: selective removal of lipoprotein particles
- *Rheopheresis*: separation of high-molecular-weight components (e.g. fibrinogen, LDL cholesterol, and IgM)
- *Thrombocytapheresis*: platelets removed

Describe how plasmapheresis works.

There are 2 methods that might be used as follows:

- *Filtration*: blood passes through filter to separate components (ICU/renal patients).
- *Centrifugation*: blood spins to separate components by density (donation).

Filtration plasmapheresis uses a similar extracorporeal set-up to RRT with the addition of a specialised filter. The circuit may be adapted for plasma exchange by allowing replacement fluid to be given back to the bloodstream.

What are the indications for therapeutic plasma exchange?

Acute liver failure is now an indication for high-volume plasma exchange. Indications are classified as first line (category I), second line (II), role not established (III), or ineffective/harmful (IV) (Table 21.1).

GUIDELINE   American Society for Apheresis 2019 Therapeutic apheresis

In which conditions is plasma exchange less helpful?

Category IV recommendations (ineffective/harmful)
- Amyotrophic lateral sclerosis
- Dermatomyositis and polymyositis
- Inclusion body myositis
- POEMS syndrome
- Rheumatoid arthritis
- Schizophrenia

Can you describe a typical treatment plan?

- 100–150% patient's plasma volume is exchanged in 1 treatment.
- Most conditions require a run of 5 exchanges but some are more intensive.
- 5% HAS is recommended for most indications.
- Thrombocytopaenic purpura (TTP) requires **solvent detergent FFP** instead.

GUIDELINE   BCSH 2015 Apheresis

What are the potential complications?

- Dilutional coagulopathy (fibrinogen monitoring required, aim > 1 g/l if bleeding risk)
- Drug dose alteration (particularly albumin-bound or continuous infusion)
- Recirculation
- Bradykinin-induced histamine release
- Hypovolaemia
- Allergy to replacement fluid
- Access related
- Anticoagulation related

Table 21.1 Some indications for therapeutic plasma exchange

	Category I (first line)	Category II (second line)
Neurological	• **Acute inflammatory demyelinating polyneuropathy (AIDP; GBS)** • **Myasthenia gravis – acute** • **NMDA antibody encephalitis** • Chronic inflammatory demyelinating polyneuropathy (CIDP)	• **Acute disseminated encephalomyelitis (ADEM)** • **Lambert-Eaton myaesthenic syndrome (LEMS)** • **Multiple sclerosis (MS) – acute/relapse** • **Hashimoto's encephalopathy** • **Voltage-gated potassium channel (VGKC) diseases** • Myasthenia gravis – long-term • Neuromyelitis optica spectrum • PANDAS – exacerbation • Refsum's disease • Age-related macular degeneration
Renal	• **Anti-glomerular basement membrane (GBM) disease** • **ANCA-associated vasculitis – rapidly progressive glomerulonephritis (RPGN) or diffuse alveolar haemorrhage:** • Microscopic polyangiitis (MPA) • Granulomatosis with polyangiitis (GPA) • Renal-limited vasculitis	• Amyloidosis – dialysis-related • Myeloma cast nephropathy
Haematological	• **Catastrophic antiphospholipid syndrome** • **TTP** • Atypical haemolytic uraemic syndrome (HUS) – factor H autoantibody • Hypergammaglobulinaemia – hyperviscosity	• Cryoglobulinaemia – severe/symptomatic • Autoimmune haemolytic anaemia (AIHA) – severe cold agglutinin disease
Transplant	• Focal segmental glomerulosclerosis – recurrence • Liver transplant – desensitisation in ABO incompatibility from living donor • Renal transplant – desensitisation in ABO incompatibility	• **Renal transplant – antibody-mediated rejection** • Haematopoietic stem cell transplant – ABO incompatibility
Other	• **ALF (high-volume plasma exchange)** • Wilson's disease – fulminant • Cutaneous T-cell lymphoma – erythrodermic	• **Thyroid storm** • SLE – severe complications • Polyarteritis nodosa – hepatitis B related • Familial hypercholesterolaemia • Mushroom poisoning

What are the indications for red cell apheresis?

- *Sickle cell disease*: acute chest, acute stroke, severe sepsis
- Severe malaria
- Polycythaemia rubra vera
- Hereditary haemochromatosis (see Chapter 143 Haemoglobinopathies)

22. REHABILITATION

What is post-intensive care syndrome?

Post-intensive care syndrome (PICS) encompasses a group of disorders that arises as sequelae of life-threatening illness and the therapies used to manage it.

It is subdivided into problems with:

- *Physical function*: weakness, pain, breathlessness, and difficulty with movement/exercise
- *Mental health*: anxiety, irritability, depression, sleep disturbance, and post-traumatic stress disorder (PTSD)
- *Cognitive function*: memory loss and difficulty thinking or concentrating

Can you give some examples of the sequelae of critical care admission?

PICS was brought to the forefront during the COVID-19 pandemic (2020) as reporting of long-term morbidity increased. The National Post-Intensive Care Rehabilitation Collaborative identified many sequelae:

- *Respiratory*: laryngeal injuries, stenosis, pulmonary deconditioning/fibrosis/embolism/hypertension, PTX, prolonged wean, and long-term tracheostomy
- *Renal*: AKI with ongoing RRT requirement
- *Neurological*: seizures, disordered consciousness, hypoxic-ischaemic injury, focal deficits, sleep-disordered breathing, and cognitive deficit
- *Cardiovascular*: LV/RV dysfunction
- *Nutritional*: anosmia, appetite loss, dysphagia, and altered bowel habit
- *Physical*: ICUAW, positioning injuries, pressure sores, joint stiffness, incontinence, and sexual dysfunction
- *Communication difficulties*: weakness and intubation-related pathology
- *Psychosocial*: 50% suffer significant symptoms during stay, and 50% of all patients have anxiety/depression/PTSD post-discharge
- *Fatigue, pain*: chronic pain in 70% survivors (new or worsening existing pain) (see Chapter 30 ICU-Acquired Weakness)

When and how would you identify patients who may need rehabilitation assistance?

Prevention of sequelae is ideal (e.g. minimising time under NMB and avoidance of benzodiazepines). Rehabilitation should start as early as possible on the ICU (e.g. passive movements of joints, nutrition plan).

NICE recommends that a short risk assessment should be carried out as soon as possible, and a comprehensive assessment should be performed in those at risk. They should have rehabilitation goals agreed within 4 days of admission or before discharge from critical care if sooner than 4 days. Reassessment should occur on the ward.

Many tools exist to assess patients' physical and non-physical status. One example is the **Post-ICU Presentation Screen (PICUPS)** tool, which was constructed using adaptations of several others. Domains assessed include medical stability, basic care and safety, cough/secretions, transfers, communication, mental health, and family distress. A rehabilitation prescription is then completed.

Further assessment and management can also be coordinated through attendance at a follow-up clinic once discharged from critical care.

GUIDELINE   NICE 2009 CG83 Rehabilitation

GUIDELINE   NICE 2017 QS158 Rehabilitation

What might you consider when assessing risk of morbidity from a critical care stay?

Physical
- Longer LOS
- Significant physical or neurological injury
- Inability to ventilate on F_1O_2 ≤0.35

- Premorbid respiratory or mobility issues
- *Risk/presence of nutritional issues*: malnutrition, pattern, appetite, enteral diet tolerance
- Assistance to transfer into/out of bed
- Inability to mobilise independently over short distances

Non-physical

- Recurrent nightmares, history of staying awake to avoid them
- Intrusive memories of events pre-admission (e.g. traffic accident) or during stay
- *Acute stress reaction*: anxiety, panic, fear, low mood, anger, irritability
- Hallucinations, delusions, excessive worry/suspiciousness
- Expressing wish not to discuss their illness or quickly changing the subject
- Lack of cognitive functioning to exercise independently

How would you plan rehabilitation goals?

- Goals can be subdivided into short, medium, and long term.
- May change throughout recovery process
- Must be achievable
- Regular assessment required throughout recovery
- Multidisciplinary input essential

For example, for a patient with reduced mobility, weakness, and fatigue:

- *Overall*: early mobilisation
- *Early*: sit on the edge of the bed with support
- *Medium*: stand aided
- *Long*: march on the spot, walk a few steps with support

Rehabilitation might include rehabilitation specialists, physiotherapists, dieticians, occupational therapists, speech and language therapists, psychologists, ENT surgeons, patient representatives, and intensive care professionals.

What should be handed over to the ward team when discharging a patient from critical care?

- Summary of stay including diagnosis and management
- Monitoring and investigation plan
- *Plan for ongoing treatment*: medications, nutrition, infection status, and limitations
- *Individualised structured rehabilitation programme*: physical, psychological, emotional, and cognitive needs
- Specific communication or language needs

What information should a critical care patient receive before discharge from hospital?

Debrief is recommended. Discussion about expectations should be held to ease the transition from hospital to home, including coverage of:

- *Physical and cognitive recovery*: including rate, based on agreed goals
- *Psychological and emotional recovery*: common symptoms
- Diet
- Other continuing treatments
- How to manage activities of daily living (ADL), self-care, re-engaging with everyday life
- Driving, returning to work, housing, and benefits
- *Support services*: statutory, non-statutory, support groups
- *General guidance (and for carers/family)*: what to expect, how to support at home

When is follow-up recommended and what would this involve?

Adults requiring critical care for more than 4 days with risk of morbidity should be followed up face-to-face 2–3 months post-discharge from critical care.

The purpose of the review includes the following:

- Assessment of new physical or non-physical problems
- Assessment of rate of recovery as per goals
- Assessment of social care or equipment needs
- Arranging support as needed

Some with shorter admissions will need review, and some may present with complications later. All patients should be able to self-refer for reassessment at any time.

Resource

- National Post-Intensive Care Rehabilitation Collaborative. Responding to COVID-19 and beyond: A framework for assessing early rehabilitation needs following treatment in intensive care, Version 1. 2020. Available from: https://www.bsrm.org.uk/downloads/2020.06.23--icsframework-for-assessing-early-reha-(1).pdf. (Accessed 14 April 2022.)

ON THE ICU

---

23. ARDS

How would you define ARDS?

Acute respiratory distress syndrome (ARDS) is syndrome of acute respiratory failure characterised by diffuse, inflammatory lung injury, which manifests with **hypoxaemia, consolidation**, and **reduced compliance**.

Definitions have changed since ARDS was first described in 1967. 'Acute lung injury' is a historical term, which has been superseded by 'mild ARDS'. Contemporary practice uses the 2012 Berlin definition. This requires the following 4 criteria, with the application of 5 cmH$_2$O PEEP/CPAP.

KEY POINT

ARDS:

1. *Hypoxaemia*: P/F ratio ≤39.9 kPa (300 mmHg)
2. *Timing*: onset ≤1 week of known insult or new/worsening respiratory symptoms
3. *Chest imaging*: bilateral lung opacities (not fully explained by effusions/collapse/nodules)
    - CXR or CT
4. *Origin of oedema*: not fully explained by cardiac failure or fluid overload
    - Exclude hydrostatic oedema with objective measure (e.g. echo/PAC) if no risk factor present.

Severity is determined by P/F ratio:

- *Mild*: 26.6–39.9 kPa (200–300 mmHg)
- *Moderate*: 13.3–26.6 kPa (100–200 mmHg)
- *Severe*: ≤13.3 kPa (≤100 mmHg)

What is the pathophysiology of ARDS?

- Acute inflammation of the alveolar membrane
- Initial increased permeability and oedema of the alveolar capillary membrane
- Inflammatory exudate and neutrophil activation inactivate surfactant
- Lung unit collapse, consolidation of distal airspaces, and loss of gas exchange surface area
- Loss of pulmonary vascular tone secondary to inflammation
- Loss of hypoxic pulmonary vasoconstriction
- Deoxygenated blood enters left heart

Histological phases:

1. *Acute/exudative (first week)*: inflammatory flooding of alveoli with protein-rich fluids, leading to a loss of pulmonary compliance
2. *Subacute/proliferative*: rapid fibroproliferation and micro-thrombus formation within the pulmonary vasculature and abnormal expression of type II pneumatocytes. Some patients recover rapidly from this phase, but others progress to a third phase.
3. *Chronic/fibrotic*: widespread lung fibrosis with remodelling and scarring (may be irreversible)

Which situations might precipitate ARDS?

Pulmonary
- Contusion
- Aspiration of gastric contents
- Drowning
- Inhalational injury

Extrapulmonary
- Non-pulmonary sepsis
- Burns
- Major trauma
- Pancreatitis
- Major blood transfusion
- CPB

How would you investigate for ARDS?

No specific investigation exists. ABG, chest imaging, and echo are usually required to fulfil diagnostic criteria.

Other useful investigations are those which:

- Consider underlying cause (e.g. sputum MC+S and PCR, and blood cultures)
- Investigate complications
- Monitor progress
- Aid prognostication

How would you manage ARDS?

Primary prevention is the key. Treatment aims to correct the underlying cause whilst avoiding further lung injury and carrying out best supportive care (e.g. nutrition, thromboprophylaxis, glycaemic control).

ARDS-specific stepwise approach
- Mild
  - LPV (strong recommendation)
  - Conservative fluid balance target
- Moderate
  - Higher PEEP (if P/F ≤27 kPa)
  - Prone positioning ≥12 h per day (if P/F ≤20 kPa) (strong recommendation)
  - NMB (cisatracurium, first 48 h, if P/F ≤20 kPa)
- Severe
  - Refer to local ECMO centre (Murray score ≥3 or pH < 7.20 on optimal management)
  - Other measures in exceptional circumstances (e.g. contraindication to ECMO)
    - ➢ Recruitment manoeuvres
    - ➢ Inhaled vasodilators (e.g. nitric oxide, nebulised prostacyclin) (recommended against)
    - ➢ High-frequency oscillatory ventilation (HFOV) (**strongly recommended against**)

Non-specific

- *Rehabilitation*: early mobilisation
- *Nutrition*: enteral, trophic acceptable initially, and consider NJ after prokinetics if absorption failure
- *Transfusion*: avoid unless absolutely indicated

GUIDELINE   FICM ICS 2018 ARDS

STUDY

ACURASYS (2010)

- Moderate-severe ARDS
- *Intervention*: cisatracurium 48 h vs placebo
- *Primary*: adjusted 90-day mortality – **significantly lower**
- *Secondary*: barotrauma, PTX – **significantly lower**; days with other organ failure – **significantly higher**; actual 90-day mortality, ICU-acquired paresis – no difference

STUDY

ROSE (2019)

- . Moderate-to-severe ARDS
- *Intervention*: cisatracurium infusion 48 h vs usual care
- *Primary*: 90-day mortality – **no difference** (around 42%)
- *Secondary*: organ dysfunction, 28-day mortality, days not in the ICU, days free of MV, and days not in hospital – no difference; patient-reported outcomes similar
- Stopped early due to futility

Relevant trials described previously:

- *HFOV*: **OSCILLATE** (2013) and **OSCAR** (2013)
- *ECMO*: **CESAR** (2009) and **EOLIA** (2018)
- *ECCO$_2$R*: **SUPERNOVA** (2019) and **REST** (2021)
- *Proning*: **PROSEVA** (2014) (see Chapter 7 Mechanical Ventilation, Chapter 8 Proning, and Chapter 9 ECMO and ECCO$_2$R)

How would you ventilate a patient with ARDS?

'Lung-protective ventilation' describes the use of ventilatory strategies that are thought to minimise ventilator-induced lung injury through avoidance of volutrauma and barotrauma. It has demonstrable mortality benefit, as supported by the **ARSDNet** trial and the 2013 meta-analysis by **Petrucci and De Feo**. No benefit has been demonstrated by using a higher PEEP strategy.

KEY POINT

Lung-protective ventilation:

- 6 ml/kg IBW
- Plateau pressure < 30 cmH$_2$O

STUDY

ARDSNet (2000)

- Acute lung injury/ARDS
- *Intervention*: low V_T (4–6 ml/kg) vs traditional V_T (10–12 ml/kg)
- *Primary*: 180-day mortality – **significantly lower**; ventilator-free days, breathing unaided by day 28 – **significantly higher**.
- *Secondary*: days without other organ failure – **significantly higher**

STUDY

ALVEOLI (2004)

- Acute lung injury and ARDS
- *Intervention*: higher vs lower PEEP (both protocolised according to F_iO_2 up to 24 cmH$_2$O)
- *Primary*: mortality before discharge home whilst breathing unaided – **no difference** (around 25%)
- *Secondary*: breathing without assistance at day 28, ventilator-free days, days not in ICU, barotrauma, and days without organ failure – no difference

What is the role of corticosteroids in ARDS?

There was some evidence supporting corticosteroid use in ARDS prior to the COVID-19 pandemic. Amongst other studies, a small RCT by **Meduri et al**. demonstrated favourable outcomes with methyl-prednisolone. Guidance recommended further research on the role of corticosteroids as an unanswered question.

The **DEXA-ARDS** trial results were published just as the COVID-19 pandemic started to unfold, showing positive outcomes with use of dexamethasone. The **RECOVERY** trial in 2021 focused specifically on patients with COVID-19 and demonstrated significantly improved outcomes with dexamethasone. Number needed to treat (NNT) was 25 in patients requiring oxygen, and 8 in those were mechanically ventilated. (See Chapter 124 COVID-19)

STUDY

Meduri et al. (2007)

- Early severe ARDS
- *Intervention*: methylprednisolone infusion (1 mg/kg/day) vs placebo
- *Primary*: 1-point reduction in lung injury score or successful extubation by day 7 – **significantly higher**
- *Secondary*: duration of MV, ICU LOS, ICU mortality, and infections – **significantly lower**

STUDY

DEXA-ARDS (2020)

- Moderate-severe ARDS
- *Intervention*: IV dexamethasone (20 mg daily for 5 days and then 10 mg daily till day 10/extubation) vs conventional treatment
- *Primary*: ventilator-free days – **significantly higher (12.3 vs 7.5)**
- *Secondary*: 60-day all-cause mortality – **significantly lower (21% vs 36%)**; ICU mortality – **significantly lower (19% vs 31%)**

Resources

- ARDS Definition Task Force. Acute respiratory distress syndrome: The Berlin Definition. JAMA. 2012;307(23):2526–2533.
- McCormack V, Tolhurst-Cleaver S. Acute respiratory distress syndrome. BJA Educ. 2017;17(5):161–5.
- Petrucci N, De Feo C. Lung protective ventilation strategy for the acute respiratory distress syndrome. Cochrane Database Syst Rev. 2013;2:CD003844.

24. OXYGEN TOXICITY

What is hyperoxia and why is it relevant to critical care?

Hyperoxia can be described as a supranormal arterial partial pressure of oxygen. Its consequences depend on the patient's individual pathology and physiology as well as the degree of hyperoxia. Its relevance is in the potential for harm alongside selected circumstances in which it may be beneficial.

What is the most common cause of serious harm secondary to oxygen therapy?

CO_2 retention may develop in some circumstances. Significant effects of hypercarbia include vasodilatation (with potential hypotension) and reduction in conscious level.

Patients at risk of hypercapnic respiratory failure include those with the following:

- COPD
- Bronchiectasis, cystic fibrosis
- Neuromuscular disease
- Chest wall deformity
- Morbid obesity

GUIDELINE   BTS 2017 Oxygen

When is hyperoxia most commonly recommended against in critical illness?

- Stroke (increased disability and mortality)
- MI (may increase infarct size)
- Post-cardiac arrest (increased mortality)
    - Highest feasible F_1O_2 recommended during CPR
    - After ROSC, target S_pO_2 94–98%, or P_aO_2 10–13 kPa

What are the other potential consequences?

- Delayed recognition of clinical deterioration
- Oxygen toxicity
- Systemic and critical organ vasoconstriction
- Reduced cardiac output
- *Neonatal*: retinopathy, bronchopulmonary dysplasia
- *Bleomycin chemotherapy*: previous exposure causes susceptibility to pulmonary oxygen toxicity even years later
- *Paraquat toxicity*: exacerbation of poisoning

Environmental

- Inappropriate use or wastage of limited resources
- Energy consumption involved in manufacturing, maintenance, and transportation of cylinders and vacuum insulated evaporator
- Fire risk surrounding supply and areas of leakage, particularly near electrical equipment
- Cost

What is the pathophysiology of oxygen toxicity?

- Reactive oxygen species (ROS) are generated by electron transport chain during respiration.
- Unpaired electrons result in highly reactive properties.
- Increased production of ROS through hyperoxia disrupts balance with antioxidants.
- Increased exposure of tissues to toxic interactions.
- ROS cause harm by:
  - Damaging DNA/RNA or processes involved in repair or transcription
  - Affecting lipid peroxidation and damaging cell membranes
  - Oxidising amino acids or enzymes and impairing protein function
- Exposure time and P_IO_2 will contribute to amount of oxidative stress

What are the effects of oxygen toxicity?

Pulmonary

- Epithelial damage in tracheobronchial tree
- Manifests with chest pain (burning/tight and dyspnoea) before reduced vital capacity at 24 h
- Inflammatory changes
- Stages of lung injury similar to ARDS (exudative, proliferative, and fibrotic)
- Permanent fibrotic changes possible
- Other pulmonary effects
  - Impaired hypoxic pulmonary vasoconstriction and worsened V/Q mismatch
  - Reduced CO_2 elimination
  - Altered control of breathing (e.g. COPD patients)
  - Absorption atelectasis
  - Reduction in mucociliary clearance

CNS

- In hyperbaric conditions (e.g. divers)
- Nausea, headache, dizziness, muscle twitching, visual disturbances, irritability, disorientation
- Seizures in more severe cases

Are there any beneficial effects of high inspired oxygen concentrations?

Normobaric

- Carbon monoxide (CO) elimination
- PTX reabsorption
- Relief of cluster headache
- Advocated during CPR to improve outcomes
- Perioperative safety net prior to airway procedures (e.g. induction of general anaesthesia)
- Possible role in preventing postoperative nausea and vomiting, surgical site infection (SSI), and anastomotic breakdown

Hyperbaric

- Treatment of decompression sickness
- Wound healing

What do you know about the evidence behind oxygenation targets?

Work is ongoing to investigate the value of a more conservative approach to oxygenation in the critical care population. Existing work includes the **ICU-ROX** and **HOT-ICU** RCTs.

ICU-ROX (2019)

- Mechanically ventilated ICU patients
- *Intervention*: conservative oxygen (target S_aO_2 90–97%) vs usual therapy (no upper limit)
- *Primary*: number of ventilator-free days – **no difference**
- *Secondary*: 180-day mortality, cognitive function, quality of life, and employment status – no difference
- *Subgroup 180-day mortality*: ischaemic hypoxic encephalopathy – **significantly lower**, sepsis – **significantly higher**, and other brain pathology – **significantly higher**

HOT-ICU (2021)

- ICU patients receiving ≥10 l/min O_2 or F_iO_2 ≥0.5 in closed system
- *Intervention*: conservative (8 kPa) vs liberal (12 kPa) oxygenation target
- *Primary*: 90-day mortality – **no difference**

What measures do we take on critical care to prevent hyperoxia?

- Treating oxygen as a drug including prescription
- Individualised target setting
- Monitoring
- Appropriate use and maintenance of equipment

How would you prescribe oxygen?

Oxygen should be prescribed on a drug chart including the following:

- Oxygen as name of drug
- Target saturation range
- Starting device
- Flow rate/concentration
- Patient details, prescriber details, and date

Resource

- Horncastle E, Lumb AB. Hyperoxia in anaesthesia and intensive care. BJA Educ. 2019;19(6): 176–182.

25. VENTILATOR-ASSOCIATED PNEUMONIA

How would you define hospital-acquired pneumonia?

HAP is a pulmonary infection contracted **after 48 h** of admission to hospital and not incubating at the time of admission. It may present up to **14 days** following discharge from hospital.

What is ventilator-associated pneumonia and why is it significant?

VAP is a healthcare-associated pulmonary infection arising more than 48 h after tracheal intubation.

VAP may have significant consequences as follows:

- Increased ICU LOS
- Increased patient ventilator days
- Increased mortality (30% increase in mortality of underlying disease)

It remains a problem partly due to the difficulty in diagnosis, with no universally agreed diagnostic criteria and significant subjectivity. Clinical, radiological, and microbiological features and overall patient context are important.

(See Chapter 115 Nosocomial Infection)

Which differential diagnoses may mimic VAP?

- ARDS
- Pulmonary oedema
- Pulmonary contusion
- Tracheobronchitis
- Thromboembolic disease

How might you approach diagnosing VAP?

A comprehensive assessment should be performed before judicious diagnosis. Scoring systems might be used to facilitate this:

Clinical Pulmonary Infection Score (CPIS)
- Score > 6 diagnostic, maximum 12. Variables score 0–3:
  - Temperature
  - Leukocytosis
  - P/F ratio
  - CXR infiltrates
  - Tracheal secretions
  - Tracheal aspirate culture
- Prone to inter-observer variability

Johannson criteria
- New/progressive infiltrates on CXR and ≥2 of the following:
  - Leukocytosis
  - Purulent secretions
  - Temperature > 38°C
- Sensitivity 69% and specificity 75%

HELICS criteria
- Clinical, radiological, and microbiological criteria
- PN1–PN5 classification based on microbiological method used
- Used in surveillance in Europe

Centers for Disease Control (CDC) definition – not intended for diagnostic use but good sensitivity and positive predictive value.

What is the pathophysiology of VAP?

Pathophysiology stems from biofilm formation within the tracheal tube and microaspiration of secretions.

- Tracheal tube disrupts protective upper airway reflexes and prevents effective coughing.
- Oropharynx colonised
- Contaminated secretions pool above cuff.
- Slow passage of secretions to trachea through folds in wall of cuff
- Bacterial biofilm forms on inner surface of tube.
- Biofilm pushed into distal airways by ventilator cycling

Risk factors
- Supine positioning
- Enteral feeding via NG tube (aspiration of gastric contents)

What is a care bundle?

A care bundle is a group of evidence-based interventions related to a condition that significantly improve patient outcome when used in combination.

How might VAP be prevented?

Ventilator care bundles are commonly used with the aim to prevent the iatrogenic effects of mechanical ventilation including the development of VAP.

The Department of Health included its '**High Impact Intervention No 5 – Care bundle for ventilated patients**' as part of its campaign, 'Saving Lives: reducing infection, delivering clean, and safe care'.

KEY POINT

Original high-impact interventions (2007):

- Daily sedation holds
- Bed head elevation (30–45°)
- Appropriate use of gastric ulcer prophylaxis
- Oral care

Additional measures (2010):

- Oral hygiene with adequate strength antiseptics
- Subglottic aspiration
- Tracheal tube pressure monitoring

Study results surrounding use of ventilator care bundles are as follows:

- Significant reduction in VAP rates, MRSA rates, and antibiotic use
- Variable demonstration of reduction in duration of mechanical ventilation and ICU LOS

Other measures under evaluation:

- *Hygiene during handling of airway equipment*: reduction in biofilm formation from handling of tracheal tube, suction devices (closed-circuit favoured), HME use, and limiting circuit changes
- Appropriate establishment of enteral feeding
- *Tracheal tube design*: cuff shape and tube coating
- Nebulised gentamicin
- *Kinetic therapy*: reduction of immobility to improve mucociliary clearance
- Probiotics
- Selective decontamination of the digestive tract (SDD)

What is the rationale for the above bundle components?

Likelihood of microaspiration will be reduced by bed head elevation, oral hygiene, and subglottic secretion aspiration.

- Sedation holds
  - Reduced duration of intubation
  - Reduction of unplanned extubations
  - Minimising reintubation rates
- Avoidance of unnecessary gastric ulcer prophylaxis
  - Acid suppression raises gastric pH
  - Bacterial overgrowth occurs.
  - Aspiration carries potential of higher bacterial load.

- Cuff pressure control avoids:
  - Passage of secretions between cuff and wall of trachea (< 20 cmH$_2$O)
  - Tracheal mucosal damage (>30 cmH$_2$O)

What are ventilator-associated events?

Multisociety universal definitions were proposed by the United States CDC in 2013 to guide surveillance and funding rather than clinical management:

- *Ventilator-associated event (VAE)*: deterioration in respiratory status after a period of stability or improvement on the ventilator (≥4 days), evidence of infection or inflammation, and laboratory evidence of respiratory infection
- *Ventilator-associated condition (VAC)*: VAE with worsening oxygenation
- *Infection-related ventilator-associated condition (IVAC)*: VAC with abnormal temperature/WCC or new antimicrobial requirement
- *Possible VAP*: VAC with possible evidence of pulmonary infection
- *Probable pneumonia*: VAC with probable evidence of pulmonary infection

Resources

- Centers for Disease Control and Prevention: National Healthcare Safety Network. January 2021. Ventilator-Associated Event (VAE). Available from https://www.cdc.gov/nhsn/pdfs/pscmanual/10-vae_final.pdf. (Accessed 25 November 2021.)
- Department of Health. Saving Lives: Reducing Infection, Delivering Clean and Safe Care: High Impact Intervention No 5: Care Bundle for Ventilated Patients (or Tracheostomy Where Appropriate). Available from: https://www.bsuh.nhs.uk/library/wp-content/uploads/sites/8/2020/09/Ventilator-care-bundle.pdf. (Accessed 24 January 2022.)
- Gunasekera P, Gratrix A. Ventilator-associated pneumonia. BJA Education. 2016;16:198–202.

26. SEPSIS

What is sepsis?

> **KEY POINT**
>
> *Sepsis-3 definition*: Sepsis is a life-threatening organ dysfunction caused by a **dysregulated host response** to infection.

The important concept is dysregulated systemic host response, which differs to local organ dysfunction from infection (e.g. pneumonia causing hypoxaemia). Severity of organ dysfunction is assessed using the SOFA (sepsis-related) score. **Organ dysfunction can be identified as an acute change in total SOFA score ≥2 points**. The features defining what was previously known as 'severe sepsis' are now present in the Sepsis-3 definition.

Septic shock is sepsis with persistent hypotension requiring vasopressors to maintain MAP ≥65 mmHg and serum lactate > 2 mmol/l.

Previous definitions of sepsis incorporated the concept of the SIRS, defined by the presence of ≥2 of the following:

- Temperature > 38 or < 36°C
- HR > 90 min^{-1}
- RR > 20 min^{-1} or P$_a$CO$_2$ < 4.3 kPa

- WCC > 12 or < 4 × 10⁹/l or > 10% immature bands (see Chapter 108 Paediatric Sepsis and Chapter 2 Scoring Systems)

Why is effective management of sepsis important?

Sepsis is the primary cause of death from infection, and early recognition and management are relevant to patient outcomes. Presentation varies according to host and pathogen factors, and organ dysfunction may be occult.

Can you describe the SOFA score in more detail?

The SOFA score assigns points according to severity of dysfunction of several organ systems using specific markers:

- *Respiratory:* P/F ratio
- *Cardiovascular:* hypotension and dose of dopamine, dobutamine, adrenaline, or NA
- *CNS:* GCS
- *Liver:* bilirubin
- *Renal:* creatinine or UO
- *Coagulation:* platelet count

A score of 0–4 is possible for each system. These are then added to give the SOFA score. Mean and highest SOFA scores have been found to correlate with mortality.

Example mortality data includes the following:

- Initial score
  - *4–5*: 20%
  - *10–11*: 50%
  - *≥12*: 95%
- Highest score
  - *4–5*: 6.7%
  - *10–11*: 45.8%
  - *12–14*: 80%
  - *≥14*: 89.7%

An increase in SOFA score of ≥2 points, as per the definition of 'organ dysfunction' above, is associated with in-hospital mortality > 10%. Septic shock is associated with hospital mortality >40%. Regardless of initial SOFA score, serial assessment showing an increase during the first 48 h of ICU admission predicts a mortality ≥ 50%.

(See Chapter 2 Scoring Systems)

What is the pathophysiology of sepsis?

Endothelium normally serves to regulate the following:

- Vasomotor tone
- Movement of cells and nutrients in/out of tissues
- Coagulation
- Balance of inflammatory/anti-inflammatory signalling

Endothelial dysfunction is profound in sepsis:

- Vasodilatation
- Loss of barrier function
- Increased leukocyte adhesion
- *Procoagulant state:* increased tissue factor expression, fibrin deposition, impaired anticoagulation, microthrombi, and plugs of WBC/RBC

What complications do these processes cause?

- *Lung interstitial oedema:* V/Q mismatch, hypoxaemia, reduced lung compliance, and ARDS

- *Circulatory failure*: increased tissue nitric oxide, decreased SVR, and cardiac output may increase
  - Decreased tissue perfusion and oxygen delivery/uptake
  - Septic shock results
  - Compounded by septic cardiomyopathy (due to impaired myocardial perfusion)
- *Encephalopathy*: BBB compromised, perivascular oedema, oxidative stress, leukoencephalopathy, and neurotransmitter alterations
- *GI permeability*: bacterial translocation and autodigestion (exacerbating inflammation)
- *Liver impairment*: hepatocyte clearance of bilirubin impaired (cholestasis)
- *AKI*: microvascular/tubular dysfunction and hypoperfusion
- *DIC*: bleeding due to consumption of platelets and clotting factors
- *Metabolic*: insulin resistance and catabolism
- *Prolonged immune dysfunction*: secondary infection

What is the glycocalyx?

The glycocalyx is a web of glycoproteins and proteoglycans which are semi-bound in the capillary membrane wall. It is usually semi-permeable to anions and impermeable to mid-/large-sized molecules (>70 kDa). It is in a state of active creating and shedding and thought to be responsible for managing mediators such as nitric oxide and protein C as well as modulating inflammatory responses.

Injury to the glycocalyx leads to increased permeability, alteration in starling forces across the capillary basement membrane, and activation of pro-inflammatory pathways. Glycocalyx dysfunction/disruption is increasingly thought to be important in the pathophysiology of sepsis.

What happens at a cellular and molecular level?

- Pathogen-associated molecular patterns (PAMPs) and damage-associated molecular patterns (DAMPs) are detected by the innate immune system.
- Epithelial cells are activated via receptors on cell surface (toll-like and C-type lectin) and in cytosol (NOD-like and RIJ-I-like).
- These cause transcription of type I interferons and pro-inflammatory cytokines (e.g. TNF-α, IL-1, and IL-6).
- Some receptors form inflammasomes that mature and secrete potent cytokines (IL-1β and IL-18).
- These can trigger caspase-mediated rapid rupture of the plasma membrane (pyropoptosis), causing cell death.

Other cytokine effects are as follows:

- Adhesion molecule and chemokine expression by endothelium
- Induction of hepatic acute phase proteins (e.g. complement and fibrinogen)
- Release of pro-inflammatory, pro-oxidant, and pro-coagulant microparticles (e.g. tissue factor, angiopoietin-2, and vWF)
- Increased tissue factor expression

Systemic injury results when a threshold is exceeded by the inflammatory response:

- ROS (e.g. hydroxyl and nitric oxide) damage cell components and DNA and impair mitochondrial function
- Complement (e.g. C5a) increases ROS generation, granulocyte enzyme release, endothelial permeability, tissue factor expression, ± adrenal medullary cell death

How should antimicrobial therapy be approached?

Supportive management should be given as indicated. Sepsis and septic shock are emergencies, and specific management should begin immediately upon identification.

The Surviving Sepsis Campaign (SSC) has developed evidence-based guidelines for sepsis management.

These have advocated time-based care bundles to improve management, which have evolved over time. The 'Sepsis Six' was drawn from this guidance by The UK Sepsis Trust to aid delivery of these recommendations:

KEY POINT

The Sepsis Six ('give 3 and take 3'):

- *Take*: serum lactate, blood cultures, and urine (accurate UO monitoring)
- *Give*: empiric antimicrobials, IV fluids, and oxygen to target saturations

KEY POINT

The SSC 1-h bundle (2018):

1. *Measure lactate*: remeasure if initially >2 mmol/l
2. Take blood cultures
3. Broad-spectrum antibiotics
4. Rapid 30 ml/kg crystalloid (if hypotensive or lactate ≥4 mmol/l)
5. Vasopressors if hypotensive during/after fluid resuscitation (target MAP ≥65 mmHg)

KEY POINT

Timing of antimicrobials (2021 update):

- Immediate, ideally **<1 h** of recognition if:
  - **Definite** or **probable** sepsis
  - Possible sepsis with **shock**
- *Possible sepsis without shock*: assess for other causes and give **<3 h** if concern persists

Other guidance:

- Procalcitonin (PCT) use not recommended in clinical decision making about commencing antimicrobials
- Empirical cover to include MRSA if high risk
- Two antimicrobials (1 Gram-negative cover) if high risk of multidrug resistance
- Antifungal if high risk
- Emergent source control intervention if appropriate

GUIDELINE   SSC 2021 Sepsis

How would you address circulatory failure in sepsis and septic shock?

- IV fluids
  - **30 ml/kg** balanced crystalloid < 3 h if sepsis-induced hypoperfusion or septic shock
  - Albumin if large volumes of crystalloid have been received
- Vasoactive agents
  - NA first-line, target **MAP ≥65 mmHg**
  - Consider peripheral vasopressors if no CVC
  - *If inadequate MAP*: consider adding vasopressin (e.g. once NA at **0.25–0.5 µg/kg/min**)

- *If cardiac dysfunction (despite adequate volume/BP)*: consider adding dobutamine or switching to adrenaline
- *Ongoing requirement for vasopressors*: add IV corticosteroids

---

STUDY

SOAP II (2010)

- Circulatory shock
- *Intervention*: dopamine vs NA
- *Primary*: 28-day mortality – **no difference**
- *Secondary*: days without vasopressor – **significantly lower**; death from refractory shock – **significantly higher**; days without ICU care and days without organ support – no difference; 28-day mortality in CS – **significantly higher**
- *Arrhythmias*: **significantly higher (24.1% vs 12.4%)**

What corticosteroid regime might you use?

The guidelines above describe using **IV hydrocortisone at 200 mg/24 h**, administered as 50 mg 6° or as a continuous infusion. The threshold for starting steroids might be the persistent requirement of adrenaline or NA infusion at doses of ≥0.25 µg/kg/min (i.e. ≥4 h after initiation).

This matches the proposed threshold for consideration of vasopressin and is equivalent to approximately 13 ml/h 'single-strength' NA (4 mg in 50 ml) in a 70-kg person.

What other interventions are recommended during monitoring and supportive care?

- *B*: high flow in preference to other NIV, lung-protective ventilation, manage ARDS as per generic guidance
- *C*: target decreasing lactate during resuscitation if initially elevated, CR as adjunct to assessment
- *D*: insulin if glucose > 10 mmol/l
- *E*: commence feed ≤72 h ideally, stress ulcer prophylaxis if risk of bleeding
- *H*: transfusion threshold Hb 70 g/l, VTE prophylaxis with LMWH
- Refer to post-hospital rehabilitation programme if ventilated >48 h or on ICU >72 h

---

STUDY

ANDROMEDA-SHOCK (2019)

- Septic shock
- *Intervention*: resuscitation aimed at normalising CR time vs decreasing lactate
- *Primary*: 28-day mortality – **no difference (34.9% vs 43.4%)**
- *Secondary*: organ dysfunction at 72 h – **significantly lower (SOFA 5.6 vs 6.6)**. 90-day mortality, support-free days, SOFA at 72 h, and LOS – no difference

---

What do you know about the evidence base for these recommendations?

Much of the early work on sepsis comes from the study by Rivers et al., who developed **early goal-directed therapy (EGDT)** in sepsis with target-driven care of the septic patient. This protocol has now been dismissed by 3 large international RCTs (**ARISE, ProMISe**, and **ProCESS**).

Other important trials are as follows:

- *BP target*: **SEPSISPAM** and **65**
- *Vasopressin use*: **VASST**
- *Corticosteroids*: **ADRENAL** and **CORTICUS** (see Chapter 148 Adrenocortical Disorders)
- *Transfusion threshold*: **TRISS** and **TRICC** (see Chapter 51 Major Haemorrhage)

- *Fluids*: **FEAST, 6S, ALBIOS**, and **SPLIT** (see Chapter 11 Fluids)
- *Glycaemic control*: **NICE-SUGAR** (see Chapter 149 Diabetes Emergencies)

Sepsis remains a complex syndrome with many contentious areas of practice. This list is not exhaustive, and many other relevant studies have been performed (e.g. those supporting recommendations against specific therapies).

STUDY

Rivers et al. (2001)

- Severe sepsis or septic shock
- *Intervention*: EGDT (6 h) vs usual care
- *Primary*: in-hospital mortality – **significantly lower (30.5% vs 46.5%)**
- *Secondary*: severity, 28-day/60-day mortality – **significantly lower**

STUDY

ARISE (2014)

- Septic shock
- *Intervention*: EGDT vs usual care
- *Primary*: 90-day all-cause mortality – **no difference**
- *Secondary*: LOS in emergency department/hospital, vasopressor duration, RRT, and MV – no difference; vasopressor requirement – **significantly higher**

STUDY

ProCESS (2014)

- Sepsis
- *Intervention*: EGDT vs usual care
- *Primary*: 60-day mortality – **no difference**
- *Secondary*: 90-day and 1-year mortality – **no difference**

STUDY

ProMISe (2015)

- Septic shock
- *Intervention*: EGDT vs usual care
- *Primary*: 90-day mortality – **no difference**
- *Secondary*: 28-day/hospital mortality and LOS – no difference; SOFA at 6 h and ICU LOS – **significantly higher**

STUDY

SEPSISPAM (2014)

- Septic shock
- *Intervention*: MAP target 80–85 vs 65–70 mmHg
- *Primary*: 28-day mortality – **no difference**
- *Secondary*: 90-day mortality and serious adverse events – no difference; new AF – **significantly higher**

STUDY

65 (2020)

- Patients older than 65 years with vasodilatory hypotension, recently commenced on vasopressors
- *Intervention*: permissive hypotension (MAP 60–65 mmHg) vs usual care
- *Primary*: 90-day mortality – **no difference (41.0% vs 43.8%)**
- *Secondary*: ICU/hospital mortality, duration of organ support, LOS, cognitive decline, and quality of life – no difference
- More pronounced morality reduction in patients with chronic hypertension

STUDY

VASST (2008)

- Septic shock
- *Intervention*: vasopressin 0.01–0.03 units/min vs NA 5–15 µg/min
- *Primary*: 28-day mortality – **no difference**
- *Secondary*: 90-day mortality, RRT, LOS, and adverse events – no difference; NA rate – **significantly lower**

What were the components of 'early goal-directed therapy' in Rivers et al.'s study?

This (now historical) treatment protocol was applied for the first 6 h and contained the following:

- Supplemental oxygen ± intubation and mechanical ventilation
- Central venous and arterial catheterisation (with ability to measure $ScvO_2$)
- Crystalloid/colloid given until CVP 8–12 mmHg
- Vasoactive agents then used to achieve $65 \leq MAP \leq 90$ mmHg
- Red cell transfusion until Hct $\geq 30\%$ and $ScvO_2 \geq 70\%$

What is activated protein C?

Activated protein C is an endogenous substance that promotes fibrinolysis and inhibits thrombosis. A recombinant form (drotrecogin alfa) was thought to offer benefit in sepsis by improving microcirculatory disruption. The **PROWESS** trial showed significant improvement in mortality with its use, and it remains the only drug that has ever been successfully licenced for sepsis.

Concern arose over serious bleeding events, and the **PROWESS-SHOCK** trial showed no improvement in mortality with its use. Subsequently, the drug was withdrawn from the market and is no longer used as a result.

Other than drugs targeting coagulopathy, others that have been investigated include anti-cytokines (e.g. etanercept), anti-virulence factors (e.g. monoclonal antibodies), and immune stimulators (e.g. G-CSF). Many supportive therapies are under evaluation (e.g. methylene blue).

STUDY

PROWESS (2001)

- Severe sepsis
- *Intervention*: drotrecogin alfa (activated) vs placebo
- *Primary*: 28-day mortality – **significantly lower (24.7% vs 30.8%)**

PROWESS-SHOCK (2012)

- Septic shock
- *Intervention*: drotrecogin alfa (activated) vs placebo
- *Primary*: 28-day mortality – **no difference**
- *Secondary*: 90-day mortality, SOFA at day 7 – no difference

Which interventions are recommended against?

The following interventions are recommended against:

- Starches and gelatin
- Terlipressin
- Levosimendan
- Polymyxin B haemoperfusion
- Vitamin C (see Chapter 148 Adrenocortical Disorders)
- Sodium bicarbonate for haemodynamic indications

CITRIS-ALI (2019)

- Sepsis and ARDS
- *Intervention*: vitamin C vs placebo
- *Primary*: modified SOFA score, CRP, thrombomodulin – **no difference**

LOVIT (2022)

- Sepsis requiring vasopressors
- *Intervention*: high-dose vitamin C vs placebo
- *Primary*: composite of 28-day mortality and persistent organ dysfunction – **significantly higher (44.5% vs 38.5%)**
- *Secondary*: days without organ dysfunction, 6-month mortality, quality of life, SOFA score, markers – no difference

What do you know about multi-organ dysfunction syndrome?

MODS (also known as multi-organ failure) is a condition in which 2 or more organ systems have altered function during an acute illness such that homeostasis cannot be maintained without intervention.

It can arise from most causes of tissue injury and may be contributed to by the following:

- Genetics
- Comorbidity
- Iatrogenesis (e.g. ventilator-induced lung injury and blood products)
- Inflammation
- Neuroendocrine dysfunction
- Mitochondrial dysfunction

Severity may depend on the nature of the insult, stage of illness, pre-existing organ reserve, and therapies provided. Aside from more common organ dysfunctions, presentation may involve cardiomyopathy, GI dysfunction, hepatic dysfunction, and bone marrow suppression.

Management is supportive, and affected patients are likely to require supranormal levels of nursing and medical intervention. It is thought to be responsible for around 50% of deaths in the ICU.

Resources

- Ferreira FL, Bota DP, Bross A, et al. Serial evaluation of the SOFA score to predict outcome in critically ill patients. JAMA. 2001;286(14):1754–1758.
- Gotts JE, Matthay MA. Sepsis: pathophysiology and clinical management. BMJ. 2016;353:i1585.
- Levy MM, Evans LE, Rhodes A. The Surviving Sepsis Campaign Bundle: 2018 Update. Intensive Care Med. 2018;44(6):925–958.
- Nickson C. Life in the Fast Lane: Multiple Organ Dysfunction Syndrome. Available from: https://litfl.com/multiple-organ-dysfunction-syndrome/. (Accessed 20 January 2022.)
- Rhodes A, Evans LE, Alhazzani W, et al. Surviving Sepsis Campaign: International Guidelines for Management of Sepsis and Septic Shock: 2016. Intensive Care Med. 2017;43(3):304–377.
- Singer M, Deutschman C, Seymour CW, et al. The Third International Consensus Definitions for Sepsis and Septic Shock (Sepsis-3). JAMA. 2016;315(8):801–810.
- The UK Sepsis Trust. Professional Resources: Clinical. Available from: https://sepsistrust.org/professional-resources/clinical/. (Accessed 20 January 2022.)

27. OUT-OF-HOSPITAL CARDIAC ARREST

What is the epidemiology of out-of-hospital cardiac arrest in the UK?

- *Annual incidence*: 55 per 100000 population
- Most occur at home (72%) or in the workplace (15%)
- 98% in adults and 33% aged 15–64 years
- 50% witnessed
- 80% cardiac in origin
- 25% initial rhythm shockable
- 70% receive bystander CPR
- <10% public defibrillator use
- <10% survive to hospital discharge when resuscitation attempted

How does this compare to in-hospital cardiac arrest?

- *Incidence*: 1–1.5 per 1000 admissions
- Average age 70 years
- *Initial rhythm*: PEA 52%, asystole 20%, and shockable 17%
- 53% ROSC when resuscitation attempted
- 23.6% survival to hospital discharge, 83% of whom have a favourable neurological outcome

What are the key concepts involved in the management of cardiac arrest in the UK?

Good cardiac arrest care has the potential to improve outcomes significantly, and all stages of the patient journey are important. The chain of survival describes stages that can be optimised to do so (Resuscitation Council UK):

- *Early recognition and call for help*: to prevent cardiac arrest
- *Early CPR*: to buy time
- *Early defibrillation*: to restart the heart
- *Post-resuscitation care*: to restore quality of life

Protocols and training courses have been developed to increase healthcare staff education and provide standardised care (i.e. the 'greatest good for the greatest number of patients'). Other strategies have included public automated external defibrillator access and education campaigns. There is significant health inequality in the management of cardiac arrest, and this might become a focus of future work.

Priorities

- *Competence at practical skills*: chest compressions, simple airway management, and safe defibrillation
- Dichotomy of 'shockable' vs 'non-shockable' cardiac arrest management
  - Defibrillation for pulseless VT and VF (± amiodarone and adrenaline)
  - Adrenaline for PEA or asystole
- *Consideration of reversible causes*: '4 Hs and 4 Ts'
  - Hypoxia, hypovolaemia, hypothermia, and hyper/hypokalaemia (other electrolytes)
  - Thrombus (PE/MI), tension PTX, toxins, and tamponade
- Human factors, teamwork, and leadership

In the UK, response to defibrillation is not checked until after 2 min of CPR, with immediate resumption of chest compressions after the shock.

Which drugs do you know of that are used in the management of cardiac arrest?

- *Adrenaline 1 mg*: non-shockable, as soon as possible; after third shock if shockable.
- *Amiodarone 300 mg*: refractory VT/VF arrest after 3 shocks (further 150 mg after fifth)
- *Lidocaine 100 mg*: alternative to amiodarone (additional bolus 50 mg)
- *Calcium chloride 10 ml 10% (6.8 mmol)*: PEA due to hyperkalaemia, hypocalcaemia, and calcium channel blocker overdose
- *Sodium bicarbonate 50 ml 8.4% (50 mmol)*: hyperkalaemia, TCA overdose
- *Alteplase 50 mg*: PE (further 50 mg if prolonged CPR, e.g. 30 min later)

Specific antidotes may be required in cases of poisoning. Standard adrenaline dosing is currently recommended in cases of cocaine toxicity. Some conditions may require specific pharmacological management.

The role of adrenaline is questionable. Early survival might be higher with its use, but favourable neurological outcome has not been demonstrated.

STUDY

PARAMEDIC2 (2018)

- OHCA
- *Intervention*: adrenaline as per ALS guidelines vs placebo
- *Primary*: 30-day survival – **significantly higher**
- *Secondary*: survival with favourable outcome – no difference; severe neurological impairment (mRS 4–5) – **significantly higher (31% vs 17.8%)**

(See Section 4: Toxicology, Chapter 42 Anaphylaxis, Chapter 120 Asthma, and Chapter 102 Obstetric Cardiac Arrest)

How would you approach a ventilated patient with a witnessed episode of VF on your unit?

- Declare cardiac arrest
- *Ensure safe use of oxygen*: can keep connected to closed circuit
- Start CPR
- Up to 3 (stacked) DC shocks as soon as possible
- Follow ALS protocol
- Amiodarone indicated after third shock if subsequent rhythm check still shows shockable rhythm
- Treat reversible causes

What is post-cardiac arrest syndrome?

This is a constellation of clinical features that often results consisting of the following:

- **Brain injury**
- **Myocardial dysfunction**
- **Systemic ischaemia-reperfusion response**

It may or may not be present, and severity can vary according to the nature of the arrest and resuscitation.

Some patients will show signs of neurological recovery (e.g. after short VF arrest), and intubation and ventilation may not be necessary.

What are the management priorities in a patient with ROSC after presumed cardiac cause?

The standard is currently to achieve coronary reperfusion in <120 min of ROSC. The time before 'wire crossing' (indicating reperfusion at the culprit lesion) usually includes significant time pre-hospital, assessment in the Emergency Department, activation and arrival of teams and porters, intra-hospital transfer, transfer to procedure table, anaesthetic and cardiology setup, arterial cannulation, and diagnostic angiography.

Management priorities in the unconscious patient are as follows:

- Secure airway and IV access if not achieved pre-hospital
- Maintenance of neuro- and cardioprotective physiology (e.g. suitable MAP using bolused vasopressors and avoidance of hyperthermia – temperature control)
- Confirmation and activation of PPCI team
- Feeding NG tube insertion, confirmation, and antiplatelet agent administration
- Transfer to cardiac catheterisation laboratory and onto procedure table

Significant delays may be caused by the following:

- Central line insertion and establishment of vasopressor infusion
- Arterial line insertion, particularly if conflict with planned cardiology access (i.e. right-sided lines)
- Attempting thorough intensive care 'housekeeping' and stability prior to definitive intervention
- CT imaging

> **GUIDELINE**   ERC ESICM 2021 Post-resuscitation care

Why is PCI time-critical?

Timely PPCI has the potential to have a significant impact on outcomes when indicated. Local and regional systems are largely streamlined to accommodate this.

Prolonged door-to-balloon times in STEMI are associated with increased mortality, and the MDT should be aware of the time-critical nature of transfer to the cardiac catheterisation laboratory. After 1 h of first medical contact, every 10-min treatment delay results in 3.3 additional deaths per 100 patients undergoing PCI with CS.

A subsequent trial, reported after the European Resuscitation Council (ERC) 2021 update, showed no difference in 30-day mortality between the use of immediate vs delayed/selective angiography in patients without ST-segment elevation.

> **STUDY**
>
> TOMAHAWK (2021)
>
> - OHCA without ST-segment elevation (age > 30 years)
> - *Intervention*: immediate angiography vs delayed/selective angiography
> - *Primary*: 30-day mortality – **no difference**

What physiological targets would you use following ROSC?

- Maximum F_IO_2 until P_aO_2 measured accurately, then avoid hypoxaemia and hyperoxaemia
- **P_aO_2 10–13 kPa**
- P_aCO_2 4.5–6.0 kPa
- Lung-protective ventilation and V_T 6–8 ml/kg IBW
- **MAP ≥65 mmHg** and target should achieve UO > 0.5 ml/kg/h
- Glucose 7.8–10 mmol/l
- Temperature ≤37.7°C for 72 h after ROSC
- temperature control and Avoidance of hyperthermia
- *Avoid seizures*: consider sodium valproate or levetiracetam if treatment required

(See Chapter 16 Temperature Control and Chapter 156 Prognostication)

When would diagnostic CT be indicated following ROSC?

The Resuscitation Council (UK) guidance advises coronary angiography before CT brain ± CT pulmonary angiography (CTPA) if there is clinical or ECG evidence of myocardial ischaemia. These investigations should follow if indicated after normal coronary angiography.

CT brain ± CTPA should be prioritised over coronary angiography if there are signs or symptoms of neurological or respiratory causes pre-arrest:

- Headache
- Seizures
- Focal neurological deficit
- SOB
- Hypoxaemia on background of known respiratory disease

CT for prognostication is a different concept. If the brain is imaged during presentation, it may occasionally support these criteria once applicable. However, repeat imaging is often required.

(See Chapter 156 Prognostication)

What is E-CPR and when might it be indicated?

E-CPR is a form of support which utilises VA-ECMO as an adjunct to ongoing conventional CPR in refractory cardiac arrest. A femoro-femoral cannulation approach is often used.

It may improve outcomes in selected circumstances. E-CPR requires prompt decision-making and rapid initiation of ECMO, so it is limited to settings in which implementation is realistic. Rapid transfer may be considered. Patient factors supporting a good outcome are considered in combination with the quality of resuscitation. E-CPR might be a bridge to specific intervention (e.g. PPCI and thrombectomy for PE).

An example of typical inclusion criteria is the French system, requiring ≥1 of the following:

- Known reversible cause
- Prolonged life support requirement anticipated
- Signs of life during CPR
- Short **no-flow (<5 min)** and **low-flow (<100 min)** durations
- Initial shockable rhythm
- **E_tCO_2 > 1.33 kPa** (10 mmHg) on arrival to hospital

Arrest-specific criteria may also include the following:

- Witnessed event
- Immediate good-quality bystander CPR
- Initial shockable rhythm
- Low-flow time (arrest to full-flow E-CPR) <60 min

GUIDELINE ELSO 2021 E-CPR

ARREST (2020)

- OHCA with initial rhythm VF/pulseless VT
- *Intervention*: early ECMO vs conventional resuscitation
- *Primary*: survival to hospital discharge – **significantly higher (43% vs 7%)**
- *Secondary*: 6-month survival – **significantly higher (43% vs 0%)**
- Posterior probability of superiority 0.9861 so trial stopped early

In which circumstances might prolonged resuscitation be anticipated?

- Drowning
- Hypothermia
- Refractory anaphylaxis
- Local anaesthetic systemic toxicity
- Drug intoxication (e.g. calcium channel blockers)
- PE requiring thrombolysis (bleeding risk relevant to cannulation for ECMO)

Resources

- Dennis M, Lal S, Forrest P, et al. In-depth extracorporeal cardiopulmonary resuscitation in adult out-of-hospital cardiac arrest. J Am Heart Assoc. 2020;9(10):e016521.
- Perkins GD, Nolan JP, Soar J, et al. Resuscitation Council UK: Epidemiology of Cardiac Arrest Guidelines. May 2021. Available from: https://www.resus.org.uk/library/2021-resuscitation-guidelines/epidemiology-cardiac-arrest-guidelines. (Accessed 20 January 2022.)
- Scholz KH, Maier SKG, Maier LS, et al. Impact of treatment delay on mortality in ST-segment elevation myocardial infarction (STEMI) patients presenting with and without haemodynamic instability: results from the German prospective, multicentre FITT-STEMI trial. Eur Heart J. 2018;39(13):1065–1074.

---

28.   PROPOFOL INFUSION SYNDROME

What is propofol infusion syndrome?

Propofol infusion syndrome (PRIS) is a condition associated with propofol use, characterised by an acute refractory bradycardia in the presence of 1 or more of the following:

- Metabolic acidosis (base deficit > 10 mmol/l)
- Rhabdomyolysis or myoglobinuria
- Lipaemia
- Enlarged or fatty liver

It was first described in 1998 in the paediatric population but has been seen in adult intensive care. The maximum safe dose of propofol sedation is thought to be **4 mg/kg/h**, but PRIS has occurred with doses as low as 1.9 mg/kg/h. Risk increases after 48 h of infusion.

How does PRIS present?

Common presenting features are as follows:

- *New onset metabolic acidosis (86%)*: renal failure and lactic acidosis
- **Cardiac dysfunction** (88%)

Other features are as follows:

- Rhabdomyolysis (45%)
- AKI (37%)

- Hypertriglyceridaemia (15%)
- Hepatomegaly
- Hyperkalaemia
- Lipaemia

What might you see on an ECG in PRIS?

- *Brugada-like changes*: coved ST-segment elevation in V1–3
- *Arrhythmias*: AF, VT, SVT, BBB
- Bradycardias progressing to asystole

What is the pathophysiology of PRIS?

- PRIS arises due to an imbalance of energy demand and utilisation.
- Mitochondrial oxidative phosphorylation and free fatty acid utilisation are impaired. This causes lactic acidosis and myocyte necrosis in both skeletal and cardiac muscle.
- As well as contributing to the lipid load, propofol is negatively inotropic through antagonism of beta-adrenergic receptors and calcium channel binding. This results in cardiovascular depression.

Why are these patients lipaemic?

- Increased sympathetic stimulation
- High circulating cortisol and GH
- Blockade of mitochondrial fatty acid oxidation
- Impaired lipid metabolism results
- High circulating levels of non-esterified fatty acids
- Raised serum triglyceride

What are the risk factors for PRIS?

High sedative requirement
- Severe TBI
- Sepsis
- High exogenous/endogenous catecholamine levels
- High exogenous/endogenous glucocorticoid levels

Fat metabolism
- Low carbohydrate-to-lipid-intake ratio
- Inborn errors of fatty acid oxidation

Why are children more prone to PRIS?

Children have a relatively low glycogen storage and high dependence on fat metabolism.

How would you manage PRIS?

- Stop propofol infusion
- Use alternative sedative agent(s)
- Ensure adequate carbohydrate load and minimise lipid intake
- Manage complications
  - Cardiovascular support
    - ➢ Chronotropic agents
    - ➢ Pacing may have limited success
    - ➢ Catecholamine resistance may occur
    - ➢ VA-ECMO
  - *RRT*: clear lactate, propofol, metabolites, and myoglobin

Prevention is ideal and may involve the following:

- Appropriate sedation score target
- Propofol dose < 4 mg/kg/h

- Monitoring CK and triglycerides
- Early suspicion in high-risk patients and prolonged propofol infusion

(See Chapter 14 Sedation)

Resource
- Loh NHW, Nair P. Propofol infusion syndrome. *CEACCP*. 2013;13(6):200–202.

---

29. DELIRIUM

What is delirium and what is its significance?

Delirium is a syndrome associated with **disturbed consciousness**, **abnormal cognitive function**, and **altered perception**. It has an acute and fluctuating course.

The incidence is approximately 29% in critical care, with half of cases manifesting within 2 days of admission. It lasts around 2–3 days in most cases but may persist for weeks or longer.

Delirium has been shown to be associated with increased hospital and ICU LOS, mortality, dementia, hospital-acquired complications (e.g. falls and pressure sores), and discharge to long-term care facilities.

GUIDELINE   NICE 2019 CG103 Delirium

What are the other clinical features of delirium?

KEY POINT

There are 3 broad types of delirium, classified by psychomotor activity:

- *Hyperactive*: heightened arousal, restless, agitated, aggressive
- *Hypoactive*: withdrawn, quiet, somnolent, reduced motor activity and speech
- *Mixed*: alternating between hypoactive and hyperactive features

Motor features of delirium may not be apparent if there are confounding factors (e.g. ICUAW).

Other features
- Inattention
- Distraction
- Sleep-wake cycle disturbance
- Disorientation
- Hallucinations
- Delusions

What are the risk factors for delirium?

Patient
- Age > 65
- Cognitive impairment
- Sensory impairment

- Drug/alcohol misuse
- Immobility
- Frailty

Drugs
- Benzodiazepines
- Opioids
- Anticholinergics
- Steroids

Physiological
- Severe illness
- Hypoxia
- Hypotension
- Dehydration
- Hunger
- Pain
- Constipation
- Sleep disturbance

How do you diagnose delirium?

This is assessed most commonly using the **CAM-ICU** tool. A patient is deemed CAM-ICU positive if they have criteria 1 + 2 + 3/4.

> **KEY POINT**
>
> CAM-ICU assessment is as follows:
>
> 1. **Altered mental state** or any fluctuation in past 24 h (GCS, RASS, and previous delirium assessment)
> 2. **Inattention test** (errors > 2): squeeze my hand when I say the letter 'A'. (SAVEAHAART/ CASABLANCA)
> 3. **Altered level of consciousness** (RASS other than 0)
> 4. **Disorganised thinking** (errors > 1)
>   - Questions
>   - Will a stone float on water?
>   - Are there fish in the sea?
>   - Does 1 pound weigh more than 2 pounds?
>   - Can you use a hammer to pound a nail?
>   - Command
>   - Hold up this many fingers (hold up 2 fingers)
>   - Now do the same with the other hand/add 1 more finger (no demonstration)

How do you manage delirium?

Prevention is ideal. High-risk patients should be identified.

Preventative strategies
- Regular assessment using a valid tool (e.g. CAM-ICU)
- Address modifiable risk factors
- Identify outpatient medications and restart as appropriate
- Assess presence/severity of pain and give analgesia if required
- Use lowest appropriate dose of sedation possible
- Sedation holds
- Pharmacological prophylaxis is not recommended

A multicomponent, non-pharmacological intervention is recommended to prevent and treat delirium:

- *Reduce or shorten delirium*: reorientation, cognitive stimulation, use of clocks
- *Improve sleep*: minimise light and noise

- *Improve wakefulness*: reduce sedation
- *Reduce immobility*: early rehabilitation
- *Reduce sensory impairment*: glasses, hearing aids

When delirium has occurred, routine pharmacological intervention is not recommended.

GUIDELINE   ICS 2014 Analgesia and Sedation

GUIDELINE   PADIS 2018

STUDY

Hope-ICU (2013)

- Mechanically ventilated adults
- *Intervention*: regular haloperidol 2.5 mg 8° vs placebo
- *Primary*: delirium-free, coma-free days in first 14 days – **no difference**
- *Secondary*: 28-day mortality, hospital LOS, long QT, extra-pyramidal symptoms) – no difference

When would you use pharmacological interventions?

Pharmacological management should be restricted to the management of agitation or psychosis. Pain should be addressed, and analgesia used before sedation. Avoidance of hyperadrenergic states (e.g. supra-normal MAP with catecholamine infusion) may be helpful.

- *Psychosis*: haloperidol first-line
- *Agitation/anxiety*: dexmedetomidine/clonidine
- *Agitation precluding weaning/extubation*: dexmedetomidine

(See Chapter 14 Sedation)

STUDY

DahLIA (2016)

- Adults remaining mechanically ventilated due to agitation
- *Intervention*: addition of dexmedetomidine vs saline
- *Primary*: median ventilator-free hours at 7 days – **significantly higher**
- *Secondary*: time to extubation, time to resolution of delirium, antipsychotic use, opioid use, and propofol dose – **significantly lower**

Resource

- van den Boogaard M, Slooter AJC. Delirium in critically ill patients: current knowledge and future perspectives. BJA Educ. 2019;19(12):398–404.

30. ICU-ACQUIRED WEAKNESS

What is ICU-acquired weakness?

ICUAW is a common secondary muscle weakness occurring during the management of life-threatening disease and is a component of the **PICS**. Prevalence is approximately 43%.

It is characterised by symmetrical, generalised lower motoneurone weakness affecting limbs and respiratory muscles predominantly. Proximal muscle groups are more greatly affected, and facial/ocular sparing is often present. There is usually reduced muscle tone.

Pathophysiology encompasses the following:

- *Critical illness myopathy (CIM)*: muscular
- *Critical illness polyneuromyopathy (CIPNM)*: mixed
- *Critical illness polyneuropathy (CIP)*: neuropathic

It is thought to differ from severe disuse muscle atrophy as differences in electrophysiology have been found. Other causes of weakness in this setting include rarer primary neuromuscular disorders such as myaesthenia gravis, GBS, amyotrophic lateral sclerosis, and MS.

What is the pathophysiology of ICUAW?

This is not fully understood, but several mechanisms have been proposed in combination as follows:

- **Muscle atrophy**
  - Immobilisation
  - Disuse
  - Unloading
  - Functional denervation
  - *Neuroendocrine alterations*: anabolism vs catabolism
- **Muscle dysfunction**
  - Structural alteration
  - Microcirculatory disturbance
  - Bioenergetic failure
  - Inadequate autophagy activation
- **Neuropathy**
  - Microvascular dysfunction
  - Oedema

What are the risk factors of ICUAW?

Modifiable
- Hyperglycaemia
- PN
- Immobility
- *Drugs*: vasoactive, steroids, NMB, antibiotics (e.g. vancomycin), and sedation

Non-modifiable
- *Disease*: higher severity score, sepsis, systemic inflammation, MODS, prolonged ventilation, and high lactate
- *Patient*: female, older, and premorbid obesity

How is ICUAW diagnosed?

Clinical quantification of muscle strength is required. This may be using a combination of different modalities:

- *Volitional functional testing*: MRC sum score, hand-held dynamometry, and 6-min walk test (6MWT)
- *Electrophysiology*: nerve conduction studies, needle EMG

- *Imaging*: MR, US, CT
- *Biopsy*: muscle, nerve

MRC sum score < 48/60 indicates significant weakness, and < 38/60 indicates severe.

Functional testing often requires more cooperation from the patient than other methods, which may be limited in critical care. Electrophysiology can differentiate between CIPNM and deconditioning.

How can respiratory muscles be assessed?

Several investigations exist to detect weakness in respiratory muscles as follows:

- **Volitional functional testing**
  - Maximal inspiratory/expiratory pressure
  - Transdiaphragmatic pressure
- **Non-volitional functional testing**
  - Transdiaphragmatic pressure in response to bilateral twitch phrenic nerve stimulation
  - Endotracheal tube pressure in response to bilateral phrenic stimulation during airway occlusion
- **Imaging**
  - *CXR*: diaphragm position
  - *US*: diaphragmatic excursion and thickening fraction

In practice, other clinical features may be more useful if these tests are not readily available.

Can you compare the electrophysiological findings in different types of ICUAW?

Electrophysiological findings differ between the types of ICUAW (Table 30.1).

What are the consequences of ICUAW?

- Higher 1-year mortality
- New functional disabilities (up to 8 years after sepsis)
- Neuromyogenic origin worse than myogenic
- At 5 years
  - Worse survival
  - Lower handgrip force
  - Shorter 6MWT
  - Lower respiratory muscle strength
  - Reduced physical quality of life

How might you prevent ICUAW?

Addressing modifiable risk factors may prevent ICUAW:

- Avoid hyperglycaemia
- Avoid early PN

Table 30.1 Electrophysiological findings in CIP and CIM

	CIP	CIM
CMAP amplitude	Low	Low
CMAP duration	Normal	High
SNAP amplitude	Low	Normal
Nerve conduction velocity	Normal	Normal
EMG at rest	Fibrillation potentials, positive sharp waves	
Motor unit potential voluntary muscle activation	Long duration, high amplitude, polyphasic	Short duration, low amplitude
Repetitive nerve stimulation	Absence of decremental response	
Direct muscle stimulation	Normal excitability	Low excitability

CMAP, compound muscle action potential; SNAP, sensory nerve action potential.

- *Avoidance of specific medications*: NMBs and steroids
- *Minimise sedation*: including use of sedation holds
- Early mobilisation

No evidence to support use of the following:

- Neuromuscular electrical stimulation
- Anabolic steroids
- Growth hormone
- Propranolol
- Immunoglobulin
- Glutamine

How is ICUAW managed?

Other than prevention, management will centre around multidisciplinary rehabilitation. This should involve early assessment, reassessment, agreement of rehabilitation goals, and appropriate follow-up.

(See Chapter 22 Rehabilitation)

Resource

- Vanhorebeek I, Latronico N, Van den Berghe G. ICU-acquired weakness. Intensive Care Med. 2020;46(4):637–653.

---

31. OPHTHALMOLOGICAL DISORDERS

What is lagophthalmos and why is this relevant to critical care?

Lagophthalmos is the incomplete closure of the eyelids graded as follows:

0 Lids completely closed
1 Any conjunctival exposure
2 Any corneal exposure

This can lead to exposure keratopathy and corneal abrasion on the critical care unit if the eyes are not protected, particularly when deeply sedated. At least 20% of ICU patients are affected; 60% patients sedated >48 h develop corneal epithelial defects.

Exposure keratopathy relates to dryness and disruption of usual regulation by tears. A corneal abrasion is a superficial scratch that removes the epithelium. Both conditions cause a red eye, and epithelial defects will stain yellow under blue light with fluorescein drops.

What is the significance of systemic fungal infection for the eye?

Systemic fungal infection can affect the eye and lead to visual loss. Ophthalmology review should be sought urgently if a patient has a positive blood or line tip culture for a fungal organism. Antimicrobials will need to penetrate the eye (e.g. fluconazole or voriconazole). (See Chapter 114 Fungal Infection)

What do you know about other eye infections?

- Eye colonisation common and time-dependent
- *Common organisms*: Pseudomonas aeruginosa, Acinetobacter spp., Staphylococcus epidermidis
- Respiratory sources implicated

Conjunctivitis
- Red and sticky eye
- Usually bacterial, infectious, and virulent
- Send swab for culture
- Clean eye with warm water and gauze and avoid cross-contamination

- Chloramphenicol 6° for 5–7 days
- *Seek expert help*: no improvement in 48 h, red eye but not sticky, or dull cornea or white patch

Microbial keratitis

- Corneal infection
- Red watery/sticky eye with ulceration
- Usually bacterial
- HSV keratitis less common (dendritic ulcer)
- Seek urgent ophthalmology review for any case

Endogenous endophthalmitis

- Red eye in septic patient and haematogenous spread
- Suspect particularly if hypopyon with white pus fluid level in anterior chamber
- Emergency which also indicates systemic sepsis
- Seek immediate ophthalmology review
- Risk of vitreous haemorrhage with tap or injection of antimicrobials (e.g. amikacin and vancomycin)

Which other sight-threatening eye conditions are you aware of in the intensive care unit?

Chemosis

- Conjunctival oedema causing bulging, associated with the following:
  - Impaired venous return (e.g. high PEEP)
  - Generalised oedema
  - Increased hydrostatic pressure
  - Capillary leak (e.g. sepsis)

Acute glaucoma

- Risk particularly if sudden rise in intra-orbital pressure (IOP)
- Retinal/optic nerve ischaemia

Ischaemic optic neuropathy

- May be caused by severe/recurrent hypotension
- Ocular perfusion pressure decreased by increased IOP
- May involve central retinal artery occlusion

How do we protect the eyes in critical care?

- Consider eyes in secondary survey, systems review, and management of infection
- Awareness of signs requiring referral to ophthalmology and emergencies
- Avoiding cross-contamination between eyes and staff/patients
- Appropriate use of eye drops and ointments
- Lagophthalmos:
  - *Grade 1*: lubrication (ointment)
  - *Grade 2*: lubrication and taping along lash margin
  - Re-lubrication every 4 h

GUIDELINE   ICS 2017 Eye care

TOXICOLOGY

How might patients present with poisoning?

Poisoning is a significant contributor to the critical care case mix and includes the following:

- *Accidental overdose*: single event, staggered, decompensation (e.g. AKI resulting in opioid toxicity), misadventure
- *Intentional overdose*: self-harm
- Recreational intoxication
- Trauma (including burns)
- *Deliberate poisoning*: intention to harm, 'date rape'
- Chemical weapon use

The patient may volunteer a description of exactly what has been taken. Alternatively, poisoning may be a differential in a patient with altered physiology or reduced conscious level. The trajectory of illness can be very variable and will depend on the patient's underlying health. All patients will benefit from early recognition and intervention, and onward referral as required.

Poisoning can affect any system and should be suspected particularly in cases involving:

- Altered consciousness
- Respiratory depression
- Cardiovascular instability
- Vomiting
- Hypothermia
- Seizures
- Trauma

How would you assess a poisoned patient?

- *Thorough history including collateral*: from paramedics, family, friends, etc.
  - Identification of potential ingested substances (e.g. usual/accessible medications)
  - Co-administered substances (e.g. alcohol)
  - Quantify doses and/or appearance of substances found
  - Timing
  - *Trigger events*: any mental health concern and need for forensic involvement
- Examination
  - **Toxidrome** features
  - *Signs of organ failure or complications requiring urgent intervention*: pulmonary oedema, aspiration, dehydration, etc.

- *Clues as to route of intoxication*: track marks, burns, cherry red facies, odours
  - *Signs of secondary trauma*: fall, head injury, wounds
- Investigations
  - Basic observations
  - FBC, U&E, LFT, glucose, clotting where appropriate, CK, osmolar gap
  - *ABG/VBG*: anion gap, methaemoglobinaemia
  - **12-lead ECG**
  - Imaging/targeted investigations pertaining to differential diagnosis or secondary trauma (e.g. CT head)
  - *Toxicology studies if available*: paracetamol and salicylate levels commonly, iron studies

Can you give an overview of the main toxidromes?

Toxidromes can be used to narrow the differential diagnosis in poisoning syndromes and guide management in the event of unknown substance ingestion. A toxidrome may be present in isolation, but often polysubstance intoxication results in mixed features (Table 32.1).

What are the main management principles in the poisoned patient?

- Reduce the effects of the toxin
  - Seek advice where necessary from specialist centres or organisations, such as the National Poisons Information Service (NPIS), TOXBASE®, and pharmacy
  - Supportive care of organ failure(s) as appropriate
- Consider other differentials and coexisting pathology
- Refer to mental health team if applicable
- Report any safeguarding or welfare concerns
- Occasional discussion with police
- *Forensic examination*: may be indicated early if suspected sexual assault, contact local sexual assault referral centre (SARC)

Table 32.1   Clinical features of common toxidromes

Toxidrome	Pupils	Neurology	Observations	Other	Common causes
Cholinergic	Miosis	Sedation Seizures	Bradycardia Hypotension	Diaphoresis SLUDGE syndrome: • Salivation • Lacrimation • Urination • Defecation • GI upset • Emesis	Organophosphates Nerve agents Neostigmine
Anticholinergic	Mydriasis	Agitation/ sedation Seizures Clonus	Tachycardia Hypertension Hyperthermia	Anti-secretory Urinary retention	Antihistamines TCAs Hyoscine Atropine Anti-parkinsonian
Sedative	Miosis	Sedation	Bradycardia Hypotension Hypoventilation Hypothermia	Constipation	Opioids Alcohols Benzodiazepines Barbiturates Antiepileptics GHB Baclofen
Stimulant	Mydriasis	Agitation Seizures Tremor	Tachycardia Hypertension Hyperventilation Hyperthermia	Anti-secretory	Cocaine Amphetamines Theophylline Caffeine

What measures can be taken to reduce the effects of a poison?

Reduce absorption

- *GI decontamination*: induced emesis, gastric lavage (not routine, airway protection a concern), whole bowel irrigation (e.g. iron poisoning), endoscopy, surgery (e.g. body packing)
- *Adsorption*: activated charcoal
- *Lipid sink*: intralipid used in some circumstances with lipophilic molecules (e.g. local anaesthetic toxicity, calcium channel blockers, cocaine)
- *Skin decontamination*: remove clothing, wash skin if topical/transdermal route of absorption, beware of opioid patches

Enhance elimination

- Fluid repletion
- Urinary alkalinisation (e.g. salicylate toxicity)
- Extracorporeal removal
- *Forced diuresis*: not recommended

Neutralise toxin/effects

- Use of specific antidotes
- Specific supportive therapies

Which drugs can be eliminated by extracorporeal methods?

RRT is more effective against substances which have the following:

- Low protein binding
- Low volume of distribution
- Low non-renal clearance
- Low molecular weight

Smaller molecules (<10 kDa) are preferentially cleared by diffusion (haemodialysis); moderate-sized molecules (<25 kDa) are better cleared with convection (CVVH). Large molecules have been known to be cleared using plasma exchange or apheresis in some circumstances.

Haemodialysis is nearly always the method of choice, but CRRT (or hybrid e.g. CVVHDF) may be favoured for specific reasons, for example, ease of use, local set-up, haemodynamic stability, drugs with slow movement from tissue to plasma. RRT may be used for support with non-dialysable toxins causing AKI (Table 32.2).

Which specific antidotes do you know of?

The majority of toxins can be alleviated with opposing supportive medicines (e.g. atropine for significant bradycardia). However, a number of specific antidotes exist for certain agents (Table 32.3).

Resources

Relevant throughout Section 4:

- Life in the Fast Lane. Toxicology Library. 2022. Available from: https://litfl.com/tox-library/. (Accessed 15 January 2022.)
- National Poisons Information Service. TOXBASE®. 2022. Available from: https://www.toxbase.org. (Accessed 15 January 2022.)
- The Internet Book of Critical Care. Approach to the Critically Ill Poisoned Patient. Available from: https://emcrit.org/ibcc/tox/. 2022. (Accessed 15 January 2022.)

Table 32.2 Drugs cleared by RRT

Haemodialysis (most toxins)		Haemofiltration	Plasmapheresis
Salicylates	Carbamazepine	Lithium	Monoclonal antibodies
Toxic alcohols	Metformin	Sympathomimetics	*Amanita phalloides*
Lithium	Aminoglycosides	Opioids	
Valproate	Theophyllines		

Table 32.3 More specific antidotes

Toxin	Antidote
Amanita phalloides	Silibinin
Amyl nitrite	Methylene blue
Arsenic, mercury, gold, and lead	Dimercaprol
Benzodiazepines	Flumazenil
Beta-blockers	Glucagon
Calcium channel blockers	Calcium
	Insulin (HIET)
Cyanide	Hydroxocobalamin (B12)
	Sodium thiosulphate
	Dicobalt edetate
	Sodium nitrite
Digoxin	Digoxin-specific antibody fragment
Iron	Desferrioxamine
Isoniazid	Pyridoxine (B6)
Methotrexate	Carboxypeptidase G2
Opioids	Naloxone
Organophosphates	Pralidoxime
Paracetamol	N-acetylcysteine (NAC)
SSRI	Cyproheptadine
Toxic alcohols	Fomepizole
	Ethanol

33. MENTAL HEALTH AND CRITICAL CARE

Why is mental health significant in critical care?

Mental health disorders are responsible for a large proportion of the critical care case mix and may also develop de novo. Consequences of such illnesses are multidimensional:

- Potential for high morbidity and mortality if untreated
- Substantial critical care caseload related to intoxication, substance dependency or chronic effects, self-harm, suicide, and assault
- Risk of recurrent admissions and reattendance with related issues
- Illicit substances evolving constantly
- High risk of delirium including withdrawal
- *Complex regular medications*: polypharmacy, interactions, withdrawal, and QTc prolongation
- Electroconvulsive therapy may be required by ICU patients (e.g. malignant catatonia)
- Potential to precipitate mental health issues in ICU patients and those close to them (e.g. depression with prolonged admission, grief)
- Refusal of medical intervention, requiring understanding of medical treatment guidance and legislation
- Staff at risk of mental health issues including burnout

What are the implications of self-harm in the critical care context on psychological management?

- Significance of attempted harm, often with high potential lethality
- Follow-up essential for risk stratification ± admission to inpatient psychiatric services
- May require detention under the Mental Health Act

When might you encounter a patient under Mental Health Section in critical care?

The Mental Health Act 1983 can facilitate preservation of safety of the patient or others due to suspected uncontrolled mental illness in which voluntary assessment and management are not possible.

- Section 136: removal from public place (including some Emergency Department areas) by police to place of safety if believed to be suffering from mental illness needing immediate care or control (risk to self or others)
- Section 5(4): permits some nurses to detain until assessment by doctor
- Section 5(2): detention by a doctor for up to 72 h for assessment
- Section 2: admission for up to 28 days for assessment ± treatment
- Section 3: admission for up to 6 months for treatment and can be renewed
- Section 17: detained patient granted leave from hospital in which they are detained

Alternatively, patients may be under voluntary admission to mental health inpatient services.

GUIDELINE   UK Legislation 1983 Mental Health Act 1983

What is a psychiatric intensive care unit?

A psychiatric ICU is a specialised area for patients suffering from an acutely disturbed phase of a serious mental disorder. Management here utilises specific psychological therapies but could involve rapid tranquilisation. Considerations to the physical environment include being on the ground floor, use of soft furnishings, and anti-ligature properties.

Admission is indicated for those who are unable to be managed safely on a psychiatric ward due to associated loss of capacity for self-control and increase in risk:

- *Externally directed aggression*: others or property
- *Internally directed aggression*: suicide risk or unresponsive to preventative measures
- *Absconding*: if severe consequences when persistent
- Unpredictability

What do you know about the Mental Capacity Act?

- The Mental Capacity Act (2005) outlines legislation which empowers and protects people who lack the capacity to make their own decisions.
- Medical and allied professionals have a duty to know how to use it.
- Capacity is decision-specific, and refusal of a specific intervention does not imply refusal of all medical treatments.

KEY POINT

Principles of the Mental Capacity Act (2005):

1. Assume capacity unless proven otherwise.
2. Maximise potential for capacity where possible.
3. Unwise decisions do not constitute a lack of capacity.
4. Make decisions in a person's best interests if lacking capacity.
5. In this context, treatment should be the least restrictive of rights and freedoms possible.

Assessed in 2 stages:

1. Does the person have an impairment of their mind or brain?
2. Does the impairment mean the person is unable to make a specific decision?
   - Understand relevant information
   - Retain information for long enough
   - Weigh up that information to make a decision

Good practice:

- Encourage participation (e.g. visual aids, correct language)
- Identify all relevant circumstances
- *Find out the person's views*: past/present wishes, beliefs, and values
- Avoid discrimination
- Assess whether capacity might be regained and delay appropriately if able

Consultation with others may be crucial and could involve family, friends, carers, any individuals named by that person, Lasting Power of Attorney, deputy of the Court of Protection, etc.

GUIDELINE UK Legislation 2005 Mental Capacity Act (2005)

What does 'DOLS' mean?

Deprivation of Liberty Safeguards (DOLS) aim to prevent unlawful restrictions to a person's freedom. A deprivation of liberty may be indicated if in the patient's or others' best interests. An application will need to be made through the local authority.

GUIDELINE BMA 2020 DOLS

When do you need a DOLS on ICU and how does this differ from treatment under the Mental Capacity Act?

Under the Mental Health Act (2005), a person lacking capacity may be **restrained** in their best interests if reasonably believed to be necessary to prevent harm to the person. Measures must be proportionate to the likelihood and seriousness of harm.

However, depriving a person who lacks capacity of their **liberty** requires a DOLS or an Order of the Court of Protection. These are more administrative systems. In reality, DOLS are rarely required in intensive care as the starting point differs to most other circumstances; patients requiring intensive care are not considered to be deprived of liberty as they are too unwell to leave of their own accord. Parents can consent to children under 16 years of age being detained.

Formal authority should be sought to prevent the patient leaving if **physically capable**, if family may remove them inappropriately, or if subject to a section 17 of the Mental Health Act (the patient is on leave of absence from hospital in which they are detained).

GUIDELINE FICM 2021 Midnight Laws

Can you describe some important withdrawal syndromes?

Withdrawal may be physical or psychological. Symptoms result from the cessation or reduction of intake of a substance to which the body has acclimatised. The withdrawal syndrome is often the inverse of the effects of the substance or features of intoxication. Sedative withdrawal may pose a greater threat to life through seizures.

Opioid withdrawal
- Anxiety
- Chills
- Myalgia
- Weakness
- Tremor

- Lethargy, drowsiness, yawning
- Restlessness, irritability, sleep disturbance
- Nausea, vomiting, diarrhoea
- Drug craving (weeks to months)

Alcohol withdrawal (benzodiazepines similar)

- Tremor
- Sweating
- Visual hallucinations
- Seizures
- Depression, anxiety
- Restlessness, irritability sleep disturbance
- Nausea

SSRI discontinuation syndrome

- Anxiety, depression
- Flu-like symptoms
- Sleep disturbance
- Impaired balance
- Sensory changes
- Nausea
- Psychosis

Features may be subclassified as neurological, psychological, and physical. (Further detail is given in subsequent topics within this section.)

Resource

- National Association of Psychiatric Intensive Care & Low Secure Units. National Minimum Standards for Psychiatric Intensive Care in Adult General Services. 2014. Available from: https://napicu.org.uk/wp-content/uploads/2014/12/NMS-2014-final.pdf. (Accessed 15 January 2022.)

34. PSYCHIATRIC MEDICATIONS

Which overdoses commonly present to critical care?

- *Often prescribed or easily accessible*: including 'over-the-counter' and others' prescriptions
- Commonly mixed ± alcohol or other intoxication
- Likely to include psychiatric medications:
  - *TCA*: more commonly prescribed in context of chronic pain than depression
  - SSRI
  - Selective noradrenaline reuptake inhibitors (SNRIs)
  - Antipsychotics

How might a patient with tricyclic antidepressant overdose present to critical care?

The most significant effects are often on the cardiovascular system. Overdose can cause the following:

- Anticholinergic toxidrome
- *Dysrhythmias*: sodium channel blockade
- *Hypotension*: vasodilatation, reduced reuptake of catecholamines
- Seizures
- Reduced consciousness, delirium

What features might be seen on an ECG?

- Tachycardia
- Right axis deviation
- Brugada Type I pattern
- Broad QRS (>100 ms seizure risk, > 160 ms VT risk)
- Long QT (torsades rare if tachycardic in this context)

What are the specific management priorities in TCA toxicity?

- Appropriate cardiac monitoring
- Pharmacological management of sodium channel blockade
  - Administration of sodium bicarbonate if:
    - ➢ Seizure
    - ➢ QRS > 100 ms
    - ➢ Hypotension not due to hypovolaemia
  - Avoidance of hypernatraemia with repeated bicarbonate infusions
  - Lidocaine indicated if refractory to bicarbonate
  - Lipid emulsion may also be used
- Early vasopressors (likely to be unresponsive to fluid)
- VT may be managed with bicarbonate, lidocaine, magnesium, or intralipid (amiodarone may cause further QTc prolongation).
- Intubation and ventilation (rarely) for:
  - Seizures
  - Significant respiratory acidosis
  - Usual indications (e.g. loss of airway reflexes)

(In addition to key principles discussed in Chapter 32 Poisoning Overview)

What is the significance of SSRI overdose?

- Overdose often benign
- Toxicity mainly relates to the development of serotonin syndrome.
- Citalopram and escitalopram exhibit dose-dependent QT prolongation and risk of torsades de pointes (at 600 mg and 300 mg, respectively).
- Effects potentiated by concomitant administration of serotonergic medications (see Chapter 36 Serotonin Syndrome)

What do you know about antipsychotic overdose?

Features of overdose of specific antipsychotic agents might aid diagnosis (Table 34.1).

Table 34.1   Key features of toxicity in antipsychotic overdose

Butyrophenones and phenothiazines (haloperidol and chlorpromazine)	Atypical (olanzapine and risperidone)	Lithium	
Fluctuant mental state CNS depression Tachycardia Hypotension Urinary retention Anticholinergic	CNS depression Hypotension Seizures (rare)	Neurological • Fine tremor • Ataxia, coarse tremor • Fasciculation • Myoclonus • Nystagmus • Hyperreflexia • Delirium • Seizure • Non-convulsive status epilepticus • Coma	GI • Nausea • Vomiting • Ileus • Diarrhoea Cardiovascular • Bradycardia • Hypotension • Long QT Hyperthermia

Key management principles
- Benzodiazepines if pharmacological management of agitation indicated
- Supportive care may necessitate intubation whilst sedatives eliminated
- *Consideration of delirium on emergence and mitigation strategies*: usual anti-delirium care ± alpha blocker (e.g. dexmedetomidine or clonidine)
- Management of withdrawal

Lithium overdose presents a specific challenge as it has a narrow therapeutic window and may be precipitated by changes in physiology or polypharmacy in ICU. Acutely, GI symptoms predominate, followed by neurological symptoms. Chronic intoxication is more common, usually due to renal dysfunction, and presents with neurological issues.

Management of lithium toxicity
- *Specific investigations*: lithium levels, thyroid function tests (TFT), and calcium (chronic endocrine suppression)
- Establishing cause of decompensation (e.g. AKI)
- Activated charcoal ineffective
- Fluid repletion
- Diuretics not recommended routinely
- *Dialysis*: guidance varies and depends on the following:
  - Lithium levels (**>4–5 mmol/l** acute and > 2.5 mmol/l chronic)
  - Extent of neurological or cardiac features
  - Trajectory
  - Tolerance of crystalloid
  - Renal dysfunction

What is the role of antidepressants in ICU patients?
Depression may develop in the critically unwell, particularly during prolonged admission. Numerous challenges accompany this, for example distinguishing between delirium and other illnesses. Depression might limit a patient's engagement with rehabilitation, feeding, etc., and therefore prolong recovery from critical illness.

Evidence-based psychological therapies are recommended first-line in the broader context. De novo prescription of antidepressants is controversial but might be a therapeutic option. The risks of ongoing depression need to be weighed against potential harms and newer agents are preferred (SSRI or SNRI). Pre-existing prescriptions should continue where suitable.

Considerations
- Modifiable factors causing low mood
- Severity of symptoms and associated risks
- Ability to engage with psychological therapies
- Drug pharmacodynamics, pharmacokinetics, interactions
- *Potential side effects*: insomnia, GI discomfort, hypertension, weight gain, appetite loss, long QT, serotonin syndrome
- *Chronicity*: weeks to months before clinical benefit, often after initial agitation and increased suicide risk
- Requirement for slow tapering and avoiding abrupt cessation

Resource
- Royal College of Psychiatrists. Position statement on depression and antidepressants. PS04/19. May 2019. Available from: https://www.rcpsych.ac.uk/docs/default-source/improving-care/better-mh-policy/position-statements/ps04_19---antidepressants-and-depression.pdf?sfvrsn=ddea9473_5. (Accessed 15 January 2022.)

What challenges might present to the critical care physician when managing patients using illicit drugs?

Illicit drug use is common in the UK, causing around 3000 deaths per year recently. Approximately 10% of adults aged 16–60 have taken illicit drugs in the last year. In England, 38% of school children aged 15 years old were found to have taken drugs in their lifetime to date (2018 government statistics). A £9.4-billion-per-year industry perpetuates this problem, and it is likely to remain a large component of the medical workload.

Presentation

- Often covert, secondary presentation with complications (e.g. trauma)
- *Potential lethality and severity of effects variable*: may not be dose related
- Mixed overdose can confound diagnosis
- *Contamination of substance taken*: bacterial, viral, other

Pharmacological

- *Pharmacodynamics unpredictable*: impure/false products, cutting agents
- *Laboratory or bedside drug tests*: availability, false positives
- Interactions with prescribed therapies (e.g. anaesthesia)
- *Evolving substances*: preparations, chemical structures, may bypass detection or policing

Other

- *Behavioural*: aggression, complications of driving intoxicated
- *Capacity issues*: non-compliance, best interests
- *Concomitant psychiatric conditions*: self-harm, addiction, anxiety, depression
- *Social issues*: legal implications, other criminal activity, safeguarding, custody, homelessness
- *Complications from long-term use*: vascular access, fistula, abscess, malnutrition, HIV, hepatitis

Which common drugs of abuse can result in intensive care admission?

Drugs of abuse are taken (or given) because of effects that are perceived to be desirable. These may be classified according to these effects:

- *Narcotics*: heroin, codeine, fentanyl, tramadol, oxycodone, carfentanil
- *Depressants*: alcohol, benzodiazepines, barbiturates, GHB, GBL, piperazines
- *Stimulants*: amphetamines, MDMA, and cocaine (Table 35.1)
- *Hallucinogens*: synthetic cannabinoids (e.g. 'Spice'), ketamine, phencyclidine
- *Anabolic steroids*: testosterones and modified derivatives (e.g. stanozolol, oxandrolone)

Use may be recreational, therapeutic, or due to physical or psychological dependence. However, there are often many associated undesirable effects. The most common to present to critical care include cocaine, alcohol, and heroin. 'Club drugs' such as MDMA and methamphetamine are a significant problem. Newly emerging drugs are increasingly involved and include synthetic cathinones ('bath salts') and synthetic cannabinoids such as 'spice'.

How would you approach the agitated, intoxicated patient?

On presentation, it may be unclear what the diagnosis is and a pragmatic approach must be undertaken in a systems review with the following priorities:

- Maintain safety towards staff and other patients
  - Security officer assistance may be required
- Continuous assessment of capacity and ability to comply with management
- Use of verbal and non-verbal de-escalation strategies

Table 35.1 CNS stimulants (including recreational drugs)

Psychomotor	Psychomimetic		Other Analeptic
Catecholamine release • Amphetamines • MDMA	Psychedelic	Serotonergic • Psilocybin • MDMA	Respiratory stimulant • Doxapram
Catecholamine/serotonin reuptake inhibition • Cocaine • Nicotine		Cannabinoidergic • Tetrahydrocannabinol (THC) • 'Spice'	Convulsant • Strychnine
Methylxanthines • Caffeine • Theophylline	Dissociative	NMDA receptor antagonists • Ketamine • Phencyclidine • Nitrous oxide	
		Opioid agonists • Salvinorin A	
	Deliriant	Anticholinergics • Atropine • Diphenhydramine	
		GABA agonists • Muscimol • Zolpidem	

- Extreme agitation may require rapid tranquilisation if a threat to self or others
  - Strategy may be based on other factors (e.g. need for imaging, likely trajectory, systemic complications, and pain)
  - General anaesthesia is indicated occasionally (e.g. head trauma requiring CT, severe hyperthermia)
  - Antipsychotics or ketamine may be suitable otherwise – with appropriate monitoring
- Manage underlying cause of agitation
  - Urinary retention (anticholinergic agents)
  - Cocaine
  - MDMA
  - Investigate important differentials as appropriate (e.g. encephalitis, thyroid storm, hypoglycaemia)
- Manage complications
  - Serotonin syndrome
  - Sympathomimetic syndrome

GUIDELINE   RCEM 2022 Acute behavioural disturbance

How would you approach the unconscious, intoxicated patient?

A similar approach may be necessary, with **stabilisation prior to diagnosis**:

- Thorough assessment of conscious state, pupillary responses, tone, reflexes, airway protection
- Suspicion of blood-borne viruses and appropriate precautions
- *Consider tracheal intubation*: high risk of aspiration, failure of gas exchange, multi-organ dysfunction, guarded trajectory, transfer indications
- Correct hypoglycaemia where present (give thiamine first if risk of Wernicke's encephalopathy)

Establish cause of impaired consciousness such as the following:

- *Opioid toxidrome*: trial of naloxone may be indicated and gradual titration prior to infusion
- Ethanol overdose and toxic alcohols
- *Intentional overdose of tablets*: often analgesics or antipsychotics (see Chapter 34 Psychiatric Medications)

Consider and manage important **differentials** – list below is not exhaustive:

- Meningoencephalitis
- Systemic sepsis
- Myxoedema coma
- Intracranial haemorrhage
- Metabolic derangement
- Non-convulsive status epilepticus
- Serotonin syndrome

Appropriate investigations might include the following:

- BM, serum glucose
- *Bloods*: VBG/ABG, biochemistry, paracetamol and salicylate levels, inflammatory markers, liver enzymes, CK, ammonia, toxic alcohol levels, blood cultures
- Urinalysis
- Pregnancy test
- Imaging: CT head
- Lumbar puncture (LP)
- *EEG*: non-convulsive status epilepticus
- Toxicology screen is of debatable use/availability, particularly after induction of anaesthesia

Tell me about toxic alcohol ingestion.

Ethanol is the most commonly abused substance in the UK and remains legal despite significant associated morbidity and mortality. Acute intoxication can result in a spectrum of conscious level changes from disinhibition to stupor and coma or death. Advanced airway support may be necessary to prevent aspiration, particularly if alcohol is combined with other intoxicants. Other complications requiring supportive care include dehydration, hypoglycaemia, ketoacidosis, lactic acidosis, hypokalaemia, and dysrhythmias. IV fluids ± glucose supplementation may be required, and IV B vitamins (e.g. Pabrinex®) should be considered if Wernicke's encephalopathy is a risk.

Other toxic alcohol ingestion should be suspected with a strong history or other clinical signs (detailed below). A toxic alcohol screen may be sent, but empirical treatment may be required if results are not available quickly. Immediate diagnosis is clinical, often involving history, signs, and markers such as biochemistry, VBG/ABG, osmolar gap, and anion gap. In the ICU, **propylene glycol** toxicity may arise from benzodiazepine infusion due to its presence as a solvent.

Ethylene glycol
- Commonly found in antifreeze, detergents, and metal polish.
- Metabolism by alcohol dehydrogenase to glycolaldehyde > glycolic acid > **glyoxylic acid** > **oxalic acid** (HAGMA produced)
- Glycolic acid may cause a spuriously high lactate.
- Urinary sodium fluorescein may be seen under Wood's lamp; oxalate under microscopy.
- *Toxic metabolites responsible for effects*: **calcium oxalate precipitates** in kidneys and brain, also resulting in hypocalcaemia
- Stages
    1 *30 min*: 2 h – similar to ethanol toxicity: GI upset, ataxia, nystagmus, coma, seizures
    2 *12–24 h*: cardiopulmonary: myocardial dysfunction, shock, MODS, ARDS
    3 *24–72 h*: renal: AKI
    4 *>72 h*: late neurological sequelae: external ocular paralysis, cranial nerve defects

Methanol
- Found in windshield wiper fluid, de-icer, antifreeze, paint remover, shoe dyes, and embalming fluid
- May be produced accidentally during home distillation
- Metabolism by alcohol dehydrogenase to formaldehyde, then by aldehyde dehydrogenase to **formic acid, a mitochondrial toxin** (HAGMA produced)
- Stages
    1 *0–6 h*: similar to ethanol toxicity: GI upset, dizziness, ataxia, confusion
    2 *6–30 h*: latent phase: may be asymptomatic

3 *6–72 h*: visual symptoms (blurring, 'snowstorm vision', optic nerve atrophy, blindness), seizures, coma, cerebral oedema, parkinsonism, transverse myelitis, basal ganglia haemorrhage, HF, respiratory arrest

Isopropyl alcohol (isopropanol)

- Found in hand sanitisers and antiseptic agents
- Metabolism by alcohol dehydrogenase to acetone (mitigates HAGMA – may not be present)
- Falsely elevated creatinine due to interference of acetone with assays
- **Direct toxic effects of isopropanol** from GABA agonism in CNS and GI irritation (± cardiovascular in high doses)
- Acetone may contribute to CNS depression.
- *Features*: profound intoxication, haemorrhagic gastritis, cerebellar signs, coma
- Management is supportive.
- Proton pump inhibitors may be helpful.

What specific treatment may be given for toxic alcohol ingestion?

- *Antidotes as detailed below*: ethanol, fomepizole (alcohol dehydrogenase inhibitor)
- Sodium bicarbonate should be used to maintain pH 7.35–7.45
- *Cofactors may be given to produce less toxic metabolites*: pyridoxine and thiamine (ethylene glycol); folate or folinic acid (methanol)

Indications for fomepizole (15 mg/kg)

- Serum concentration > 20 mg/dl
- Ingestion confirmed/suspected plus 2 of:
  - Osmolar gap > 10 mOsm
  - Arterial pH < 7.30
  - HCO_3^- > 20 mmol/l
  - Presence of urinary oxalate crystals

Indications for haemodialysis (metabolite clearance)

- Serum concentration > 50 mg/dl
- Arterial pH < 7.25
- Visual disturbance
- AKI
- Refractory electrolyte abnormalities
- Refractory haemodynamic instability

What do you know about GHB?

Gamma-hydroxybutyrate is a drug which causes euphoria followed by a rapid onset of CNS and respiratory depression, before a rapid elimination and recovery. Metabolism is by alcohol dehydrogenase and is impaired by concomitant alcohol intoxication. Withdrawal can include hallucinations, insomnia, paranoia, agitation, and anxiety.

A high-profile conviction took place in 2020 in Manchester, UK, when one individual was suspected to have sexually assaulted over 195 men over 2½ years using GHB and similar substances.

What relevant drugs legislation is there in the UK?

- **The Medicines Act (1968)**
  - Governs manufacture and supply of medicine with or without prescription
- **The Misuse of Drugs Act (1971)**
  - Controls drugs to prevent non-medical use
  - Changed over time
  - Classification A–C and 'temporary class' guide penalties
  - Penalties for possession, supply (selling, dealing, and sharing), and production
    - ➤ A: crack cocaine, cocaine, MDMA, heroin, lysergic acid diethylamide, magic mushrooms, methadone, methamphetamine
    - ➤ B: amphetamines, barbiturates, cannabis, codeine, ketamine, methylphenidate, synthetic cannabinoids, synthetic cathinones

> *C*: anabolic steroids, benzodiazepines, GHB (due to be reclassified to 'B' after above case), GBL, piperazines, khat

> *Temporary class*: some methylphenidate substances and derivatives

- **The Psychoactive Substances Act (2016)**
  - Newer legislation to restrict production, sale, and supply of 'new psychoactive substances,' originally termed 'legal highs'.
  - A psychoactive substance is defined as "any substance which is capable of producing a psychoactive effect in a person who consumes it" and is not exempted.
  - Exemptions include food, alcohol, nicotine, caffeine, medicines, and drugs already regulated under the Misuse of Drugs Act (1971).

Resources

- Black C. Review of Drugs Executive Summary. February 2020. Available from: https://www.drugsandalcohol.ie/31655/1/UKSummaryPhaseOne-Review_of_drugs.pdf. (Accessed 15 January 2022.)
- Farkas J. The Internet Book of Critical Care. Ethylene Glycol & Methanol Poisoning. Available from: https://emcrit.org/ibcc/alcohols/. (Accessed 15 January 2022.)
- Legislation.gov.uk. Medicines Act 1968. Chapter 67. Available from: https://www.legislation.gov.uk/ukpga/1968/67/contents. (Accessed 15 January 2022.)
- Legislation.gov.uk. Misuse of Drugs Act 1971. Chapter 38. Available from: https://www.legislation.gov.uk/ukpga/1971/38/contents. (Accessed 15 January 2022.)
- Legislation.gov.uk. Psychoactive Substances Act 2016. Chapter 2. Available from: https://www.legislation.gov.uk/ukpga/2016/2/contents. (Accessed 15 January 2022.)
- Long N. Life in the Fast Lane. Isopropanol. Available from: https://litfl.com/isopropanol/. (Accessed 15 January 2022.)
- Public Health England. United Kingdom Drug Situation 2019: Focal Point Annual Report. Available from: https://www.gov.uk/government/publications/united-kingdom-drug-situation-focal-point-annual-report/united-kingdom-drug-situation-focal-point-annual-report-2019. (Accessed 15 January 2022.)

36. SEROTONIN SYNDROME

What is serotonin syndrome?

Serotonin syndrome is a potentially life-threatening state that results from a **systemic excess of the neurotransmitter serotonin**.

KEY POINT

Serotonin syndrome manifests as a triad of the following:

- **Altered mental status**
- **Autonomic instability**
- **Neuromuscular hyperexcitability**

What is the pathophysiology of serotonin syndrome?

Serotonin, or 5-hydroxytryptamine (5-HT), is an endogenous substance, produced by metabolism of tryptophan. It acts as a neurotransmitter and is then subject to reuptake or inactivation by monoamine oxidase (MAO) to 5-hydroxyindoleacetic acid before renal excretion.

Several receptors are involved in mediating the effects of serotonin. Most are G-protein coupled. Serotonin acts to modulate thermoregulation, behaviour, and attention in the CNS and peripheral effects in the GI tract, uterus, vasculature, and bronchi. It also promotes platelet aggregation.

Serotonin syndrome or toxicity is classically drug induced, involving a combination of 2 or more agents, but may occur in susceptible individuals with 1 agent.

It can happen through a variety of mechanisms as follows:

- *Excessive formation/precursors*: L-tryptophan, L-dihydroxyphenylalanine (L-DOPA)
- *Increased release*: cocaine, MDMA, amphetamines, alcohol, pethidine, methadone, mirtazapine
- *Receptor stimulation*: TCA, pethidine, fentanyl, ondansetron, St John's Wort, lower severe disability (LSD), lithium, sumatriptan
- *Decreased reuptake*: SSRI, SNRI, tramadol, pethidine, fentanyl, TCA, ondansetron, St John's Wort
- *Decreased metabolism*: monoamine oxidase inhibitors (MAOI), linezolid, methylene blue

Effects may be potentiated by changes in pharmacokinetics of the above agents (e.g. cytochrome P450 enzyme system).

How might serotonin syndrome present?

This condition typically develops over 24 h and may occur up to 6 weeks after cessation of a causative agent (e.g. some MAOIs and SSRIs). A thorough toxicology history is indicated where possible including drug timings. MAOI involvement is associated with greater severity. Effects range from relatively benign to life-threatening, and a patient may present with multi-organ dysfunction. Clinical features include the following:

Altered mental state
- Akathisia (restlessness)
- Hypomania
- Agitation, hypervigilance
- Hallucinations, delirium

Neuromuscular excitability (lower limbs predominantly)
- Tremor
- Hyperreflexia
- *Clonus*: spontaneous/inducible
- *Ocular clonus*: slow and continuous horizontal movement
- Babinski sign
- Muscle rigidity
- Mydriasis

Autonomic dysfunction
- Labile BP and HR
- Flushing, diaphoresis
- Hyperthermia
- Dry mucous membranes
- GI hypermotility, diarrhoea

How would you diagnose serotonin syndrome?

Serotonin syndrome requires a high index of suspicion clinically, and the gold standard is diagnosis by a medical toxicologist. The **Hunter Serotonin Toxicity Criteria** may be helpful (84% sensitivity and 97% specificity). The presence of 1 point with a history of at least 1 serotonergic agent indicates a positive result:

- Spontaneous clonus
- Inducible clonus + agitation/diaphoresis
- Ocular clonus + agitation/diaphoresis
- Tremor + hyperreflexia
- Hyperthermia + temperature > 38°C + ocular/inducible clonus

What are the important differentials?

- Neuroleptic malignant syndrome (NMS)
- MH
- Sympathomimetic intoxication
- Anticholinergic intoxication

- Sedative withdrawal
- CNS infection
- Thyroid storm

What are the key management steps in a critically ill patient with serotonin syndrome?

- **Resuscitation**
  - *Intubation and ventilation*: sedation ± paralysis if severe hyperthermia (>41.1°C), agitation, status epilepticus, chest wall rigidity
  - *Benzodiazepines*: if severe agitation, seizures, mild increases in BP/HR
  - *Volume replacement*: high insensible loss from pyrexia, rhabdomyolysis
  - Cardiovascular
    - ➤ *Hypotension*: direct-acting (e.g. NA, adrenaline, phenylephrine)
    - ➤ *Hypertension*: short-acting (e.g. esmolol, sodium nitroprusside)
  - Cooling to normothermia
- **Remove the cause**
  - Stop causative medication and those acting on serotonin where possible
  - Avoid starting serotonergic agents and consider alternatives
- **Specific therapies**
  - *Serotonin antagonists*: cyproheptadine (if failure to improve with sedation), chlorpromazine, olanzapine
  - Lipid emulsion has been used for lipophilic drugs (e.g. cocaine, SSRIs)
  - Dexmedetomidine may have some advantage against serotonin activity
- **Medications to avoid**
  - *Bromocriptine*: serotonin agonist
  - *Antipyretic agents (e.g. paracetamol)*: ineffective as hyperthermia is not mediated by hypothalamus
  - *Propranolol*: may cause prolonged hypotension and mask tachycardia used in monitoring response to treatment
  - *Dantrolene*: may be considered in muscular hyperactivity (no effect on survival in animal models)
- **Other**
  - Liaison with pharmacy
  - Communication with other care providers (e.g. general practitioner [GP])

What is NMS?

NMS is a condition that arises due to a **systemic deficit of dopamine**. It is an idiosyncratic reaction to neuroleptic antipsychotic medications (dopamine blockade) or withdrawal of dopamine receptor agonists.

KEY POINT

NMS manifests as a tetrad of:

- **Altered mental state**
- **Autonomic instability**
- **Muscle rigidity**
- **Hyperthermia**

What is the difference between neuroleptic malignant syndrome and serotonin syndrome?

NMS is an important differential of serotonin syndrome, and it may be difficult to distinguish between them. Clinically, the significance of extrapyramidal signs such as muscle rigidity is greater in NMS;

hyperreflexia and myoclonus are rare. It may progress to a catatonic state, severe encephalopathy, and coma. The presentation is more insidious over days to weeks and may also result in rhabdomyolysis and multi-organ dysfunction, resolving over a much longer course.

Management priorities are similar to those in serotonin syndrome (see above). EEG may be indicated to rule out non-convulsive status epilepticus. There is little evidence on specific therapies, but these may include benzodiazepines and dantrolene, before dopamine agonists (e.g. bromocriptine and amantadine) in extreme cases. Electroconvulsive therapy has also been used in refractory cases. The causative agent should not be restarted for 2 weeks.

Resources
- Boyer EW. UpToDate: Serotonin Syndrome (Serotonin Toxicity). 2022. Available from: https://www.uptodate.com/contents/serotonin-syndrome-serotonin-toxicity. (Accessed 15 January 2022.)
- Wijdicks EFM. UpToDate: Neuroleptic Malignant Syndrome. 2022. Available from: https://www.uptodate.com/contents/neuroleptic-malignant-syndrome?search=neuroleptic%20malignant%20syndrome&source=search_result&selectedTitle=1~68&usage_type=default&display_rank=1. (Accessed 15 January 2022.)

37. CARDIOVASCULAR MEDICINES

What are the specific concerns surrounding calcium channel blocker overdose?

Calcium channel blockers include dihydropyridines (e.g. nifedipine, amlodipine, nimodipine) and non-dihydropyridines (e.g. verapamil, diltiazem).

Toxicity may be difficult to treat due to the following:

- Concomitant cardiovascular disease
- Long-acting preparations
- Refractory cardiovascular instability

What effects would you expect?

- *Hypotension*: may be from vasodilation or myocardial suppression
- Bradycardia and heart block
- Effects of multi-organ hypoperfusion (e.g. ileus, delirium, loss of consciousness [LOC], and AKI)
- Cardiac arrest

What specific management interventions would you consider?

Pharmacological
- Early vasoactive medications, dependent on cause of hypotension (low SVR vs myocardial suppression)
  - *Catecholamines*: positive inotropy and chronotropy ideal (e.g. adrenaline, isoprenaline)
  - *Phosphodiesterase inhibitors*: less ideal as potential to worsen hypotension (e.g. milrinone, enoximone)
  - Specific to calcium channel blocker toxicity
    - *Calcium chloride/gluconate*: positive inotropy and temporising measure
    - α-*agonists*: vasoconstriction increasing SVR to improve BP (e.g. NA and phenylephrine)
    - *Vasopressin*: vasoconstriction
- Avoidance of fluid overload
- *Hyperinsulinaemic (or 'high dose insulin') euglycaemia therapy (HIET)*: increasingly advocated for early use
- *High-dose glucagon*: positive inotropy and chronotropy

- Second-line therapies
  - IV lipid emulsion
  - *Levosimendan*: vasodilatation may be problematic
  - Methylene blue
- Atropine is unlikely to be significantly effective but can be tried as a temporising measure.

General
- *Echo helpful in assessment*: vasodilatation vs pump failure
- *Early intubation*: avoidance of profound hypotension post-induction
- *Decontamination*: may be of more benefit with modified release preparations if patient intubated already
- *Pacing*: capture unpredictable, BP may not improve alongside HR
- VA-ECMO may be indicated in CS

What is HIET?
HIET is indicated in myocardial dysfunction and is thought to be of more benefit in calcium channel blocker toxicity. Care needs to be taken to avoid hypoglycaemia. HIET facilitates intracellular transport of substrate and oxygen. Insulin also causes calcium-dependent inotropy and terminal arteriolar vasodilatation. HIET can facilitate the weaning of high-dose catecholamine (and other) infusions and mitigate their deleterious effects. It should be started early where indicated.

Insulin
- Bolus 1 unit/kg
- Followed by infusion (e.g. 1 unit/kg/h)
- Titrated every 10–15 min (e.g. to HR > 50 bpm, systolic BP > 90 mmHg)
- Usual rate 1–10 units/kg/h

50% dextrose
- 50–100 ml is administered concurrently
- Followed by concentrated infusion (e.g. 1 ml/kg/h 50% dextrose)
- Close monitoring of blood glucose is essential, with a moderately high target, until stability is reached

How do glucagon and milrinone work in beta-blocker overdose?
Indirect sympathomimetic effects (i.e. not reliant on beta adrenergic receptors):

- Increase myocardial cAMP
- Positive inotropy and chronotropy

They are most effective in those with bradycardia and myocardial suppression and less helpful in vasodilatory shock (such as in calcium channel blocker overdose). Glucagon is emetogenic, so it should be factored into assessment of aspiration risk.

Milrinone is an inodilator, and concern exists surrounding its potential to worsen hypotension. It may be more useful in refractory bradycardia or whilst glucagon is being sourced.

Many management principles are common to calcium channel blocker and beta-blocker toxicity. Beta-blockers may be amenable to haemodialysis if hydrophilic (e.g. sotalol, atenolol).

What do you know about salicylate toxicity?
Salicylates (e.g. aspirin) are readily available analgesics. Toxicity causes an initial respiratory alkalosis before a HAGMA due to uncoupled oxidative phosphorylation. Early signs include nausea, vomiting, and tinnitus.

Supportive care may be required for seizures, impaired consciousness, hypotension, or pulmonary oedema. Other complications include hyperthermia, cerebral oedema, impaired glucose regulation, and hypokalaemia.

Specific management will involve urinary alkalinisation with sodium bicarbonate. Haemodialysis is indicated if:

- Failure of urinary alkalinisation
- Increasing serum levels despite other management
- End-organ impairment
- Very high serum levels (e.g. >100 mg/dl acutely)

What are the features of digoxin toxicity?

Digoxin can be problematic due to its narrow therapeutic index and tricky patient population. Levels will also be affected by altered renal clearance or metabolic enzyme inhibition/induction.

Acutely, GI upset precedes neurological symptoms. Chronic toxicity usually manifests with gradually worsening neurological symptoms.

GI
- Nausea and vomiting
- Diarrhoea
- Abdominal pain

Cardiovascular
- Bradycardia
- AV block
- AF, junctional escape rhythm
- Junctional tachycardia
- Bigeminy, VT, and VF more common in chronic toxicity

Neurological
- *Visual disturbance*: colour alteration, blurred vision, diplopia
- Delirium
- Seizures

What specific management may be required?

- Measurement of digoxin level (post-distribution level, i.e. 6 h post-dose)
- Reduce absorption (<1 h)
- Digoxin-specific antibody fragments (DSFab) (e.g. Digibind® or Digifab®)

Resources
- Farkas J. The Internet Book of Critical Care. Calcium Channel Blocker (CCB) & Beta-Blocker (BBl) Overdose. April 2021. Available from: https://emcrit.org/ibcc/ccb/. (Accessed 15 January 2022.)
- Graudins A, Lee HM, Druda D. Calcium channel antagonist and beta-blocker overdose: antidotes and adjunct therapies. Br J Clin Pharmacol. 2016;81:452–461.
- National Poisons Information Service. TOXBASE®: High Dose Insulin Euglycaemic Therapy. 2021. Available from: https://www.toxbase.org/Chemical-incidents/Miscellaneous/High-Dose-Insulin-Euglycaemic-Therapy-Adults-only/. (Accessed 14 January 2022.)

38. LOCAL ANAESTHETIC SYSTEMIC TOXICITY

When might you encounter patients with local anaesthetic systemic toxicity?

- Overdose of local anaesthetic infusion via wound catheter
- Overdose of intentional IV lidocaine infusion (e.g. scoliosis correction, laparotomy)
- Inadvertent intravascular injection of local anaesthetic (e.g. regional anaesthesia in orthopaedic theatres, delivery suite)
- Overdose during other procedures (e.g. chest drain insertion)

Presentation may be delayed by some time from initial injection. It may be difficult to recognise and should be suspected with any unusual cardiovascular or neurological signs after local anaesthetic administration.

What are the clinical features of severe local anaesthetic toxicity?

Neurological
- Altered mental status
- Severe agitation
- LOC
- Tonic clonic seizures
- Respiratory arrest

Cardiovascular
- Bradycardia
- Heart block
- Asystole
- VT

Early signs might include dysphoria, tinnitus, perioral numbness, metallic taste, and dysarthria.

What is the pathophysiology of systemic toxicity?

Local anaesthetic is circulated after being absorbed from soft tissues or by inadvertent injection to the circulation. Systemic absorption often presents in a more delayed manner. Effects will depend on the route of administration, choice of agent, dose, and patient pharmacodynamics/pharmacokinetics.

The mechanism is not fully understood. Effects usually relate to interference with conduction in the heart and brain as local anaesthetic crosses cell membranes or blocks ion channels, causing an imbalance of various pathways.

Procedure-related risk factors
- Longer-acting agents (e.g. bupivacaine, ropivacaine)
- More vasoactive agents (e.g. bupivacaine more than levobupivacaine)
- 'CC/CNS ratio': dose required to produce cardiovascular collapse vs induction of seizures (e.g. bupivacaine lower than lidocaine so will more readily lead to cardiovascular collapse after CNS signs)
- More proximal regional block
- Continuous infusion

What mechanisms exist to reduce the risk of toxicity?

- *Pre-procedure*: thorough patient assessment, safe dosing
- *During regional block*: frequent aspiration, incremental injection, test dose, US guidance
- *Post-procedure*: clear labelling of catheters, non-Luer lock connections
- *Institutional*: readily available lipid emulsion

Once suspected, how would you manage severe local anaesthetic systemic toxicity?

The AoA has produced a guideline and flow chart to facilitate emergency management.

Key principles
- Stop injection
- Administer lipid emulsion intravenously
- Advanced airway support is likely to be required
- Resuscitation may be prolonged

Other measures
- Hyperventilation to reduce acidosis may improve contractility.
- Seizures may be managed with benzodiazepines, thiopental, or propofol.
- Antiarrhythmics can be used as usual with the avoidance of relevant agents (e.g. lidocaine).

- Large doses of adrenaline and any vasopressin may be better avoided.
- E-CPR may have some value.
- *Follow-up*: monitor for pancreatitis as high risk, report locally and to lipid registries

AoA 2010 Severe Local Anaesthetic Toxicity

What dose of intravenous lipid emulsion would you use?

KEY POINT

20% lipid emulsion (e.g. Intralipid®):

- Bolus **1.5 ml/kg** (over 1 min)
- Infusion 15 ml/kg/h

Repeat bolus after 5 min if cardiovascular stability is not restored or adequate circulation deteriorates. A maximum of 3 boluses may be given in total. The infusion should also be doubled after 5 min in these circumstances to 20 ml/kg/h.

Infusion can be discontinued when adequate circulation is restored or when the maximum dose is reached. The maximum cumulative dose is 12 ml/kg.

Propofol is not a suitable substitute as the lipid sink; it will cause significant cardiovascular depression.

Resources

- Association of Anaesthetists. Quick Reference Handbook: Guidelines for Crises in Anaesthesia. 2021. Available from: https://anaesthetists.org/Portals/0/PDFs/Guidelines%20PDFs/QRH_complete_October%202021.pdf?ver= 2021-11-09-135429-103. (Accessed 15 January 2022.)
- Christie LE, Picard J, Weinberg GL. Local anaesthetic systemic toxicity. BJA Educ. 2015;15(3):136–142.

39. ENVIRONMENTAL POISONS

Why is corrosive ingestion relevant to critical care?

- Readily available household items
- May occur through 'off gassing' (e.g. formaldehyde in paint, chlorine if mixing household cleaning agents)
- Potentially life-threatening
  - *Airway compromise*: oedema, laryngeal injury
  - GI perforation
  - Specific effects

Depending on the agent involved, complications can include GI stricture, perforation, shock, haemorrhage, mediastinitis, and multi-organ failure. Long-term morbidity may relate to psychosocial implications, airway incompetence, GI failure, and increased risk of oesophageal malignancy.

Specific care may include the following:

- Decontamination with oral rinse only
- Avoidance of blind GI procedures
- Early airway intervention
- Endoscopy
- Surgical review

What features might you expect following petroleum ingestion?

- Dysrhythmias
- CNS depression
- Hepatotoxicity
- Chemical pneumonitis if aspirated

What effects may result from acute heavy metal ingestion?

Heavy metals will cause GI irritation (vomiting, diarrhoea, large fluid loss, electrolyte abnormalities, and haemorrhage) and dose-related systemic toxicity and multi-organ failure. In addition:

Iron
- ALF
- Cirrhosis

Lead
- Acute lead encephalopathy
- Hypertension may be associated with chronic exposure.

Arsenic
- Hypersalivation, garlic odour sensation
- Encephalopathy, seizures
- Acute myopathy
- Bone marrow failure
- Ascending peripheral neuropathy

What specific management is there for heavy metal poisoning?

- X-ray imaging may be helpful
- Whole bowel irrigation with polyethylene glycol
- Prokinetics
- Endoscopy
- *Iron*: chelation with desferrioxamine
- *Arsenic*: chelation with succimer (dimercaptosuccinic acid [DMSA]) or dimercaprol

What is the significance of chemical weapons to critical care?

Exposure to environmental hazards may be weaponised or non-weaponised, through many potential routes. Chemical, biological, radiological, and nuclear materials can cause great harm, and critical care physicians may be involved in the management of those exposed. Mass casualty incidents may evolve.

These agents may be classified according to potential harm:

- *Damaging*: impact on resources (e.g. mustard gas, low-dose radiation)
- *Incapacitating*: temporary inability to function
- Lethal (e.g. cyanide, nerve agents, phosgene, anthrax, high-dose radiation)

A chemical weapon may be defined as a 'substance which is intended for use in military operations to kill, seriously injure, or incapacitate people due to its physiological effects'.

What chemical weapons do you know of?

Nerve agents
- Rapid-acting organophosphates
- Irreversibly bind to anticholinesterase (e.g. sarin)
- Cholinergic (muscarinic and nicotinic) toxidrome
- Managed with antagonist anticholinergic medications (e.g. atropine IV infusion)
- Specific treatment: cholinesterase reactivator (e.g. pralidoxime chloride, obidoxime)

Cyanides
- Inhibit cytochrome oxidase impairing aerobic respiration (i.e. asphyxiation), causing severe refractory lactic acidosis

- e.g. *hydrogen cyanide*: volatile, most significant in enclosed spaces, inhalational route
- Managed with supportive oxygenation
- Specific antidotes (see next question)

Others include **vesicants or blistering agents** (e.g. mustard gas) and **pulmonary or choking agents** (e.g. chlorine and phosgene). Management of associated poisoning is supportive.

Novichok agents are a specific group of nerve gases, or their precursors, which were designed to be undetectable with high lethality. They were implicated in several deaths in the south of England in 2018.

What other inhaled toxins are you aware of?

CO
- Released during incomplete combustion (e.g. faulty boiler, barbecue with poor ventilation)
- *Severe*: HbCO > 30%, neurological signs, ECG ischaemia, metabolic acidosis
- Manage with high F_1O_2 (e.g. 1.0 until HbCO < 5%)
- Hyperbaric oxygen not recommended by NPIS

Cyanide
- Found in pesticides, tobacco smoke, and fruit seeds
- Released during combustion (e.g. of polyurethane and vinyl) and breakdown of sodium nitroprusside
- Suspect in burns patient with worsening metabolic acidosis
- *Severe*: lactate > 7, HAGMA, low arteriovenous oxygen gradient, neurological signs, cardiovascular compromise
- Manage with high F_1O_2
- First-line antidote is hydroxocobalamin (B12)
- *Alternatives antidotes*: sodium thiosulphate, dicobalt edetate, sodium nitrite

What weaponised biological agents do you know of?

Anthrax
- *Bacillus anthracis*: Gram-positive, spore-forming, aerobic bacillus
- Multisystem effects depending on exposure site
- Most lethal are pulmonary anthrax and meningitis

Ricin
- Glycoprotein extract of beans from the castor plant
- Inhibits protein synthesis causing cell death
- Significant pulmonary toxicity when inhaled
- Ingestion causes rapid and severe GI upset with death several days later

Others include **botulinum toxin, smallpox** (orthopoxvirus), and **plague** (*Yersinia pestis*).

Strychnine, a plant derivative, has potential for abuse due to its availability as a rodenticide. Glycine antagonism causes unopposed neuromuscular stimulation similar to that seen in tetanus.

(See Chapter 91 Tetanus and Botulism)

Can you describe acute radiation syndrome?
Acute radiation syndrome is an illness caused by whole-body irradiation and may be diagnosed with a significant history alongside lymphopaenia. It is dose dependent, and onset may vary from several hours to weeks following exposure.

Criteria
- Large dose (>0.7 Gray [Gy] or 70 rads)
- External source
- Penetrating
- Entire body (or significant portion) exposed
- Delivered in a short time

Stages
- *Prodromal*: nausea, vomiting, anorexia, diarrhoea (minutes to days)
- *Latent*: appearance of health (hours to weeks)
- *Manifest illness*: syndromic symptoms as below (hours to months)
- *Recovery or death*: most deaths within several months, recovery takes up to 2 years

Manifestations
- **Bone marrow syndrome** (>0.7 Gy)
  - Bone marrow destruction
  - Infection and haemorrhage
  - Dose-dependent increase in mortality
- **GI syndrome** (>10 Gy)
  - GI destruction
  - Infection, dehydration, electrolyte disorders
  - Survival extremely unlikely, death within 2 weeks
- **Cardiovascular/CNS syndrome** (>50 Gy)
  - Circulatory collapse
  - High ICP secondary to oedema, vasculitis, meningitis
  - Death inevitable within 3 days

Management priorities
- Appropriate triage, identification, and supportive care
- Treat contamination.
- Management of concomitant major trauma, burns, and respiratory injury
- Investigations to include lymphocyte count and HLA tissue typing pre-transfusion
- Expectant management and appropriate palliative care may be necessary.

What is the difference between poisoning and envenomation?

Poisons and venoms are toxic substances that can cause harm. The difference lies in the mode of entry to the body. A venom is a substance that has evolved specifically to harm and must enter the bloodstream from a wound (i.e. a bite or sting). Poisons have a more passive role, entering the body through other routes (e.g. ingestion, topical absorption).

Envenomation may result from contact with animals including snakes, spiders, insects, jellyfish, and octopi. Most effects are due to neurotoxin activity, rhabdomyolysis, and anticoagulation.

Management centres on the following:

- Prompt recognition, investigation, and supportive care
- Application of pressure-immobilisation first-aid bandage (most venom subcutaneous)
- Antivenom administration
  - Haemodynamic support may be required (cardiovascular collapse more likely with non-specific antivenom)
- Transfusion as required for haemorrhage and coagulopathy
- Analgesia
- Antibiotics and tetanus prophylaxis as appropriate if contaminated

Resources

- Berstein AD, Handy JM. (Eds.) Oh's Intensive Care Manual, 8th ed. Amsterdam: Elsevier Limited; 2019.
- Centers for Disease Control and Prevention. A Brochure for Physicians: Acute Radiation Syndrome. Available from: https://www.cdc.gov/nceh/radiation/emergencies/pdf/ars.pdf. (Accessed 15 January 2022.)
- Long N. Life in the Fast Lane. Paracetamol Toxicity. November 2020. Available from: https://litfl.com/paracetamol-toxicity/. (Accessed 15 January 2022.)
- Long N. Life in the Fast Lane. Salicylate toxicity. November 2020. Available from: https://litfl.com/salicylate-toxicity/. (Accessed 15 January 2022.)

AIRWAY

40. DIFFICULT INTUBATION

What is the significance of airway complications in critical care?

Failure of intubation is much more likely in the critically ill than during anaesthetic practice. The report and findings of the fourth National Audit Project of the Royal College of Anaesthetists (NAP4) found that 20% of all airway incidents occurred in the ICU. A large proportion of incidents involved tracheostomies.

Patients suffered a disproportionately high degree of harm than those elsewhere: 61% of incidents caused neurological damage or death (compared with 14% in anaesthesia and 33% in the Emergency Department). Cardiac arrest during intubation occurs in around 2% of cases, with most experiencing severe hypoxaemia.

Problems
- Unrecognised oesophageal intubation (due to absence of/misinterpreted waveform capnography)
- Displacement of devices, particularly in the obese and on moving for care
- Delayed recognition of displacement
- Lack of advanced airway equipment and skills
- Failure to identify high-risk airways
- Ineffective airway planning

What factors might limit airway assessment in the critically ill?

- Reduced patient capacity to comply with history-taking and examination
- Urgency
- Patient agitation/distress
- Oxygen dependency precluding oral examination (e.g. CPAP, NIV, hoods, or high-flow oxygen)
- Distraction (e.g. major trauma management)
- Cognitive overload
- Inadequate lighting
- Availability of clinical records
- *Skill mix*: variable airway expertise

What could help to inform your assessment?

- Consideration of risks to patient of difficult intubation/rescue and aspiration
- Specific assessment tools (e.g. MACOCHA – validated in critically ill: Mallampati score III/IV, Apnoea syndrome [obstructive], Cervical spine limitation, Opening mouth < 3 cm, Coma, Hypoxia, and 'Anaesthesiologist nontrained')
- Thorough use of collateral information, e.g. handover details
- Brief removal of face mask for examination may be worthwhile.
- Nasendoscopy could be useful.

What other factors might increase the difficulty of intubation in critically unwell patients?

Pathology
- Airway disease (e.g. trauma, oedema, or recent intubation/surgery)
- Reduced physiological reserve
- Increased oxygen demand (e.g. sepsis)
- Involvement of tracheostomy (e.g. obstruction or false tract)

Environment
- 'Sterile cockpit' may need to be created or difficult to achieve
- Ergonomically non-specific for airway management (e.g. wide ICU beds)
- Crowding by equipment
- Difference in experience between ICU, Emergency Department, and theatre staff typically

Intubation
- Limited equipment in some locations
- Instability can mean potentially inappropriate drug dosing, resulting in poor conditions
- Use of wider 'ICU tube' with subglottic suction port
- Requirement for lung isolation (e.g. with double-lumen tube)
- Requirement for immobilisation (e.g. cervical spine fracture)

Can you describe some interventions that might positively influence intubation?

Human factors
- Good teamwork including leadership and followership
- Checklist use
- Display and follow algorithm for unanticipated difficult intubation
- Training

Patient optimisation
- Timing of intubation
- Haemodynamics (e.g. fluid resuscitation in asthma)
- Adjuncts (e.g. nebulised adrenaline and steroids in stridulous patient)
- Analgesia (may avoid overdose of hypnotic where appropriate)

Procedure
- Optimising positioning (e.g. mattress on firm setting)
- Consider pre-oxygenation with NIV or HFNO
- Delayed sequence induction may be beneficial in agitated patients
- 'Peroxygenation' (oxygenation during intubation)
- Precautions against aspiration attempts
- Use of videolaryngoscopy

GUIDELINE   DAS 2017 Critically ill

What is the significance of the phrase 'can't intubate, can't oxygenate'?

'Can't intubate, can't oxygenate' (CICO) is a declaration of a state of emergency with potentially life-threatening consequences after failed primary upper airway management.

It was previously termed 'can't intubate, can't ventilate' but this was updated to better reflect emergency priorities. It implies failure of optimisation of laryngoscopy, supraglottic airway use, and bag mask ventilation, involving Plans A, B, and C on the Difficult Airway Society (DAS) algorithm. After failed intubation, specific to the critically ill, Plans B and C are merged as 'rescue oxygenation'.

Plan B/C

- Second-generation supraglottic airway rotated with 2-person face mask ventilation with adjuncts
- Maximum of 3 attempts at each
- Changes in device/size/operator as indicated
- Front of neck airway (FONA) kit should be opened during Plans B/C.
- If Plan B/C fails, CICO should be declared.

CICO should trigger a progression to Plan D, FONA, and a call for expert help.

The 'Vortex' tool is used in some regions, whereby failure of the best attempt at the 3 'lifelines' (endotracheal tube, supraglottic airway, and face mask) triggers CICO rescue.

How would you perform FONA in the critically ill?

Indications
- CICO
- Marginal oxygenation
- Aspiration
- Difficult ventilation
- Impossible intubation via supraglottic airway

Preparation
- Exclude oxygen failure and blocked circuit
- Neck extension
- Adequate NMB
- Ongoing rescue oxygenation attempts

Equipment
- Scalpel blade (wide, e.g. size 10 or 20)
- Bougie (≤14 French gauge)
- Tube (5.0–6.0 mm internal diameter cuffed)

KEY POINT

Scalpel cricothyroidotomy:

- Laryngeal handshake
- Palpate cricothyroid membrane
- (If impalpable, make large midline vertical incision followed by blunt dissection to larynx)
- Transverse stab
- Turn blade 90°, sharp edge towards feet
- Insert bougie along trachea
- Railroad lubricated tube and remove bougie
- Inflate cuff and confirm position

Aftercare
- Tracheal suction
- Recruitment
- CXR
- *Surgical review*: definitive airway (usually tracheostomy) must be secured for adequate ventilation. A 6.0-mm tube via cricothyroidotomy is a temporary solution for short-term oxygenation only
- Agree airway plan
- Documentation

What other techniques are there?

Needle or Seldinger cricothyroidotomy is no longer recommended first-line. A narrow-bore rescue airway is not considered definitive, requiring conversion, with transtracheal jet ventilation in the interim. This has a high risk of failure (42%), barotrauma (32%), and other complications (51%). Further intervention will be required to convert it to a more appropriate airway.

An experienced operator may choose to insert a percutaneous/surgical tracheostomy instead of scalpel cricothyroidotomy. However, the default in nearly all situations of CICO is emergency surgical cricothyroidotomy.

What do you know about failed FONA?

Front-of-neck access may not be the solution to an airway disaster, and failure of FONA is possible.

- Cardiac arrest usually occurs.
- FONA may be attempted lower in the trachea.
- Tracheostomy or non-scalpel FONA may be performed by an experienced operator.

Can you describe some other situations in which airway complications might occur in the intensive care unit?

- Tracheal tube exchange
- Tracheostomy insertion
- During routine care (e.g. roll and proning)
  - *Airway displacement*: unplanned extubation or dislodged tracheostomy
  - *Airway occlusion*: mucus plug or clot
  - *Device malfunction*: pilot tube rupture or tube kinking
- Planned extubation
  - May be appropriate to perform in theatre but delayed complications not avoided

Resources

- Chrimes N. The vortex: a universal 'high-acuity implementation tool' for emergency airway management. Br J Anaesth. 2016;117(S1):i20–i27.
- Harper J, Cook T, Rangasami J, Intensive care. In: Cook T, Woodall N, Frerk C, eds., 4th National Audit Project of the Royal College of Anaesthetists and the Difficult Airway Society: Major Complications of Airway Management in the United Kingdom: Report and Findings. March 2011. Available from: https://www.national-auditprojects.org.uk/downloads/NAP4%20Full%20Report.pdf. (Accessed 17 January 2022.)
- Higgs A, Cook TM, McGrath BA. Airway management in the critically ill: the same, but different. Br J Anaesth. 2016;117(S1):i9–i13.

---

41. STRIDOR

What is stridor?

Stridor is an abnormal breath sound associated with partial airway obstruction (there is no sound with complete obstruction). It is not a diagnosis but a sign of underlying pathology. The turbulent airflow causes characteristically harsh, high-pitched sounds.

It can be described by timing with the respiratory cycle:

- *Inspiratory stridor*: at/above the level of the vocal cords (classical picture)
- *Expiratory stridor*: below the level of the vocal cords (intrathoracic)
- Biphasic stridor

Stertor is an abnormal breath sound associated with partial obstruction of the upper airways at the level of the pharynx/nasopharynx. It is characteristically lower-pitched than stridor.

What are the likeliest scenarios in which to encounter stridor in the critically ill?

- Anaphylaxis
- Trauma

- Infection
- Laryngeal swelling from airway devices and intubation trauma

What is the significance of post-extubation stridor in adult critical care?

Post-extubation stridor is a common complication in the critical care unit. There are numerous potential causes, including laryngospasm, arytenoid cartilage dislocation, laryngeal nerve palsy, and granulation tissue. However, laryngeal oedema is by far the most common.

Significant morbidity may result from ensuing respiratory failure as a relatively late sign of partial airway obstruction.

Extubation is a resource-demanding intervention which ideally reduces dependency on the critical care unit. Reintubation will add to demand and will require some redistribution of resources. It may be more time-critical than most other intubations in critical care, carrying additional pressure.

(See Chapter 48 Laryngeal Injury)

Which patients are at risk of post-extubation laryngeal oedema and how are they managed?

Risk factors
- Relatively large tube size
- Prolonged intubation (>48 h)
- High cuff pressure
- Difficult or repeated translaryngeal intubation
- Obesity ± gastro-oesophageal reflux
- Infections affecting the upper airway (e.g. severe acute respiratory syndrome coronavirus 2 [SARS-CoV-2])

These risk factors are not reliable in isolation. A multimodal approach to assessing airway patency should be used: clinical assessment, then additional tools such as the cuff-leak test, videolaryngoscopy, or ultrasonography.

Targeted treatment of 'high-risk' individuals with prophylactic steroids or proton pump inhibitors has been proposed, but evidence is lacking, and this is not routine practice.

What is a cuff-leak test?

A cuff-leak test is an easy-to-perform, bedside test which may provide additional information about likelihood of laryngeal oedema. Deflating the cuff of a tracheal tube should allow gas to escape around the tube and out via the upper airways. Leak may be detected by auditory signs or measurement of the cuff-leak volume by the ventilator. Other criteria exist, and the test performs differently depending on baseline settings.

KEY POINT

Example cuff-leak test method:

- *Preparation*: explain to patient and suction secretions
- Record inspiratory and expiratory V_T
- Deflate cuff slowly
- Listen/feel for gas escaping via the upper airways
- Record expiratory V_T over 6 breathing cycles
- Average 3 lowest values
- Cuff-leak volume = (inspiratory V_T at start of test) − (average expiratory V_T)
- A cuff-leak volume of less than a predefined threshold concerning.
- Examples of threshold values studied: **110 ml** or **10–18% V_T**

Any concerns should delay extubation attempts and prompt consideration of visualising the airway (nasendoscopy) and treating pathology.

How would you manage a patient with post-extubation stridor?

Clinical situations vary greatly. Always consider extubation problems and plan accordingly. Respiratory distress is likely to require urgent reintubation, which may be difficult.

In the absence of indications for immediate reintubation, a proposed strategy is to try salvage manoeuvres such as the following, before reintubation in a timely manner (e.g. in 1 h) if these don't lead to improvement:

- *IV corticosteroid (dexamethasone/methylprednisolone)*: continue 24–48 h
- Nebulised budesonide 1 mg
- Nebulised adrenaline 1 mg in 5 ml 0.9% NaCl
- *NIV and HFNO*: may buy time and prevent reintubation in some patients, associated with increased mortality (suggested to be due to delayed reintubation when indicated)

Avoid in this setting the following:

- *Nasendoscopy*: may occlude an already compromised airway and unlikely to be tolerated
- *Heliox*: may decrease work of breathing but F_IO_2 limited, not readily available, training issues

Name some common causes of stridor in children.

- *Inspiratory*: croup or epiglottitis
- *Expiratory*: foreign body
- *Biphasic*: bacterial tracheitis

Which clinical features are suggestive of severe croup?

Viral croup (laryngotracheobronchitis) is usually due to infection with parainfluenza, influenza, RSV, or rhinovirus. Around 2% of children with croup require hospital admission; 0.5–1.5% of those require invasive ventilation. Assessment of severity can be assessed using scoring systems – several 'croup scores' exist (e.g. Westley or Downes).

More severe features are as follows:

- Stridor
- Barking cough
- Delayed breath sounds
- Flaring, suprasternal, and intercostal recession
- $F_IO_2 \geq 0.4$

Can you name some other signs of increased work of breathing in children?

- Distress or agitation and later exhaustion
- Head bobbing
- Nasal flaring
- Subcostal, sternal, and intercostal recession
- Grunting in infants
- Tripod or arched posturing
- See-saw movement of chest and abdomen

What are the principles of managing the stridulous child?

- Avoidance of distressing child further through cannulation or oral examination (tolerance of IV cannulation may herald exhaustion)
- Treatment of underlying cause (e.g. infection)
- Reducing airway oedema:
  - Nebulised/oral/IV steroid (e.g. budesonide 2 mg and dexamethasone 0.6 mg/kg)
  - Nebulised adrenaline (0.5 ml/kg to maximum 5 ml 1:1000)
- If intubation likely to be required (e.g. croup score ≥7), early movement to place of relative safety with appropriate senior and specialty support
- Involvement of paediatric intensive care and/or transfer teams

How might intubation be carried out if required in this setting?

This is a scenario that requires specialised paediatric airway anaesthetic experience. Broadly speaking, the choice of technique is between IV induction and paralysis, or inhalational induction. The latter should only be performed by experienced experts. The following preparation should be considered:

- Induction in theatre environment with anaesthesia, intensive care, and ENT consultants present (Emergency Department may be suitable in some hospitals)
- Rigid bronchoscopy and surgical tracheostomy kit ready in addition to difficult airway trolley
- Appropriate preparation of parent if accompanying
- Team brief and intubation checklist

Inhalational induction is slower but provides bronchodilatation and, in some cases, spontaneous ventilation may prevent occlusion of the airway where over-ventilation would not.

Often, IV access has been established by the time the child requires intubation – agitation often gives way to apathy and exhaustion. IV induction allows rapid control with a familiar technique and maintained depth of anaesthesia. F_1O_2 1.0 can be administered.

Resources
- Davies I, Jenkins I. Paediatric airway infections. BJA Educ. 2017;17(10):341–345.
- Maloney E, Meakin GH. Acute stridor in children. CEACCP. 2007;7(6):183–186.
- Pluijms WA, van Mook WNKA, Wittekamp BHJ, et al. Postextubation laryngeal edema and stridor resulting in respiratory failure in critically ill adult patients: updated review. Crit Care. 2015;19(1):295.

---

42. ANAPHYLAXIS

What is anaphylaxis?

KEY POINT

Anaphylaxis has been defined by the World Allergy Organization (WAO) Anaphylaxis Committee as follows:

- A serious systemic hypersensitivity reaction
- That is usually rapid in onset
- And may cause death.

Severe anaphylaxis is characterised by potentially life-threatening compromise in A, B, or C. Typical skin features or circulatory shock may be absent.

Features
- *A*: facial swelling, sensation of throat closing, hoarseness, stridor, and loss of airway
- *B*: breathlessness, increased work of breathing, bronchospasm/wheeze, cough, fatigue, hypoxaemia, and respiratory arrest
- *C*: shock – pallor, tachycardia, clammy skin, hypotension, dizziness, loss of consciousness (LOC), arrhythmia, and cardiac arrest
- *Skin*: patchy erythema, generalised rash, and urticaria
- *GI*: abdominal pain, incontinence, and vomiting

How is anaphylaxis diagnosed?

Anaphylaxis is an immediate clinical diagnosis. The WAO suggests that anaphylaxis is highly likely when either of 2 criteria is fulfilled:

KEY POINT

WAO anaphylaxis criteria:

1. Acute onset (minutes to hours), simultaneously involving **skin/mucosal tissue/both**, and ≥1 of the following:
   1. Respiratory compromise
   2. Reduced BP or associated symptoms of end-organ dysfunction
   3. Severe GI symptoms (especially after exposure to non-food allergen)
2. Acute onset of any of the following, after **exposure to known/highly probable allergen** for that patient:
   1. *Hypotension*: systolic BP > 30% decrease in baseline or low for age (< 90 mmHg in adults)
   2. Bronchospasm
   3. *Laryngeal involvement*: stridor, vocal changes, or odynophagia (painful swallowing)

How is anaphylaxis graded?

The WAO systemic allergic reaction grading system is divided into non-anaphylaxis reactions (Grades 1–2) and anaphylaxis (**Grades 3–5**):

Grade 1 (1 organ system)
- *Cutaneous*: urticaria, erythema-warmth, pruritus, tingling/itching lips, or angioedema
- *Upper respiratory tract*: nasal (sneezing, rhinorrhoea, pruritus, or congestion), itchy throat, or non-bronchospasm cough
- *Conjunctival*: erythema, pruritus, or tearing
- *Other*: nausea or metallic taste

Grade 2 (≥2 organ systems as above)

Grade 3
- *Lower airway*: mild bronchospasm – cough/wheeze/SOB responding to treatment
- *GI*: abdominal cramps and/or vomiting/diarrhoea
- *Other*: uterine cramps or any features from Grade 1

Grade 4
- *Lower airway*: severe bronchospasm – not responding or deteriorating
- *Upper airway*: laryngeal oedema with stridor

Grade 5
- Respiratory failure
- Cardiovascular collapse/hypotension
- LOC (excluding vasovagal)

GUIDELINE   WAO 2020 Anaphylaxis

What are the most common causes of anaphylaxis?

In the UK general population:

- *Food*: peanut, tree nuts, and cow's milk
- *Drugs*: antibiotics and chemotherapeutic agents
- *Venom*: insect stings

Perioperatively, from the NAP6 report:

- **Antibiotics** (47%): co-amoxiclav (23% of these) and teicoplanin (18%)
- **NMBs** (33%)
- **Chlorhexidine** (9%)

What is the pathophysiology of anaphylactic shock?

This was classically described as 'distributive' shock due to capillary leak. Inflammatory pathway activation causes the following:

- Fluid extravasation
- Vasodilatation
- Reduced venous return
- Reduced cardiac output
- Complicated further by reduced coronary perfusion

Bronchospasm further reduces pulmonary blood flow and exacerbates hypoxia. Inadequate tissue perfusion results.

What are the priorities in the immediate management of anaphylaxis?

The focus of current guidance is on a systematic A–E approach with appropriate assistance (a senior anaesthetist may be required), prioritising the following:

- Removal of trigger/cause (e.g. stopping infusion of antibiotic or decontamination of skin)
- Supine positioning (± straight leg raise)
- Early administration of adrenaline (IM to the mid-thigh for non-experts)

Further measures
- High-flow oxygen
- Repeat adrenaline dose after 5 min if no response
- *IV crystalloid bolus*: child 10 ml/kg or adult 500–1000 ml (may require large volumes)
- Progression to refractory anaphylaxis algorithm if progression/no improvement after 2 doses of adrenaline

> **GUIDELINE**   Resuscitation Council UK 2021 Anaphylaxis

What dose of adrenaline would you use initially?

Trained experts may choose to use IV adrenaline in the non-arrested patient with anaphylaxis (often 10–100 μg boluses depending on severity). IM adrenaline is familiar to non-expert clinicians, but its immediate effect may be unpredictable in shocked states.

IM adrenaline 1:1000 (1 mg/ml)

- Adult or child > 12 years: 500 μg (0.5 ml)
- *Child 6–12 years*: 300 μg (0.3 ml)
- *Child 6 months–6 years*: 150 μg (0.15 ml)
- *Child < 6 months*: 100–150 μg (0.1–0.15 ml)

Partial airway obstruction may be temporised with nebulised adrenaline 5 mg (5 ml of 1 mg/ml).

Cardiac arrest IV dosing
- Pre-made adrenaline strength 1:10000 (100 μg/ml)
- *Adults*: 1 mg (10 ml)
- *Paediatrics*: 10 μg/kg (often diluted to 10 ml total volume with 0.9% NaCl)

What is refractory anaphylaxis and how is it managed?

Refractory anaphylaxis occurs when there has been no improvement in respiratory or cardiovascular symptoms despite 2 appropriate doses of IM adrenaline.

- Dedicated IV/IO access; seek expert help early
- Rapid IV fluid bolus + start adrenaline infusion
- IM adrenaline bolus every 5 min until infusion started

- High-flow oxygen to target S_pO_2 94–98%
- Monitor HR, BP, S_pO_2, and ECG
- Take blood for mast cell tryptase

Peripheral adrenaline infusion:

- 1 mg adrenaline in 100 ml 0.9% NaCl
- 0.5–1 ml/kg/h starting rate
- Titrate to response

What is the role of other pharmacological agents?

Chlorphenamine and hydrocortisone were featured previously on the treatment algorithm.

- Non-sedating antihistamines are now advocated as third-line treatment, after stabilisation, and do not feature on the algorithm. They may be beneficial if skin symptoms persist.
- Corticosteroids and antihistamines are no longer recommended during routine management. They may be given in refractory bronchospasm/shock but should not be used in preference to adrenaline.

Severe bronchospasm may be managed with nebulised **bronchodilators**, IV **salbutamol/aminophylline**, or **inhaled anaesthetic agents**.

If refractory to infused adrenaline, a second vasopressor may be used under expert supervision and extra-corporeal support may be indicated. Resuscitation from cardiac arrest may be prolonged, and E-CPR should be considered.

The Resuscitation Council UK advises the use of **NA**, **vasopressin**, or **metaraminol** second line. The AoA Quick Reference Handbook details the use of **glucagon** (1 mg bolus repeat as necessary) or vasopressin (2 units repeat as necessary/IV infusion) in perioperative anaphylaxis.

What follow-up should be offered?

- Patient education before discharge and information about support groups
- Specialist allergy clinic appointment
- Adrenaline injector as interim measure (unless drug-induced) + training
- Report reaction to The Anaphylaxis Registry
- Yellow Card report of medication triggers
- Local reporting

Mast cell tryptase sampling is now recommended where the diagnosis is uncertain. It should not delay resuscitation. A minimum of 1 sample should be taken within 2 h (max 4 h) of onset. Ideally:

- Initial sample as soon as possible
- Second at 1–2 h (max 4 h)
- Third (>24 h resolution, or in convalescence, e.g. at clinic – for baseline)

What other conditions may mimic airway swelling in anaphylaxis?

Angioedema is swelling of the deeper tissues in the subdermis, and facial/airway involvement is not specific to anaphylaxis.

Urticaria ± angioedema may be due to the following:

- *Chronic inducible urticaria*: majority idiopathic, may be triggered by heat, cold, pressure, sunlight, vibration, ACh release, and water
- *Autoimmune disorders*: SLE and Hashimoto's thyroiditis
- Exercise-induced 'anaphylaxis'
- Urticaria pigmentosa
- Systemic mastocytosis

Causes of angioedema without urticaria are as follows:

- Idiopathic
- Autoimmune disorders
- *Hereditary angioedema*: C1-esterase inhibitor deficiency or dysfunction

- ACE-I-induced angioedema
- Drug-related angioedema
- Systemic capillary leak syndrome
- Insect bites
- Food

Hereditary angioedema typically presents with recurrent episodes of an evolving angioedema that is unresponsive to adrenaline and where there is no clear allergen.

Specific therapy
- C1-esterase inhibitor concentrate
- Plasma kallikrein inhibitors (e.g. ecallantide)
- Bradykinin B2 receptor antagonists (e.g. icatibant)
- FFP may be given if these are unavailable and balanced against requirement for respiratory support.
- Long-term prophylaxis may involve attenuated androgens (e.g. danazol) or TXA.

Resources
- Association of Anaesthetists. Quick Reference Handbook: Guidelines for Crises in Anaesthesia. 2021. Available from: https://anaesthetists.org/Portals/0/PDFs/Guidelines%20PDFs/QRH_complete_October%202021.pdf?ver=2021-11-09-135429-103. (Accessed 15 January 2022.)
- Bernstein J. 2022. BMJ Best Practice: Urticaria and Angio-Oedema. Available from: https://bestpractice.bmj.com/topics/en-gb/844. (Accessed 17 January 2022.)
- Cook T, Harper N. (Eds.) Anaesthesia, Surgery and Life-Threatening Allergic Reactions: Report and Findings of the Royal College of Anaesthetists' 6th National Audit Project: Perioperative Anaphylaxis. May 2018. Available from: https://www.nationalauditprojects.org.uk/downloads/NAP6%20Report%202018.pdf. (Accessed 17 January 2022.)
- The Anaphylaxis Registry. 2020. Available from: https://www.anaphylaxie.net/en/. (Accessed 17 January 2022.)

---

43. ASPIRATION AND CHOKING

When would you suspect choking?
Choking is the partial or complete airway obstruction by a foreign body, causing impaired breathing.

Suspect choking with a sudden inability to talk or speak, particularly when eating or taking medication. In children, choking is also common during play. If unwitnessed, sudden onset respiratory symptoms with no preceding illness should trigger suspicion.

How would you manage somebody who is choking?
As per Basic Life Support (BLS) guidelines:

- Encourage coughing if conscious
- *If coughing ineffective*: up to 5 back blows
- *If back blows ineffective*: up to 5 abdominal thrusts
- Continue alternating these until choking relieved
- If patient unresponsive, start CPR

Paediatrics
- Infant
  - Head-down, prone position on rescuer's lap
  - Support the head at the angle of the lower jaw, avoiding soft tissues
  - Up to 5 back blows
  - Head-down, supine position for up to 5 chest thrusts (similar to chest compressions but sharper and slower)

- Child > 1 year
  - Head down if possible or leaning forward
  - Up to 5 back blows
  - Up to 5 abdominal thrusts
- If unconscious, perform paediatric BLS (initially 5 rescue breaths, then 15:2 CPR)

GUIDELINE Resuscitation Council UK 2021 Adult BLS

GUIDELINE Resuscitation Council UK 2021 Paediatric BLS

What is acute aspiration?

Acute aspiration is the inhalation of foreign material below the vocal cords.

Solid or liquid material may be inhaled and lead to aspiration pneumonitis or aspiration pneumonia

- *Pneumonitis*: chemical injury (Mendelson syndrome)
- *Pneumonia*: infection from colonised orogastric contents

These may be complicated by a severe inflammatory response, ARDS, or abscess formation.

What are the risk factors for aspiration in critical care?

- **Patient factors**
  - Full stomach
  - Delayed gastric emptying (opioids, pain, neuropathy, pregnancy, and motility disorders)
  - High BMI
  - Hiatus hernia
- **Iatrogenic factors**
  - Head down/supine positioning
  - Sedation or paralysis
- **Disease factors**
  - Decreased level of consciousness
  - GI disease
  - ICUAW

Bacterial colonisation is more likely if:

- *Drugs*: antacids, H_2 receptor antagonists, or proton pump inhibitors
- Enterally fed
- GI motility disorder present
- Elderly

Aspiration pneumonitis may be more significant with increased gastric content acidity.

How might aspiration present in critical care?

- Witnessed or reported choking or aspiration (most common)
- *Peri-intubation*: de novo, signs of previous aspiration (e.g. after intentional overdose)
- Airway obstruction
  - Note early signs (e.g. disproportionate distress, hypertension, and tachycardia)
  - Beware previous blood in upper airway and subsequent clot migration (e.g. surgical or epistaxis)
- Post-obstructive pulmonary oedema
- Hypoxaemia

- VAP
- Lobar collapse

How would you manage acute aspiration in the ICU?

- ABCDE approach
- Choking management as indicated
- Prevent further aspiration
  - Recovery position if own airway
  - Suction contaminants
  - *Decompress stomach*: aspirate feed from existing NG tube, insert wide-bore (Ryle's) NG tube
  - Invasive airway support as required
- Expectorate aspirated material
  - Chest physiotherapy
  - Bronchoscopy may be required
- Supportive therapy for complications (e.g. ARDS or hypotension)
- Antimicrobials may be indicated in pneumonia (e.g. broad spectrum including anaerobic cover empirically).

Antimicrobial prophylaxis is not recommended in uncomplicated pneumonitis. In the intubated patient, some of the above measures may minimise morbidity (e.g. prevention of further aspiration and need for bronchoscopy).

How might aspiration be prevented?

- Tracheal intubation if indicated (e.g. low GCS or absent airway reflexes)
- Intubation strategy should be optimised in high-risk patients, RSI (and adaptations) being the most common method.
- *Avoidance of GI stasis with full stomach*: regular assessment and adjustment of enteral feeding as required and prokinetics as indicated
- Fasting and/or aspiration of NG feed prior to planned procedures (balanced with nutritional demands)
- *Management of nausea*: anti-emetics and minimising precipitants
- Avoidance of excessive sedation
- Subglottic and oral suction and other components of ventilator care bundle

(See Chapter 25 Ventilator-Associated Pneumonia)

Resources

- 19. Cook T, Frerk C, Aspiration of gastric contents and of blood. In: Cook T, Woodall N, Frerk C, eds., 4th National Audit Project of the Royal College of Anaesthetists and the Difficult Airway Society: Major Complications of Airway Management in the United Kingdom: Report and Findings. March 2011. Available from: https://www.nationalauditprojects.org.uk/downloads/NAP4%20Full%20Report.pdf. (Accessed 17 January 2022.)
- d'Escrivan T, Guery B. Prevention and treatment of aspiration pneumonia in intensive care units. Treat Respir Med. 2005;4(5):317–324.

44. INHALATIONAL INJURY

What is smoke inhalation injury?

Smoke inhalation injury is the damage caused by breathing harmful gases, vapours, and particulate matter found in smoke. A variable amount with many possible components will be produced depending on fire temperature, materials involved, and oxygen supply.

It is more common in those presenting after fire/explosion and those with facial burns. Over 70% will suffer respiratory complications, with 20% developing ARDS. Effects may be thermal, chemical, or cause systemic toxicity.

What is the pathophysiology of smoke inhalation injury?

Heat
- Burns to nasal or oropharyngeal mucosa
- Superheated steam may injure lower airways
- Progressive oedema in first 36 h

Particulate matter/irritants
- Mechanical obstruction and oedema/inflammation of lower airways
- Increased airway resistance, decreased compliance, and increased work of breathing
- Specific irritant effects
  - *Water-soluble*: acid/alkali damage to airway mucosa
  - *Fat-soluble*: absorbed by mucosa leading to delayed damage
- Inflammatory cascade
- ROS cause further cell necrosis
- Exacerbating factors
  - *Nitrogen oxide*: vasodilatation and V/Q mismatch
  - *Tissue injury also increases vascular permeability*: worsening diffusion, V/Q mismatch, and oedema
  - *Airway casts formed by neutrophils and fibrinogen*: further obstruction

Asphyxiation/systemic toxicity
- Low F_IO_2 (as little as 0.1) as a result of combustion in enclosed space
- CO intoxication
  - Competitive binding with Hb
  - Shift in oxygen dissociation curve
  - Competitive inhibition of oxygen binding to cytochrome oxidase in mitochondria
- Hydrogen cyanide
  - 20 times more toxic than CO
  - Combines with ferric ion in mitochondrial cytochrome a3 oxidase
  - Impaired cellular respiration results

(See Chapter 39 Environmental Poisons)

When might you suspect smoke inhalation injury?

History
- Fire in confined space
- LOC at scene
- Fatalities in same incident
- Dyspnoea

Examination
- Cough
- Voice change, hoarseness, and stridor
- Facial/oral/nasal burns, soot, and singed hair
- Respiratory distress
- Hypoxaemia (might be masked by falsely elevated S_pO_2 measurement in by HbCO)

What would your approach to the airway be in such patients?
A thorough history and examination will facilitate decision-making. There should be a low threshold for intubation and ventilation (and despite a reassuring first assessment) due to the potential for progressive airway oedema and increasing difficulty of intubation. This is more significant in children who have narrower native airways.

Indications for intubation are as follows:

- Any concern about a threat to the airway
- Concerning features on assessment
- *Humanitarian*: extreme pain
- *Facilitation of imaging*: trauma series
- Emergency surgery

Fibre-optic nasendoscopy may be useful in borderline cases with a history of smoke inhalation.

Concerning findings in these patients include the following:

- Oedema of true or false cords
- Soot in oral cavity
- Facial burns
- Body burns

Procedure

- Experienced operator, ideally a senior anaesthetist
- Aim to intubate on first attempt with minimal trauma.
- Uncut tube with low-pressure cuff should be used as swelling can be severe.
- Consider haemodynamic stability in induction drug choice.
- Avoid suxamethonium (contraindicated outwith first 24 h due to risk of hyperkalaemia).
- Bed head should be elevated to facilitate venous and lymphatic drainage post-intubation.

Why might tracheal intubation be difficult?

- **Risk of airway loss**
  - *Difficult pre-oxygenation*: distress and hypoxia
  - *Difficult bag mask ventilation*: oedema and loss of skin
  - *Difficult laryngoscopy*: anatomical distortion by oedema
  - More significant consequences of traumatic intubation
- **Risk of hypoxaemia**
  - Hypermetabolic state
  - V/Q mismatch
  - Hypovolaemia
  - Toxic compounds (e.g. CO or cyanide)
- **Risk of cardiovascular collapse**
- **Associated issues** (e.g. c-spine injury requiring immobilisation or dental trauma)

How might respiratory support be tailored to manage smoke inhalation injury?

Ventilation:

- LPV
- *Bronchoscopy*: diagnosis, grading, or lavage
- *Nebulisers*: heparin in saline, 20% NAC, or salbutamol
- Chest physiotherapy and respiratory hygiene
- May require extracorporeal support

Toxicity from carbon monoxide ± cyanide should be considered and addressed. Distinguishing between under-resuscitation and cyanide toxicity in persistent metabolic acidosis can be tricky. Treatment will involve a balance of risks due to differing mechanisms of treatment options.

(See Chapter 54 Burns and Chapter 39 Environmental Poisons)

What do you know about bronchial clearance in severe burns?

Bronchial clearance is more pertinent in inhalational injury as effective expectoration becomes more challenging, risking atelectasis, acute lung injury, and pneumonia.

Contributing factors
- Increased mucus production
- Inactivation of surfactant
- Bronchial cast sloughing
- Injury to mucociliary escalator
- Sedation

Clearance techniques may be mechanical, involve pharmacotherapy such as nebulisers, or a combination of these techniques in the form of bronchoalveolar lavage (BAL). Bronchoscopy is often performed soon after admission for assessment and initial bronchial clearance. It may be continued daily until clinical improvement is shown. Prophylactic antibiotics and corticosteroids are not used routinely.

Nebulisers
- *Salbutamol*: bronchodilator, increasing alveolar water clearance
- *NAC (3 ml of 20%, 8°)*: mucolytic but causes bronchospasm
- Sodium bicarbonate (10 ml of 1.4%, 4°)
- *Heparin*: inhibits fibrin cast formation and reduces impact of ROS
- *Other*: dornase alfa, ipratropium, adrenaline, or prostacyclin

BAL
- *NaCl (0.9%, up to 250 ml)*: during bronchoscopy
- *Sodium bicarbonate (10 ml of 1.26%)*: non-directed bronchial lavage (NBL) during physiotherapy

Mechanical
- Postural drainage in selected cases
- Physiotherapy (e.g. percussion)

Resources
- Gill P, Martin RV. Smoke inhalation injury. BJA Educ. 2015;15(3):143–148.
- Prior K, Nordmann G, Sim K, et al. Management of inhalational injuries in burns centres – a questionnaire survey. J Intensive Care Soc. 2009;10(2):141–144.
- Spinou A, Koulouris NG. Current clinical management of smoke inhalation injuries: a reality check. Eur Respir J. 2018;52(6):1802163.

45.   LUDWIG'S ANGINA

What is Ludwig's angina and why is it significant to critical care?

- Gangrenous cellulitis affecting the soft tissues of the neck and floor of mouth
- Described by Karl Friedrich Wilhelm von Ludwig in 1836
- May cause profound sepsis and airway compromise

What causes Ludwig's angina?

- Dental abscess
- Parapharyngeal abscess
- Mandibular fracture
- Oral laceration/piercing
- Submandibular sialadenitis

Ludwig's angina is usually caused by mixed aerobes and anaerobes, usually mouth flora (e.g. *Staphylococcus* and *Streptococcus* species).

Predisposing conditions
- Immunocompromise
- Poor dentition
- Recent dental treatment
- Trauma

What are the concerning airway features in Ludwig's angina?
- Potential for **airway obstruction/occlusion**
  - *Oedema*: generalised, increased soft tissue bulk, or laryngeal oedema
  - Drooling or inability to swallow
  - *SOL*: collections
  - Anterior distribution of infection over neck, reducing effect of laryngoscopy
- Potentially **difficult intubation** if required
  - Distortion of normal anatomy by above
  - Soft tissues less mobile, particularly if infection established
  - Sick patient, severe sepsis likely, and commonly immunocompromised
- Potentially **difficult front of neck access** due to location of infection
- Risks associated with **poor dentition**
  - Sharp teeth may tear cuff.
  - Loose teeth may obstruct airway.

Airway obstruction is the leading cause of death in this disease.

How would you manage a patient with this condition?
- **Early diagnosis and specialist review**: ENT and anaesthesia
  - Flexible nasendoscopy may be possible to assess airway
  - CT imaging not essential but will aid assessment of spread
  - Observation in selected cases
  - Planning for surgical and anaesthetic intervention with difficult airway
- **Chemical decompression**
  - Dexamethasone 48 h
  - Nebulised adrenaline to native airway
- **Source control**
  - Surgical debridement
  - Antimicrobials (e.g. empirical broad-spectrum anaerobic and aerobic cover)
- **Airway management**
  - Regular monitoring
  - Avoid lying flat if airway threatened pre-intubation
  - May required prolonged airway support on ICU
  - Additional expertise may be required for difficult tracheostomy
- **Other supportive care** (e.g. vasopressors for sepsis)

What is Lemierre's syndrome?
Lemierre's syndrome is a condition in which infection with *Fusobacterium necrophorum* (necrobacillosis) spreads to the deep tissues of the neck, resulting in septic thrombophlebitis of the IJVs.

Septic emboli may cause effects in other organs, typically lung abscesses. Lemierre's syndrome predominantly affects young adults, usually following a bacterial throat infection. Mortality is around 5%.

Resources
- Riordan T, Wilson M. Lemierre's syndrome: more than a historical curiosa. Postgrad Med J. 2004;80(944):328–334.
- Saifeldeen K, Evans R. Ludwig's angina. Emerg Med J. 2004;21(2):242–243.

46. MASSIVE HAEMOPTYSIS

What is massive haemoptysis and why is it relevant to critical care?

Haemoptysis is the production of blood from the respiratory tract, usually during coughing. There are numerous causes, and severity can involve anything from blood-streaked sputum to catastrophic haemorrhage.

There is no universally accepted definition. Massive haemoptysis can be defined by quantity of blood expectorated, but clinical significance might be more useful. Examples are as follows:

- 100 ml in 1 episode
- 1000 ml/24 h
- Volume that is life-threatening due to airway obstruction or blood loss (anatomical dead space of large airways is approximately 100–200 ml)

Massive haemoptysis can be one of the most challenging presentations to manage in critical care due to its simultaneous effects on airway patency, respiration, and circulation. Often, patients are awake and aware of their symptoms before they deteriorate, causing significant distress that requires sensitive management.

Mortality is estimated at 30–85% in non-traumatic cases, with death usually secondary to asphyxia rather than exsanguination. If loss exceeds 1000 ml/24 h, mortality is around 58%.

Give some possible causes of massive haemoptysis.

Massive haemoptysis may arise from any lesion in the respiratory tract or a presentation of GI bleeding or epistaxis ± aspiration.

Bronchial sites are largely responsible (90%), in comparison with pulmonary aetiology (5%). Bronchial vessels are under higher pressure and so more likely to be implicated in severe bleeding. Alveolar vessels are subjected to lower pressures but may pool a significant volume in the alveolar space. Diffuse alveolar haemorrhage relates to origin from the pulmonary vasculature.

Any of the causes below will be exacerbated by coagulopathy (not detailed here):

- Vascular
  - Arteriobronchial fistula (may arise from aorta)
  - Bronchial telangiectasia
  - PE/infarct
  - Arteriovenous malformation
  - Mitral stenosis
  - Left ventricular failure (LVF)
- Infective
  - Mycobacteria (e.g. TB)
  - Lung abscess
  - Necrotising pneumonia (e.g. *Klebsiella*, *Staphylococcus*, and *Legionella* spp.)
  - Aspergilloma
  - Hydatid cyst
- Inflammatory
  - Behçet's disease (PA aneurysm)
  - GPA (formerly Wegener's granulomatosis)
  - Anti-glomerular basement membrane (GBM) disease (formerly Goodpasture's syndrome)
  - Bronchiectasis or cystic fibrosis
- Traumatic
  - Blunt/penetrating injury
  - Foreign body aspiration
- Iatrogenic
  - PA catheterisation
  - Bronchoscopy
  - Transbronchial biopsy

- Ulceration related to suction catheter
- Tracheo-innominate artery fistula
- Neoplastic
  - Bronchial carcinoma/adenoma
  - Pulmonary metastases
  - Sarcoma
  - Lymphangioleiomyomatosis (LAM)
- Other
  - Catamenial haemoptysis
  - Munchausen's syndrome (e.g. unwitnessed episodes of bloodletting)
  - Self-harm

What are the immediate priorities in resuscitation and stabilisation of the patient with massive haemoptysis?

- Determine suitability for potential interventions (multisystem or malignant disease often present)
- Evaluate coagulation profile (may be reversible)
- **Airway protection** (see question below)
  - Intubation and ventilation if asphyxiation risk
  - *Bronchoscopy*: suction, lavage, and topical agents (e.g. adrenaline)
- **Localising site of bleeding**
  - Surgical consultation if unstable
  - Respiratory consultation
  - *Investigation depending on stability*: flexible/rigid bronchoscopy, angiography, or CT thorax
- **Definitive management**
  - May be amenable to bronchial artery embolisation or angiographic technique
  - Thoracotomy might be required
  - *Vasculitis*: steroids, IVIg, or plasma exchange may be appropriate
- **Supportive care**
  - Appropriate oxygenation
  - *Haemorrhage*: appropriate access, cross-match, transfusion, and adjuncts (e.g. TXA and management of coagulopathy)
  - Antimicrobials if suspected/confirmed infection
  - *Sensitive communication*: patient may not be obtunded
  - Ongoing investigation often before discharge from hospital

Unusual cases

- *ECMO patient*: tracheal tube may need to be clamped to tamponade bleeding
- *Tracheo-innominate artery fistula*: tamponade by overinflating tracheostomy tube cuff, intubation of top end and tube/cuff manipulation, and digital compression of stoma
- *PAC complication*: temporise by withdrawing slightly and reinflating balloon

How might you intubate and ventilate such a patient?

Early protection of the airway will eliminate one of the major concerns in achieving stability. However, there are significant challenges in doing so, and senior anaesthetic and critical care input would be prudent. If possible, move to a place of relative safety with optimal intubating conditions (e.g. theatre). Priorities include facilitating bronchoscopy and suction as well as protection of non-soiled sites.

Issues

- *Visual field easily obscured by frank blood*: use 2 suction devices.
- Haemodynamic instability possible due to bleeding
- *Distressing scenario with dramatic visual load for the patient and staff*: human factors and the environment may be difficult to manage.
- *Catecholamine drive significant*: haemodynamics even more vulnerable at induction of anaesthesia
- Salvage is the main priority, but it may be possible to improve outcome with skilled operation.

Adaptations
- **Positioning**
  - Bleeding side down if possible (e.g. unilateral lung cancer)
  - Right-sided intubation may be facilitated by the right lateral position
- **Tube choice**
  - Wide, single-lumen tube until lesion identified (facilitates bronchoscopy and suction)
- **Ventilation**
  - Selective intubation of contralateral bronchus
    - ➤ Selective bronchoscopic intubation
    - ➤ Occlusive catheterisation of bleeding side (e.g. Fogarty catheter 14 French/100 cm length alongside tracheal tube)
    - ➤ *Right lung (i.e. left bleeding)*: can advance single-lumen tube, which may occlude RUL bronchus
  - *Differential lung ventilation using double-lumen tube*: less suitable unless experienced operator as tube positioning is crucial with small margin for error

What other ongoing investigations might be indicated?

- ABG, viscoelastic testing, and coagulation screen
- *Specific bloods*: anti-GBM, ANCA, ANA, beta-D-glucan, and galactomannan
- *Echo*: unusual causes of bleeding and functional assessment
- *Sputum*: microscopy, cytology, and bacterial/fungal culture
- Urinalysis
- *CXR*: lesion, infiltrates, and localisation occasionally
- High-resolution CT thorax
- *PFT*: risk/benefit as forced expiration relatively contraindicated

Resources

- Grant CA, Dempsey G, Harrison J, et al. Tracheo-innominate artery fistula after percutaneous tracheostomy: three case reports and a clinical review. Br J Anaesth. 2006;96(1):127–131.
- Håkanson E, Konstantinov IE, Fransson S-G, et al. Management of life-threatening haemoptysis. Br J Anaesth. 2002;88(2):291–295.
- Lordan JL, Gascoigne A, Corris PA. The pulmonary physician in critical care * Illustrative case 7: Assessment and management of massive haemoptysis. Thorax. 2003;58(9):814–819.

---

47. TRACHEOSTOMY EMERGENCIES

What are the most common tracheostomy emergencies?

There are many possible complications of tracheostomy insertion and maintenance. Several of these have the potential to be immediately life-threatening. The vast majority of tracheostomy emergencies occur after insertion although peri-procedural problems are well described.

- **Loss of airway** (complete or partial)
  - Obstruction
  - Displacement
- **Haemorrhage**
  - At time of insertion
  - *Delayed*: trauma to mucosa/vessels or tracheo-innominate artery fistula
- **Other**
  - Severe air leak (e.g. surgical emphysema, PTX, or pneumomediastinum) causing respiratory or other organ failure
  - Cuff leak resulting in ineffective ventilation

Emergencies might arise in the ICU or outwith critical care in the ward or home environment. Patients may present to hospital because occasionally of this or, more commonly, have been admitted due to another reason.

How might you recognise a tracheostomy emergency?

The patient themselves may be able to detect that something is wrong. Occasionally, tracheostomy emergencies may manifest with respiratory or cardiac arrest.

Red flag signs can be categorised as follows:

- **Airway** (with cuffed tracheostomy)
  - Vocalising
  - Audible air leak
  - Bubbles of saliva
  - Grunting
  - Snoring
  - Stridor
- **Breathing**
  - Respiratory distress
  - Higher airway pressures
  - Lower V_T
  - Noisy breathing
  - Hypoxia
  - *Apnoea*: clinical or on capnography
- **Specific** tracheostomy flags
  - Visible displacement
  - Blood or blood-stained secretions around tube
  - Increased discomfort/pain
  - High volume of air to maintain cuff inflation
- **General**
  - Physiological sign derangement (e.g. RR, HR, BP, or GCS)
  - Anxiety, restlessness, agitation, and confusion may indicate airway obstruction

How would you manage a tracheostomy emergency?

The National Tracheostomy Safety Project (NTSP) has produced a set of algorithms for use during a tracheostomy and laryngectomy emergencies. The relevant algorithm and patient-specific airway information should be present on an airway poster at the head of the bed.

Often, another party will have called for your help as an airway expert.

Stages in resuscitation
- Assessment
  - Look, listen, and feel
  - Mapleson C circuit and waveform capnography may help assessment
- If breathing, apply high-flow oxygen to both face and tracheostomy. If not, start CPR
- Assess tracheostomy patency in stages
  - Remove inner tube (and speaking valve or cap if present)
  - Attempt to pass suction catheter (if patent, perform suction and ventilate)
  - Deflate cuff (if effective, tube was partially obstructed or displaced)
- If not patent despite above, remove the tracheostomy tube
- Reassess
- If still no signs of life, start CPR
- *Primary emergency oxygenation*: oral airway manoeuvres (cover stoma)
  - If ineffective, ventilate via stoma with laryngeal mask or paediatric face mask
- *Secondary emergency oxygenation*: oral intubation to beyond stoma
  - If unsuccessful, intubate stoma

Stoma intubation may be performed with a small tracheostomy tube or 6.0-mm cuffed tracheal tube. An airway exchange catheter, bougie, or fibre-optic scope may be helpful.

GUIDELINE   NTSP 2012 Tracheostomy emergencies

How would you classify tracheostomy-related bleeding?

- **Early** (≤4 days)
  - Skin related
  - Thyroid related
  - Anticoagulant or antiplatelet therapy related
- **Late** (>4 days)
  - Erosion (e.g. tracheo-innominate artery fistula)
  - Granulation
  - Mucosal trauma (e.g. from suction catheter)

Significance may range from negligible bleeding to catastrophic haemorrhage. Tracheo-innominate artery erosion is rare, occurring in <1% tracheostomy cases but with high mortality. A pulsating tracheostomy tube may indicate proximity to a major vessel. Risk factors are as follows:

- Low placement of tracheostomy
- Excessive movement of tube
- Overinflation of cuff
- Suboptimal tracheostomy tube position

How would you manage tracheostomy-related bleeding?

- Experienced clinician involvement at early stage
- Sit patient up.
- Administer supplemental oxygen.
- Consider as an emergency if >10 ml fresh blood (e.g. dressing soaked).
- Notify appropriate head and neck surgeon (e.g. parent team listed on bedhead sign).
- Major arterial erosion may be managed with cuff hyper-inflation or direct digital tamponade.
- Manage major blood loss.

Minor bleeding might be managed using regular dressing changes and/or topical coagulants. Anticoagulant therapy and coagulopathy should be evaluated to prevent bleeding.

(See Chapter 46 Massive Haemoptysis and Chapter 51 Major Haemorrhage)

What is the significance of airway emergencies in patients with previous laryngectomy?

A separate algorithm exists for laryngectomy management due to the absence of an upper airway. There may be questions surrounding suitability for escalation, but many patients will have had curative surgery. Previous radiotherapy and neck dissection may complicate airway management.

KEY POINT

Patients with laryngectomies have **no connection** between their upper airways (nose/mouth) and their lungs.

Main differences in resuscitation are as follows:

- Apply high-flow oxygen to stoma (if any doubt, apply to face also)
- Assessment of patency is as follows:
  - Same staged approach, but with initial removal of stoma cover if present
  - Most laryngectomies will not have a tube in situ

- *Primary emergency oxygenation*: ventilate via stoma
- *Secondary emergency oxygenation*: intubate stoma

What is a TEP valve?

A tracheo-oesophageal puncture (TEP) valve is a prosthetic device that may have been inserted to allow 1-way passage of gas from the trachea to the oesophagus to facilitate speech (effectively by controlled burping). Expired gas can be forced from the trachea into the oesophagus via the TEP valve by occluding the laryngectomy stoma during expiration. TEP valves should not be removed during initial attempts at resuscitation as the fistula is easily damaged. They will not occlude the airway.

What equipment should be available for patients with tracheostomies and laryngectomies?

Bedside
- Humidification equipment
- Suction with selection of appropriate catheters
- Spare tracheostomy tubes (1 same size and 1 smaller)
- Clean pot for spare inner cannula
- Sterile water for cleaning suction tube
- Scissors (± stitch cutter)
- Water-soluble lubricating jelly
- Sterile dressing pack
- Tracheostomy dressings
- Tracheostomy tapes
- Personal protective equipment (PPE)
- Sterile gloves for performing deep suction
- Nurse call bell

Emergency
- Basic airway equipment
- Advanced airway equipment
- Capnography
- Fibre-optic scope
- Tracheal dilators
- Bougies

What systems are in place to try and prevent or reduce the severity of tracheostomy emergencies?

- **Training**
  - Regular training and updates for staff caring for patients with tracheostomies
  - Patient care in appropriate environment with trained staff
  - Multidisciplinary simulation
- **Patient care**
  - Regular patient review and assessment
  - Equipment available as above
  - Appropriate monitoring (waveform E_tCO_2 should be available)
  - Scheduled tube changes
  - Secretion management
  - Care of stoma site and neck
  - Difficult airway trolley availability
  - Emergency airway responder availability
- **Communication**
  - Appropriate documentation in notes
  - Airway sign
  - Accurate handover of information

Resources

- National Tracheostomy Safety Project. Complications, Red Flags & Emergencies. 2021. Available from: https://www.tracheostomy.org.uk/storage/files/Red%20flags.pdf. (Accessed 30 December 2021.)
- National Tracheostomy Safety Project. Tracheostomy Emergencies: Bleeding. 2021. https://www.tracheostomy.org.uk/storage/files/Bleeding.pdf. (Accessed 30 December 2021.)

48. LARYNGEAL INJURY

Why are the laryngeal complications of airway management important in critical care?

Critical care patients often require prolonged intubation. Tracheostomy is required in about 10–15% of all intubated ICU patients. Airway injuries and dysfunction are common and can cause significant morbidity. Most are minor, but more significant injuries can occur.

Effects include delay or failure of the following:

- Primary extubation
- Decannulation
- Recovery of speech
- Recovery of swallowing
- Recovery of functional cough

Complications include the following:

- Impaired secretion management and airway protection
- Aspiration pneumonia
- Dysphagia
- Prolonged hospital stay
- Increased mortality
- Financial burden

What laryngeal complications might occur after intubation or tracheostomy?

- Oedema
- *Dislocation*: arytenoid cartilages (during intubation/extubation)
- Ulceration
- *Necrosis*: submucosa, perichondrium, or cartilage
- Atrophy
- Granulation
- Stenosis
- Polyp formation
- Anterior glottic web
- *Nerve palsy*: hoarseness or desensitisation
- Laryngo-/tracheomalacia
- Dysphonia

Tracheostomy (all above plus)

- Stoma infection, wound breakdown, or granulation
- Incoordinated glottic closure with mechanical ventilatory airflow
- Vocal cord tremor

Prolonged cuff inflation causes the following: desensitisation, secretion stasis, uncoordinated glottic closure, poor cough strength, and aspiration risk.

Which structures are most vulnerable?

- Arytenoid cartilages
- Vocal processes
- Cricoarytenoid joints
- Posterior glottis
- Vocal folds
- Subglottis

How might the recurrent laryngeal nerve be damaged during airway management?

- Cuff inflation
- Tracheostomy insertion
- Other front of neck access

When would a patient be at high risk of laryngeal injury?

Patient

- Age (≥50 years 3 × risk cord paralysis)
- Female
- High BMI
- Diabetes mellitus or hypertension (× 2 risk)
- Laryngopharyngeal reflux
- Malnutrition and renal/hepatic failure

Intubation/tube related

- Cardiothoracic surgery
- Heart/lung transplant
- Thyroid surgery
- Emergency intubation (particularly if no NMB)
- Skill level of operator
- Intubating conditions
- Bougie/stylet use
- Larger diameter-to-patient-height ratio
- Tube/cuff design

Post-intubation

- Prolonged intubation (>6 h × 15 risk)
  - 3–5 days 2% risk laryngeal stenosis (two thirds require long-term tracheostomy)
  - 6–10 days 5% risk
- Agitation
- Poor humidification
- Local infection
- High mean cuff pressure/volume
- Number of reintubations required

What signs might indicate laryngeal complications post-extubation?

- *Stridor*: laryngeal oedema
- *Hoarseness*: vocal cord motility disorder, ulceration, or granulation
- Vocal fatigue
- Sore throat
- Hoarseness
- Difficulty clearing secretions
- Retention of saliva in upper airway
- Poor cough
- Absent/impaired swallowing
- Aspiration

More significant injury is suggested by persistence of symptoms beyond a few days.

(See Chapter 41 Stridor)

What is dysphonia?

Dysphonia is the term used to describe impaired voice quality. It can result from many conditions and may result in communication difficulties and low mood.

Aphonia is the complete loss of voice.

What is the pathophysiology of post-extubation dysphagia?

Post-extubation dysphagia occurs in 60% of ICU patients requiring intubation and persists in up to a third of patients discharged from hospital. This might be contributed to by cognitive impairment, residual effects of medications, sepsis, and mechanical factors as follows:

- Duration of intubation
- Tracheal tube size
- Mucosal inflammation
- Disuse muscle atrophy
- Diminished proprioception
- Laryngeal desensitisation
- Laryngeal injury

What is the pathophysiology of dysphagia following tracheostomy insertion?

- Tracheostomy tube results in absent/abnormal gas flow across larynx
- Desensitisation and disuse atrophy
- Glottic closure becomes uncoordinated
- Swallowing impairment results

What is the role of speech and language therapists in this setting?

A speech and language therapist can detect, assess, and rehabilitate laryngeal complications. Similarly to any rehabilitation in critical care, earlier intervention has the potential to improve outcomes. GPICS recommend early and timely SLT assessment.

They may use fibre-optic endoscopic evaluation of swallowing (FEES) by the bedside to aid assessment by detecting certain pathology (e.g. silent aspiration) and determining optimal individualised treatment.

What is 'above cuff vocalisation'?

Above-cuff vocalisation is vocalisation facilitated by the delivery of retrograde gas flow above the tracheostomy cuff and out of the mouth via the vocal cords. The technique requires a well-positioned subglottic suction tracheostomy tube. Specific 'talking tubes' are also available with dedicated above-cuff ports for additional gas flow.

How might laryngeal complications be managed?

Multidisciplinary input is essential, utilising skills of SLT, respiratory physiotherapists, nursing, and medical staff.

The most obvious intervention is to facilitate weaning and extubation. Others focus on reducing risk factors, secretion management, and rehabilitation of the larynx. Rehabilitation might include specific voice exercises or newer interventions such as pharyngeal electrical stimulation.

Specific therapies
- *Laryngeal oedema*: corticosteroids (see Chapter 41 Stridor)
- *Excessive salivation (if simple measures fail)*: hyoscine patch, glycopyrrolate, sublingual atropine, botulinum toxin to salivary glands, and radiotherapy
- *Altered translaryngeal gas flow*: speaking valve and above-cuff vocalisation

Surgery is indicated in some circumstances (e.g. stenosis dilation, tracheal stenting, vocal fold injection, and arytenoid adduction procedures).

What is tracheal stenosis?

Tracheal stenosis is the narrowing of part of the trachea. The term 'subglottic stenosis' is used to describe airway narrowing below the vocal cords and may or may not include tracheal stenosis.

Translaryngeal intubation is a recognised cause of airway stenosis. Around 11% of intubated patients will develop this complication. Mucosal ischaemia and ulceration result from the pressure of parts of airway devices (e.g. tube wall or cuff). As this heals, fibrous scarring reduces the diameter of the airway.

Typical symptoms include SOB, inspiratory stridor, and expiratory wheeze (classically monophonic). Approximately 30% stenosis can take place before symptoms occur at rest.

Therapeutic options include bronchoscopic dilatation and stenting, with a minority of patients requiring reconstructive surgery. The use of high-volume, low-pressure cuffs in critical care aims to prevent this complication.

Resources

- Spittle N, McCluskey A. Lesson of the week: tracheal stenosis after intubation. BMJ. 2000;321(7267):1000–1002.
- Wallace S, McGrath BA. Laryngeal complications after tracheal intubation and tracheostomy. BJA Educ. 2021;21(7):250–257.

RESUSCITATION

What is major trauma?

Major trauma refers to an injury or combination of injuries that are life-threatening and could be life changing because they may result in long-term disability. Major trauma can be retrospectively defined by an ISS > 15.

Major trauma is responsible for approximately 15000 deaths per year in the UK. The management of the severely injured patient has evolved over the last decade. It is now delivered by an MDT, usually following pre-hospital bypass to a major trauma centre (MTC), resulting in a systematic, multidisciplinary, parallel approach to assessment and treatment.

What is a major trauma centre?

A major trauma centre is a hospital providing tertiary trauma care, characterised by certain features:

- Training
- 24/7 trauma lead and team
- Specific specialties
- Appropriate network setup
- Ability to perform resuscitative thoracotomy
- Massive haemorrhage protocol
- Available relevant diagnostics
- Rehabilitation services

Specialties with consultant presence within 30 min if required:

- *Surgery*: neurosurgery, spinal, vascular, general, trauma and orthopaedics, plastic, oral and maxillofacial, ENT
- Anaesthetics
- IR
- ICM

The optimal destination for patients with major trauma is usually an MTC. Other hospitals may function as trauma units and provide emergency care if the MTC is not accessible (e.g. within 45 min) or 'pitstop' care for urgent stabilisation if airway threat or cardiac arrest has occurred.

GUIDELINE   NICE 2016 NG39 Major trauma

What is the role of TARN?

The **Trauma Audit and Research Network (TARN)** carries out independent clinical audit for traumatic injuries in the UK and serves as the largest European Trauma Registry. Local coordinators submit anonymised data which is used to analyse and report performance in order to improve trauma care, reinforced by financial implications. Survival rates are calculated and compared against predicted probability of survival.

Example standards are as follows:

- RSI ≤ 45 min of initial call to emergency services if GCS < 9
- TXA administration within 1 h of arrival at scene if ≥1 injury associated with significant bleeding
- Consultant review ≤ 5 min of arrival if ISS > 15
- CT imaging within 60 min of arrival for head injury with GCS < 13
- Provisional written radiology report ≤ 60 min of scan
- Clinical frailty score completed ≤ 72 h of admission by a geriatrician in patients ≥ 65 years old
- Fixation of open fractures of long bones and definitive soft tissue cover ≤72 h of injury
- Rehabilitation prescription if ISS > 8

Can you describe the Injury Severity Score in more detail?

The ISS is an anatomical score used to classify severity of trauma.

The body is divided into 6 regions:

1 Face
2 Head and neck
3 Chest
4 Abdomen and pelvis
5 Extremities and pelvic girdle
6 External

Each region then has a score applied to its injuries – Abbreviated Injury Scale (AIS):

1 Minor
2 Moderate
3 Serious
4 Severe
5 Critical
6 Maximal (untreatable)

The 3 most injured regions' scores are then squared and added together to give the ISS (maximum 75).

Notes:

- A score of 6 in any region automatically gives an ISS of 75 (unsurvivable).
- *Non-linear*: certain scores are unobtainable, whereas others are common (e.g. 9, 16).
- Scores are assigned according to a dictionary of injuries based on investigation, operative and post-mortem findings.

How would you approach a patient presenting to hospital following major trauma?

Early management has huge potential to influence outcomes and is front-loaded within a short space of time. This is the concept behind the 'golden hour' of trauma.

- MTC pre-alerted to the arrival of a severely injured patient
- *Team assembled*: introductions, allocation of roles, brief, major haemorrhage protocol activation, often referred to as the **zero point survey**
- *On arrival*: patient handover, primary survey conducted in tandem with any urgent resuscitation measures
- Initial ongoing treatment as indicated
- Review

- Further treatment (e.g. time-critical intervention – transfer to theatre, IR)
- Secondary survey
- *Ongoing plan*: command huddle, confirm drugs given, inform family, transfer

Team members (may vary from institution to institution):

- Trauma team leader
- Anaesthetist
- Primary survey clinician
- General surgeon
- Orthopaedic surgeon
- Experienced nurse

Additionally:

- Radiologist/radiographer
- Neurosurgeon
- Intensive care clinician

What is meant by primary, secondary and tertiary survey?

The traditional 'surveys' serve different purposes:

- *Primary*: identification of life-threatening injuries amenable to immediate management
- *Secondary*: meticulous head-to-toe examination for other potential causes of severe illness
- *Tertiary*: documentation of all injuries post investigation to ensure no injuries have been missed

The **primary survey** is often carried out horizontally, with different team members assessing systems and reporting findings back to the team leader. It is used largely to identify any of the 6 life-threatening injuries (the 'lethal 6'). It involves the **<c>A+CBCDE** approach. '<c>' refers to catastrophic haemorrhage assessment and management.

The **secondary survey** guides the need for additional imaging, for example knee and ankle X-rays, and to ensure injuries such as lacerations are addressed promptly.

The **tertiary survey** often occurs 48–72 h after initial admission, when the patient is awake and orientated and all major injuries have been managed effectively. Clinical and radiological findings are compared. This also ensures that 'minor' injuries (e.g. fractures to the digits), which may have an enormous impact on function and quality of life, are addressed.

How would you assess and manage catastrophic haemorrhage?

- Assessment usually obvious
- Application of direct pressure, pressure dressings
- *Indirect pressure if unsuccessful*: proximal arterial compression (e.g. groin for lower leg haemorrhage)
- *Tourniquets to extremities*: note time of application

What are the priorities in the 'A + C' part of the primary survey?

Cervical spine protection is prioritised alongside airway patency. A pragmatic approach may be required (i.e. not worsening agitation).

Indications for RSI
- Actual/impending airway loss
- Ventilatory failure
- *Low/declining GCS*: particularly motor score
- Significant agitation
- *Humanitarian*: painful injury requiring further intervention

Challenges
- *Manual in-line stabilisation of cervical spine (MILS)*: mitigated by video laryngoscope, adjuncts
- Orofacial disruption or haemorrhage
- Laryngeal disruption
- Systemic decompensation

What are the 'lethal 6' injuries?

The 'lethal 6' injuries are those which are immediately life-threatening and often require intervention during the primary survey (Figure 49.1). These are as follows:

1 *Airway obstruction*
2 *Tension PTX*: finger thoracostomy/needle decompression, intercostal drain
3 *Open PTX*: 3-way dressing, intercostal drain
4 *Massive haemothorax (HTX)*: intercostal drain, transfusion, consideration of thoracotomy if unstable
5 *Flail chest*: multimodal analgesia (e.g. paravertebral/erector spinae block), rib fixation
6 *Cardiac tamponade*: echo helpful, thoracotomy (percutaneous drainage less useful)

What would you consider in the rest of your primary survey?

C – Circulation

- *Wide-bore access*: IV/IO (central wide-bore in some circumstances)
- *Significant sites*: 'blood on the floor plus 4 more' – chest, abdomen, pelvis, long bones
- *Damage control resuscitation*: including medical management of coagulopathy (see Chapter 51 Major Haemorrhage)
- *TXA*: if not already given (1 g ≤ 3 h of injury, 1 g over subsequent 8 h)

Differentials of shock in trauma:

- *Hypoxic*: airway compromise, hypoventilation, pulmonary contusion, aspiration, high sympathetic drive
- *Anaemic*: haemorrhage
- *Stagnant*: myocardial contusion, MI, tension PTX, tamponade, hypovolaemia through insensible loss, neurogenic
- *Histotoxic*: cyanide, sepsis

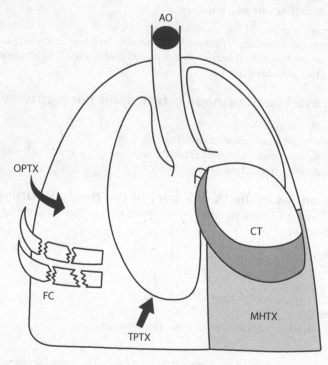

Figure 49.1 The 'Lethal 6' injuries.

AO, airway obstruction; OPTX, open pneumothorax; FC, flail chest; TPTX, tension pneumothorax; MHTX, massive haemothorax; CT, cardiac tamponade.

D – Disability
- Assess GCS, pupillary reaction to light, other neurological signs for injury to brain or spinal cord (see Chapter 83 Traumatic Brain Injury)
- *Note breakdown of score*: initial, arrival to hospital, prior to RSI if indicated

E – Everything else
- Other injuries that are immediately life-threatening
- Log roll to examine back
- Control environment and temperature – avoid hypothermia

Which interventions should be carried out in the pre-hospital setting?

Pre-hospital care focuses on appropriate triage, management of immediate threats to life, and prevention of significant complications. Timely transfer is key. Response will vary depending on the crew attending an incident. Helicopter emergency medical services (HEMS) are becoming increasingly available and patients may have received a number of critical care interventions prior to arrival.

Appropriate interventions might include the following:

- *Measures to mitigate haemorrhage*: direct pressure, tourniquet, pelvic binder, TXA (<3 h of injury)
- *Intubation*: if unable to maintain airway and/or ventilation
- *Decompression of suspected tension PTX*: haemodynamically unstable, respiratory compromise
- Covering open PTX
- Peripheral IV or IO access
- Titration of volume resuscitation to palpable central pulse (blood components or crystalloid)

NICE recommend that RSI should be performed as soon as possible where indicated, **within 45 min** of initial call to emergency services. If this is not possible, the patient should be transported to an MTC (if ≤60 min journey time). Divert to a trauma unit for RSI if MTC > 60 min away.

Which surgical interventions might be necessary to control catastrophic haemorrhage?

Occasionally, uncompressible catastrophic haemorrhage may require surgical access by an experienced operator exposing vessels proximal to the immediate zone of injury for clamping/tying or packing. Pulses may be unreliable, making anatomical landmarks important. Examples include longitudinal incision along anterior border of sternocleidomastoid (ABSCM), clam shell thoracotomy, and longitudinal groin incisions for leg vessel access.

The role of retrograde endovascular balloon occlusion of the aorta (REBOA) is unclear at present. IR is not recommended for genuine catastrophic haemorrhage in the unstable patient.

> **GUIDELINE** NHS 2020 Major Incidents

What is the role of CT imaging in major trauma?

Whole body CT scanning (vertex to toes 'scan-o-gram') followed by CT from vertex to mid-thigh should be performed in all patients aged 16 or older with suspected multiple injuries.

A provisional written report should be available within 60 mins. Plain X-rays and focused assessment with sonography for trauma (FAST) scans should not delay the transfer to CT scan. Diagnostic imaging may also be used to guide IR techniques in patients with solid-organ (spleen, liver, or kidney) arterial haemorrhage.

The decision whether to perform CT imaging in haemodynamically unstable patients will require multidisciplinary input and consideration of factors, including local geography and expertise available. The potential gain from additional information for targeted management will need to be balanced against the risk of further decompensation by delaying intervention.

What are the critical care priorities following major trauma?

Initial priorities
- Immediate assessment and resuscitation
- Correct macrovascular instability
- Restore circulating volume
- Correct coagulopathy
- Begin to reverse oxygen debt

Ongoing priorities
- Repeat assessment
- Optimise fluid status
- Ensuring definitive haemostasis
- *Correct microvascular status*: endothelial injury and glycocalyx dysfunction likely
- Correct acid-base status
- Correct nutritional status
- *Remain vigilant for sequelae*: sepsis, electrolyte disorder, transfusion-associated circulatory overload (TACO), transfusion-related acute lung injury (TRALI)

Resources
- Reid C, Brindley P, Hicks C, et al. Zero point survey: a multidisciplinary idea to STEP UP resuscitation effectiveness. Clin Exp Emerg Med. 2018;5(3):139–143.
- TARN: The Trauma Audit & Research Network. The Injury Severity Score (ISS). Available from: https://www.tarn.ac.uk/Home.aspx?c=3117. (Accessed 15 April 2022.)

50.   COMPLEX INJURIES

How would you manage pelvic trauma?

Pelvic trauma usually results from blunt injury with high energy transfer. It can result in massive (concealed) haemorrhage into the pelvis and retroperitoneum due to shearing of the iliac vessels. Mortality can be as high as 15% in the shocked patient with unstable pelvic trauma.

Fractures may be described anatomically by the Tile classification, in which injuries falling into categories A-C are each scored 1–3. The alternative Young-Burgess classification uses mechanism of injury.

Tile categories
A Stable
B Rotationally unstable, vertically stable ('open book' fractures in the category)
C Rotationally and vertically unstable

Young-Burgess categories
- Anteroposterior compression
- Lateral compression
- Vertical shear injuries
- Combined mechanism

Specific management
- Avoid log roll if possible
- *Use of a pelvic binder*: first-line treatment, reduces pelvic volume, brings fractures into approximation
    - Consider reduction or skeletal traction in vertical shear fractures, prior to placement
    - Place over the greater trochanters, internally rotating the toes
    - Aim to remove as soon as possible and no later than 24 h after application

- CT with angiography
- External fixation
- Intervention radiology to embolise bleeding vessel
- Open surgical packing of the pelvis

How would you manage the patient with concomitant haemorrhagic shock and traumatic brain injury?

This is a common dilemma in immediate trauma management. There is an apparent conflict in ideal strategies for management of circulation in haemorrhagic shock (restrictive) and TBI (high MAP to maintain cerebral perfusion).

This requires a careful judgement of the potential sequelae of each strategy for the individual patient: would the consequences of secondary brain injury-exacerbated hypotension outweigh those of massive transfusion, or is the threat to life from exsanguination so severe that secondary brain injury is an acceptable outcome?

Guidelines suggest deciding which condition is dominant and prioritising accordingly.

(See Chapter 51 Major Haemorrhage and Chapter 83 Traumatic Brain Injury)

Can you describe the pathophysiology of blast injuries?

An explosive is a material that can undergo an exothermic reaction from solid or liquid to gas very rapidly using its own energy. Injury is caused by the blast wave: a rapidly expanding and then contracting wave of energy.

Blast injuries
- *Primary*: direct effect of abnormal ambient pressure
- *Secondary*: air around blast displaced, high velocity blast winds, surrounding objects turned into projectiles, resultant blunt/penetrating injuries
- *Tertiary*: result due to the impact of people themselves against surrounding objects – usually blunt injuries
- *Quaternary*: not directly attributable to the blast (e.g. burns)

Secondary and tertiary blast injuries often result in multisystem trauma due to shearing effects at tissue interfaces (e.g. blast lung, visceral injury) and direct injury (e.g. TBI, traumatic fracture/amputation).

What is blast lung?

In blast lung, forces are propagated through the lung parenchyma, disrupting the alveolar capillary membrane and tearing alveolar septae. In situ haemorrhage causes a proinflammatory and pro-coagulant response. Toxin and smoke exposures may be significant.

Features
- *ARDS*
- *Bleeding*: haemoptysis, catastrophic haemorrhage
- *Air leak*: PTX, bronchopleural fistula

This results in **gas exchange failure** and **systemic gas embolism** with subsequent sequelae:

- CNS/focal defects due to spinal or central obstruction
- *Cardiovascular instability*: coronary artery obstruction
- Ischaemia in peripheral arterial tree
- Visual field defects due to retinal artery involvement

Treatment is supportive with oxygen and mechanical ventilation. Permissive hypercapnia and treatment of PTX may be required. Blast injury combined with haemorrhage is particularly life-threatening.

GUIDELINE   NHS 2020 Major Incidents

What do you know about penetrating injuries?

Assault with a sharp object is the most common method of sustaining a non-accidental penetrating injury in the UK (gunshot wounds being significantly less common).

Rapid transport to hospital is important to allow definitive haemorrhage control. Trauma resuscitation principles should be followed. Upon arrival to hospital, a patient may be haemodynamically stable, unstable, or in cardiac arrest. Large volume transfusion may be required.

- *Stable*: primary survey, CT imaging
- *Unstable*: emergency transfer to theatre
- *Cardiac arrest*: resuscitative thoracotomy may be indicated

How is traumatic cardiac arrest approached?

Adaptation of resuscitation might be indicated in traumatic mechanisms of cardiac arrest. Common reversible traumatic causes of cardiac arrest include hypoxia, tension PTX, tamponade, and hypovolaemia. Medical causes (e.g. MI prior to traumatic fall) should be considered and standard resuscitation algorithms followed in such cases.

Once confirmed, initial life-saving interventions should be carried out. Resuscitative thoracotomy might be indicated if improvement is not made. After circulation is restored, consideration should be made of transfer to theatre for damage control surgery, CT imaging, and admission to critical care. Vasopressors might be indicated before surgery in cases of head injury.

Initial priorities
- Stop catastrophic external haemorrhage
- Adequate oxygenation and ventilation
- Bilateral thoracostomies
- Minimising internal haemorrhage (e.g. pelvic binder)
- Rapid blood transfusion (warmed)
- (*De-prioritise*: external chest compressions, vasopressors, defibrillation)

Indications to stop resuscitation
- Cardiac standstill on US (in absence of tamponade and ROSC)
- Lack of response to life-saving interventions
- Persistently low E_tCO_2
- Prolonged arrest

GUIDELINE   RCEM 2019 Traumatic cardiac arrest

When is immediate resuscitative thoracotomy indicated?

Evidence is sparse and guidelines vary. Some refer to signs of life other than presence of a pulse (e.g. pupillary response, spontaneous ventilation, extremity movement, cardiac electrical activity, i.e. PEA).

Outcomes of this procedure are poor but better in penetrating injuries than blunt chest trauma. It should be commenced **within 10 min** of cardiac arrest if indicated. A non-surgical operator is often required. Survival is approximately 15% in penetrating injuries; 35% if cardiac. If performed after blunt trauma, survival is in the range of 0–2%.

Indications (and conditional indications in brackets)
- Penetrating chest trauma
  - *Peri-arrest*: **unable to tolerate transfer to theatre**, requires adapted RSI
  - *Established cardiac arrest*: **other signs of life**
  - (*Established cardiac arrest*: no other signs of life, short downtime)
- Blunt chest trauma
  - (*Established cardiac arrest*: other signs of life)
  - (Recommended against if established cardiac arrest and no other signs of life)

Unlikely to be successful if
- *Penetrating trauma*: CPR > 15 min
- *Blunt trauma*: CPR > 10 min

GUIDELINE   EAST 2015 Emergency department thoracotomy

GUIDELINE   ERC 2015 Special circumstances

What does the technique involve?

- Position supine with 360° access.
- *Simultaneous interventions to prevent delay*: IV access, intubation, ventilation
- *Pragmatic asepsis*: sterile gloves, aseptic non-touch technique (ANTT), rapid application of skin preparation solution
- *Open chest*: bilateral thoracostomies, joined by clamshell incision in fourth intercostal space, extend posteriorly to posterior axillary line, attach self-retaining rib spreader
  - *Release cardiac tamponade*: vertical incision on 'tent' of anterior pericardium, evacuate by hand
  - *Cardiac repair*: finger occlusion, suture/staple
  - *Cardiac massage*: attempt capture by flicking with finger, two-handed massage avoids kinking
  - Remove rib spreader before defibrillation if required
- If successful, will require immediate anaesthesia
- *Manage subsequent bleeding*: clamp internal mammary/intercostal arteries, repair in theatre

Resources

- Weatherford B. Pelvic Ring Fractures. Available from: https://www.orthobullets.com/trauma/1030/pelvic-ring-fractures. (Accessed 17 January 2022.)
- Nickson C. Life in the Fast Lane: Classification of Pelvic Fractures. November 2020. Available from: https://litfl.com/classification-of-pelvic-fractures/. (Accessed 15 April 2022.)
- Tompkins A. RCEM Learning: Blast Injuries. Available from: https://www.rcemlearning.co.uk/reference/blast-injuries/#1568201150912-c69dabd0-8340. (Accessed 17 January 2022.)
- Sheffy N, Chemsian RV, Grabinsky A, et al. Anaesthesia considerations in penetrating trauma. Br J Anaesth. 2014;113(2):276–285.
- Paulich S, Lockey D. Resuscitative thoracotomy. BJA Educ. 2017;20(7):242–248.

51.   MAJOR HAEMORRHAGE

When might you encounter major haemorrhage?

Common scenarios
- Major trauma
- GI bleeding
- Ruptured AAA
- Perioperatively
- Major obstetric haemorrhage (MOH)

(See Chapter 49 Major Trauma, Chapter 141 Bleeding and Clotting Disorders, Chapter 66 Abdominal Aortic Aneurysm, Chapter 139 Gastrointestinal Haemorrhage, and Chapter 99 Major Obstetric Haemorrhage)

How would you define major haemorrhage?

No single definition exists to quantify blood loss – volume or rate may be used. Examples:

- Whole blood volume in 24 h
- Half blood volume in 2 h
- 150 ml/min
- Bleeding with evidence of hypotension or tachycardia

Haemorrhagic shock has been classified by physiological signs historically but this is of limited use clinically. It may be helpful to identify how much a patient has decompensated on presentation.

What is damage control resuscitation?

Damage control resuscitation is a concept used in traumatic haemorrhage but it has been applied elsewhere.

KEY POINT

Key components of damage control resuscitation:

- *Permissive hypotension*: titrate circulatory support to central pulse
- *Haemostatic resuscitation*: early blood products, minimise crystalloid, prevent coagulopathy
- *Damage control surgery*: temporising attenuation of internal bleeding points through packing/resection/vascular intervention (without definitive surgical procedure)

What are the aims of damage control surgery?

This is emergency surgery (or IR) to save life or limb in trauma. Its goal is to achieve physiological and metabolic, rather than anatomical, stability.

Priorities
- **Haemorrhage control**
- **Decompression of compartments**: cranium, abdomen, limbs, thorax
- **Decontamination** of wounds and ruptured viscera
- **Fracture splintage**

Operative time should be kept below **90 min**. Anatomical correction can be performed on planned return to theatre after a period of stability on the critical care unit. Prolonged primary surgery carries significant risk and is likely to increase morbidity. It may also lead to more complex procedures being undertaken. Definitive surgery can be considered in patients responding to resuscitation.

GUIDELINE   NICE 2016 NG39 Major trauma

Define massive transfusion

Again, many definitions exist. Examples:

- Transfusion of >1 blood volume in 24 h
- Transfusion of >50% blood volume in 4 h
- > 40 ml/kg transfusion in paediatrics

What is trauma-induced coagulopathy?

Trauma-induced coagulopathy results from the imbalance of pro- and anticoagulant factors in major trauma, with hyperfibrinolysis, raised levels of systemic anticoagulant factors, and platelet dysfunction.

It is further exacerbated by hypothermia, citrate in blood products, and dilution by resuscitation fluids. **INR > 1.2** is an accepted definition of trauma-induced coagulopathy.

Describe the pathophysiology of the trauma 'diamond of death'.

This term refers to potentially avoidable conditions in trauma that may spiral out of control through positive feedback loops, rapidly leading to death.

> **KEY POINT**
>
> The 'diamond of death':
>
> - **Acidaemia**
> - **Hypothermia**
> - **Coagulopathy**
> - **Hypocalcaemia**

The pathophysiology does not just involve the exacerbation of bleeding. Reduced oxygen delivery can exacerbate hypothermia. Acidaemia will further impair cardiac output and oxygen delivery. Coagulopathy will prevent binding of substrate and contribute to anaerobic respiration and lactic acidosis. Hypocalcaemia results from trauma itself and transfusion. It will exacerbate acidosis and bleeding, alongside its negative effects on myocyte contractility.

How would you investigate a patient with major haemorrhage?

Major haemorrhage is a dynamic situation, requiring emergency care based on clinical signs. In trauma, the shock index may be used to assess hypovolaemia alongside other physiological markers, mechanism, injury pattern, and response to resuscitation.

An urgent blood group and crossmatch should be requested but this should not delay emergency blood product administration when indicated.

Imaging may be required, balanced against haemodynamic stability and necessity to transfer to theatre. (See Chapter 49 Major Trauma)

Caution should be exercised with investigations which are specific to a particular point in time if the situation has since changed. Components of circulating volume may not be accurately represented in haemorrhage and measurement will depend on dilutional or concentrating factors. The time taken for results to appear will limit these investigations' usefulness in this setting. Investigations may have uses in specific contexts:

- *ABG*: rough point-of-care Hb, ionised calcium, K^+, extent of decompensation (lactate, acid-base status)
- *Viscoelastic haemostatic assay (VHA) testing*: point of care assessment of clotting deficiency (see **ITACTIC**)
- *FBC*: baseline Hb, platelet count (may be normal early in trauma, does not represent dysfunction)
- *Clotting profile*: useful later to target specific coagulation factors, limited by time to result
- *Clauss fibrinogen assay*: more reliable than value derived from PT

What is the value of viscoelastic testing?

Viscoelastic testing allows point-of-care assessment of a patient's clotting. Information can be ascertained in around 30 min about deficiency of clotting factors, platelet function, or fibrinolysis. This can guide blood product administration in a timely manner in those with coagulopathy following haemorrhage. Two commonly used methods are thromboelastography (TEG®) and rotational thromboelastometry (ROTEM®).

Survival benefit has not been demonstrated definitively in traumatic haemorrhage but it may have a role in TBI. Near patient testing is advocated by the British Society for Haematology (BSH) and

Joint UK Blood Transfusion and Tissue Transplantation Services Professional Advisory Committee (JPAC).

How would you manage severe bleeding specifically?

Trauma principles can be transferred to most settings involving haemorrhage. (See Chapter 49 Major Trauma)

Source control
- Resuscitative (e.g. direct pressure)
- Surgical
- IR

General measures
- Avoid dilutional anaemia
- Permissive hypotension where indicated
- Appropriate transfusion thresholds
- Normothermia
- Correction of acidaemia
- *Avoidance of vasodilatation*: hypercarbia, drugs
- Note contraindications to blood products (e.g. cultural)

Blood products: ratio 1:1 of plasma:red cells (**PROPPR**), appropriate device (e.g. rapid infuser)

- *Packed red cells*: anaemia, major haemorrhage
  - Whole blood has some use in trauma resuscitation depending on availability
- *FFP*: single/multiple clotting factor deficiencies, major haemorrhage (dose 15–20 ml/kg)
  - *Octaplas (solvent/detergent-washed FFP)*: lower risk of TRALI, lacks vWF/VIII
  - Pathogen-reduced plasma (methylene blue with FFP)
- Platelets
- Other components
  - *Cryoprecipitate (factor VIII, XIII, vWF, fibronectin, fibrinogen)*: following the **CRYOSTAT-1** feasibility study, **CRYOSTAT-2** is underway at the time of writing
  - Fibrinogen concentrate
  - Cryosupernatant (vWF, factor XIII, fibronectin)
  - *Coagulation factor concentrates (PCC / XIII / VIIa)*: trauma, cirrhosis, drugs
  - *PCC (factors II, VII, IX, X)*: acquired coagulopathy
- **Pharmacological**
  - *Desmopressin*: 1-deamino-8-D-arginine vasopressin (DDAVP) – 0.3 µg/kg
  - *Antifibrinolytics*: aproptinin, lysine analogies (TXA, aminocaproic acid)
  - Reversal of anticoagulants

GUIDELINE   European Guideline 2019 Major bleeding and coagulopathy following trauma

STUDY

PROPPR (2015)

- Severe trauma predicted to require massive transfusion
- *Intervention*: 1:1:1 ratio vs 1:1:2 control (plasma:platelets:red cells)
- *Primary*: 24 h mortality, 30 day mortality – **no difference**
- *Secondary*: time to haemostasis, complications, transfusion, functional status – no difference
- Does not provide evidence of benefit for platelets

STUDY

CRYOSTAT-1 (2015)

- Major haemorrhage in trauma
- *Intervention*: addition of 2 early pools of cryoprecipitate vs standard care
- *Primary*: feasibility – receipt of cryoprecipitate within 90 min in associated arm of study (achieved in 85%, median time 60 min)

What is the role of tranexamic acid in major haemorrhage?

TXA is indicated early in trauma (**CRASH-2**) including TBI (**CRASH-3**). It should be considered in non-traumatic contexts. It may be harmful in hyperfibrinolytic states (e.g. DIC).

STUDY

CRASH-2 (2010)

- Trauma with/at risk of significant haemorrhage
- *Intervention*: early TXA vs placebo
- *Primary*: death in hospital within 4 weeks of injury – **significant reduction (14.5% vs 16%)**
- *Secondary*: transfusion requirement, vaso-occlusive events – no difference

STUDY

CRASH-3 (2019)

- TBI within 3 h of injury
- *Intervention*: TXA vs placebo
- *Primary*: 28-day in-hospital head injury associated mortality – **no difference**
- *Secondary*: vaso-occlusive events, seizures – no difference

Do you know of any specific reversal agents that might be indicated in patients taking direct oral anticoagulants?

Specific reversal agents for direct oral anticoagulants (DOACs):

- *Dabigatran*: **idarucizumab** (Praxbind®)
- *Rivaroxaban, apixaban*: **andexanet alfa** (Ondexxya®, Andexxa®)

Often, the use of non-specific agents will be advised in addition to these (e.g. PCC), or if no specific agent exists, such as with edoxaban.

Which reversal agents might be used to reverse other drugs affecting coagulation?

- *Heparin (including LMWH)*: protamine sulphate
- *Warfarin*: vitamin K, PCC (FFP less desirable)
- *Antiplatelet agents*: platelet transfusion, DDAVP

Can you describe some transfusion targets that might be used in ongoing care?

- Stable Hb
- Platelets ≥ 50–75×10^9/l (differs between guidelines)
- APTT and/or PT ratio ≤ 1.5
- Fibrinogen > 1.5 g/l
- Ionised calcium within normal limits

GUIDELINE   BSH 2015 Major haemorrhage

What are the complications of major haemorrhage?

These may be caused by the insult of the initial bleed, consequence of transfusion, or combination of both.

- **Hypoperfusion**
  - *Individual organ failure*: MI, AKI, brain injury, GI ischaemia, liver infarction
  - MODS
- **Hypothermia**
- **Coagulopathy**
  - Trauma-induced (see above)
  - *Dilutional*: infusion of crystalloid or packed red cells without clotting factors
  - *Consumptive*: clot formation uses up clotting factors
- **Biochemical**
  - *Hypocalcaemia*: consumed as co-factor in clotting cascade
  - *Hyperkalaemia*: packed red cells
  - *Acidosis*: hypothermia, lactic acidosis, hyperchloraemic acidosis with 0.9% NaCl
  - *Alkalosis*: citrate from packed red cells
- **Transfusion reactions** (see Chapter 52 Transfusion Reactions)

Which important organisational and human factors may facilitate the management of major haemorrhage?

Organisational factors

- Trust-wide major haemorrhage protocol (dictates and streamlines pathways in an emergency)
- Emergency call number (alerting laboratory and porters to support major haemorrhage protocol)
- 'Code red' alert system (allows pre-hospital activation of major haemorrhage protocol)
- Access to O negative emergency blood in key clinical areas
- Shock packs (sets of blood products dictated by major haemorrhage protocol) (support correct administration, vary nationally, often contain 4 units of packed red cells and 4 bags (1 dose) FFP ± platelets)
- Protocols for use of blood products (checking, monitoring)
- Templates to support documentation
- Staff training

Human factors

- Clear team communication, working, and leadership
- *Team briefing*: supports role allocation

- *Pauses*: clarify circumstances
- *Situation reports*: brief, every 10–15 min, allow all teams to remain informed

When else might transfusion be indicated in critical care scenarios?

Many trials have compared transfusion thresholds in different stable patient groups. These have been consolidated in recent European guidelines.

A restrictive transfusion threshold (70 g/l vs 90 g/l) is recommended in the general ICU population. This includes those with:

- Prolonged weaning from mechanical ventilation
- Sepsis and septic shock
- Cardiac surgery (75 g/l)

Liberal transfusion threshold of 80–90 g/l is conditionally recommended in **critically ill adults with acute coronary syndromes (ACS)** only. Applying this threshold to critically ill patients with chronic cardiovascular disease is controversial.

No recommendation between restrictive/liberal thresholds:

- *Acute neurologic injury*: TBI, SAH, stroke (**SAHaRA** and **HEMOTION** trials underway at time of writing)
- Patients undergoing ECMO
- *Malignancy*: haematological or solid tumour
- Elderly patients

Other recommendations:

- Target Hb or Hct (not SvO_2, pH, rhythm, ECG changes)
- Avoid using iron/erythropoietin/combination to reduce red cell transfusion
- Use small volume blood sampling tubes
- Use blood conservation devices for sampling
- (Further research required surrounding platelet/plasma transfusion for procedures)

GUIDELINE   ESICM 2020 Transfusion

STUDY

TRICC (1999)

- Patients admitted to ICU
- *Intervention*: restrictive (Hb 70 g/l) vs liberal (100 g/l) transfusion threshold
- *Primary*: 30-day mortality – **no difference**
- *Secondary*: in-hospital mortality – **significantly lower (22% vs 28%)**

STUDY

TRISS (2014)

- Patients with septic shock
- *Intervention*: transfusion threshold of ≤70 g/l vs 90 g/l
- *Primary*: 90-day mortality – **no difference**
- *Secondary*: median number of transfusions – **significantly lower**; patients not undergoing transfusion – **significantly higher**

TRICS-III (2017)

- Patients undergoing cardiac surgery with moderate-to-high risk of death (EuroSCORE ≥ 1)
- *Intervention*: transfusion threshold of 75 g/l vs 95 g/l intra-/post-op or 85 g/l on ward
- *Primary*: in-hospital composite of death, MI, new-onset AKI requiring dialysis – **non-inferior**
- *Secondary*: LOS, duration of ventilation, AKI, seizures, delirium – no difference

Resources

- Centre for Trauma Sciences. CRYOSTAT 1 & 2. Available from: https://www.c4ts.qmul.ac.uk/research-programmes/cryostat. (Accessed 19 April 2022.)
- ClinicalTrials.gov. HEMOglobin Transfusion Threshold in Traumatic Brain Injury OptimizatioN: The HEMOTION Trial (HEMOTION). Available from: https://clinicaltrials.gov/ct2/show/NCT03260478. (Accessed 19 April 2022.)
- Docherty AB, O'Donnell Rb, Brunskill S, et al. Effect of restrictive versus liberal transfusion strategies on outcomes in patients with cardiovascular disease in a non-cardiac surgery setting: systematic review and meta-analysis. BMJ. 2016;352:i1351.
- English SW, Fergusson D, Chassé M, et al. Aneurysmal SubArachnoid Haemorrhage – Red Blood Cell Transfusion and Outcome (SAHaRA): a pilot randomised controlled trial protocol. BMJ Open. 2016; 6(12):e012623.
- Gaunt C, Woolley T. Management of haemorrhage in major trauma. CEACCP. 2014;14(6):251–255.
- Joint United Kingdom (UK) Blood Transfusion and Tissue Transplantation Services Professional Advisory Committee. Transfusion Handbook: 7.3: Transfusion Management of Major Haemorrhage. Available from: https://www.transfusionguidelines.org/transfusion-handbook/7-effective-transfusion-in-surgery-and-critical-care/7-3-transfusion-management-of-major-haemorrhage.pdf. (Accessed 17 January 2022.)
- Klein AA, Arnold P, Bingham K, et al. AAGBI guidelines: the use of blood components and their alternatives 2016. Anaesthesia 2016;71(7):829–842.
- Wray JP, Bridwell RE, Schauer SG, et al. The diamond of death: hypocalcemia in trauma and resuscitation. Am J Emerg Med. 2021;41:104–109.

52.   TRANSFUSION REACTIONS

What is the significance of transfusion reactions in critical care?

Transfusion reactions may be acute or delayed and can range from mild to life-threatening illness with significant morbidity and mortality.

- *Acute transfusion reaction*: reaction occurring within 24 h of receiving transfusion
- *Delayed transfusion reaction*: reaction occurring > 24 h after transfusion

Symptoms and signs can overlap significantly and mimic other illnesses.

How might a transfusion reaction present?

- *Non-specific symptoms*: high temperature, chills/rigors, GI upset, rash/pruritus, wheeze, pain
- Angioedema
- Respiratory failure
- Cardiovascular collapse
- Bleeding

Severity
- *Mild*: isolated temperature > 38°C or pruritis/urticaria only

- *Moderate*: temperature > 39°C and/or rash or other non-severe features
- *Severe/life-threatening*: respiratory distress, airway compromise, cardiovascular compromise, bleeding

What are the different types of transfusion reaction?

Acute
- Febrile non-haemolytic reaction
- Allergic reaction
- Acute haemolytic reaction
- TACO
- TRALI
- Biochemical abnormalities
- Bacterial contamination
- Hypothermia
- Dilutional coagulopathy

Delayed
- Infective
    - *Viral*: HBV, HCV, HIV, CMV
    - *Bacterial*: syphilis (from donor at time of collection)
    - Variant CJD
- Transfusion-associated graft-versus-host disease (TA-GvHD)
- Post-transfusion purpura
- Iron overload

How would you manage a transfusion reaction?

Early detection may be facilitated by transfusion with an appropriate environment, monitoring, equipment, and trained staff. Systematic A–E assessment should be performed and severity stratified once a reaction is identified.

Priorities
- Recheck patient identity, blood product details, compatibility
- Inspect the blood product
- Stop transfusion, disconnect the giving set from patient (for all moderate and severe reactions)
- Keep all blood product bags and labelling – often require return to laboratory for investigation
- Instigate specific investigation and management
- *Reporting*: Medicines and Healthcare products Regulatory Agency (MHRA) and Serious Hazards of Transfusion (SHOT) collect data on adverse events from transfusion and provide recommendations to improve safety.

Prevention is ideal if possible, for example:

- Strict protocols to avoid 'wrong blood in tube' – multiple samples, identity checks
- Decontamination
- Leukodepletion
- Donor screening

GUIDELINE   BSH 2012 Transfusion reactions

Can you describe the management of some life-threatening transfusion reactions?

Anaphylaxis
- Manage as per anaphylaxis guidelines. (See Chapter 42 Anaphylaxis)

- Can present in patient with IgA deficiency as they develop IgA antibodies which react to transfused blood – may require IgA level checking
- Refer to immunology.

TRALI
- ARDS-like picture either during or within 6 h of transfusion
- Immune or non-immune mediated (reactive lipid products from donor cells)
- 6–9% mortality, over 2/3 require mechanical ventilation
- Supportive management
- Difficult to differentiate from TACO – diuresis may increase mortality in TRALI

TACO
- Acute/worsening pulmonary oedema within 6 h of transfusion
- Risk factors
    - *Patient*: increasing age, renal impairment, HF, low albumin, pre-existing fluid overload
    - *Transfusion*: large volume, rapid, red blood cells
- Supportive management including diuresis

Haemolytic reaction due to ABO incompatibility
- Acute (<24 h) or delayed
- Donor antigen and recipient antibodies produce a complex that leads to haemolysis and breakdown of donated blood.
- Presents with fever, chest/flank pain, flushing, rigors, urticaria, respiratory distress, and hypotension
- *Investigations*: falling Hb, elevated bilirubin and LDH, positive direct antiglobulin test
- Supportive management including RRT – risk of Hb deposition and thrombosis in the distal convoluted tubule. Significant haemodynamic support may be required.

Resources
- Maxwell MJ, Wilson MJA. Complications of blood transfusion. CEACCP. 2006;6(6):225–229.
- Norfolk D. United Kingdom Blood Services: Handbook of Transfusion Medicine. 5th ed. Norwich: Stationery Office; 2013. Available from: https://www.transfusionguidelines.org/document-library/documents/transfusion-handbook-5th-edition. (Accessed 17 January 2022.)
- SHOT. 2020 Annual SHOT Report – Individual Chapters. Available from: https://www.shotuk.org/shot-reports/report-summary-and-supplement-2020/2020-annual-shot-report-individual-chapters/. (Accessed 17 January 2022.)

53.   DROWNING

What is drowning?
Drowning is the process in which submersion or immersion in a liquid medium results in **primary respiratory impairment**.

- *Immersion*: airway above surface, patient usually floating face-up (e.g. wearing life-jacket)
- *Submersion*: whole body underwater (i.e. including airway)

The definition of drowning was updated by WHO in 2002 to include what used to be called 'near-drowning' (i.e. drowning does not necessarily result in death).

What is the epidemiology of drowning?
- 236000 drowning deaths per year globally
- 7% of all injury-related deaths
- Third leading cause of unintentional injury death worldwide
- 80% incidents thought to be preventable

Risk factors

- Children
- *Males*: related to exposure to water, risk-taking behaviour, alcohol, boating
- *Increased access to water*: fishing, small boat use
- Flood disasters
- Travelling on water
- Other
  - Lower socioeconomic status
  - Ethnic minority
  - Medical conditions (e.g. epilepsy)
  - Tourists unfamiliar with local water risks and features

Paediatrics

- Associated with lapse in supervision and living near open water sources
- One of the top 5 causes of death in young people in many countries
- 43% of all paediatric deaths in ages 1–4 years in Bangladesh

Can you name any measures that might prevent drowning?

- Flotation devices
- Swimming education
- Safety and rescue plans on vehicles
- Survival campaigns (e.g. promoting attempts to lie back and float)

What is the pathophysiology of cold water shock?

Cold water shock (or cold water immersion syndrome) is the syndrome of respiratory and autonomic responses to sudden immersion in cold water. It has 4 pathophysiological stages which may each result in death:

1 **Cold shock** (0–3 min)
   - Water < 25°C (all UK fresh waters)
   - Reflexes initiated by thermoreceptors sensing rapid skin cooling in order to increase cardiac output:
     - Risk of decompensation of pre-existing vascular disease
     - Inhalational gasp (torso reflex)
     - Tachpnoea > 60/min
     - Impaired breath-holding ability, increased likelihood of aspiration
     - Centrally-mediated tachycardia and peripheral vasoconstriction
     - 'Autonomic conflict' causing dysrhythmias, cardiac arrest
   - Different to diving reflex (for oxygen conservation) which involves
     - Bradycardia
     - Expiratory apnoea
     - Peripheral vasoconstriction
     - Adrenal catecholamine release
     - Vascular splenic contraction
2 **Short-term immersion** (3–15 min)
   - Coordination loss
     - Extremity cooling
     - Hyperventilation-induced tetany
     - Shivering thermogenesis
   - Slower nerve conduction with cooling
   - Loss of tactility and weakness
   - Life-saving tasks impaired
   - Swimming failure
3 **Long-term immersion** (>30 min)
   - *Hypothermia*: core temperature < 35°C
   - Ataxia, shivering, dysarthria, apathy, amnesia first signs to develop
   (See Chapter 58 Hypothermia)

4 Circumrescue collapse
- *Hypovolaemia*: cold diuresis, loss of hydrostatic cephalad blood displacement ('hydrostatic squeeze')
- *Sympathetic 'slump'*: decreased circulating catecholamines
- *Core afterdrop*: dysrhythmias from sudden cardiac cooling

What is the pathophysiology of submersion injuries?

Loss of protective measures:
- Initial breath hold
- Swallowing
- Loss of breath hold (20 s–5 min) causing inhalation
- Laryngospasm
- Laryngeal muscle relaxation
- Mass aspiration

Effects of aspiration:
- Hypoxia and hypercapnia from water in alveolar spaces preventing gas transport
- Uncontrolled respiration
- Hypoxaemic LOC, apnoea, cardiac arrest
- Other contributing mechanisms
  - Surfactant washout, alveolar collapse
  - Bronchospasm
  - Alveolar toxicity, oedema
  - V/Q mismatch
  - ARDS

How would you resuscitate a drowned patient?

General resuscitation
- *Dynamic risk assessment*: rescuer safety, chances of survival
- Manage as trauma patient depending on likely mechanism
- Rescue lying down not upright (avoid circulatory collapse on removal from water)
- Remove clothing if minimal displacement possible, avoid massage
- Dry and warm patient as required
- Highest F_IO_2 until titration possible with reliable S_pO_2 (94–95%) or P_aO_2 (10–13 kPa)

Cardiac arrest
- Five rescue breaths/ventilations first using 100% oxygen if available
- *CPR 30:2*: compression only technique inappropriate
- Intubate trachea if safe to do so (high risk of aspiration from water-filled stomach)
- *Consideration of hypothermia if core temperature < 35°C*: warming, adjustment of drug dosing intervals/defibrillation
- Consider E-CPR

(See Chapter 58 Hypothermia)

What are the priorities in ongoing management?

- Secondary survey
- Supportive care
  - LPV
  - *Optimise haemodynamics*: may require significant volume replacement
  - Neuroprotection
  - Management of electrolyte abnormalities occasionally
- Management of underlying condition that may have led to drowning (e.g. intoxication)
- Consider antimicrobials if contaminated water or signs of pneumonia
- Safeguarding reporting where required
- Police involvement may be required

What is the prognosis in drowning?

Drowning is preventable but, once it has occurred, its prognosis depends on **time to rescue** and **water temperature** amongst other factors. These features are used in determining appropriate search durations. Salinity of water has an inconsistent effect on outcome.

At scene
- 0°C: death within 1 h
- 15°C: survival up to 5 h
- Higher chance of survival ≥ 16°C

Poor prognostic indicators – from paediatrics:

- Immersion > 10 min – poor neurological recovery
- Time to BLS > 10 min after arrest
- Persisting GCS < 5
- Core temperature > 33°C on arrival
- Water temperature > 10°C (if survival to rescue)
- Persistent pH < 7.1 or P_aO_2 < 8 kPa despite treatment

Resources
- Brooks CJ. Survival in cold water: a report Prepared for Transport Canada. August 2001. Available from: https://www.dco.uscg.mil/Portals/9/DCO%20Documents/5p/CG-5PC/CG-CVC/CVC3/notice/flyers/Cold_Water_Survival_Hypothermia.pdf. (Accessed 17 January 2022.)
- Deakin CD, Soar J, Davies R, et al. Resuscitation Council UK: Special Circumstances Guidelines. May 2021. Available from: https://www.resus.org.uk/library/2021-resuscitation-guidelines/special-circumstances-guidelines. (Accessed 17 January 2022.)
- Farstad DJ, Dunn JA. Cold water immersion syndrome and whitewater recreation fatalities. Wilderness Environ Med. 2019;30(3):321–327.
- The child with an electrical injury or drowning. In: Samuels M, Wieteska S (Eds.) Advanced Paediatric Life Support: A Practical Approach to Emergencies, 6th ed. Chichester: John Wiley & Sons; 2016:161–166.
- World Health Organisation. Global Report on Drowning: Preventing a Leading Killer. November 2014. Available from: https://www.who.int/publications/i/item/global-report-on-drowning-preventing-a-leading-killer. (Accessed 17 January 2022.)

---

54. BURNS

In which situations might a patient sustain burns?

- Scalds (54% of those admitted to hospital)
- Contact burns (23%)
- *Other (16%)*: fires, explosions

Mechanisms include thermal, chemical, electrical, cold, and radiation injuries (e.g. sunburn).

(See Chapter 49 Major Trauma and Chapter 55 Electrical Injury)

What are the main concerns when managing patients presenting with burns?

General
- Safety for first responders to approach
- Possibility of multiple casualties including children
- May require transfer to tertiary centre
- Police involvement
- Safeguarding issues

Patient

- Trauma patient, may have other injuries – blast, jumping to escape fire
- External vs internal (airway) burns, inhalational injury
- Potential difficult airway
- Inhaled substance toxicity (e.g. CO, cyanide)
- Loss of skin integrity, susceptibility to infection
- Significant fluid shifts
- Pain
- Cause of burn or fire (e.g. intoxication, collapse from another cause)
- Mental health concerns (e.g. self-harm)

How is the extent of skin burns assessed?

Body surface area (BSA) may be assessed in different ways. The Wallace Rule of Nines is described below. Regions are allocated a percentage BSA, which are then totalled. Simple erythema is excluded. Alternatives include the use of Lund-Browder charts, palm area 1% rule, or smartphone apps.

> **KEY POINT**
>
> Wallace Rule of Nines (%):
>
> - *Adult*: Head 9, Anterior torso 18, Back 18, Arm 9, Arm 9, Leg 18, Leg 18, Perineum 1
> - *Child*: **Head 18**, Anterior torso 18, Back 18, Arm 9, Arm 9, **Leg 13.5, Leg 13.5**, Perineum 1

Depth (previously first, second, third degree)

- *Superficial (epidermis only)*: erythema
- **Partial-thickness**
  - *Superficial (touches dermis)*: pale, painful, blistering, rapid CR
  - *Deep (extension into dermis)*: blotchy, cherry red, ± pain, blistering, sluggish CR or non-blanching
- *Full-thickness (entire dermis)*: dry, white/brown/black, no blisters, leathery/waxy, painless, non-blanching

What is the pathophysiology behind the sequelae of major burns?

'Major burns' involve **>15% total BSA**. The pathophysiology largely depends on the extent of tissue affected.

Local effects

- **Zone of coagulation**
  - Direct injury resulting in dead tissue
- **Zone of stasis**
  - Injury results in vasoconstriction and hypoperfusion
  - Vulnerability to ischaemia, infection, necrosis
  - Burn wound may expand and deepen
- **Zone of hyperaemia**
  - Inflammation triggered by necrotic tissue
  - Vasodilatation, increased vascular permeability, oedema
  - Hypovolaemia exacerbated by fluid shift
  - Further tissue hypoperfusion

Systemic effects

- *SIRS*: associated with burns >25% BSA
- *Burns shock*: hypovolaemia, myocardial depression
- *Rhabdomyolysis*: significant direct and indirect muscle injury
- *Hypermetabolic phase*: from around 48 h to 1 year post injury

Concomitant inhalational injury may also be significant. (See Chapter 44 Inhalational Injury)

How would you manage the intubated patient with major burns?

- **Respiratory support** (see Chapter 44 Inhalational Injury)
- **Cardiovascular support**
  - Fluid resuscitation using **Parkland formula** if >15% BSA (10% in children)
  - Prevent moisture loss with emollient and 'cling film' dressing
  - Consider deresuscitation with HAS and diuresis in later stage of admission
- **Immediate surgery** may be indicated
  - Fasciotomy
  - *Escharotomy*: large or circumferential chest/neck burns
- **Metabolic modulation** – to attenuate hypermetabolism and hypercatabolism
  - Analgesia
  - Warm ambient temperature (28–30°C)
  - *Early excision surgery*: deep burn debridement reduces necrotic load, infection risk, SIRS
  - *Oxandrolone*: stimulates protein synthesis
  - GH might be of value in children with > 60% burns
- **Management of toxins** (see Chapter 44 Inhalational Injury and Chapter 39 Environmental Poisons)

What is the Parkland formula?

This is a formula used to calculate the fluid volume requirement for burns resuscitation in the first 24 h (from time of injury).

> **KEY POINT**
>
> Parkland Formula
>
> - Volume (ml) = 4 ml × %BSA × actual body weight (kg)
> - Give half in 8 h, half in subsequent 16 h

Crystalloid should be used initially, with evidence suggesting harm from HAS in the early phase. Third space loss will be significant and HAS may be considered later.

A modified formula has been suggested, with the aim to limit excessive fluid administration. Conversely, many patients will require larger volumes and under-resuscitation carries significant problems. Individual circumstances and the evolving clinical picture should be taken into consideration. Hct and UO (ideally 0.5–1 ml/kg/h by IBW) can be used to guide ongoing resuscitation. (See Chapter 11 Fluids)

What is the mortality of major burns?

The revised Baux score is used most widely to predict mortality.

> **KEY POINT**
>
> Revised Baux score = age + %BSA (+17 if inhalational injury present)

The '**point of futility**' was originally defined as a score of 100, whereby predicted mortality approaches 100%. However, improvements in burn care have meant that this now overestimates mortality. This point has been increased to 160. The 'Baux50' describes the score at which predicted mortality is 50%, approximately 110. Using the Baux score, all children are deemed potential survivors.

Mortality aside, the morbidity of major burns is significant and will require intensive aftercare for years to come.

Give some examples of the ongoing issues in the care of burns patients on the critical care unit.

- Complex dressings and emollient routine
- Difficulty monitoring with loss of skin integrity, dressings

- High nutritional requirement
- Capillary leak and positive fluid balance
- Difficult diagnosis of complications such as sepsis
- Requirement for reconstructive surgery
- Pain
- Psychological trauma
- Significant LOS

What considerations are made to nutrition in major burns?

Nutritional requirements are significant to counteract hypermetabolism, wound healing, and fluid shifts/exudate.

Protein

- Higher requirement in this patient group, around **1.5–2.0 g/kg/day** (1.5–3.0 g/kg/day in children)
- Enteral, high-protein nutrition should be initiated **within 12 h of injury**.
- Carbohydrate should not exceed 60% total energy intake (or 5 mg/kg/min), targeting a glucose level of 4.5–8 mmol/l.
- **Glutamine** or ornithine alpha-ketoglutarate supplementation is recommended.
- Methods to increase protein synthesis
  - Oxandrolone
  - Non-selective beta-blockers (e.g. propranolol)
  - Recombinant human GH in children

Micronutrient supplementation

- Zinc
- Copper
- Selenium
- Vitamins B1, C, D, E

Additional supplementation might include the following:

- Magnesium
- Phosphate
- Folate

GUIDELINE   ESPEN 2013 Major burns

(See Chapter 17 Nutrition)

How would you approach burn sepsis?

There are many confounding factors in diagnosing burn sepsis. Pyrexia, inflammation, and a hypermetabolic state are common to both processes. Specific criteria have been designed, but diagnosis remains difficult. Most clinicians would consider regular microbiological surveillance, prevention of infection where possible, and use of focused antimicrobials for confirmed infection.

Resources

- Gill P, Martin RV. Smoke inhalation injury. BJA Educ. 2015;15(3):143–148.
- McCann C, Watson A, Barnes D. Major burns: Part 1. Epidemiology, pathophysiology and initial management. BJA Educ. 2022;22(3):94–103.
- McGovern C, Puxty K, Paton L. Major burns: Part 2. Anaesthesia, intensive care and pain management. BJA Educ. 2022;22(4):138–145.

55.   ELECTRICAL INJURY

What is the significance of electrical injury in critical care?

- Patients with electrical injuries may be critically unwell.
- Electricity used therapeutically carries significant risk.
- Electrical equipment in an oxygen-rich environment poses a hazard to staff.
- Uncommon; team experience may be limited.
- Often coexisting acute pathology requires consideration.
- Mass casualty incidents are possible.

What sources might be implicated in electrocution?

- Faulty equipment or inadequate safety precautions
  - External (e.g. mains supply to ventilator)
  - Internal (e.g. CVC microshock)
- Complication of therapeutic electricity (e.g. DCCV, DC shock, electroconvulsive therapy, dia-thermy, ICD)
  - Short-circuit during contact
  - Arcing through ionised air
  - Mistimed electricity (e.g. R on T phenomenon during cardioversion)
- Intentional harm (e.g. taser shock)
- Lightning strike

What are the risk factors for electrical injury?

- *Age < 6 years*: accidental play with electrical equipment
- *Construction work*: electricians, painters
- *Male sex*: largely due to occupational demographic
- *Outdoor sports*: lightning strike

What are the main mechanisms of injury from electricity?

Current sources
- *Resistive coupling*: tissue path completes a circuit
- *Capacitive coupling*: tissue acting as a plate of a capacitor

Processes
- Electrocution
- Electrical burns (direct)
- Burns from electrical fire
- Traumatic complications: falls, blast injury, tetanic contraction
- Power failure elsewhere following surge

What factors influence the severity of electrical injury?

Current
- Amplitude high
  - Resistance low (see path)
  - Voltage high
- Path
  - Presence of earthing pad
  - Direction of travel and proximity to significant tissue (e.g. myocardium)
  - Impedance from other tissue (e.g. thickness of fat layer)
- Density
- *Type*: AC worse at low current than DC
- Duration

Environment
- Ambient oxygen concentration
- Humidity
- Ventilation

Patient
- Body habitus
- Other pre-morbid state
- Medications altering electrical conduction (e.g. seizure threshold)
- Factors affecting heat distribution (e.g. volume status)

What is the pathophysiology of electrocution?

- Intrinsic electrical currents responsible for cell processes
  - Neuronal impulse transmission
  - Myocardial conduction
  - Voltage-gated ion channels
- Additional current can disrupt these functions
- Thermal injury to tissues occurs when electrical energy is converted to heat

What are the clinical effects or complications of electrocution?

Effects may vary from mild to multi-organ dysfunction and death. Those relevant to critical care include the following:

- *A*: laryngospasm, aspiration
- *B*: ventilatory failure
- *C*: VF, asystole, myocardial injury and dysfunction
- *D*: coma, encephalopathy, autonomic dysfunction, peripheral nerve injury, seizures
- *E*: tetany, fractures and other musculoskeletal injury, pain, burns, tympanic rupture, cateracts
- *F*: rhabdomyolysis, effects of oedema on nearby tissues, compartment syndrome
- *G*: bowel contusion, ileus
- *H*: thrombosis

Burns with a small contact wound may be extensive internally. The psychological impact may be significant.

What are the priorities in clinical management of the electrically injured patient?

- Rescuer safety, including avoidance of wet areas
- Stopping current flow and burning
- Consideration of major trauma including cervical spine injury
- Seeking location of entry and exit wounds (may assist in anticipation of injuries)
- Patient extrication to place of safety
- Potential for prolonged resuscitation
- Management of burns
- Tetanus management and antibiotics as indicated
- Reporting and retirement/replacement of faulty equipment

Can you describe some specific resuscitation measures?

- *A*: intubation and ventilation if unconscious or significant systemic injury/taken to theatre
- *B*: LPV, management of airway burns
- *C*: fluid resuscitation for burns, vasoactive drugs for SIRS/myocardial dysfunction
- *D*: neuroprotective measures, normoglycaemia
- *E*: injury surveys, burns dressings
- *F*: fluid and electrolyte management for rhabdomyolysis

How might electrical injury be prevented?

Electrical safety is the mainstay in preventing injuries:

- Earthing
- Fuses

- Circuit breakers
- Equipment classification
- System checks
- Training

What do you know about lightning strike?

- Lightning strike is a high-tension electrical injury with voltage much higher than that found in domestic circumstances.
- Lightning might cause injury from direct contact, side-flash, or ground current electrocution.
  - Most damage caused by heat from high amplitude current
  - Heat may ignite clothes
  - Severe muscle contraction may cause a person to be 'thrown'
- Spider-like appearance of entrance and exit sites
- Initial LOC common with neurological stunning (e.g. fixed pupils)
- Despite this, prognosis may be good with 80–90% survival
- Survivors may suffer from cardiovascular complications and neurological sequelae including weakness, tingling, muscle spasms, blindness, autonomic disruption (e.g. dry eyes), pain and psychological issues.

Resources

- Critchley LAH, Electrical safety and injuries. In: Bersten AD, Handy JM, (Eds.) Oh's Intensive Care Manual, 8th ed. Amsterdam: Elsevier Limited; 2019:999–1005.
- Dheansa B, Berner JE. BMJ Best Practice: Electrical Injury. Available from: https://bestpractice.bmj.com/topics/en-gb/655. (Accessed 18 January 2022.)
- Nickson C. Life in the Fast Lane: Electrical Injury. Available from: https://litfl.com/electrical-injury/. (Accessed 17 January 2022.)
- Nickson C. Life in the Fast Lane: Lightning injury. Available from: https://litfl.com/lightning-injury/. (Accessed 17 January 2022.)

56. GAS EMBOLISM

What is vascular gas embolism?

Vascular gas embolism (VGE) is the entrainment of gas from the environment into the circulation with systemic effects. Effects may vary from mild to rapid deterioration with permanent neurological injury or cardiac arrest. Several gases can be implicated: air, oxygen, CO_2 (laparoscopy), helium (IABP).

Arterial gas embolism

- Gas enters arterial circulation
- Emboli travel to distal capillary beds
- Ischaemic effects
- Notable in coronary or cerebral circulations

Venous gas embolism

- Gas enters venous circulation
- Embolises to RA, RV, lungs
- Large amounts will cause obstructive shock, right HF, and cardiac arrest
- May embolise to the RCA causing dysrhythmias

GUIDELINE ICS 2019 Gas embolism

How might gas enter the circulation?

Arterial
- Cardiovascular procedures (e.g. imaging, interventional, surgical)
- Pulmonary veins
  - Barotrauma during positive-pressure ventilation
  - Chest trauma
  - Decompression sickness (e.g. diving ascent, aircraft pressure change)
  - Blast injury
- Paradoxical embolism
  - Intracardiac right-left shunt
  - Pulmonary arterio-venous malformation
  - Overwhelmed pulmonary filter mechanism

Venous
- Venous line insertion, manipulation, removal
- Insufflation of body cavities with open venous channels (e.g. pneumoperitoneum)

Retrograde cerebral venous gas embolism (RCVGE)
- Venous gas bubbles float upwards to cerebral venous system

Which procedures carry the highest risk for VGE?

- Sitting position craniotomy
- Posterior fossa/neck surgery
- Laparoscopy
- Total hip arthroplasty
- Caesarean delivery
- CVC insertion/removal
- Craniosynostosis repair

Other significant aetiologies include other cranial/spinal surgery, prostatectomy, GI endoscopy, contrast radiography, blood product transfusion, coronary/open heart surgery, lung biopsy, and hydrogen peroxide ingestion.

What is the pathophysiology of gas embolism?

Gas bubbles acting as a foreign substance
- Coagulation cascade activated
- Increased C3a and C5a
- Prostaglandin and leukotriene synthesis
- Platelet and leukocyte activation
- Ongoing microcirculation impairment
- Fibrin release, adhesion to endothelium
- Vasospasm then vasodilatation

Cerebral effects
- Damage to blood-brain barrier
- Cerebral oedema
- Raised ICP and sequelae

Arterial
- *Large volume*: immediate coronary or cerebral embolism, death
- **0.02 ml/kg** potentially fatal
- *Smaller volume*: peripheral capillary bed involvement, organ ischaemia

Venous
- *Large volume*: cardiac output cessation, circulatory collapse, refractory arrest
- *Smaller volume*: filtered by lung bed, full recovery possible
  - May travel to brain in retrograde manner
  - May arterialise with ischaemic effects

How is gas embolism prevented?

- Staff training and awareness
- Careful counselling for awake procedures
- Priming of equipment
- Use of appropriate clamps, valves, caps on lines
- Infusion pumps with air-in-line sensors and alarms
- *CVC*: secure well, remove safely, avoid sitting position and short entry path during insertion

How should a central venous catheter be removed to prevent VGE?

- Trendelenberg position
- Firm digital pressure for 5 min after haemostasis
- Occlusive dressing
- Patient advised to lie flat for 60 min after removal

How is VGE diagnosed?

VGE is a clinical diagnosis and a high index of suspicion is required. Gas bubbles or effects may be seen on imaging: TTE, TOE, CT, MR. It should be suspected in any periprocedural stroke or neurological event.

- Cardiovascular
  - Dyspnoea, chest pain
  - Dysrhythmias, hypotension, shock, JVP distension
  - **'Mill wheel murmur'**
  - Cardiac arrest
- Neurological
  - Restlessness, anxiety, feeling of impending doom
  - Altered mental state, seizures, hemiparesis, coma
- Subtle signs
  - **Cutis marmorata** (marble skin)
  - Retinal gas bubbles
  - **Liebermeister's sign** (tongue pallor)
- Sucking noise reported during gas entrainment

What are the management priorities in a patient with gas embolism?

Overcoming mechanical obstruction, limiting gas effects, and supportive care are the mainstays of treatment.

- **Minimise further gas entry**
  - *Check intravascular devices and recent removal sites*: connections, valves, air in lines, dressings/wounds
  - Notify surgeon to occlude entry sites (e.g. stop pneumoperitoneum, damp swab over cranial surgical field)
  - Lower surgical field to below the heart (short period only, then lie flat)
- **Reduce embolism size**
  - Highest possible F_1O_2
  - If CVC in situ, attempt aspiration
- **Resuscitation and supportive care**
  - Consider **Durant manoeuvre** (left lateral decubitus position)
  - CPR best supine and flat, may force air out of pulmonary outflow tract
  - Avoid prolonged Trendelenberg position to minimise cerebral oedema
  - Early vasopressors/inotropes
- **Consider differentials and evaluate extent of effects**
  - Neurological assessment
  - TTE/TOE
  - CT head and chest as soon as possible
- **Consider suitability for transfer for hyperbaric oxygen**

When is hyperbaric oxygen indicated?

Urgent hyperbaric oxygen is the most effective treatment and is ideal **within 6–7 h**, particularly if neurologically compromised. Delayed treatment might be considered and regular reassessment for transfer should be carried out. Transfer should occur at low altitude <1000 ft. In the UK, the nearest British Hyperbaric Association chamber and National Diving Accident Helpline should be contacted.

Contraindications include bullous lung disease and undrained PTX in which air leaks might be caused or exacerbated by hyperbaric conditions.

How does hyperbaric oxygen work in VGE?

- Reduces size of emboli (Boyle's law)
- Denitrogenation causes further embolus reduction
- Improves oxygen delivery to ischaemic penumbra
- Decreases ICP by cerebral arteriolar constriction
- Improves microcirculation
  - Inhibits membrane guanylate cyclase
  - This inhibits B2 integrin adherence
  - Decreases leukocyte 'stickiness'

57.   FAT EMBOLISM SYNDROME

What is fat embolism syndrome?

- **Fat embolism syndrome (FES)** is the clinical syndrome which follows an identifiable insult associated with release of fat into the circulation.
- **Fat embolism** is the presence of fat globules in the pulmonary microcirculation.

In which settings does FES occur?

- *Orthopaedic trauma*: closed long bone fractures in areas with high yellow marrow content
  - Femoral (0.5% incidence if isolated, increases with multiple fractures)
  - Pelvic
- Other (rare)
  - Pancreatitis
  - Sickle crisis
  - Alcoholic liver disease
  - Bone marrow harvest/transplant
  - Liposuction

What is the pathophysiology of FES?

The mechanisms of FES have not been fully elucidated. It is thought to be the result of 2 main processes and features may result from differing combinations of each:

Mechanical theory (obstructive)
- Small emboli
  - Fat migrates to venous sinusoids
  - Local platelet aggregation and accelerated fibrin generation (coagulation theory)
  - Complexes lodge in PA circulation
  - Pulmonary capillary obstruction
  - Interstitial haemorrhage, oedema, alveolar collapse, hypoxaemic vasoconstriction
- Large emboli:
  - Macrovascular obstruction
  - Shock

Biochemical theory (inflammatory):
- Fat is broken down by tissue lipases.
- Glycerol and toxic free fatty acids are released.
- In the lung, endothelial damage triggers proinflammatory cytokine cascade.
  - Phospholipase A2, TNF-a, IL-1, IL-6, ROS levels are elevated.
  - Progression to ARDS
- Other end-organ damage occurs.

Fat may cross the pulmonary to systemic circulation in 2 ways:

- Paradoxical embolism through intracardiac defect
- Traversing pulmonary capillary bed completely

How does FES manifest?

- Presentation is often 12–72 h post-insult.
- *Classic triad*: **hypoxaemia** (96%), **neurological features** (86%), **petechiae** (60%)
- Presentation may vary from subclinical to multi-organ dysfunction and death.
- High prevalence of subclinical fat embolism in trauma patients and those receiving CPR
- Potentially fully reversible, mortality < 10%

Systemic features
- *A/B*: dyspnoea, tachypnoea, hypoxaemia, ARDS
- *C*: RV dysfunction, biventricular failure, shock
- *D*: confusion, lethargy, agitation, coma, Purtscher's retinopathy, seizures, focal deficit
- *E*: petechial rash in non-dependent regions (conjunctivae, head, neck, axillae, thorax), pyrexia
- *F*: AKI, lipiduria, proteinuria, haematuria
- *G*: jaundice
- *H*: DIC

How would you diagnose FES?

- Can be difficult to diagnose, based on clinical features, requires high index of suspicion
- Does not require confirmation by sample containing fat globules
- Multiple scoring systems exist: Gurd, Lindeque, Schonfeld criteria

Specific investigations
- Biochemistry
  - May present with unexplained anaemia and thrombocytopaenia
  - Hypocalaemia possible (FFA binding to calcium)
  - Serum lipid concentration does not correlate with severity
    - ➢ PAC sampling lacks sensitivity and specificity
  - *Urine*: as above
- Cytology (blood, urine, sputum)
  - Free fat globules, fat within macrophages
  - BAL has been used
- Some characteristic radiological findings but none diagnostic
  - *CXR*: normal, ARDS, air space consolidation at periphery/bases from haemorrhage
  - *CT chest*: focal ground glass opacification, interlobular septal thickening
  - *MR brain*: high-intensity T2 signals (does correlate with degree of clinical impairment), 'starfield' appearance
  - Echo features as above

What are the Gurd criteria?
1 major + 4 minor criteria required for diagnosis of FES:

- Major
  - Petechial rash
  - Respiratory symptoms with radiographic changes
  - CNS signs unrelated to trauma/other

- Minor
  - Tachycardia
  - Pyrexia
  - Retinal changes
  - Renal abnormalities
  - Acute thrombocytopaenia
  - Acute decrease in Hb
  - High ESR
  - Fat globules in sputum

What are the management priorities in the critically unwell patient in whom you suspect FES?

Supportive care
- Respiratory support
- Fluid resuscitation often required
  - Crystalloid commonly
  - Albumin controversial in neurological injury but lowers circulating free fatty acids in animal models
- Vasoactive infusions ± pulmonary vasodilators
- Careful neurological monitoring, neuroprotection ± seizure prophylaxis
- Mechanical or extracorporeal support may be indicated

Anticoagulation
- May be difficult in this population
- Heparin thought to clear lipaemic serum but no benefit demonstrated
  - Lipase activation by heparin also potentially harmful
  - Therapeutic dose not used routinely
- Aspirin may have a role in embolic neurological deficit

Corticosteroids
- No benefit shown once syndrome established
- May have a role in fulminant FES

(Other—hypertonic glucose, NAC, aliskiren [renin inhibitor] also studied but not widely accepted.)

What do you know about prevention of FES?

- Some evidence for prophylactic corticosteroids in long bone fractures, consider if high risk
- Early surgical fixation (<24 h trauma) lowers risk
- Surgical technique may be important (e.g. limiting intramedullary pressure)
- Primary prevention of injuries would reduce prevalence

Resources
- Gupta A, Reilly CS. Fat embolism. CEACCP. 2007;7(5):148–151.
- Kosova E, Bermark B, Piazza G. Fat embolism syndrome. Circulation. 2015;131(3):317–320.
- Luff D, Hewson DW. Fat embolism syndrome. BJA Educ. 2021;21(9):322–328.

58. HYPOTHERMIA

What is hypothermia and how is it classified?

Hypothermia is a core body temperature of <35°C:

- *32–35°C*: mild

- *28–32°C*: moderate
- *<28°C*: severe

Swiss staging

  I Clearly conscious, shivering
  II Impaired consciousness without shivering
  III Unconscious
  IV Not breathing
  V Death due to irreversible hypothermia

What causes hypothermia?

- *Excess heat loss*: trauma, surgery, environmental, skin disease, iatrogenic
- *Insufficient heat production*: hypometabolic states (e.g. hypothyroidism)
- *Disordered thermoregulation*: hypothalamic disease, behavioural (e.g. intoxication)

What are the clinical effects and complications of hypothermia?

Hypothermia causes multisystem effects as demonstrated below (Table 58.1). The cardiovascular, neurological and immunological responses are significant in critical care.

ECG findings

- Broadening of the PR interval, QRS complex, QT interval
- Subsequent presence of Osborn/J waves <33°C

How would you adapt resuscitation for a hypothermic patient in cardiac arrest?

- Pulse check for 1 min
- 3 × DC shock for VF, then no more until >30°C
- <30°C: no drugs

Table 58.1 Effects of hypothermia at different temperatures (°C)

	<35	<33	<30	<28	<24	<20
A	Loss of cough reflex Bronchorrhoea					
B	Depression Bradypnoea			Apnoea		
C	Vasoconstriction Hypertension Tachycardia Then bradycardia	Bradycardia AF		VF VT		Asystole
D	Depression ↓ CMR, protective		Fixed dilated pupils	Loss of deep tendon reflexes		Isoelectric EEG
E	7% BMR drop per 1°C Shivering max 35°C	Shiver lost < 32°C				
F	Diuresis – vasoconstriction, ADH resistance Metabolic acidosis ↑ K⁺, Mg²⁺					
G	↓ GI motility ↓ hepatic blood flow (and drug metabolism) ↓ glu/fat metabolism, hyperglycaemia					
H	↑ viscosity Thrombocytopaenia					
I	↓ WCC Impaired immunity					

- *30–35°C*: double drug dose interval
- Must be > 30–32°C to diagnose death

How might you warm a hypothermic patient?

- *Passive*: dry, warm environment, insulate
- *Active*
  - *Less invasive*: encourage movement, forced air warmer, warm pads
  - *Invasive*: warmed inhaled gases, IV fluids, body cavity lavage (thoracic, urinary, gastric, peritoneal)

(See Chapter 16 Temperature Control and Chapter 53 Drowning)

Resources

- Deakin CD, Soar J, Davies R, et al. Resuscitation Council UK: Special Circumstances Guidelines. May 2021. Available from: https://www.resus.org.uk/library/2021-resuscitation-guidelines/special-circumstances-guidelines. (Accessed 17 January 2022.)
- Nickson C. Life in the Fast Lane: Hypothermia. Available from: https://litfl.com/hypothermia/. (Accessed 17 January 2022.)

59. MALIGNANT HYPERTHERMIA

How do core and peripheral temperature differ?

Core temperature is usually 1–2°C higher than peripheral temperature but might be more markedly different on a cold day. The 'core' includes deeper structures such as the brain, intra-thoracic and intra-abdominal and pelvic organs. Core temperature is more useful in most clinical situations.

Time of day and hormonal cycles will affect a person's temperature, and this will vary by 0.5–1.0°C between individuals.

What are the different types of elevated body temperature and how do they differ?

Hyperthermia and fever are the main types of elevated body temperature above 37.5°C. Definitions vary with the threshold anywhere from 37.5 to 38.3°C.

> **KEY POINT**
>
> **Hyperthermia** results from an imbalance of heat production, regulation and loss. Some patients may be more at risk (e.g. extremes of age, high BMI).
> Fever and pyrexia are used interchangeably although subtly different:
>
> - *Fever*: condition in which the hypothalamic set point is raised
> - *Pyrexia*: elevated measured temperature

'Hyperpyrexia' refers to a body temperature >41°C. It is a misnomer as this state is more common in hyperthermic conditions (Table 59.1).

What are the differential diagnoses of perioperative hyperthermia?

- *Excessive heating/environmental*: particularly in infants or children
- Surgical devices (e.g. diathermy)
- Prolonged epidural anaesthesia

Table 59.1 Comparison of hyperthermia and fever

	Hyperthermia	Fever
Hypothalamic set point	Normal	Raised
Response to antipyretics	No	Yes
Extreme elevation	More common	Less common
Examples	Environmental • Heat stroke (>40.6°C) Endocrine • Thyrotoxicosis • Phaeochromocytoma • Adrenal crisis Drug reaction • NMS • MH • Serotonin syndrome	Infectious Non-infectious • Drug reaction (e.g. toxic epidermal necrolysis [TEN]) • VTE • Neurological injury • Pancreatitis • Autoimmune (e.g. SLE) • Neoplastic • Drug withdrawal • Transfusion reaction

- 'Septic shower' (e.g. during manipulation of urological stent)
- Transfusion reaction
- Allergic reaction

What is malignant hyperthermia?

MH is a progressive, idiosyncratic drug reaction caused by specific anaesthetic agents. MH susceptibility is the genetic predisposition to develop MH when in contact with a trigger.

- Incidence 1:50000 UK population (1:3000–1:100000 MH susceptibility)
- 40–50 positive tests for MH susceptibility per year
- Autosomal dominant
- Defect in RYR1 or CACNA1S genes coding for ryanodine and dihydropyridine (DHPR) receptors

Trigger agents
- Suxamethonium
- Volatile anaesthetic agents: halothane, isoflurane, sevoflurane, enflurane, desflurane, ether, methoxyflurane

How does the pathophysiology of MH compare to normal muscle activity?

Normal excitation-contraction coupling (ECC) (conversion of electrical energy to muscle contraction)

- Action potential spreads across the muscle cell membrane
- DHPR receptors in the membrane T-tubules and ryanodine receptors in the sarcoplasmic reticulum interact to release calcium into the cytosol
- Calcium binds to troponin C on myofilaments causing cross bridge formation between actin and myosin, using ATP
- Muscle contraction occurs, using oxygen and releasing CO_2
- This interaction loses 60% energy supplied as heat

MH
- Dysregulated ECC causes sustained calcium release
- Increases metabolic demand for ATP
- Increased CO_2 production stimulates SNS resulting in tachycardia
- Muscle contraction follows increasing calcium release, followed by rigidity
- Excess heat is produced
- Rhabdomyolysis results from sustained contraction

How does MH present?

Characteristics
- Unexplained tachycardia

- Rising E_tCO_2
- Rise in core body temperature
- Muscle rigidity

Classified into 8 presentations:

1 Fulminant MH
2 Moderate features (resolved before life-threatening or diagnosis confirmed)
3 Mild features (1 or more metabolic signs)
4 Masseter spasm
5 Masseter spasm with rhabdomyolysis
6 Masseter spasm with metabolic disturbance
7 Unexplained perioperative death or arrest
8 Other: post-op pyrexia (commonest reason for referral), post-op rhabdomyolysis

Volatile anaesthetic agents are not limited to anaesthetic use in theatre and intensivists may become involved in a variety of contexts in addition to attendance in theatre:

- Pre-hospital analgesia (methoxyflurane inhalers)
- Refractory bronchospasm in ventilated patients (sevoflurane, isoflurane)
- Difficult sedation in paediatric intensive care (sevoflurane has been used)

What is the immediate management of a MH crisis?

- **Call for help**, extra personnel, declare incident
- **Minimise exposure** to trigger
  - Finish or abandon surgery as soon as possible
  - Remove vaporisers
  - Insert charcoal filters on the anaesthetic machine if available
  - If not, consider manual ventilation before a replacement ventilator
- **Reduce effects** of existing exposure
  - Increase fresh gas flow and hyperventilate with F_IO_2 1.0
  - Maintain anaesthesia with IV agent
- **Reduce metabolic demand**
  - Switch off active warming, expose patient
  - Paralyse with non-depolarising neuromuscular agent
  - Give dantrolene (2–3 mg/kg bolus, repeat every 5 min 1 mg/kg)
    - ➤ Target E_tCO_2 < 6 kPa, T < 38.5°C, normal MV
  - Active cooling
- **Monitoring/investigation**
  - Core and peripheral temperature, arterial BP, CVP
  - Group and save/cross match if not already done
  - Send every 30 min: U&E, CK, FBC, coagulation
  - Urinary myoglobin
- **Treat complications**
  - *Hyperkalaemia*: calcium, glucose/insulin, bicarbonate
  - *Arrhythmias*: magnesium, amiodarone, metoprolol
  - *Metabolic acidosis*: sodium bicarbonate
  - *Myoglobinaemia*: target UO ml/kg/h with crystalloid, consider forced alkaline diuresis ± RRT
  - *DIC*: transfusion

GUIDELINE   AoA 2020 Malignant hyperthermia

Can you describe the main difficulties in managing a MH crisis?

The above management will be **labour intensive** and roles should be delegated. The following is suggested by the AoA:

- *Nurse/ODP 1*: Runner: collect dantrolene, cold saline, insulin. Prepare lines.
- *Nurse/ODP 2*: Prepare dantrolene, documentation
- *Surgeon*: Finish surgery, catheterise, commence cooling
- *Anaesthetist 1*: Lead team
- *Anaesthetist 2*: Give dantrolene, start total intravenous anaesthesia (TIVA), manage complications
- *Anaesthetist 3*: Arterial line, send bloods, CVC, monitor temperature

Dantrolene is very difficult to mix as it is relatively insoluble and large volumes will be needed per dose. This may be done in a large sterile bowl by the scrub nurse.

The metabolic reaction **may return** up to 14 h after initial resolution.

What later actions will need to be taken?

- Explanation to patient ± family
- Local incident reporting
- Notify GP
- Referral for MH susceptibility investigation

What do you know about cooling in this context?

Cooling is key to preventing myocyte cell death. Active cooling measures include the following:

- *Environmental*: reducing ambient temperature, removing clothing/bedding
- *Non-invasive*: cooling blankets and ice packs to vascular areas (groin, axillae, anterior neck)
- *Lavage with cold water*: bladder, gastric, peritoneal
- *Extracorporeal devices*: CVVH, ECMO, CPB

(See Chapter 16 Temperature Control)

Resources

- Association of Anaesthetists. Quick Reference Handbook: Guidelines for Crises in Anaesthesia. 2021. Available from: https://anaesthetists.org/Portals/0/PDFs/Guidelines%20PDFs/QRII_complete_October%202021.pdf?ver=2021-11-09-135429-103. (Accessed 15 January 2022.)
- Gupta PK, Hopkins PM. Diagnosis and management of malignant hyperthermia. BJA Educ. 2017;17(7):249–254.
- Niven DJ, Laupland KB. Pyrexia: aetiology in the ICU. Crit Care. 2016;20(1):247.

SURGERY

60. EMERGENCY LAPAROTOMY

Can you name some common pathologies that may require an emergency laparotomy?

- Ischaemic bowel
- Small or large bowel obstruction
- Perforated duodenal ulcer
- Uncontrollable haemorrhage (e.g. traumatic, post-operative)
- Intra-abdominal sepsis with collection

Do you know of any pathologies in which early laparotomy is associated with worse outcome?

Patients with acute pancreatitis should be managed conservatively where possible in the first 2 weeks as early surgery is associated with high mortality. Any relook laparotomy carries significant risk of morbidity.

What makes surgery high-risk?

Surgery may be deemed 'high-risk' for many reasons involving a combination of patient, anaesthetic, surgical and institutional factors. The risk usually relates to intra- or post-operative morbidity and mortality.

Assessment of risk is complex and requires a judicious multi-disciplinary effort involving history-taking, examination, investigation, and knowledge of available options. Shared decision-making is key and consent surrounding the balance of acceptable quality of life and use of resources is sometimes tricky to navigate. The subjective communication and interpretation of risk makes this all the more difficult and the value of scoring systems in these discussions is controversial.

Relating to emergency laparotomy, one of the most widely used scores is P-POSSUM. A threshold of 5% 30-day mortality is used to determine 'high-risk' cases and often influences the decision for post-operative admission to critical care. In addition, any indicator of frailty may deem a patient 'high-risk'.

Ancillary investigations that may be helpful include echo, previous cardiopulmonary exercise or stress test results, and anaesthetic charts.

In summary, 'high-risk' is a subjective assessment of an individual's situation in which there is expected to be a high burden of an indicated operation, which may compromise outcomes important to the patient.

Which parameters are included in the P-POSSUM score?

Physiological (highest scoring criteria in brackets)
- General
  - Age (> 70 years)

- Cardiac failure (raised JVP, cardiomegaly)
- Dyspnoea (at rest, pulmonary fibrosis, or consolidation on CXR)
- Observations
  - Systolic BP (< 90 mmHg)
  - HR (< 40 or > 120/min)
  - GCS (< 9)
- Serum bloods
  - Hb (< 100 or > 180 g/l)
  - WCC (> 20 or < 3 × 10⁹/l)
  - Urea (> 15 mg/dl)
  - Sodium (< 126 mmol/l)
  - Potassium (< 2.9 or > 5.9 mmol/l)
- Presence of ECG abnormality (abnormal rhythm except AF with rate 60–90, > 4 ectopics per minute, Q waves, or ST-segment/T-wave changes)

Operative
- Operation type (complex major)
- Number of procedures (>2)
- Blood loss (>1000 ml)
- Peritoneal contamination (free bowel content, pus, or blood)
- Malignancy status (malignancy with distant metastases)
- NCEPOD classification (emergency within 2 h)

What is pre-operative patient optimisation?

Optimisation is the correction of physiological derangement prior to surgery with a view to improving outcomes. It is more time-sensitive if the procedure is not arranged electively.

An individualised balance of intervention load and surgical timing must be struck. This may involve management of haemodynamics, electrolytes, blood glucose, and transfusion, amongst other parameters. Issues surrounding consent may need to be managed concomitantly.

Optimisation requires multi-disciplinary input and is often led by the anaesthetist in more urgent cases. Interventions may occur in a variety of locations including the emergency department, ward, theatre recovery (or high dependency area), critical care, anaesthetic room, or theatre itself.

What is 'National Emergency Laparotomy Audit (NELA)'?

NELA is a centrally funded clinical project in the UK, founded in 2012, which aims to improve the quality of care for patients undergoing emergency laparotomy through the provision of high-quality comparative data. Some patient groups are excluded from analysis (e.g. children, trauma/vascular laparotomy).

Can you name any examples of quality standards in emergency laparotomy?

- Time to consultant review
- Time to first dose of antibiotics
- Elapsed time between decision to operate and entry to theatre
- Proportion of patients with documented pre-operative objective assessment of risk of mortality and morbidity, carried out at time of consent
- Proportion of patients in which goal-directed fluid therapy was utilised
- Proportion of patients in which seniority of surgeon/anaesthetist was appropriate to the risk of death (consultant if ≥5% unless junior staff have adequate experience and manpower with no competing responsibilities; all cases ≥ 10%)
- Proportion of eligible patients reviewed by elderly medicine specialist post-operatively

Which outcome measures are recorded?

- Short-term mortality (30 days)
- Unplanned escalation of care from ward

- Proportion of patients with unplanned return to theatre in same admission
- Length of post-operative hospital stay
- Thirty-day unplanned readmission

What is 'Enhanced Recovery After Surgery (ERAS)'?

The ERAS Society have developed guidelines to provide a multimodal perioperative care pathway, designed to achieve early recovery for patients undergoing major surgery.

This initiative has demonstrated benefit in LOS, complications, and costs of some elective surgical procedures.

GUIDELINE   ERAS 2018 Colorectal surgery

Some principles are transferable to the emergency laparotomy and are relevant to critical care. This involves a balance of appropriate continuation of therapy vs 'de-medicalising' patients, alongside specific interventions to promote recovery. Examples include the following:

- Removal of indwelling devices
- Optimal fluid management
- Recommencing EN
- Early mobilisation
- Physiotherapy

Resource

- National Emergency Laparotomy Audit. Principle Standards Reported by the National Emergency Laparotomy Audit (NELA). Available from: https://www.nela.org.uk/Standards-Documents. (Accessed 19 January 2022.)

---

61. SPLENIC INJURY

Give some common causes of splenic injury

- Polytrauma (e.g. road traffic collision)
- Blunt force injury (e.g. fighting, sports, handlebar injury)
- Penetrating trauma (e.g. abdominal stabbing)
- Post-procedural (e.g. colonic resection)
- Spontaneous rupture (e.g. infectious mononucleosis)

What is the significance of splenic laceration?

- Can cause significant blood loss and instability
- Asplenism and associated complications

What is asplenism?

Asplenism is the loss of functioning spleen. The spleen may be absent (i.e. splenectomy) or still present with 'functional asplenism' in which tissue does not work well (e.g. sickle cell, coeliac disease). Consequences include immunocompromise and a prothrombotic tendency.

How is splenic laceration graded?

Splenic laceration is graded by size, significance of haematoma, and vascular injury. If there are multiple splenic injuries (up to grade 3), grade should increase by 1 (Table 61.1).

Table 61.1   Summary of splenic laceration classification

Grade	Parenchymal laceration	Haematoma
1	<1 cm	Subcapsular < 10% surface area Capsular tear
2	1–3 cm	Subcapsular 10–50% surface area Intraparenchymal < 5 cm
3	>3 cm	Subcapsular > 50% surface area Ruptured subcapsular/intraparenchymal haematoma ≥ 5 cm
4	>25% devascularisation (segmental/hilar)	
	Any splenic vascular injury Active bleeding confined within splenic capsule	
5	Any splenic vascular injury with active bleeding beyond spleen into peritoneum	

What are the main therapeutic options for the trauma patient with splenic laceration?

- *Conservative management*: non-interventional (e.g. transfusion) in less extensive injuries
- *IR*: embolisation often attempted first line
- *Laparotomy*: emergency splenectomy if failed IR or other priorities

(See Chapter 49 Major Trauma)

What is overwhelming post-splenectomy infection (OPSI)?

OPSI is rare but rapidly fatal unless treated. It is often caused by encapsulated organisms against which the spleen usually protects:

- *Yersinia pestis*
- *Escherichia coli*
- *Salmonella typhi*
- *Streptococcus pneumoniae/pyogenes*
- *Neisseria meningitidis*
- *Klebsiella pneumoniae*
- *Haemophilus influenzae type b*
- *Pseudomonas aeruginosa*
- *Bordatella pertussis, Bacillus anthracis*
- *Cryptococcus neoformans*

How are asplenic patients managed pharmacologically?

- Antibiotic prophylaxis in high risk of pneumococcal infection (oral phenoxymethylpenicillin or erythromycin):
  - Extremes of age
  - Poor response to vaccination
  - Previous invasive pneumococcal disease
  - Underlying haematological malignancy as indication for splenectomy
- Immunisation

Which immunisations are recommended?

- Vaccination against Meningitis C (*N. meningitidis*) and *H. influenzae* type b is recommended. This should take place 2 weeks prior to elective splenectomy or in convalescence after emergency procedures.
- **Meningococcal groups A, C, W, Y, and B** may be offered
- Pneumococcal vaccination (*S. pneumoniae*) with booster every 5 years
- Annual **Influenza** vaccination

Resources

- Davies JM, Lewis MP, Wimperis J, et al. Review of guidelines for the prevention and treatment of infection in patients with an absent or dysfunctional spleen: prepared on behalf of the British Committee for Standards in Haematology by a Working Party of the Haemato-Oncology Task Force. Br J Haematol. 2011;155(3):308–317.
- Kozar RA, Crandall M, Shanmuganathan K, et al. Organ injury scaling 2018 update: spleen, liver, and kidney. J Trauma Acute Care Surg. 2018;85(6):1119–1122.

---

62. ACUTE PANCREATITIS

What is acute pancreatitis?

Acute pancreatitis is an inflammatory condition of the pancreas.

It is caused by gallstones and alcohol excess most commonly. Other causes include ischaemia, drugs (e.g. steroids), hypothermia, hypercalcaemia, trauma (including ERCP), cystic fibrosis, primary sclerosing cholangitis and viral disease (e.g. EBV, HIV, CMV, possibly SARS-CoV-2).

How is acute pancreatitis diagnosed?

Diagnosis involves both the clinical and biochemical pictures, with serum pancreatic enzyme measurement – the gold standard tool. **Serum lipase** is more reliable than serum amylase as a diagnostic marker and is recommended as such.

Scoring tools include the Ranson and Glasgow criteria, requiring 48 h of assessment. If there is no history of gallstones or alcohol excess, serum triglycerides and calcium should be measured (triglycerides > 11.3 mmol/l diagnostic). Severity should be stratified within 48 h of diagnosis to guide management.

Imaging
- US should be performed on admission
- CT if doubt about presence of pancreatitis
- SAP should be assessed with CT
    - Ideally 72–96 h after onset of symptoms
    - Follow-up 7–10 days after initial CT
    - Additional imaging if clinical deterioration, failure to improve, or for intervention
- Magnetic resonance cholangiopancreatography (MRCP) or endoscopic US indicated if idiopathic to rule out occult biliary disease (then MRI)

GUIDELINE   UK WPAP 2005 Acute pancreatitis

How is acute pancreatitis classified?

The **Revised Atlanta Classification (RAC)** was described in 1992 and revised in 2012. RAC is the recommended severity index. The Detriment-Based Classification of Acute Pancreatitis Severity (DBC) is also used and includes 'critical acute pancreatitis'. It notes the duration of organ failure and presence of necrosis with or without infection. The Balthazar CT Severity Index grades pancreatitis radiologically (based on inflammation, collections, and necrosis) with associated mortality values.

RAC severity grading
- Mild < 1 week
    - No organ failure
    - No local or systemic complications

- Moderate
  - Transient organ failure (<48 h)
  - Local or systemic complications
- Severe
  - Persistent single or multiple organ failure (>48 h)

Peripancreatic collections
- Acute necrotic collection (ANC)
  - Fluid and necrotic tissue
  - First 4 weeks
- Walled-off necrosis (WON)
  - Mature, encapsulated collection
  - >4 weeks after onset

GUIDELINE WSES 2019 Severe pancreatitis

How might severe acute pancreatitis be predicted?
The **Bedside Index of Severity of Acute Pancreatitis (BISAP)** score and **APACHE-II** scores are the best available at predicting severity.

Predictors of complications/severity
- Clinical impression of severity
- Obesity
- APACHE II > 8 in first 24 h admission
- Glasgow > 3
- CRP ≥ 150 mg/l at day 3 (severity)
- Urea > 30 mg/dl (mortality)
- Hct > 44% (necrosis)
- PCT (pancreatic infection, low value has strong negative prediction)
- BISAP 3–5 (>15% mortality)

Describe the epidemiology and prognosis of acute pancreatitis

Mild disease
- 80–85% of cases
- 1–3% mortality

SAP
- 20–30% of cases
- 15% hospital mortality

Infected necrosis
- 20–40% of severe cases
- 35% mortality if severe (i.e. organ failure present)
  - vs 20% with sterile necrosis
  - vs 1.4% without organ failure

How would you manage acute pancreatitis as an intensivist?

- **Manage underlying condition**
  - Surgical parent team guidance
  - Multi-disciplinary input
- **Decision to admit**
  - Monitor in HDU environment if organ dysfunction occurs
  - ICU if persistent organ dysfunction or failure despite adequate fluid

- **Fluid resuscitation**
  - Early isotonic crystalloid
  - *Avoid overload*: worse outcomes
- **Oxygenation**
  - HFNO or CPAP appropriate
  - Invasive ventilation where ineffective (e.g. tachypnoea, dyspnoea, high secretion load, tiring)
- **Antibiotics**
  - Indicated in infected SAP (14-day maximum course length if no positive culture)
  - Prophylaxis not recommended
  - Must penetrate tissue/collection appropriately
  - Serial PCT may be valuable
  - CT-guided fine needle aspiration can help to guide therapy but no longer routine
- **Analgesia**
  - Multimodal approach
  - Consider epidural or PCA
- **Nutrition**
  - Enteral preferred where tolerated
- **Management of intra-abdominal hypertension**
  - Prevention ideal
- **Consider transfer to tertiary unit (commonly when intervention indicated)**
  - Embolisation in bleeding
  - Stenting to drain collection (e.g. AXIOS™ stent)
  - Necrosectomy

(See Chapter 67 Compartment Syndromes)

When might IR be indicated?

- Percutaneous drainage of collection (first line for infected necrosis)
- Fine needle aspiration of collection for MC + S
- Embolisation or other procedure for bleeding

What are the indications for surgery?

Early surgical intervention has a negative effect on survival. There are very specific indications:

- Step-up after percutaneous/endoscopic procedure
- Abdominal compartment syndrome
- Unsuccessful endovascular intervention for bleeding
- Bowel ischaemia
- Acute necrotising cholecystitis
- Bowel fistula to peripancreatic collection

Minimally invasive procedures cause less post-operative organ dysfunction than open procedures but require repeated intervention (e.g. transgastric endoscopic necrosectomy).

Laparoscopic cholecystectomy is indicated in mild acute gallstone pancreatitis. Otherwise, it should be deferred until collections and inflammation stabilise/resolve.

---

63. BOWEL OBSTRUCTION AND ILEUS

What causes acute bowel obstruction?

Acute bowel obstruction is the mechanical interruption of the flow of GI contents. It presents with crampy, intermittent abdominal pain and distention, nausea, vomiting, and apparent constipation. There may be an intolerance of enteral feeding. There is a risk of perforation of distended bowel and subsequent peritonitis and systemic illness.

Common causes
- Malignancy
- Volvulus
- Stricture
- Foreign body

What is feeding intolerance?

Feeding intolerance often presents with GI symptoms related to delayed gastric emptying when enteral feed is introduced or built up (e.g. vomiting, high gastric residual volume, gastric distension, constipation, diarrhoea). It may be a sign of underlying ileus.

What is ileus and what causes it?

Ileus is a **slowing of GI motility without mechanical obstruction**. It presents similarly to bowel obstruction but is a diagnosis of exclusion. Causes include the following:

- **GI pathology**
  - Post-operative ileus
  - Acute peritonitis
  - Intra-abdominal collection
  - Ischaemia
  - Pancreatitis
- **Metabolic imbalance**
  - Hypokalaemia
  - Hyponatraemia
  - Hyperglycaemia
  - Uraemia
- **Medications**
  - Sedatives (e.g. opioids, alpha agonists)
  - Anti-diarrhoeals (e.g. loperamide)
  - Anti-cholinergics (e.g. TCA)
  - Smooth muscle relaxants (e.g. baclofen, calcium channel blockers)
  - NMB
- **Other**
  - Dehydration/oedema
  - Neurological (e.g. TBI, spinal cord injury, stroke)
  - Mechanical ventilation
  - Severe illness, hypoxaemia, hypotension

Acute colonic pseudo-obstruction is a paralytic ileus of the large intestine, also known as Olgilvie's syndrome.

How would you manage a patient with ileus on the critical care unit?

- **Detection**
  - Gastric residual volume 'aspirates' often used in monitoring but little evidence to support this
  - Should not be aspirated more than 6°
- **Measures to prevent aspiration**
  - Avoid lying flat, deprone if required
  - Consideration of airway support early if reduced level of consciousness
- **Reduce GI load**
  - NG decompression (e.g. Ryle's tube, suction)
  - May require trophic feed if tolerated
  - IV hydration
- **Treat underlying cause**
  - Rule out bowel obstruction
  - Reduction/replacement of opioid analgesia
  - Involve surgical team as indicated
  - Address reversible causes of GI dysmotility

- **Supportive care**
  - Allow time to resolve
  - PN if prolonged
  - Consider delaying discharge from critical care
- **Facilitate GI motility**
  - Prokinetics metoclopramide/erythromycin used commonly but no strong evidence
    - Erythromycin 250 mg 6° + metoclopramide 10 mg 8° (IV)
    - More effective in combination, use ≤5 days
  - Neostigmine may be considered in post-operative ileus

How might feed be adjusted?
Local protocol should be used. Example:

- Reduce infusion rate by 50% for 4–6 h
- Progressively increase rate over next 1–2 days
- Once gastric residual volume < 200 ml, reinstill and continue normal feeding regime

Resource
- Nickson C. Life in the Fast Lane: Ileus. Available from: https://litfl.com/ileus/. (Accessed 19 January 2022.)

64. NECROTISING FASCIITIS

What is necrotising fasciitis?
Necrotising fasciitis is an infection of the subcutaneous tissue. This includes the superficial and deep fascia and subdermal fat and associated structures. It may progress rapidly to multi-organ dysfunction and death.

KEY POINT

Type (microbial classification):

  I. *Polymicrobial*: mixed aerobes and anaerobes (bowel flora)
  II. *Monomicrobial*: Group A β-haemolytic *Streptococcus* (GAS), *Staphylococcus aureus*
  III. *Gram-negative*: *Vibrio* spp. (marine-related)
  IV. *Trauma-associated*: *Candida* spp., *Zygomycetes*

Can you name some other diseases caused by 'Group A *Strep.*'?

- Streptococcal toxic shock syndrome (TSS)
- '*Strep.* throat'/tonsillitis
- Impetigo
- Rheumatic fever
- Scarlet fever
- Post-streptococcal glomerulonephritis

(See Chapter 111 Toxic Shock Syndrome)

What is the pathophysiology of necrotising fasciitis?

- Infection from contaminated site (e.g. wound, perforated viscus, abscess)
- Spread through fascial planes
  - Poor microcirculation
  - Local ischaemia, necrosis

- Thrombosis of traversing vessels
  - Skin ischaemia
- Endotoxin and exotoxin release
  - Inflammation

What are the clinical features?

Dermatological stages
1 Defined, erythema, tenderness beyond erythema, swelling, warmth
2 Bullae, blisters, skin fluctuation
3 Haemorrhagic bullae, crepitus, skin necrosis, gangrene

Other features
- Skin may appear normal initially
- Pain disproportionate to physical findings
- Septic shock
- TSS
- Multi-organ dysfunction

How would you investigate a patient for necrotising fasciitis?

- *Clinical diagnosis*: may see visible spread across body surface
- *Risk scoring*: Laboratory Risk Indicator for Necrotising Fasciitis (LRINEC) involves CRP, WCC, Hb, Na+, creatinine, glucose
- *CT/MR imaging*: may help but should not delay emergency surgery

How is necrotising fasciitis managed in the critically unwell patient?
Management is likely to involve close liaison between Emergency Medicine, General Surgery, Anaesthesia, Intensive Care, Microbiology, and Plastic Surgery teams:

- *Aggressive resuscitation*
  - Intubation and ventilation if for theatre, compromised airway or significant multi-organ dysfunction/shock (often all 3)
  - Fluid resuscitation
  - Early vasopressors
  - Consider cardiac output monitoring
- *Early adequate surgical debridement*
  - May necessitate limb amputation
  - Significant blood loss common
- *Antimicrobials*: broad spectrum (e.g. piperacillin-tazobactam) plus antitoxin (e.g. clindamycin)
- *IVIg*: limited evidence, consider in group A *Streptococcus* or staphylococcal infection
- *Analgesia*
- *Wound management*
  - Wounds often not closed (± vacuum dressings)
  - Multiple debridements may be required
  - May require defunctioning stoma to prevent contamination
  - Hyperbaric oxygen to inhibit toxin production
  - Reconstructive surgery in quiescence

Resource
- Davoudian P, Flint NJ. Necrotizing fasciitis. CEACCP. 2012;12(5):245–250.

65. BOERHAAVE SYNDROME

What is Boerhaave syndrome?

Boerhaave syndrome is the condition in which there is spontaneous effort rupture of the oesophagus.

What is the pathophysiology of this condition?

- Oesophagus often normal pre-morbidly
- Precipitating event (e.g. vomiting, severe straining, seizure)
- Sudden increase in intraoesophageal pressure combined with negative intrathoracic pressure
- Oesophageal tear occurs
- Passage of GI contents, secretions, and air into mediastinum

Oesophageal perforation may also arise from iatrogenesis (e.g. endoscopy) or trauma (e.g. foreign body/caustic substance ingestion, penetrating trauma). A Boerhaave syndrome-like picture can both necessitate oesophageal surgery and result from planned oesophageal intervention.

Can you describe some eponymous findings in this condition?

Mackler's triad (present in < 1/3 cases)
- Thoracic pain (chest pain may be worse on neck flexion and swallowing and radiate to left shoulder)
- Vomiting
- Subcutaneous emphysema

Hamman's sign
- Abnormal precordial sound, synchronous with the apex beat
- Crunching or rasping in nature
- Due to mediastinal emphysema, other (e.g. tracheobronchial injury)

How might Boerhaave syndrome be investigated?

- In precipitous cases, clinical findings and radiographs will suffice until stable
- *CXR*: PTX, widened mediastinum, left-sided pleural effusion
- *CT chest (± oral contrast)*: leak site, extent of contamination, inflammation, abscess
- *Gastrografin oesophagography*: contrast leak if perforation present (10% false negative)
- *OGD*: may be valuable but risk of worsening lesion
- *Pleural tap*: pH < 6.0, raised salivary amylase, frank presence of undigested food

What are the major complications of this condition?

- Mediastinitis
- Multi-organ dysfunction
- Massive pleural effusion
- Empyema
- Subcutaneous emphysema
- Pneumomediastinum (see Chapter 81 Air Leak Syndrome)
- Cardiac tamponade
- ARDS
- Death

What are the priorities in initial clinical management?

- Early diagnosis and stabilisation
- Surgical review
  - May require transfer to tertiary centre
  - Non-contained leak may require primary repair, controlled fistula, or resection (oesophagectomy)
  - Lung isolation usually necessitated intraoperatively
  - Conservative management may involve stent placement
- Judicious fluid management
- Analgesia as appropriate (e.g. early epidural, paravertebral blocks or wound catheters)
- Antimicrobials
- Alternative nutritional support, avoidance of blind NG tube insertion

What is the prognosis of Boerhaave syndrome?

- Mortality up to 40%
- Better outcomes if treated early
- Likely to require prolonged organ support
- Further contrast studies may be indicated when inflammation settled (e.g. 2–3 weeks after repair)
- Long-term adaptations may affect quality of life (e.g. cervical oesophagostomy and feeding jejunostomy)

What does oesophagectomy involve?

Oesophagectomy involves excising a portion of oesophagus and forming an anastomosis in the mediastinum, the 'gastric conduit'. Access is tricky and the surgical field can be hostile. Significant incisions will impact on post-operative recovery. Anaesthesia will involve a degree of lung isolation to facilitate surgical access (with right lung collapse most commonly).

Approaches
- **Ivor Lewis** (right thoracotomy + midline laparotomy)
- **Minimally invasive oesophagectomy** (thoracoscopic + laparoscopic)
- Ivor Lewis with rooftop abdominal incision(right thoracotomy + transverse upper abdominal incision)
- Tri-incisional(Ivor Lewis + left neck incision)
- Transdiaphragmatic (extensive left thoracotomy)
- Transhiatal (supraumbilical midline laparotomy + left neck incision)

Why are oesophagectomy patients at significant risk of morbidity and mortality?

The most common indication for oesophagectomy is malignancy. Risk factors for adverse outcomes are common in this group:

- Advanced age
- Poor cardiopulmonary function
- Advanced tumour stage
- Diabetes mellitus
- Impaired general health
- Hepatic dysfunction
- Peripheral vascular disease
- Smoking
- Chronic steroid use

Prehabilitation may mitigate some of these (e.g. smoking cessation, nutritional support, exercise) but time is limited before surgery should take place.

The anastomosis is also particularly vulnerable as it is formed at the extreme end of the foregut's blood supply.

What might the care of a patient who has undergone oesophagectomy include?

Care centres around minimising dependency on organ support and care of the anastomosis.

Anastomotic protection
- Avoidance of CPAP/HFNO immediately post-operatively – theoretical risk
- Optimal perfusion (see Chapter 69 The Post-Op Free Flap Patient)
  - Appropriate BP
  - Neutral fluid balance
    - ➤ *Avoidance of overload*: venous congestion
    - ➤ *Avoidance of underfilling*: excessive vasoconstrictor use
  - *Cardiac output monitoring tricky*: echo limited, oesophageal Doppler contraindicated
- *NG decompression*: positioned intraoperatively
- Proton pump inhibitors
- Early nutrition
- *Vigilant monitoring*: gastric secretions, bleeding

Other supportive care
- *Ventilation*: early extubation, often in theatre unless additional concern
- Multimodal analgesia
  - Regional techniques associated with better outcomes
  - e.g. thoracic epidural, paravertebral catheters ± PCA, ketamine IV infusion
- *Normothermia*: prevention of pneumonia
- Enhanced recovery
  - Early mobilisation
  - Chest physiotherapy
  - Appropriate removal of invasive devices
- Monitoring for and addressing complications

What are the early complications of oesophagectomy?

Respiratory (17–51%)
- Recurrent laryngeal nerve palsy (4–67%)
- Air leak
- *Thoracic duct injury*: chylothorax
- Pneumonia
- ARDS

Cardiovascular
- *Arrhythmias*: AF very common
- Haemorrhage
- Pericardial injury

GI
- Ileus
- **Anastomotic leak (10–37%)**
  - Responsible for 35% perioperative mortality
  - Presents typically within first 5 days with severe sepsis
  - Smaller leaks may present later, more occult

How is an anastomotic leak managed?

- *GI tract protection*: nil by mouth, monitoring with contrast studies
- *Alternative nutrition*: may require PN, high-protein feed
- Antibiotics
- Chest physiotherapy
- *Collections*: radiologically guided drainage
- *Major leak*: surgical exploration ± revision

Resources
- Howells P, Bieker M, Yeung J. Oesophageal cancer and the anaesthetist. BJA Educ. 2017;17(2):68–73.
- King WD. Oesophageal injury. BJA Educ. 2015;15(5):265–270.

66.   ABDOMINAL AORTIC ANEURYSM

What is an abdominal aortic aneurysm?

AAA is a dilatation or widening of the abdominal aorta of **3 cm** or more based on US imaging (approximately 2 SD above the mean in men).

AAA is more prevalent with age (negligible < 55 y). Risk factors include the following:

- Smoking
- Male sex
- Age
- Atherosclerosis
- Hypertension
- Ethnicity
- Family history of AAA

Risk of AAA in diabetics is half of that in non-diabetics.

What are the clinical features of an abdominal aortic aneurysm?

Intact aneurysm
- Majority clinically silent, often detected incidentally or on screening programme
- Pulsatile mass palpation < 50% sensitivity, not reliable
- Tenderness on palpation
- Abdominal pain radiating to back/groin
- Symptoms of compression (e.g. bowel obstruction, lower limb oedema)

Rupture
- Haemodynamic compromise
- More significant abdominal/back pain
- Abdominal distension
- Primary aorto-enteric or arterio-venous fistula

How is aneurysm rupture diagnosed?

- *CT angiography*: gold standard for suspected rupture, stability permitting
- *US*: useful in detection of AAA but low sensitivity for haemorrhage
- *Clinical features*: only 50% will have the triad of hypotension, pain, and pulsatile mass
- *Differentials*: ureteric colic and MI are common erroneous diagnoses

How might the intensivist be involved in the care of these patients?

- Post-operative care in elective repair
- Post-operative care from emergency repair
- Management of unstable patient in ruptured aneurysm as part of MDT
- MDT decision for non-operative repair and palliation
- Management of patient with complications of aneurysm or repair

What are the initial management priorities in patients with a ruptured abdominal aortic aneurysm?

- **Haemodynamic stabilisation**
  - **Permissive hypotension** vs 'hypotensive haemostasis'
  - Transfusion ratio 1:1 plasma to red cells, avoid crystalloid
  - Target adequate conscious level, systolic BP 70–90 mmHg
- **Prevention and management of coagulopathy**
- **MDT discussion** of risk and expectations with patient ± family if possible
- **Aneurysm repair where suitable**
  - Early vascular surgery and anaesthesia opinions
  - May require transfer to tertiary centre

What are the risk factors for increased perioperative mortality in ruptured AAA?

- **Pre-operative**
  - Severe haemodynamic instability
  - Cardiac arrest
  - LOC
  - Renal impairment
  - CCF
  - Significant anaemia
- **Intraoperative**
  - Intraperitoneal rupture
  - Aortofemoral reconstruction
  - Adjunctive vascular procedures
  - Total operating time
- **Post-operative**
  - Multi-organ failure
  - Respiratory and renal failure
  - Bleeding
  - CVA

What is the prognosis of a ruptured abdominal aortic aneurysm?

Emergency repair of rupture
- **Open surgical**
  - >50% mortality historically
  - 39.5% in-hospital mortalityin 2019, 50% in 2020
  - 59% immediate post-op mortality in patients > 80 years old
  - Almost 100% mortality if CPR required before surgery
    - ➤ Higher survival in those undergoing endovascular aneurysm repair (EVAR) in 1 small study
    - *Vascular Surgery Quality Improvement Project (VSQIP)*: in-hospital mortality 39.5% (2019), 50% (2020)
- **EVAR**
  - RCTs and meta-analyses show no difference in mortality at 30 and 90 days post-op between choice of repair.
  - Selection bias may be responsible for some data suggesting better immediate outcome with EVAR (due to stability for CT angiography).
  - VSQIP in-hospital mortality 20% (2019, 2020)

Elective repair (comparison)
- 7% mortality if 'unfit'
- 1–2% mortality if 'fit'

When might patients be considered for endovascular repair vs open surgery?

- Advantages of endovascular repair
  - Shorter LOS in hospital
  - Lower immediate risk at time of intervention
  - Less risk associated with post-op CT monitoring
- Disadvantages
  - 20–30% patients not suitable for endovascular repair (e.g. anatomical abnormalities, organ position and arterial supply, access and 'runoff' vessels)
  - Ongoing monitoring
  - May require additional surgery to repair or prevent failure of stent

There is evidence suggesting that repair of ruptured AAA under local anaesthesia may have better outcomes than under general anaesthesia. It is recommended to attempt repair of a ruptured AAA with EVAR under local anaesthesia where possible.

GUIDELINE   NICE 2020 NG156 AAA

STUDY

IMPROVE (2014)

- Ruptured AAA
- *Intervention*: EVAR vs open repair
- *Primary*: 30-day mortality – **no difference** (around 35%)
- LA vs GA for EVAR associated with **4-fold reduction in 30-day mortality**

What complications might be anticipated in this patient group?

- **Hypoperfusion**
  - ACS
  - AKI
  - Bowel ischaemia, ileus
  - Abdominal compartment syndrome
  - Spinal cord ischaemia, paraplegia, sexual dysfunction
  - Liver dysfunction
  - Lower limb ischaemia, compartment syndrome
- **Post-operative recovery**
  - Pain
  - Respiratory failure, prolonged wean
  - Transfusion-related
  - Wound-related (e.g. herniae, infection)
  - VTE
- **Graft/stent**
  - Endoleak
  - Lower limb ischaemia
  - Distal embolisation
  - Infection

- Occlusion
- Secondary aorto-enteric fistula
- Pseudoaneurysm

(See Chapter 67 Compartment Syndromes)

How would you manage the post-operative patient on the critical care unit?

- Supportive care including optimisation of haemodynamics and normothermia
- Analgesia (e.g. wound infiltration of local anaesthetic, PCA)
- Monitoring for complications (e.g. drain output, U&E, acid-base balance, abdominal pressures)
- Prevention and management of complications, including use of:
  - RRT
  - Lumbar spinal drain
  - PN

Resources

- Clinical Effectiveness Unit, the Royal College of Surgeons of England, Vascular Society of Great Britain and Ireland, British Society of Interventional Radiology. National Vascular Registry: 2021 Annual Report. Available from: https://www.vsqip.org.uk/content/uploads/2021/11/NVR-2021-Annual-Report-Main-Report.pdf. (Accessed 20 January 2022.)
- Faizer R, Weinhandl E, El Hag S, et al. Decreased mortality with local versus general anesthesia in endovascular aneurysm repair for ruptured abdominal aortic aneurysm in the Vascular Quality Initiative database. J Vasc Surg. 2019;70(1):92–101.E1.

67. COMPARTMENT SYNDROMES

What compartment syndromes are you aware of and why do they occur?

A compartment syndrome is the process in which pressure within a body compartment rises enough to restrict perfusion to and viability of the contents of that compartment.

These compartments are usually restricted by tight boundaries (e.g. fascia, bone). Other processes fitting this description include intracranial hypertension and cardiac tamponade (although more complex). 'Polycompartment syndrome' describes the simultaneous, often related, involvement of several areas of the body.

Compartment syndromes
- **Extremity**
- **Abdominal**
- Orbital
- Intracranial
- Thoracic
- Cardiac
- Hepatic
- Renal
- Pelvic

(See Chapter 133 Rhabdomyolysis)

What is the pathophysiology of a compartment syndrome?

Perfusion pressure = MAP − compartment pressure

A specific perfusion pressure will be required to achieve adequate oxygenation of the compartment tissues. From first principles, this will differ where pressure autoregulation ranges and processes are affected (e.g. in chronic hypertension). Therefore, this is compromised by:

Inadequate MAP
- Shock
- Elevation (e.g. limb raised)
- Drugs (e.g. sedation, antihypertensives)

Elevated compartment pressure
- Increased content
  - Ascites
  - Inadequate venous drainage
  - SOL
  - Vasodilatation
  - Bleeding
  - Other viscus contents (e.g. bowel)
- Decreased size/compliance
  - Restrictive dressing
  - Scarring (e.g. post-operative, eschar)
  - Surgical closure
  - External compression (e.g. equipment – cooling blanket, bedding)
  - Pericardial effusion
  - PEEP

Subsequent tissue necrosis/lysis and oedema worsens compartment perfusion. Specific compartments will have other complications. Eschars from burns may also cause issues other than deficiency in perfusion (e.g. ventilatory restriction).

What is abdominal compartment syndrome?
IAH is an IAP > **12 mmHg**. Grading of IAH (mmHg):

1 12–15
2 16–20
3 21–25
4 ≥26

Abdominal compartment syndrome:

- Sustained increase in IAP > **20 mmHg***, with
- New organ dysfunction

(*i.e. Grade 3–4 IAH)

Abdominal compartment syndrome is more common in certain scenarios (e.g. SAP, traumatic bowel contusion, post-operative ruptured AAA repair).

What are the complications of abdominal compartment syndrome?

- *A/B*: ventilatory compromise, reduced FRC, aspiration risk
- *C*: increased afterload, reduced venous return, fall in cardiac output
- *D*: impaired venous drainage, raised ICP
- *G*: ischaemia, translocation of bacteria, ileus, obstructive liver dysfunction, biliary stasis
- *F*: obstructive uropathy, prerenal AKI, RAS activation

How is abdominal compartment syndrome managed in critical care?

Prevention is key. Management aims to optimise perfusion by removing factors contributing towards compartment syndrome.

A step-wise approach is presented by the World Society of the Abdominal Compartment Syndrome (WSACS), advocating strong consideration of surgical decompression when medical management is refractory (Table 67.1). Specific to aneurysm repair, **IAP > 30 mmHg** is an indication for abdominal decompression.

GUIDELINE	WSACS 2013 Abdominal compartment syndrome

What is an open abdomen?

This is the state in which an abdominal wound is left open to decompress IAP.

It is the equivalent to a fasciotomy for limb compartment syndrome. Surgical decompression may be performed in a standalone laparotomy, or prophylactically at the end of a complex procedure.

Specialised dressings are used for antisepsis and specific precautions must be taken including management of temperature, fluid balance, and prevention of injury to intra-abdominal contents.

What is orbital compartment syndrome?

Orbital compartment syndrome is a raised intraocular pressure resulting in reduced retinal and optic nerve perfusion. It is a sight-threatening condition and a surgical emergency. It may be encountered by the intensivist in several scenarios and can drastically change a patient's long-term outcome.

Orbital compartment syndrome may occur through retrobulbar haemorrhage or traumatic optic neuropathy, alongside other causes of raised ICP and associated raised intraocular pressure (e.g. venous sinus thrombosis).

Table 67.1   Step-wise IAH management by pathophysiological mechanism

		Reduce compartment pressure		
		Improve compliance	Reduce contents	
	Increase MAP (aim APP > 60 mmHg)		Intraluminal	Extraluminal (SOL)
1	Fluid resuscitation Avoid overload Aim 0 to negative balance by day 3	Adequate sedation Adequate analgesia Remove constriction	NG ± rectal tube Prokinetics	US abdomen
2	Haemodynamic monitoring, drugs Hypertonic fluids/colloids Judicious fluid removal (diuresis)	Reverse Trendelenberg position	Reduce enteral feed Enemas	CT abdomen ± percutaneous drainage
3	Dialysis/filtration	NMB	Colonoscopic decompression Stop enteral feed	Surgical evacuation
4		Laparotomy		

Features
- Acute reduction in vision
- Tense, swollen eyelids
- Orbital congestion
- Proptosis
- ± Relative afferent pupillary defect (RAPD)
- ± Fixed dilated pupil

How would you manage this once suspected?

- Immediate decompression: **lateral canthotomy and cantholysis**
  - Local anaesthetic injection at lateral canthus
  - Grasp lower lid with toothed forceps
  - Divide lateral canthal tendon using long, horizontal, full-thickness cut with blunt-ended straight scissors
  - Divide restricting bands of septum between lower lid and orbital rim
  - Spontaneous healing and closure
- Monitoring: distance visual acuity, colour vision, pupillary reflexes/RAPD, orbital pressure by palpation, intraocular pressure
- Ophthalmology review
- Manage underlying cause where able

This procedure may need to be performed under remote ophthalmology guidance whilst awaiting emergency review.

Resources
- Malbrain MLNG, Roberts DJ, Sugrue M, et al. The polycompartment syndrome: a concise state-of-the-art review. Anaesthesiol Intensive Ther. 2014;46(5):433–450.
- Timlin H, Manisali M, Verity D, et al. Traumatic Orbital Emergencies. The Royal College of Ophthalmologists FOCUS, 2015. Available from: https://www.rcophth.ac.uk/wp-content/uploads/2015/02/Focus-Autumn-2015.pdf. (Accessed 09 June 2021.)

68.   INTESTINAL FAILURE

What is intestinal failure?
Intestinal failure is the state of reduced gut absorption requiring supplementation of macronutrients and/or water and electrolytes to maintain health or growth.

Severity can be classified by degree of supplementation required:

- *Mild*: oral nutritional fluids
- *Moderate*: EN
- *Severe*: PN

Causes
- Acute
  - Fistula/obstruction
  - *Small bowel dysfunction*: ileus, enteritis (chemotherapy, infection)
- Chronic
  - Short bowel
  - Gut bypass
  - *Small bowel dysfunction*: enteritis (irradiation, Crohn's), dysmotility

What is 'short bowel'?

'Short bowel' refers to a remaining (post-operative) length of bowel of **under 2 m**, which is significant as nutritional supplementation is likely to be required. Women are more at risk than men, possibly due to shorter starting bowel length.

Clinical categories
- *Jejunum-colon*: jejunoileal resection and jejunocolic anastomosis
- *Jejunum-ileum*: predominantly jejunal resection, >10 cm ileum remaining, colon remaining
- *Jejunostomy*: jejunoileal resection, colectomy, stoma

Can you name some indications for surgery resulting in short bowel?

- Crohn's disease
- Superior mesenteric artery thrombosis
- Irradiation damage
- Other: small bowel volvulus, adhesions, ulcerative colitis (UC), desmoid

What physiological consequences might intestinal resection have?

- Altered motility
- Water and salt loss, reduced reabsorption
- Gastric acid hypersecretion (first 2 weeks)
- Malabsorption (B_{12}, fat, fat-soluble vitamins)
- Hypomagnesaemia, decreased parathormone, decreased 1,25-hydroxy-vitamin D manufacture
- Increased hepatic synthesis of bile salts
- Hyperphagia
- D-lactic acidosis

Short bowel may manifest with weight loss, diarrhoea, prerenal failure, confusion, poor drug absorption, gallstones, renal stones, social difficulties (diarrhoea, treatment-dependency).

Seventy percent of PN-related deaths are due to indwelling line sepsis. Risk factors include high-dose opioid treatment and presence of a stoma.

What are the main goals of management in patients with short bowel syndrome?

- Provide nutrition, water, and electrolytes necessary to maintain health
- Use oral/enteral in preference to PN if suitable
- Reduce complications from underlying condition, intestinal failure, or supplementation
- Achieve good quality of life

How should a high output stoma be managed?

- *Exclude causes other than short bowel*: intra-abdominal sepsis, obstruction, enteritis, underlying disease recurrence, drug withdrawal, prokinetic prescription
- Correct dehydration
- Reduce oral hypotonic fluids (and use replacement solutions)
- Drugs to reduce motility
- Drugs to reduce gastric acid secretion if secretory element

What do you know about intestinal transplantation?

- Not yet recommended as an alternative when stable on supportive therapy (PN), unlike other transplantable organs
- Difficult due to immunogenicity, non-sterile contents
- 80% 1-year survival, 50% at 5 years
- Survivors mostly free from PN, increased quality of life reported

- Referral
  - Complications of PN (liver disease, vascular access limited, significant central line sepsis, inadequate maintenance)
  - High risk conditions (extensive evisceration: desmoid tumour, trauma)
- There are only 3 centres in the UK (Leeds, Cambridge, Birmingham – paediatrics). Fourteen intestinal grafts have been performed to date on adults in the UK.

GUIDELINE   Small Bowel and Nutrition Committee 2006 Short bowel

69.   THE POST-OP FREE FLAP PATIENT

What kinds of flap surgery are you aware of?

Flap surgery is indicated to provide reconstruction for cosmesis as well as deep wound coverage. It can be classified by blood supply, tissue, and donor site location. Common reconstructive sites include breast and orofacial areas, with the latter group often being admitted to critical care post-operatively.

There are 2 main types of autologous flaps:

- *Free flap*: completely disconnected and anastomosed at new site
  - Deep inferior epigastric perforator (DIEP)
  - Transverse rectus abdominis myocutaneous (TRAM)
  - Fibula free flap
  - Anterolateral thigh free flap
  - Radial forearm free flap
- *Pedicled flap*: own arterial and venous supply, subclassification of local/regional/distant
  - Pectoralis major myocutaneous (PMMC)

What are the main concerns in free flap patients?

Viability of the flap is paramount. Microvascular anastomoses are used to perfuse and drain a free flap and any ischaemia and subsequent inflammatory mediator release may threaten the surgical outcome.

Free flaps will be denervated, with a loss of intrinsic sympathetic tone. Lymphatics will be compromised, risking oedema. Other stimuli may still cause vascular changes: cold, catecholamines, drugs.

Other issues
- Underlying pathology to be considered (e.g. malignancy)
- Difficult airway might be encountered ± tracheostomy involvement

What are significant stages for flap viability?

KEY POINT

- **Primary ischaemia**
  - Cessation of blood flow intraoperatively during flap transfer
  - Severity proportional to duration of ischaemia
- **Reperfusion**
  - When vessels unclamped after anastomosis
  - Ischaemia/reperfusion injury may occur
- **Secondary ischaemia**
  - After flap transfer and reperfusion
  - More harmful than primary ischaemia
  - May cause massive intravascular thrombosis and interstitial oedema

Which physiological measures can be applied to post-operative care to optimise perfusion of free flaps?

Physiological goals will centre around the Hagen-Pouiselle equation applied to microvascular blood flow (Q), which then translates to perfusion of the flap:

$$Q = \frac{\pi(\Delta P)r^4}{8\eta l}$$

- *Radius(r)*: avoidance of vasoconstriction
  - Appropriate temperature
  - Normovolaemia
  - Adequate analgesia
  - Some surgeons advocate avoidance of specific vasoconstrictors (e.g. metaraminol or NA) but there is no evidence that vasopressors cause adverse outcomes.
- Pressure gradient (ΔP)
  - Adequate perfusion pressure
  - Low SVR
  - *Adequate venous drainage*: careful positioning, avoidance of compression
  - *Antiemetics*: avoid pressure fluctuations
- *Viscosity (η)*: Hct within target range: 0.30–0.35
- *Length (l)*: vessel used in anastomosis

What causes free flap failure?

These usually relate to 1 or more of the above factors affecting perfusion. Examples:

- Anastomotic breakdown
- Vasospasm
- Thrombosis due to vessel injury
- Compression from haematoma/other
- Reperfusion injury
- Oedema
- Hypercoagulable states

How is ischaemia identified in critical care?

- Regular surgical review
- Perfusion observations
  - Flap colour
  - CR time
  - Skin turgor
  - Skin temperature
  - Bleeding on pinprick
- Transcutaneous Doppler monitor (site marked or implanted by surgeon) – arterial and venous phases

Arterial pathology results in cool, pale tissue with slow CR and absence of bleeding on pinprick. Venous defects cause a warm, blue, congested appearance with brisk CR and dark bleeding.

How would you manage suspected ischaemia?

- Inform the surgical team
- May need to prepare patient for emergency theatre
- Optimise physiology as above
- Specialised measures for venous congestion (e.g. application of leeches)

Resource

- Nimalan N. Anaesthesia for free flap breast reconstruction. BJA Educ. 2016;16(5):162–166.

Why might transplant patients be admitted to critical care?

- Related to transplant
  - Immediate post-operative care
  - Early complications
  - Late complications
- Related to immunosuppression
  - Side effects of medications
  - Infection
- Related to underlying disease (i.e. relapse)
- Unrelated condition (e.g. trauma)

Describe some challenges of providing critical care to transplant patients.

- Availability of expertise limited to tertiary centres
- Recovery from lengthy surgery and anaesthetic
- Analgesia often difficult, combined with metabolic dysfunction
- Significant comorbid illness possible
- End-stage vascular access (e.g. renal patients)
- Marginal donors becoming increasingly common, impact on graft recovery
- Difficult fluid and electrolyte management
- Uncommon surgical complications with specific syndromes
- Polypharmacy, absorption issues
- Opportunistic infections (including fungal) with immunosuppression
- Donor may be known to the patient and may have stormier post-operative recovery (e.g. directed living donor kidney transplant)

What management strategies will be required immediately post-operatively?

General:
- Analgesia (e.g. epidural, PCA)
- Thromboprophylaxis
- Graft optimisation measures
  - Adequate perfusion
  - Avoidance of anastomosis disruption (e.g. by retching)
  - Liaison with surgical and transplant MDT
- Immunosuppression
  - Commonly scheduled by transplant team
  - Drug level monitoring
  - Steroid management
  - Antibiotic prophylaxis
- Vigilance for complications
  - Regular blood sampling
  - Post transfusion care – may have received significant quantities in theatre

Organ-specific:
- **Heart**
  - Early extubation < 24 h
  - Furosemide to offload RV

- Low-dose inotropic support 24 h
- Physiological manipulation to lower PVR
- **Lung**
  - LPV
  - Early extubation
  - Fluid restriction
  - May require differential lung ventilation
- **Liver**
  - Management of coagulopathy, hypocalcaemia
  - Monitoring for liver and renal dysfunction
- **Kidney**
  - Close monitoring of UO
  - Avoidance of hypovolaemia
- **Pancreas**
  - Highest complication rate of solid organ transplants: 40% require relaparotomy
  - Euglycaemia with variable rate insulin infusion

What is primary graft dysfunction?

Primary graft dysfunction (PGD) is a term which describes **poor initial function of a transplanted organ** and will present with an organ-specific insufficiency syndrome as well as possible systemic features. It may be related to ischaemia-reperfusion injury.

- *Heart*: mechanical support or LVEF < 45% despite high-dose inotropes (<24 h post-op)
- *Lung*: impaired oxygenation with diffuse alveolar opacities on CXR
- *Liver*: lactataemia, hypoglycaemia, hyperbilirubinaemia, raised INR, ALT, AST
- *Kidney*: hyperkalaemia, poor UO
- *Pancreas*: hyperglycaemia

What other complications of transplantation are you aware of?

There are many potential complications of transplantation other than PGD (Table 70.1).

Can you name some immunosuppressive medications and any common, significant side effects?

- *Steroids*: hypertension, delirium, mood change, diabetes, Cushing's syndrome, peptic ulcer disease
- **Calcineurin inhibitors**
  - *Ciclosporin*: nephrotoxicity, drug interactions
  - *Tacrolimus*: diabetes
- *Azathioprine* (antimetabolite): irritant IV
- *Mycophenolate* (IMPDH inhibitor): increased likelihood of opportunistic infection
- *Biologics* (lymphocytedepleting vs non-depleting)
  - Basalixumab
  - Alemtuzumab

Side effects of biologics are as follows:

- Infusion-related fever, nausea, vomiting
- Anaphylaxis
- Angina, HF
- Stevens-Johnson syndrome (SJS), TEN
- Hepatitis B, TB reactivation
- Progressive multifocal leukoencephalopathy (PML)

Table 70.1   Complications of solid organ transplantation

	Early	Late
Generic	Haemorrhage Ischaemia-reperfusion injury Primary allograft dysfunction Primary allograft non-function Secondary graft dysfunction Graft thrombosis Infection AKI Death Post-op recovery of living donor	Immunosuppressant side effects Graft rejection Recurrent primary disease CMV infection Susceptibility to intracellular bacteria
Heart	PGD in ⅓ (6% 30-day mortality) Vasoplegia Cardiac tamponade Pulmonary hypertension Stroke	Donor coronary artery disease Dysrhythmias Altered physiology from denervation
Lung	PGD in 30% (6% require VV-ECMO) Mucus plugging, atelectasis HTX PTX Bronchial anastomotic leak PE Dynamic hyperinflation RV dysfunction Stroke Aspergillus infection	Pulmonary infarction Post-transplant lymphoproliferative disease Lung cancer Osteoporosis Bronchiolitis obliterans
Liver	IVC and hepatic vein thrombosis	Biliary tree obstruction
Kidney	Hypovolaemia Hyponatraemia, hyperkalaemia (mannitol)	
Pancreas	Inflammatory storm Hyperglycaemia 'Graft pancreatitis' Enzyme / enteric leak Bladder problems Collections	Pseudoaneurysm

Resources

- Buckwell E, Vickery B, Sidebotham D. Anaesthesia for lung transplantation. BJA Educ. 2020;20(11):368–376.
- Edwards S, Allen S, Sidebotham D. Anaesthesia for heart transplantation. BJA Educ. 2021;21(8):284–291.
- Kashimutt S, Kotzé A. Anaesthesia for liver transplantation. BJA Educ. 2016;17(1):35–40.
- Morgan-Hughes N, Hood G. Anaesthesia for a patient with a cardiac transplant. BJA CEPD Rev. 2002;2(3):74–78.
- Mayhew D, Ridgway D, Hunter JM. Update on the intraoperative management of adult cadaveric renal transplantation. BJA Educ. 2016;16(2):53–57.
- Pichel AC, Macnab WR. Anaesthesia for pancreas transplantation. CEACCP. 2005;5(5):149–152.

CARDIOTHORACICS

71. CARDIAC ADVANCED LIFE SUPPORT

When might you suspect deterioration in the cardiothoracic post-operative setting?

- Failure to follow usual post-operative course
- Signs of an underlying problem (e.g. hypotension)
- Signs of organ hypoperfusion (e.g. reduced UO)
- Metabolic disturbance, increasing lactate/failure to improve

Describe some causes of cardiac arrest in the cardiothoracic critical care unit.

- *Hypovolaemia*
  - Capillary leakage
  - Haemodilution
  - Redistribution
  - Polyuria
- *Bleeding*
  - *'Medical'*: coagulopathy: heparin, platelet dysfunction, clotting factor deficiency
  - *'Surgical'*: consider if high drain output (e.g. 400 ml/h first hour, 200 ml/h 2 consecutive hours, 100 ml/h consecutive hours)
- *Low output* (ventricular dysfunction)
  - Myocardial stunning (e.g. prior cardioplegia use)
  - Myocardial oedema following CPB
  - Metabolic dysfunction
  - Reperfusion injury
  - Ischaemia
  - Hypocalcaemia
  - Presence of air in coronary artery (e.g. RCA following valve surgery)
- *Vasoplegia*
  - Rewarming
  - Sepsis
  - Anaphylaxis
  - Vasoplegic syndrome
  - Unopposed inodilator use
  - Adrenal insufficiency
- *Graft/valve failure*: new ECG changes with low output
- *Tamponade*
- *Dysrhythmias*: AF, pacing issues

What is CALS and when does it apply?

CALS, or Cardiac (Surgery) Advanced Life Support, is a protocol designed for use in all cardiothoracic ICUs for cardiac surgical patients suffering cardiac arrest. It is less applicable to those who have undergone pulmonary surgery.

Cardiac arrest may present unconventionally in those already intubated and ventilated and the following may also trigger the protocol:

- Absence of pulsatile arterial trace
- Flat CVP/PAP trace
- Reduction in E_tCO_2

Describe the main features of the CALS protocol.

The protocol begins with a rhythm assessment, as in conventional ALS.

Subsequent initial management:

- *VF/VT*: DC shock (×3) > BLS > amiodarone
- *Asystole/bradycardia*: pace if wires available > BLS > external pacing
- *PEA*: BLS> turn off pacing to exclude VF

Preparation for **resternotomy** should occur once the interventions above have been tried. A DC shock should be delivered every 2 min for ongoing VF/VT.

Adjunctive measures:
- F_iO_2 1.0
- 0 PEEP
- Change to bag/valve circuit, verify tube position and cuff inflation
- Exclude PTX/HTX, decompress tension
- Change IABP from ECG to pressure trigger if present

What are the key concepts underlying the modifications in cardiac advanced life support?

There is questionable benefit of external chest compressions and use of adrenaline in this specific context.

- Surgical complications are significant and may be worsened by mechanical injury to the surgical site or elsewhere in the heart. The protocol allows BLS to be delayed by 1 min as a result.
- Defibrillation and pacing institution/adjustment are prioritised as myocardium is presumed to be viable.
- Adrenaline is not given unless an experienced clinician advises this.

How might you allocate roles during CALS?

There are lots of tasks to consider in a CALS scenario. Recommended roles to be delegated:

- External cardiac massage
- Airway and breathing
- Defibrillation
- Team leader
- Drugs and syringe drivers
- ICU coordinator
- Resternotomy will require a main operator and an assistant.

Describe resternotomy.

- Full sterile scrub may be sacrificed in the interest of time – often skin is decontaminated, sterile drapes used, and operators wear sterile gloves and gown without handwashing.
- A changeover from non-sterile to sterile cardiac massage will require careful coordination.
- The main operator will use a scalpel to reopen the median sternotomy wound.
- The assistant will hold the wire taut whilst the operator cuts.
- The assistant pulls the sternal wires out.
- Internal cardiac massage and other interventions may be performed.

Resources

- Brand J, McDonald A, Dunning J. Management of cardiac arrest following cardiac surgery. BJA Educ. 2018;18(1):16–22.
- Dunning J, Nandi J, Ariffin S, et al. The Cardiac Surgery Advanced Life Support Course (CALS): delivering significant improvements in emergency cardiothoracic care. Ann Thorac Surg. 2006;81(5):1767–1772.

72.   CARDIAC TAMPONADE

What is cardiac tamponade?

Cardiac tamponade is the condition in which compression of the heart causes increased intrapericardial pressure. This results in impaired diastolic filling and cardiac output.

It may be caused by slow or rapid accumulation of a substance in the pericardial space (e.g. exudate, pus, blood, or gas).

What is the aetiology of cardiac tamponade?

There is an extensive list of causes but some are more likely to result in tamponade than others:

- Neoplastic disease
- Infection (e.g. EBV, CMV, HIV, TB)
- Iatrogenic (e.g. PCI, TAVI, PPM/ICD implantation, ablation, biopsy)
- Post-traumatic pericardial effusion
- Post-cardiotomy syndrome
- Haemopericardium in aortic dissection and rupture of the heart after acute MI
- Renal failure

Decompensation may be precipitated by other factors (e.g. drugs, sepsis, dehydration).

Some causes of effusion are unlikely to progress to tamponade:

- Autoimmune disease
- Thyroid disease
- Dressler's syndrome
- Other pericardial disease (e.g. chylopericardium)
- HF
- Pulmonary hypertension
- Pregnancy

How is cardiac tamponade diagnosed?

This condition may present in a spectrum ranging from preclinical signs (pericardial pressure = RA pressure < LA pressure) to haemodynamic shock and cardiac arrest.

Clinical signs:
- Hypotension, tachycardia
- Tachypnoea/dyspnoea
- JVP distension – steep x descent, loss of y descent
- Pulsus parodoxus

Other:
- *ECG*: low voltage QRS, electrical alternans
- *CXR*: enlarged cardiac silhouette
- *Echo*: pericardial effusion, RA ± RV diastolic collapse

Differentials include constrictive pericarditis, CCF, and advanced liver disease with cirrhosis.

What is pulsus paradoxus?

Pulsus paradoxus is a drop of **>10 mmHg** in systolic BP during inspiration.

How do the haemodynamics of constrictive pericarditis and cardiac tamponade compare?

Similarities
- Diastolic dysfunction and preserved ventricular ejection fraction
- Increased ventricular interdependence
- Increased respiratory variation of ventricular inflow/outflow (as pulsus paradoxus)
- Equalisation of pressures during diastole (RA, RV, PCWP)
- Pulmonary hypertension

Timing
- In constrictive pericarditis, there is reduction in diastolic filling by reaching the elastic limit of the pericardium. Early diastole is not affected. This manifests as a rapid y descent in the CVP.
- In cardiac tamponade, there is impaired filling throughout diastole ('holodiastolic').

Pressure dissociation
- Constrictive pericarditis prevents transmission of negative intrathoracic pressure at inspiration to the cardiac chambers. RA pressure remains constant and PCWP decreases. JVP does not decrease with inspiration (Kussmaul's sign). Friedrich's sign describes the associated steep y descent.
- RA pressure will decrease during inspiration in cardiac tamponade. There is preserved inspiratory increase in systemic venous return.

When is pericardial drainage indicated?

Timing
- If stable, within 12–24 h after FBC, etc.
- If haemodynamic shock – urgent pericardiocentesis

Indications for surgical drainage
- Haemopericardium from Type A aortic dissection
- Ventricular free wall rupture in acute MI
- Trauma
- Purulent effusion in unstable septic patient
- Loculated effusion not amenable to percutaneous drainage

Due to the range of manifestations of cardiac tamponade and potential for deterioration, a scoring system may be used (score ≥ 6 supporting urgent pericardiocentesis). Features scoring highly include the following:

- *Aetiology*: malignancy, TB
- *Presentation*: orthopnoea without crepitations, pulsus parodoxus, rapid deterioration
- *Imaging*: circumferential effusion, LA collapse, IVC inspiratory collapse, RV collapse

What are the main contraindications to immediate/urgent pericardiocentesis?

- Uncorrected coagulopathy
- INR > 1.5 from anticoagulant therapy
- Platelets < 50 × 10^9/l
- Small/posterior/loculated effusion

What specific supportive measures might help in a patient with cardiac tamponade?

- Avoidance of excessive heat and dehydration
- Avoidance of surges in catecholamine release (e.g. stress, pain)
- Transfer to a tertiary institution is recommended if limited experience available or contraindications are present, allowing for stability

In which other situations might you encounter the concept of tamponade in intensive care medicine?

Tamponade is otherwise most frequently encountered in the context of bleeding. Examples include the management of variceal haemorrhage, epistaxis, and trauma. Pressurised occlusion of a defect can be helpful in these situations:

- Balloon tamponade in **refractory variceal bleeding** – occludes venous blood flow, bides time to definitive management (e.g. TIPSS)
- Balloon tamponade in **epistaxis** (e.g. RAPID RHINO™ device in the post-cardiac arrest patient on anticoagulants)
- Surgical packing to prevent ongoing bleeding where source is difficult to manage (e.g. liver injury)
- Application of direct pressure to source of catastrophic haemorrhage – prevents exsanguination before definitive management

Deleterious tamponade also occurs in obstructive uropathy and compartment syndromes. (See Chapter 67 Compartment Syndromes)

Resources

- Doshi S, Ramakrishnan S, Gupta S. Invasive hemodynamics of constrictive pericarditis. Indian Heart J. 2015;67(2):175–182.
- Ristić AD, Imazio M, Adler Y. Triage strategy for urgent management of cardiac tamponade: a position statement of the European Society of Cardiology Working Group on Myocardial and Pericardial Diseases. Eur Heart J. 2014;35(34):2279–2284.

73. HYPERTENSION

What is hypertension?

> **KEY POINT**
>
> Hypertension is defined as an office **SBP ≥ 140 and/or DBP ≥ 90 mmHg** (Table 73.1).
>
> - **Optimal** BP < 120/80 (mmHg)
> - **Normal** < 130/90
> - **High-normal** 130/90 to 140/90
> - **Isolated systolic hypertension** SBP ≥ 140 and DBP < 90

Resistant hypertension occurs when hypertension is refractory to treatment and adherence to therapy is confirmed.

> **GUIDELINE**   ESC ESH 2018 Hypertension

Table 73.1   Classification of hypertension (systolic and/or diastolic BP criteria, mmHg)

Grade	Systolic BP	Diastolic BP
1	140–159	90–99
2	160–179	100–109
3	≥180	≥110

What are the causes of secondary hypertension?

- **OSA** (5–10%)
- **Renal**
  - Parenchymal disease (2–10%)
  - *Renovascular disease (1–10%)*: fibromuscular dysplasia, renal artery stenosis
- Endocrine
  - **Primary aldosteronism** (5–15%)
  - Thyroid disease (1–2%)
  - Phaeochromocytoma (<1%)
  - Cushing's syndrome (<1%)
  - Hyperparathyroidism (<1%)
- Coarctation of the aorta (<1%)

When might you suspect secondary hypertension?

- Young patient
- Acute worsening in stable patient
- Resistant hypertension
- Severe (grade 3) hypertension or hypertension emergency
- Extensive **hypertension-mediated organ damage (HMOD)**
- Features of other causes listed above

What hypertension emergencies are there?

Hypertension emergencies are situations in which **severe hypertension** (grade 3, ≥180/110 mmHg) is associated with **acute HMOD**. Rate and magnitude of BP increase is important.

- Malignant hypertension
- Sudden severe hypertension due to phaeochromocytoma
- Pregnancy with severe hypertension or pre-eclampsia
- Severe hypertension associated with other clinical conditions likely to require urgent reduction of BP
  - Acute aortic dissection
  - Acute MI
  - Acute HF

'Hypertension urgency' describes an acute presentation of severe hypertension **without HMOD**.

What are the symptoms of a hypertension emergency?

Hypertensive encephalopathy
- Headache
- Somnolence
- Lethargy
- Seizures
- Visual disturbance, cortical blindness
- LOC

Other features
- Chest pain
- Dyspnoea
- Dizziness

Focal neurology is rare and should prompt investigation for stroke. Features of organ dysfunction or an underlying condition may be apparent.

What is PRES?

Posterior reversible encephalopathy syndrome (PRES) is a clinico-radiological diagnosis:

- Features of **hypertensive encephalopathy** (headache, altered mental state, seizures, visual disturbance)

- Imaging demonstrating **white matter vasogenic oedema**, predominantly in the occipital and posterior parietal lobes

What is malignant hypertension?

Malignant hypertension is severe hypertension associated with:

- *Fundoscopic changes*: flame haemorrhages, papilloedema
- *Microangiopathy*
- *DIC*

Other possible associations are as follows:

- Encephalopathy (15%)
- Acute HF
- AKI

It is characterised by **small artery fibrinoid necrosis** in the kidneys, retinas, and brain, and has a poor prognosis if untreated.

How would you investigate a suspected hypertension emergency?

All

- Fundoscopy
- ECG
- *Bloods*: Hb, platelets, fibrinogen, U&E, LDH, haptoglobin
- Urine albumin-to-creatinine ratio (ACR), microscopy
- Pregnancy test in women of child-bearing age

Specific indications
- *Troponins*: cardiac involvement
- *CXR*: congestion
- *Echo*: dissection, HF, ischaemia
- *CT angiography*: acute aortic disease
- *CT/MR brain*: CNS involvement
- *US renal tract*: impairment or underlying cause
- *Urine toxicology screen*: methamphetamines, cocaine

What are the management priorities in a suspected hypertension emergency?

- Establishing target organs affected, supportive care as indicated
- Establish if precipitating cause may affect management (e.g. pregnancy)

Table 73.2 BP targets in hypertension emergencies (excluding stroke)

Condition	Target reduction	Timescale	First-line therapy (alternative)
Malignant hypertension	20–25% of MAP	Hours	Labetalol/nicardipine (sodium nitroprusside, urapidil)
Hypertensive encephalopathy	20–25% of MAP	Immediate	Labetalol/nicardipine (sodium nitroprusside)
ACS	Systolic BP < 140 mmHg	Immediate	GTN/labetalol (Urapidil)
Acute cardiogenic pulmonary oedema	Systolic BP < 140 mmHg	Immediate	Sodium nitroprusside/GTN (urapidil) with loop diuretic
Acute aortic dissection	Systolic BP < 120 mmHg, HR < 60 bpm	Immediate	Esmolol with Sodium nitroprusside/ GTN/nicardipine (Labetolol/metoprolol)
Eclampsia, severe pre-eclampsia, HELLP	Systolic BP < 160 mmHg, Diastolic BP < 105 mmHg	Immediate	Labetolol/nicardipine and $MgSO_4$ (Delivery)

- BP lowering in recommended timescale/magnitude with appropriate monitoring
- Manage underlying condition (e.g. thyrotoxicosis, aortic dissection)

What BP target would you aim for when managing a hypertension emergency?

Some emergencies require specific BP targets (Table 73.2).

Hypertension in **acute stroke** is a different concept to true hypertension emergencies, whereby it is more significant in terms of bleeding risk. Antihypertensive management is indicated in ICH and patients undergoing thrombolysis, or if another hypertension emergency is present. European Society of Cardiology (ESC) guidelines recommend clinical judgement in extreme BP elevation, suggesting that antihypertensive therapy might be appropriate ≥ **220/120 mmHg**, with a target reduction of **15%**. (See Chapter 84 Ischaemic Stroke)

74. INFECTIVE ENDOCARDITIS

What is infective endocarditis?

Infective endocarditis (IE) is an infection of the endocardium which may be mural/valvular.

What is the pathophysiology of IE?

- Haematogenous spread of infection results in seeding at a vulnerable site in the heart.
- The endocardium may have been damaged by high-velocity blood or mechanical damage, or altered by the presence of foreign bodies (e.g. prosthetic valve).
- Sterile thrombotic vegetation formed (mass attached to the endocardium or implanted cardiac material)
- Organisms adhere during transient bacteraemia, facilitated by platelets and fibrin.

What are the clinical features of IE?

Common features on presentation are as follows:

- **Fever** (90%)
- **Murmur** (85%)
- **Embolic phenomena** (25% at time of diagnosis)
- Chills
- Loss of appetite
- Weight loss
- Vascular/immunological phenomena

Features of underlying disease are as follows:

- Indwelling devices
- Congenital heart disease
- Stigmata of IV drug use

What are the complications of IE?

Local
- HF
- Myocarditis
- Abscess
- Pseudoaneurysm
- Mycotic aneurysm
- Fistulation
- Perivalvular extension
- Conduction disorders

Systemic
- Persistent sepsis
- Sequelae of shock (e.g. AKI)
- *Septic emboli*: CVA, ICH, splenic infarct, abscesses, PE, myocardial ischaemia, discitis, osteomyelitis

How is it diagnosed?

IE requires a high index of suspicion as it has a broad range of presentations, often over a protracted period of time, and sometimes atypically. A multidisciplinary approach should be used with the team potentially involving cardiology, neurology, microbiology, infectious diseases, intensive care, anaesthesia, cardiothoracic surgery, and allied professionals.

After clinical suspicion, the modified Duke criteria may be used to aid diagnosis and IE can be confirmed/rejected at this stage. In indeterminate cases, further investigations are advised. The ESC 2015 modified diagnostic criteria then divide cases into definite/possible/rejected IE. The key criteria centre on echo and blood culture findings but other imaging or bloods (e.g. IgG antibodies) may assist with diagnosis.

Echo
- TTE (70/50% sensitivity for native/prosthetic valve vegetations)
- TOE recommended (96/92%) where non-diagnostic or negative
- TOE also recommended if prosthetic valve/device present and with positive TTE
- Repeat 5–7 days later if initially negative

Blood cultures
- ≥3 sets to be taken 30 min apart.
- Repeat at 48–72 hours to assess response.
- No rationale to delay for episodes of fever
- Blood culture negative infective endocarditis (BCNIE) occurs in 31%.

GUIDELINE ESC 2015 Infective endocarditis

What are the modified Duke criteria?

These diagnostic criteria include clinical, echocardiographic, and biological findings (Table 74.1). In practice, clinical criteria will be the most familiar but it may also be diagnosed using pathological criteria. Approximately 80% sensitivity can be achieved. The diagnosis can be rejected if there is a firm alternative diagnosis, symptoms resolve within 4 days of antibiotic commencement, no pathological evidence is obtained in that time, or the criteria are not met.

KEY POINT

Definite IE (both of):

- **Pathological criteria**
  - *Microorganisms demonstrated*: culture, vegetation histology, embolus, or intracardiac abscess, or
  - *Pathological lesion*: active endocarditis in vegetation/intracardiac abscess on histology
- **Clinical criteria** (Table 74.1):
  - 2 major/(1 major + 3 minor)/5 minor

Possible IE:

- (1 major + 1 minor) or 3 minor clinical criteria

Table 74.1 Adaptation of ESC 2015 modified criteria for the diagnosis of IE

Major criteria	Minor criteria		

1 Blood cultures
• Typical organism × 2 samples
• Consistent organism, persistently positive
   • ≥ 2 at 12 h apart
   • All of 3/majority ≥ 4 with ≥ 1 h over whole set
	1 Predisposition (heart condition, IV drug use)		

	2 Fever (>38°C)		
	3 Vascular phenomena • Major arterial emboli • Septic pulmonary infarcts • Infectious (mycotic aneurysm) • ICH • Conjunctival haemorrhages • Janeway's lesions		

2 Imaging
• Echo
  • Vegetation
  • Abscess, pseudoaneurysm, intracardiac fistula
  • Valvular perforation/aneurysm
  • New partial dehiscence of prosthetic valve
• Abnormal prosthesis implantation on nuclear imaging/CT
	4 Immunological phenomena
	• Glomerulonephritis
	• Osler's nodes
	• Roth's spots
	• Rheumatoid factor		

	5 Microbiological evidence • Blood culture not meeting major criteria • Serological evidence of active infection with consistent organism		

What do you know about the microorganisms involved in IE?

Typical microorganisms
- *Strep. viridans*
- *Strep. bovis (gallolyticus)*
- *Strep. aureus*
- Community-acquired *Enterococci*
- HACEK group
  - ***Haemophilus*** *parainfluenzae, H. aphrophilus, H. paraphrophilus, H. influenzae*
  - ***Actinobacillus*** *actinomycetemcomitans*
  - ***Cardiobacterium*** *hominis*
  - ***Eikenella*** *corodens*
  - ***Kingella*** *kingae, K. denitrificans*

Blood culture-negative IE
- *Brucella* spp.
- *Coxiella burnetii*
- *Bartonella* spp.
- *Mycoplasma* spp.
- *Legionella* spp.
- Fungi

What do you know about prevention of IE?

Antibiotic prophylaxis during procedures involving bacteraemia was introduced based on animal models and observational studies but has since been discouraged after risk-benefit analyses.

Bacteraemia during specific procedures (e.g. dental extraction) has not been linked to IE directly. Antibiotic prophylaxis has not been shown to improve bacteraemia in humans.

Current guidelines recommend prophylaxis in high-risk cases:

- Any prosthetic valve (including TAVI)
- Patients with previous episode of IE
- *Congenital heart disease*: cyanotic or repaired with prosthesis

Other preventative measures:

- Good oral hygiene
- Disinfection of wounds

- Eradication of chronic bacterial disease (e.g. urine/skin)
- Curative antibiotics for bacterial infection
- Avoidance of patient self-medication with antibiotics
- Strict infection control procedures
- Avoidance of tattooing and piercing
- Limitation and monitoring/changing of indwelling devices when appropriate

What are the management priorities in the critical care context?

- Supportive care as indicated
- MDT involvement
- Appropriate investigation, diagnostic workup, and monitoring
- Early antimicrobials (e.g. flucloxacillin + gentamicin), long course (4–6 weeks)
- Management of affected indwelling devices – may require replacement/removal
- Management of comorbidity (e.g. drug withdrawal, congenital heart disease)
- Medium term IV access (e.g. PICC)

What are the indications for surgical intervention?

Decision-making should be individualised and will often involve high-risk features. Indications in left-sided lesions are listed below (urgent within days unless otherwise specified):

- **Heart failure:** severe aortic/mitral regurgitation, obstruction, or fistula resulting in any of:
  - Refractory pulmonary oedema (emergency, <24 h)
  - CS (emergency)
  - Symptomatic HF
  - Echo signs of poor haemodynamic tolerance
- **Uncontrolled infection**
  - *Local*: abscess (lengthening PR interval), false aneurysm, fistula, enlarging vegetation
  - Fungi or multiresistant organisms (urgent/elective, i.e. 'scheduled')
  - Persisting positive blood cultures despite medical management of source/emboli
  - Prosthetic valve with Staphylococcus or non-HACEK gram negative bacteria (urgent/elective)
- **Prevention of embolism**
  - Persistent vegetation > 10mm after ≥ 1 embolic episode despite antimicrobials
  - Vegetation > 10 mm with severe valve stenosis/regurgitation and low operative risk
  - Very large vegetation > 30 mm
  - Isolated large vegetation > 15 mm

Resource

- Martinez G, Valchanov K. Infective endocarditis. CEACCP. 2012;12(3):134–139.

---

75.   ACUTE CORONARY SYNDROMES

Why are ACS relevant to critical care?

ACS may present with varying severity and overlap with critical care in many ways, with significant effects on patient outcomes in certain situations. Hospital infrastructure is not standardised, with services variably distributed between cardiology wards, coronary care units, high dependency, and intensive care depending on the institution.

Intensivists may be involved in the management of (or decisions relating to):

- Resultant organ failure
  - CS '
  - Pulmonary oedema
  - Cardiorenal syndrome
  - Ischaemic cardiomyopathy
- High-dependency care following PPCI
- Post resuscitation care after cardiac arrest
- Perioperative MI
- New presentation of ACS in existing critical care patients
- Unrelated conditions in patients with history of ACS

What are the acute coronary syndromes?

KEY POINT

The term 'acute coronary syndrome' (ACS) encompasses a broad range of conditions of varying severity, including the following:

- **Cardiac arrest**
- **Electrical or haemodynamic instability** with CS (due to ongoing ischaemia or mechanical complications)
- MI
  - STEMI
  - Non-ST segment elevation MI (NSTEMI)
- **Unstable angina** (UA)

Where acute chest discomfort is present, ACS are subclassified to guide management:

- **ST-segment elevation ACS** (STE-ACS)
- **Non-ST segment elevation ACS** (NSTE-ACS)
  - *NSTEMI*: biomarker change
  - *UA*: no biomarker change

GUIDELINE   ESC 2017 STEMI

GUIDELINE   ESC 2020 NSTE-ACS

GUIDELINE   NICE 2020 NG185 ACS

(See Chapter 27 Out-of-Hospital Cardiac Arrest)

How is MI diagnosed?

Diagnosis may be ongoing during the period of stabilisation and resuscitation. European guidelines recommend diagnosis within 10 min of first medical contact.

History

- *May be asymptomatic*
- *Chest discomfort > 15 min*: easy to misdiagnose as musculoskeletal/GI
  - May have upper limb, mandibular, epigastric discomfort
  - Usually > 20 min, diffuse, not affected by movement/position
  - Caution in certain groups: female, elderly, diabetic, post-op, critically ill
  - Do not diagnose using response to GTN
- *Other*: dyspnoea, fatigue, nausea, vomiting, syncope, palpitations

Examination

- Tachypnoea, crepitations, hypoxia
- Diaphoresis, change in complexion
- Hypotension
- Complications (e.g. mitral regurgitation, decreased UO)

Investigations

- *Twelve lead ECG*: significant changes
- *Biomarker assays*: high sensitivity troponin I or T
  - If low risk, single test acceptable at presentation to rule out MI, second test only if positive
  - Otherwise, second test as per specific assay requirements
- U&E, glucose
- *Echo*: functional impairment, effusion, valvular incompetence

What ECG changes might indicate STEMI?

ST-segment elevation in ≥2 contiguous leads:

- ≥2 mm in V2–3 in men over 40 years
- ≥2.5 mm in V2–3 in men under 40 years
- ≥1.5 mm in V2–3 in women
- ≥1 mm in other leads

New LBBB is also suggestive. If pre-existant LBBB or pacing are present, Smith-Modified Sgarbossa Criteria may be used, which involve the concordance or proportionally excessive discordance of ST changes.

Which other conditions might be associated with a troponin rise?

Primary cardiac

- Tachyarrhythmias
- HF
- Myocarditis
- Takotsubo cardiomyopathy
- Valvular heart disease

- Cardiac contusion
- Procedural (e.g. CABG, PCI, ablation, pacing, cardioversion)

Other
- Hypertension emergencies
- Critical illness
- Aortic dissection
- PE, pulmonary hypertension
- Renal dysfunction with associated cardiac disease
- Acute neurological event (e.g. stroke, SAH)
- Extreme endurance efforts
- Hypo-/hyperthyroidism
- Infiltrative disease (e.g. amyloidosis, haemochromatosis, sarcoidosis)
- Drug toxicity (e.g. doxorubicin)
- Rhabdomyolysis

How is MI classified?

The third international definition includes a **universal classification** by aetiology.

KEY POINT

MI Types

1. Spontaneous
2. Secondary to **ischaemic imbalance** (e.g. coronary spasm/embolism, hypotension, dysrhythmias, anaemia, respiratory failure)
3. Resulting in death when biomarkers unavailable
4. a. Related to PCI
   b. Related to stent thrombosis
5. Related to CABG

The term 'MINOCA' refers to MI with non-obstructive coronary arteries on angiography.

Outline the initial management when suspecting a patient of STEMI/STE-ACS.

- *A*: may require invasive ventilation if obtunded/severely agitated before PPCI
- *B*: target appropriate oxygenation (S_pO_2 90%, P_aO_2 8.0 kPa), avoid hyperoxia
- *C*: prevent further ischaemia, optimise coronary perfusion
  - Nitrates (e.g. GTN)
  - *Reperfusion*: PCI vs fibrinolysis, time-critical
  - CS may require inotrope/inodilator infusion, mechanical support, vasoconstrictors in the interim.
  - Arterial line should not delay PCI (avoid right radial/femoral sites if required).
- *D*: titrated IV opioid (e.g. diamorphine), consider mild sedative if very anxious
- *E*: explore concomitant issues (e.g. injury following a collapse)
- *F*: may require RRT (e.g. in MODS)
- *G*: NG tube if unable to swallow, avoid hyperglycaemia (target < 11)
- *H*: anticoagulation

(See Chapter 78 Heart Failure)

How is coronary reperfusion achieved in STE-ACS and when are different therapies indicated?

Definitive management should be carried out as soon as possible to minimise total ischaemic time. This is guided by pathways and networks which often start pre-hospitally.

- **Coronary angiography ± follow on PPCI**
  - STEMI presenting <12 h of symptom onset (if PPCI can be delivered within 120 min of time fibrinolysis could have been given)
  - STEMI with CS presenting <12 h
  - STEMI presenting >12 h in selected cases with ongoing ischaemia
- **Coronary angiography with a view to coronary revascularisation**
  - STEMI with CS presenting >12 h (or developing CS later)
- **Fibrinolysis**
  - If PPCI cannot be delivered within 120 min of time it could have been given
  - Give an antithrombin simultaneously
  - *ECG after 60–90 min*: if ongoing ischaemia, for angiography ± rescue PCI

During angiography, culprit vessel (if CS present) vs complete revascularisation (no CS) will be considered in multivessel disease. Stenting may be indicated with preference of drug-eluting stents.

STUDY

ISIS-2 (1988)

- Acute MI with in 24 h of symptom onset
- *Interventions*: streptokinase/aspirin/both vs placebo
- *Primary*: 5-week vascular mortality – **significantly lower** (reduced by 23% and 20%, 40% in combination)

STUDY

NORDISTEMI (2010)

- STEMI post-thrombolysis
- *Intervention*: immediate PCI vs PCI for rescue/deterioration
- *Primary*: 12-month composite death, stroke, reinfarction – **significantly lower (6% vs 16%)**

How would you manage antithrombotic therapy in STE-ACS?

Antiplatelet agents
- Dual antiplatelet therapy (DAPT)
  - **Aspirin** 300 mg per os (PO)/NG/PR immediately for all patients unless clear evidence of allergy
  - **Prasugrel** (if not already anticoagulated, risk vs benefit in age >75y)
    - Clopidogrel if already taking oral anticoagulant
    - Ticagrelor if not for PPCI (unless high bleeding risk – use clopidogrel)
- If PPCI
  - Not for glycoprotein IIb/IIIa or fibrinolytics before arrival at catheter laboratory
  - During PPCI: **glycoprotein IIb/IIIa inhibitor** (e.g. tirofiban)

Anticoagulation
- **Unfractionated heparin (UFH), bivalirudin, or enoxaparin IV**
- Fondaparinux contraindicated in context of PPCI – potential harm

Doses might be specific to indication (Table 75.1).

Outline the cardiology management of NSTE-ACS.

- *Aspirin loading*
- *Fondaparinux*
  - Avoid if high bleeding risk or immediate angiography.
  - If renal impairment, consider UFH.

Table 75.1 Anticoagulant and antiplatelet agents used in ACS

	Drug	Dose (enteral unless specified)	Maintenance dose/infusion
Antiplatelet	Aspirin	300 mg (can give PR)	75 mg OD
	Prasugrel	60 mg (delay until PCI if NSTE-ACS)	5 mg (<60 kg or ≥ 75 y) or 10 mg (>60 kg, <75 y) OD
	Clopidogrel	300/600 mg	75 mg OD
	Ticagrelor	180 mg	90 mg BD
Glycoprotein IIb/ IIIa inhibitors	Tirofiban	25 µg/kg over 3 min IV at start of PPCI 400 ng/kg/min over 30 min IV infusion in NSTEACS with planned PCI	150 ng/kg/min up to 48 h total (STEMI) 150 ng/kg/min for 12–24 h, max 48 h total (NSTE-ACS) 100 ng/kg/min at least 48 h, continue 12–48 h post PCI, max 108 h
	Eptifibatide	180 µg/kg IV	
	Abciximab	0.25 mg/kg IV	
Antithrombin	Bivalirudin (direct thrombin inhibitor)	750 µg/kg IV in PPCI 100 µg/kgIV in NSTE-ACS with planned intervention	1.75 mg/kg/h during procedure (further dose reduction 4–12 h post-procedure if required) 250 µg/kg/h (duration depends on timing of intervention)
	UFH (indirect thrombin inhibitor)	5000 units or 75 units/kg IV	18 units/kg/h (with laboratory monitoring)
Fibrinolytic	Alteplase	15 mg IV	0.75 mg/kg (< 65 kg) or 50 mg (>65 kg) over 30 min IV infusion then 0.5 mg/kg (<65 kg) or 35 mg (>65 kg) over 60 min IV infusion (max total 100 mg over 90 min)
	Streptokinase	1500000 units over 60 min IV infusion	
	Tenecteplase	30–50mg over 10 seconds IV	

- *DAPT*: add second agent once diagnosis confirmed.
- Risk assessment for future adverse cardiovascular events (e.g. Global Registry of Acute Coronary Events (GRACE) score – caution in younger patients)
- *Diagnosis of culprit lesion(s)*: angiography depending on risk:
  - *Immediate invasive (<2 h)*: very high risk: unstable, shock, refractory pain, arrhythmias, mechanical complications, acute HF, significant ST-segment changes
  - *Early invasive (<24 h)*: high risk: established NSTEMI, dynamic ST-segment/T-wave changes, post-arrest without ST-segment elevation or shock, GRACE score > 140
  - *Selective invasive*: low risk: absence of above features

What might specific ongoing management in critical care include?

- *Further cardiology input*
  - If received fibrinolysis, consider coronary angiography during same admission.
  - May require urgent CABG.
  - Liaison regarding secondary prevention, risk evaluation, and follow–up
  - Planning suitable location for step down of care
- *Secondary prevention* after MI
  - *ACE-I*: as soon as haemodynamically stable, facilitates remodelling
  - *DAPT*: up to 12 months, aspirin indefinitely

- *Beta-blocker*: as soon as haemodynamically stable
- Statin or alternative
- *Aldosterone antagonist*: if HF with reduced EF
- *Supportive care* for complications
  - *Prolonged wean*: tracheostomy may be required
  - *Epistaxis*: ENT input, balloon tamponade, cautery
  - *Dysrhythmias*: aim K$^+$ 4.0–4.5 mmol/l, may require PPM/ICD
  - *HF*: pharmacological/mechanical support, workup for transplant (see Chapter 78 Heart Failure and Chapter 12 Mechanical Circulatory Support)
  - *GI bleeding*: often supportive, consider ruling out other causes
- *Investigations*
  - *Echo*: LV function assessment before discharge from hospital
  - Ischaemia testing if conservatively managed
  - HbA1c if not known to have diabetes
  - Fasting glucose > 4/7 after onset
- *Other*: liaison with GP, health education, referral to cardiac rehabilitation

Resources

- Cardiology Trials.org: Explaining the Most important Trials in Cardiology. Available from: http://cardiology-trials.org. (Accessed 24 January 2022.)
- National Institute for Health and Care Excellence. British National Formulary. Available from: https://bnf.nice.org.uk. (Accessed 24 January 2022.)
- Thygesen K, Alpert JS, Jaffe AS, et al. Third universal definition of myocardial infarction. Circulation. 2012;126:2020–2035.

76. ARRHYTHMIAS

What is the significance of atrial fibrillation in critical care?

AF is the most common arrhythmia encountered in critical care due to high prevalence in populations at risk of critical illness and critical illness itself.

It is more prevalent in patients with:

- Electrolyte disturbances
- Greater disease severity
- Vasoactive agent use – dopamine and adrenaline (chronotropic)
- Greater illness severity
- Larger atrial size on echo

AF is often accompanied by a high ventricular rate and may lead to a reduced cardiac output. The 'atrial kick' is lost, which usually assists ventricular filling during diastole. Outcomes are difficult to assess as AF is often an indicator of severe disease.

In critically ill patients with new-onset AF:

- 37% develop haemodynamic instability
- 11% exhibit new signs of ischaemia/HF
- 86% resolution prior to hospital discharge
- ×2 incidence of in-hospital ischaemic stroke

What are the causes of AF in critical illness?

The mechanism of AF in critical care is thought to involve a combination of arrhythmogenic atrial substrate and arrhythmogenic trigger. There may be chronic structural/electrical remodelling due to age, diabetes, HF, CKD, or tachycardia.

Remodelling in critical illness may be due to:

- *Inflammation*: surgery, infection
- *Accelerated fibrosis*: infection
- *Atrial stretch*: volume overload
- *Altered ion channel expression*: sustained tachycardia, bacterial toxins
- *Altered intracellular ion handling*: thyroid storm, antiarrhythmics

Triggers include the following:

- *Excessive adrenergic stimulation*: vasoactive substances, sepsis, ventilator dyssynchrony
- *Myocyte trauma/injury*: uraemia, myocardial ischaemia, right heart catheterisation
- *Altered intracellular ion handling*: electrolyte derangements

How would you manage new-onset AF in the ICU?

- **DCCV** if haemodynamic compromise – ischaemia, HF, hypotension (systolic BP < 90), syncope, extreme HR (>150 or <40)
- **Address cause** if identifiable (e.g. stop beta-agonists, use alternative vasoactive agent)
- **Correct reversible factors**
  - Electrolytes
  - Ventilation
  - Myocardial ischaemia
  - Volume status
  - Infection
- **Manage ongoing instability**
  - *Rate-related*: beta-blocker, non-dihydropyridine calcium channel blocker, digoxin
  - *Rhythm-related*: magnesium, amiodarone
- **Anticoagulation** for stroke prevention not usually commenced during the acute phase of critical illness

Would you continue a patient's beta-blocker during critical care admission?

Rate control is ideal in certain circumstances to optimise diastolic filling time and reduce myocardial oxygen demand, potentially preventing AF and perioperative MI.

However, routine use of beta-blockers has been linked to adverse events, as shown by the **POISE** trial. The **DECREASE** trials, with findings including a 91% reduction in cardiac death and MI, were discredited due to misconduct. Subsequent meta-analyses found that perioperative initiation of beta-blockers increases mortality (by around 27%).

Most clinicians would not start beta blockade de novo in this context. It may be appropriate to continue existing prescriptions in haemodynamically stable patients.

POISE (2008)

- Patients undergoing non-cardiac surgery
- *Intervention*: metoprolol succinate pre- and post-op vs placebo
- *Primary*: 30-day composite cardiovascular death, non-fatal MI, non-fatal cardiac arrest – **significantly lower**
- *Secondary*: 30-day mortality, stroke – **significantly higher**. Clinically significant hypotension, bradycardia – **significantly higher**

How would you approach other tachycardias?

Tachycardias can be managed as per ALS protocols. Synchronised DCCV is recommended if compromised (as above).

Broad complex
- Regular
  - *VT*: amiodarone
  - *SVT with BBB*: treat as narrow complex
- Irregular
  - *AF with BBB*: treat as narrow-complex
  - *Pre-excited AF*: amiodarone

Narrow complex
- Regular
  - Vagal manoeuvres (e.g. modified Valsalva if suitable)
  - Adenosine 6 mg > 12 mg > 18 mg
    - ➤ Rapid IV bolus, pacing defibrillator attached
    - ➤ *Avoid in asthma/COPD*: causes bronchospasm
  - *Second line*: verapamil 2.5–5mg IV over 2 min
  - Rate control may be required if refractory (e.g. beta-blockade)
- *Irregular*: AF (see above)

How would you perform DCCV?

Synchronised DCCV should be performed as per recommended life support guidance. In the UK:

- Safety measures as with any defibrillation (e.g. oxygen management)
- *Apply pads*: anteroposterior pad position ideal in AF/flutter
- Sedation required if conscious
- Synchronise defibrillator
- Charge.
  - *Broad-complex tachycardia or AF*: 120–150 J, increase if fails
  - *Other narrow complex tachycardia or atrial flutter*: 70–120 J initially
- *Shock*: button may need to be held until correct point in ECG cycle achieved
- Check for cardiac output
- If delivering subsequent shocks, ensure defibrillator synchronised again

What is Wolff-Parkinson-White syndrome?

Wolff-Parkinson-White syndrome is characterised by a congenital accessory conducting pathway and may give rise to a narrow-complex SVT. It is characterised by pre-excitation: short PR-interval/delta wave, broad QRS complex, and T-wave abnormalities on resting ECG.

Drug choice is significant:

- Adenosine is first line
- Verapamil is contraindicated
- Amiodarone may be used safely

What is long QT syndrome?

The QT interval is measured from the start of the QRS complex to the end of the T wave on an ECG. It is affected by HR (shorter if rate higher) and so the corrected QT interval (QTc) can be calculated using the RR interval (60/HR). Many formulae exist – the original was the Bazett Formula:

$$QTc = QT / \sqrt{RR}$$

A normal QTc interval is <430 ms in men and <450 ms in women. Definite prolongation is present if >**450 ms** and >**470 ms**, respectively.

Long QT Syndrome (LQTS) is the presence of a prolonged QT interval in the absence of secondary causes and is usually inherited:

- *Autosomal dominant*: Romano-Ward, Andersen-Tawil, Timothy syndromes
- *Autosomal recessive*: Jervell and Lange-Nielsen syndrome

Diagnostic criteria for LQTS are as follows:

- QTc ≥ 480 ms in repeated 12-lead ECGs, or
- Schwartz LQTS risk score > 3

The risk score utilises the following criteria:

- *ECG*: QTc duration, QTc response to exercise, torsades de pointes, T-wave alternans, notched T wave in 3 leads, low resting HR < 2nd percentile for age
- *Clinical*: syncope, congenital deafness
- *Family history*: definite LQTS, unexplained sudden cardiac death < 30 years in immediate family

Short QT (≤ 340 ms) is rare but highly lethal. It may result from hypercalcaemia, digoxin use, and genetic mutations. Over 40% of those with inherited disease will have a cardiac arrest before 40 years of age.

GUIDELINES ESC 2015 Ventricular Arrhythmias

What are the causes of long QT in critical care?

KEY POINT

- **Electrolyte abnormalities**
  - Hypokalaemia
  - Hypomagnaesaemia
  - Hypocalcaemia
- **Hypothermia**
- **Myocardial ischaemia**
- **Raised ICP**
- **Drugs**
  - *Antipsychotics*: haloperidol, droperidol, quetiapine, olanzapine, chlorpromazine
  - *Antiarrhythmics*: quinidine, procainamide, flecainide, sotalol, amiodarone
  - *TCA*: amitriptyline, imipramine, nortriptyline
  - *Other antidepressants*: citalopram, escitalopram, venlafaxine
  - *Antihistamines*: diphenhydramine, loratidine
  - *Other*: macrolides, quinine, chloroquine, hydroxychloroquine

How would you manage torsades de pointes?

Torsades de pointes is a form of polymorphic VT (multiple ventricular foci resulting in variable QRS amplitude, axis, duration) that occurs with QT prolongation. It may degenerate into VF. This condition arises when a premature ventricular complex occurs on the preceding T wave, the 'R on T' phenomenon.

Management:
- Address precipitating cause
- May be self-limiting
- Magnesium infusion (2 g over 10 min, repeated as appropriate)
- Overdrive pacing
- *If compromised but pulse present*: synchronised DCCV
- *Pulseless*: defibrillation

What is 'electrical storm' and how is it managed?

Electrical storm is a state of electrical instability characterised by multiple episodes of VT/VF. It may present with haemodynamic instability or multiple shocks in patients with ICDs. It is distressing for patients and families, with significant psychological consequences.

- **Electrical storm** is diagnosed when ≥3 separate episodes occur in 24 h resulting in ICD therapy.
- **Incessant VT** is where sustained VT resumes within 5 min of a successful shock and continues for >12 h.

Management
- *Sedation*: reduces sympathetic tone and potentially distress
- *Correct reversible factors*: majority have no identifiable cause
  - Electrolyte imbalance
  - *Acute ischaemia*: treat flow-limiting coronary artery disease
  - *Exacerbation of HF*: correct volume overload
  - Adjustment or non-compliance with antiarrhythmic medication
  - Recent introduction to biventricular pacing
- *Device programming*: consider temporarily disabling shock therapy in conscious patient
- *Antiarrhythmics*
  - Beta-blockers first line
  - Amiodarone in structural heart disease (30% refractory despite amiodarone)
  - Lidocaine
- *Overdrive (atrial) pacing*
- *Radiofrequency catheter ablation*
- *Surgery*: left cardiac sympathetic denervation

Resources
- Bosch NA, Cimini J, Walkey AJ. Atrial fibrillation in the ICU. Chest. 2018;154(6):1424–1434.
- Burns E. 2021 Life in the Fast Lane. Drugs Causing QT Prolongation. Available from: https://litfl.com/drugs-causing-qt-prolongation/. (Accessed 18 December 2021.)
- Cole G, Grancis D. Perioperative β-blockade: guidelines do not reflect the problems with the evidence from the DECREASE trials. BMJ. 2014;349:g5210.
- Hendriks AA, Szili-Torok T. Editor's Choice – The treatment of electrical storm: an educational review. Eur Heart J Acute Cardiovasc Care. 2018;7(5):478–483.
- Soar J, Clarke AB, Gwinnutt C, et al. (Eds.) Advanced Life Support, 8th ed. London: Resuscitation Council (UK); 2021.

---

77. CARDIOMYOPATHIES

What is a cardiomyopathy?

KEY POINT

A cardiomyopathy is a condition of the myocardium in which

- The heart muscle is **structurally and functionally abnormal**
- In the absence of coronary artery disease/hypertension/valvular/congenital heart disease sufficient to cause the observed myocardial abnormality.

Which types of cardiomyopathy are you aware of?

The classification of cardiomyopathies is complicated, largely due to the varying pathophysiology amongst a broad range of conditions, with differing influence of any concomitant disease.

The most recent classification from the ESC is by phenotype:

- *Hypertrophic cardiomyopathy (HCM)*: myocardial hypertrophy in absence of haemodynamic stress
- *Dilated cardiomyopathy (DCM)*: LV dilatation and LV systolic dysfunction in absence of abnormal loading conditions
- *Arrhythmogenic right ventricular cardiomyopathy (ARVC)*: progressive replacement of RV myocardium with adipose and fibrous tissue, confined to triangle of dysplasia (apex, RV inflow/outflow tracts)
- *Restrictive cardiomyopathy (RCM)*: restrictive ventricular pathology with normal/decreased systolic and diastolic volumes and normal ventricular wall thickness
- *Unclassified*

Each phenotype is subclassified into familial and non-familial forms. Within each of these, conditions are then classified into those with an unidentified gene defect, and those of a disease subtype.

Previous classification by WHO/International Society and Federation of Cardiology (ISFC) had involved LV dysfunction from coronary artery disease, hypertension, valvular disease, and congenital heart disease. However, these have not been included as they are thought to involve different issues to the rest of the cardiomyopathies.

Can you name some causes of cardiomyopathy?

Causes of cardiomyopathy may be classified by phenotype (Table 77.1).

What is Takotsubo cardiomyopathy?

Takotsubo cardiomyopathy is a potentially reversible cause of acute HF. It is characterised by transient regional LV **apical or mid-ventricular** systolic dysfunction without obstructive coronary disease on angiography (this is required for diagnosis).

'Takotsubo' originates from the Japanese name for an octopus trap, which the echocardiographic appearance is thought to resemble (Figure 77.1).

Presentation may mimic ACS:
- Abrupt, severe chest pain
- Diffuse T-wave inversion
- Mild cardiac enzyme elevation

The pathophysiology is thought to relate to elevated NA concentrations related to emotional or physical stress, hence the alternative name 'broken heart syndrome'. Other names include apical ballooning

Table 77.1   Causes of cardiomyopathies

	Non-familial	Familial
HCM	Obesity Athletic training Amyloid Infants of diabetic mothers	Glycogen storage disease Noonan's syndrome Friedrich's ataxia Beckwith-Wiedermann syndrome
DCM	Myocarditis Kawasaki disease Pregnancy Alcohol Eosinophilic Endocrine	Mutations in genes coding different components of sarcomere/myocytes
ARVC	Inflammation (possible)	Mutations in genes coding different components of sarcomere/myocytes
RCM	Amyloid Scleroderma Medications (e.g. busulfan, methysergide) Carcinoid Radiation	Pseudoxanthoma elasticum Haemochromatosis Desminopathy
Unclassified	Takotsubo	Causes of LV non-compaction

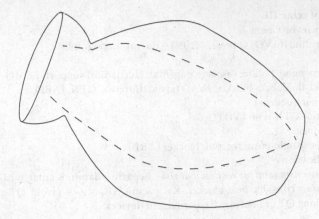

Figure 77.1 The octopus pot appearance in Takotsubo cardiomyopathy (solid line) vs normal left ventricular shape (dashed line).

syndrome and acute stress-induced cardiomyopathy. Takotsubo cardiomyopathy is most prevalent in post-menopausal women.

Stress-induced cardiomyopathy may also be caused by neurogenic myocardial stunning following acute cerebral accidents such as SAH, phaeochromocytoma crisis, exogenous catecholamine administration, and critical illness such as sepsis or post-cardiac arrest syndrome.

How would you investigate suspected Takotsubo cardiomyopathy?

- *ECG*: **ST-segment elevation** in 44%
- *Echo*: apical ballooning, other variants possible
- *Diagnostic*
  - Coronary angiography with left ventriculography to exclude acute MI – depends on ST-segment elevation, risk scoring (e.g. InterTAK Diagnostic Score)
  - Coronary CT angiography can be performed in some stable patients instead.
- *Biomarkers*
  - Troponin is usually comparable to ACS.
  - Increased BNP and N-terminal-proBNP (peak 24–48 h after onset)

What complications might arise from Takotsubo cardiomyopathy?

Frequent (highest incidence in brackets)
- Acute HF (45%)
- LV outflow tract obstruction (LVOTO) (25%)
- Mitral regurgitation (25%)
- CS (20%)

Moderate
- AF (15%)
- LV thrombus (8%)
- Cardiac arrest (6%)
- AV block (5%)

Rare: other dysrhythmias, torsades de pointes, acute VSD. Death occurs in around 4.5% of cases.

What are the priorities in managing the patient with Takotsubo cardiomyopathy requiring critical care?

- **High index of suspicion**
  - May present to critical care undiagnosed (e.g. CS in 'ACS', post-cardiac arrest syndrome)
  - TTE/TOE may be the first indicator of Takotsubo

- **Management of acute HF**
  - Cardiology involvement
  - First, determine if LVOTO present (20%) – during angiography
  - CS
    - ➤ *Primary pump failure*: vasoactive agents*, mechanical support, ECMO
    - ➤ *LVOTO*: fluid, beta-blocker, LVAD (avoid diuretics, GTN, IABP)
  - HF/pulmonary oedema
    - ➤ Diuretics/GTN if no LVOTO
    - ➤ Beta-blocker
    - ➤ ACE-I or angiotensin receptor blocker (ARB)
- **Manage complications**
  - *Thromboembolism (and prevention if at risk)*: heparin/vitamin K antagonist/DOAC
  - *Dysrhythmias*: consider beta-blocker, RV pacing, DC shock (avoid QT prolongation, beta-blocker in long QT or bradycardia, permanent devices)

*Choice of vasoactive agent:

- Guidelines suggest avoiding adrenaline, NA, dobutamine, milrinone, isoprenaline where possible due to 20% mortality in those treated with catecholamines – potential selection bias.
- Levosimendan (calcium sensitiser) might be beneficial.

Further management after discharge may involve targeting other underlying disorders (coronary artery disease, anxiety/depression) and prevention of recurrence – hormone replacement may be indicated.

(See Chapter 78 Heart Failure)

What is peripartum cardiomyopathy?

Peripartum cardiomyopathy (PPCM) is a rare, idiopathic cardiomyopathy characterised by systolic dysfunction presenting in late pregnancy or the early post-partum period. Incidence varies globally. Definitions differ in terms of the timeframe affected.

KEY POINT

ESC 2010 definition of PPCM:

- HF secondary to LV systolic dysfunction, **LVEF < 45%**,
- towards end of pregnancy or in the months following delivery (mostly in the first month), with
- no other identifiable cause of HF.

The pathophysiology is unclear but is thought to involve the combination of systemic angiogenic imbalance and host susceptibility. Risk factors may include the following:

- Multiparity
- Multiple pregnancies
- Family history
- *Ethnicity*: African, African-American
- Smoking
- Diabetes
- Hypertension
- Pre-eclampsia
- Malnutrition
- Advanced maternal age
- Prolonged use of tocolytic beta-agonists

Resource

- Bauersachs J, König T, van der Meer P, et al. Pathophysiology, diagnosis and management of peripartum cardio-myopathy: a position statement from the Heart Failure Association of the European Society of Cardiology Study Group on peripartum cardiomyopathy. Eur J Heart Fail. 2019;21(7):827–843.

- Elliott P, Andersson B, Arbustini E, et al. Classification of the cardiomyopathies: a position statement from the European Society of Cardiology working group on myocardial and pericardial diseases. Eur Heart J. 2008;29(2):270–276.
- Ghadri J-R, Wittstein IS, Prasad A, et al. International Expert Consensus Document on Takotsubo Syndrome (Part II): diagnostic workup, outcome, and management. Eur Heart J. 2018;39(22):2047–2062.
- Richard C. Stress-related cardiomyopathies. Ann Intensive Care. 2011;1(1):39.

78.   HEART FAILURE

What is heart failure and how is it classified?

> **KEY POINT**
>
> Heart failure (HF) is
>
> - A clinical syndrome
> - Due to a structural/functional abnormality of the heart,
> - Resulting in **elevated intracardiac pressures** and/or **inadequate cardiac output**
> - At rest and/or during exercise.

It is most commonly the result of myocardial dysfunction: systolic/diastolic/mixed. Valvular, pericardial, and endocardial pathology, and rhythm disturbances can also contribute to HF.

HF may be classified according to the nature of the LVEF:

- *Preserved (HF with preserved ejection fraction [HFpEF]):* ≥50%
- *Mildly reduced (HFmrEF):* 41–49%
- *Reduced (HFrEF):* ≤40%

It may also be described in terms of its onset as acute vs chronic HF. Chronic HF can also present acutely and is termed 'decompensated HF'.

RV dysfunction may also result in HF. (See Chapter 79 Pulmonary Hypertension)

> **GUIDELINE**   ESC 2021 Heart failure

What are the risk factors for HF?

- Sedentary lifestyle
- Smoking
- Obesity
- Excessive alcohol intake
- Influenza, other viruses
- Other microbes: *Trypanosoma cruzi, Streptococci*
- Cardiotoxic drugs
- Chest radiation
- Hypertension

- Dyslipidaemia
- Diabetes mellitus
- Coronary artery disease

How is chronic HF managed?

Pharmacological therapies reducing the risk of hospitalisation/death in HFrEF:

- *ACE-I*
  - Alternatively angiotensin receptor-neprilysin inhibitor (ARNI) – sacubitril/valsartan
- *Beta-blocker*
- *Mineralocorticoid receptor antagonists*: spironolactone, eplerenone
- *Sodium-glucose co-transporter-2 (SGLT2) inhibitors*: dapagliflozin, empagliflozin

Other pharmacological therapies are as follows:

- *Loop diuretics*: reduce congestive symptoms, improve exercise capacity, reduce hospitalisation
- *ARB*: if unable to have ACE-I or ARNI
- *I$_f$-channel inhibitor (ivabradine)*: If LVEF ≤ 35%, sinus rhythm, HR ≥ 70 despite above or unable to tolerate beta-blocker
- *Soluble guanylate cyclase receptor stimulator (vericiguat)*: worsening despite above
- *Hydralazine, isosorbide dinitrate*: selected ethnicities
- *Digoxin*: selected patients with symptoms despite above

Non-pharmacological

- *Management of underlying disease*: coronary artery disease, iron deficiency, arrhythmias, valve disease
- *Modifying risk factors* (e.g. smoking cessation, immunisation, exercise rehabilitation)
- *Education* (e.g. avoidance of large fluid intake, lifestyle adaptations)
- *Cardiac resynchronisation therapy* pacemaker/defibrillator (see Chapter 13 Pacing)
- *Mechanical support*: bridge to recovery, candidacy, or transplantation
- *Heart transplantation*

STUDY

REMATCH (2001)

- End-stage HF
- *Intervention*: LVAD vs medical management
- *Primary*: all-cause mortality – **significantly lower at 1 year (52% vs 25%) and 2 years (23% vs 8%)**
- *Secondary*: serious adverse events – **significantly higher**

(See Chapter 12 Mechanical Circulatory Support)

What is advanced HF?

Advanced HF is characterised by the persistence of HF symptoms despite maximal therapy. It is defined by the following criteria:

- **NYHA III or IV** symptoms
- **Severe cardiac dysfunction** (1 of:)
  - EF ≤ 30%
  - Isolated RV failure
  - Non-operable severe valve/congenital abnormality
  - Persistently high or rising BNP/NT-proBNP and severe LV diastolic dysfunction or structural abnormalities
- **Decompensation**
  - Episodes of pulmonary/systemic congestion requiring high-dose IV diuretics, or

- Episodes of low output requiring inotropes/vasoactive drugs, or
- Malignant arrhythmias causing > 1 unplanned hospital visit in last 12 months
- **Severe impairment of exercise capacity** (1 of:)
  - Inability to exercise
  - Low 6 MWT distance (<300 m)
  - pVO_2 < 12 ml/kg/min or < 50% predicted and of cardiac origin

What are the causes of acute HF?

Acute HF is characterised by symptoms severe enough that a patient seeks urgent medical attention (i.e. unplanned hospital attendance/admission). It may be due to the decompensation of chronic HF or de novo:

CHAMPIT

- *Coronary*: ACS
- *Hypertensive crisis*
- *Arrhythmia*
- *Mechanical cause*: myocardial rupture, trauma (e.g. contusion), iatrogenic, valve incompetence, aortic dissection, thrombosis
- *PE*
- *Infection*: myocarditis, sepsis
- *Tamponade*

Drug toxicity (e.g. calcium channel blockers, beta-blockers) may also be implicated.

How might patients with acute HF present?

The clinical profiles in acute HF were described by the ESC in 2016 based on the presence or absence of **congestion** and/or **hypoperfusion** (Table 78.1).

Features of hypoperfusion

- *Clinical*: cold sweaty extremities, oliguria, altered consciousness, dizziness, narrow pulse pressure
- *Laboratory*: metabolic acidosis, hyperlactataemia, elevated serum creatinine

Features of congestion

- Pulmonary congestion
- Orthopnoea/paroxysmal nocturnal dyspnoea
- Peripheral oedema
- Jugular venous distention
- Congested hepatomegaly
- Hepatojugular reflux
- Gut congestion
- Ascites

More recently, major clinical presentations have been described:

- **Acute decompensated HF** (wet and warm, or dry and cold)
- **Acute pulmonary oedema** (wet and warm)
- **Isolated RV failure** (dry and cold, or wet and cold)
- **CS** (wet and cold)

How is cardiogenic shock defined?

CS is a syndrome of life-threatening tissue hypoperfusion due to inadequate cardiac output from primary cardiac dysfunction.

Table 78.1 ESC clinical profiles of acute HF

	No congestion	Congestion
No hypoperfusion	Warm-dry	Warm-wet
Hypoperfusion	Cold-dry	Cold-wet

Diagnosis of CS:

- Hypotension (SBP < 90 mmHg)
- Despite adequate filling status
- With signs of hypoperfusion (see above)

Classification

A. *At risk for CS*: no signs or symptoms but at risk,
B. *Beginning shock*: relative hypotension or tachycardia without hypoperfusion.
C. *Classic CS*: hypoperfusion requiring intervention beyond volume resuscitation.
D. *Deteriorating*: failure to respond to initial interventions (e.g. on multiple vasopressors or requirement for mechanical support).
E. *Extremis*: cardiac arrest with ongoing CPR and/or ECMO, supported by multiple interventions.

What is critical cardiogenic shock?

Critical CS describes a patient with the 'crash and burn' presentation:

- Life-threatening hypotension despite rapidly escalating inotropic support
- Critical organ hypoperfusion
- Worsening acidosis and/or lactate levels

What are the INTERMACS profiles?

The Interagency Registry for Mechanical Assisted Circulatory Support (INTERMACS) profiles classify patients with potential indications for mechanical support devices according to clinical features. This classification is also used in prognostication in those undergoing urgent heart transplantation or LVAD implantation.

INTERMACS profile:

1. Critical CS
2. Progressive decline
3. Stable on inotrope or inotrope-dependent
4. Frequent flyer
5. Housebound
6. Exertion limited
7. Advanced NYHA class III symptoms

INTERMACS profiles 1–4 may be suitable for short-term mechanical support as a bridge to bridge, decision, recovery, candidacy, or transplantation. Those in profiles 5–7 are termed 'stable ambulatory' patients.

How would you manage a patient in acute left HF?

Cardiovascular
- **Manage myocardial hypoperfusion**
  - **Increase myocardial oxygen delivery**
    - ➢ *Oxygenation to target S_pO_2 90% or P_aO_2 8 kPa*: high flow, CPAP, invasive ventilation
    - ➢ *Increase perfusion*: **inopressors** (NA, adrenaline), IABP
    - ➢ *Inodilators* (milrinone, enoximone)
  - **Reduce myocardial oxygen demand**
    - ➢ *Reduce HR*: beta-blocker
    - ➢ *Reduce afterload*: loop diuretic, **vasodilators** (nitrates, SNP), RRT

- **Improve myocardial function**
  - *Inotropes (levosimendan, dobutamine)*: if symptomatic hypotension with hypoperfusion
  - *Revascularisation*: if CS
  - *Alternative pump*: VAD, VA-ECMO

Other
- *Specialist input*: cardiology, cardiothoracic surgery, cardiothoracic critical care
- Consideration of transfer to tertiary centre
- *Addressing treatment limitations*: palliative care might be appropriate
- Optimisation of medical therapy
- Relief of dyspnoea/anxiety (e.g. opioids)
- Thromboembolism prophylaxis

STUDY

SHOCK (1999)

- Shock due to LV failure complicating MI
- *Intervention*: emergency revascularisation vs initial medical stabilisation
- *Primary*: 30-day mortality – **no difference** (46.7% vs 56.0%)
- *Secondary*: 6-month survival – **significantly lower (50.3% vs 63.1%)**

When might an intra-aortic balloon pump be indicated in circulatory failure?

- Prior to surgical correction of specific mechanical issues (e.g. mitral regurgitation, septal rupture)
- Severe acute myocarditis
- *Acute myocardial ischaemia/infarction*: peri-revascularisation (routine use not recommended as benefit not demonstrated)

STUDY

IABP-SHOCK II (2012)

- Acute MI and CS
- *Intervention*: IABP vs medical therapy
- *Primary*: 30-day all-cause mortality – **no difference**
- *Secondary*: re-infarction, peripheral ischaemia, bleeding, sepsis – no difference

Which vasopressors are useful in acute HF?

Peripheral arterial vasoconstrictors are used in marked hypotension to increase BP and redistribute blood flow to vital organs. However LV afterload will increase.

- *NA*: first line
- *Dopamine* (> 5 µg/kg/min): can be used, associated with more side effects (e.g. tachycardia, arrhythmias), higher mortality
- *Adrenaline*: may be indicated in persistent hypotension despite adequate filling pressures and use of other agents, or in emergency resuscitation protocols

(See Chapter 79 Pulmonary Hypertension)

What do you know about HF with preserved ejection fraction?

HFpEF is the more contemporary terminology for what was previously known as 'diastolic HF'.

Understanding of the pathophysiology of HF has changed over time. As HF was observed in patients with normal ejection fractions, diastolic dysfunction became increasingly recognised as a causative factor. Diastole, or ventricular relaxation, involves passive and active processes to achieve ventricular filling.

With increasing research into HF, the term 'HFpEF' was adopted as it more accurately reflected this group of syndromes. The term 'diastolic HF' implied causation by myocardial pathology.

Patients are more often older and female, with AF, CKD, and non-cardiovascular comorbidities. Presentation is often with effort intolerance and dyspnoea/fatigue on activity of reducing amounts as the condition progresses.

KEY POINT

Diagnosis of HFpEF:

- Symptoms and signs of HF
- LVEF ≥ 50%
- Objective evidence of structural/functional abnormalities consistent with LV diastolic dysfunction or raised LV filling pressures

---

Management surrounds screening for and management of underlying cardiovascular conditions (e.g. hypertension, coronary artery disease) and other comorbidities. Diuretics are recommended if congestive symptoms are present but disease-modifying pharmacotherapy remains under evaluation.

What are cardiorenal syndromes?

Cardiorenal syndromes are disorders of the heart and kidneys in which dysfunction in one may induce dysfunction of the other. They are characterised by the presence of AKI, refractory HF with congestion, and worsening renal function during HF management. They may be classified by pathogenesis:

Type
1 Acute decompensated HF → AKI
2 Chronic HF → CKD
3 AKI → acute HF
4 CKD → chronic HF
5 Codevelopment of HF and CKD

Patients with cytokine release syndrome (CRS) types 1 and 3 often present to critical care. Existing evidence does not support the use of RRT in this setting.

STUDY

CARRESS-HF (2012)

- Acute decompensated HF and cardiorenal syndrome.
- *Intervention*: ultrafiltration vs medical management.
- *Primary*: change in serum creatinine and weight at day 4 – **creatinine worse, no difference in weight**.
- *Secondary*: 60-day all-cause mortality, weight loss, and renal improvement – no difference.

Resources

- Baran DA, Grines CL, Bailey S, et al. SCAI clinical expert consensus statement on the classification of cardiogenic shock. Catheter Cardiovasc Interv. 2019;94(1):29–37.
- Nickson C. Life in the Fast Lane: Cardiorenal syndrome. Available from: https://litfl.com/cardiorenal-syndrome/. (Accessed 24 January 2022.)
- Pfeffer MA, Shah AM, Borlaug BA. Heart failure with preserved ejection fraction in perspective. Circ Res. 2019;124(11):1598–1617.
- Ponikowski P, Voors AA, Anker SD, et al. 2016 ESC Guidelines for the diagnosis and treatment of acute and chronic heart failure. Eur J Heart Fail. 2016;18(8):891–975.

What is pulmonary hypertension?

KEY POINT

Pulmonary hypertension is an increase in **mean pulmonary arterial pressure ≥ 25 mmHg** at rest as assessed by right heart catheterisation.
(Normal pressure: 14 ± 3 mmHg; significance unclear between 21 and 24 mmHg)

GUIDELINE   ECS ERS 2015 Pulmonary hypertension

What are the causes of pulmonary hypertension?

Pulmonary hypertension is classified by aetiology.

KEY POINT

Pulmonary hypertension class

1. **Pulmonary arterial hypertension** (PAH)
2. *Pulmonary hypertension due to **left heart disease***: systolic/diastolic dysfunction, valvular, congenital
3. *Pulmonary hypertension due to **lung diseases***: COPD, ILD, sleep-disordered breathing, altitude
4. ***Chronic thromboembolic** pulmonary hypertension (CTEPH)*: VTE, arteritis, tumours, parasitic
5. *Pulmonary hypertension with **unclear and/or multifactorial** mechanisms*: haemolysis, myeloproliferative, splenectomy, sarcoidosis, histiocytosis, LAM, neurofibromatosis, glycogen storage disease, Gaucher disease, thyroid diseases, CKD, fibrosing mediastinitis

(WHO, 2003)

PAH is characterised by pre-capillary pulmonary hypertension:

- PAWP ≤ 15 mmHg and PVR > 3 Wood units
- In the absence of other causes of pre-capillary pulmonary hypertension

'**Cor pulmonale**' is a term describing right HF secondary to pulmonary hypertension due to lung disease.

What is the pathophysiology of pulmonary hypertension?

Common to all aetiologies, increased PVR requires increased work by the right heart.

Specific mechanisms by class:

1. *PAH*: smooth muscle hypertrophy, vessel fibrosis
2. *Left heart disease*: diastolic dysfunction causes back pressure, mitral regurgitation, loss of LA compliance
3. *Lung disease*: increased intrathoracic pressure, hypoxic pulmonary vasoconstriction, inflammation
4. *CTEPH*: obstruction of pulmonary vascular bed

Chronic RV dysfunction or failure may result from LV dysfunction-induced pulmonary hypertension. Other causes of RVF include MI, ARVC, and valvular disease.

What is Eisenmenger's syndrome?

Eisenmenger's syndrome is a condition resulting from the reversal of a previous left-to-right shunt due to the development of pulmonary hypertension (pulmonary pressure > systemic pressure). Subsequent right-to-left shunting causes arterial hypoxaemia and hyperviscosity secondary to increased erythropoiesis. Lung or heart-lung transplantation is curative in selected cases.

What is platypnoea-orthodeoxia syndrome?

Platypnoea-orthodeoxia syndrome is a rare condition characterised by hypoxaemic dyspnoea induced by upright posture. Right to left intracardiac shunting occurs in the presence of normal right-sided cardiac pressures in some individuals, usually on the background of an atrial septal defect (e.g. patent foramen ovale). It should be suspected in patients with disproportional hypoxaemia to underlying disease and can be cured surgically.

What might the diagnostic workup of pulmonary hypertension include?

History
- SOB on exertion
- Fatigue, weakness
- Angina
- Syncope
- RV failure (e.g. ankle swelling, abdominal distension)

Examination
- Left parasternal heave
- Loud S2, S3, pansystolic murmur (tricuspid regurgitation), diastolic murmur (pulmonary regurgitation)
- *Advanced disease*: elevated JVP, hepatomegaly, ascites, peripheral oedema, cool peripheries
- Absence of wheeze/crepitations

Bloods
- FBC, U&E, LFT, TFT
- ABG
- Others (e.g. HIV serology, thrombophilia screen, other antibodies e.g. anti-centromere, double-stranded DNA, Ro)

Imaging
- *ECG*: may be normal, P pulmonale, R axis, RVH, RV strain, RBBB, long QT
- *CXR*: central pulmonary arterial dilatation, 'pruning' of peripheral vessels, large RA/RV
- *Echo*: estimate of PAP, cardiac disease, signs of pulmonary hypertension, e.g. flat septum, wide PA/IVC
- *PFT*: underlying lung disease
- *US abdomen*: liver disease
- *V/Q scan, CTPA*: CTEPH if unexplained pulmonary hypertension
- *High-resolution CT*: lung disease
- *Right heart catheterisation ± pulmonary angiography*: pressures in PAH and CTEPH

How is PAH managed outside the ICU?

- *General measures*: rehabilitation, infection prevention, psychosocial support, etc.
  - Pregnancy is associated with high mortality (12–17%) – prevention and termination may be advocated
  - Baseline established and monitored using functional tests (e.g. 6MWT)
- *Calcium channel blockade* (e.g. nifedipine, diltiazem)
- *Other specific drugs*:
  - Endothelin receptor antagonists (e.g. bosentan, ambrisentan, macitentan)
  - Phosphodiesterase-5 inhibitors and guanylate cyclase stimulators (e.g. sildenafil, riociguat)
  - Prostacyclin analogues and receptor agonists (e.g. epoprostenol, iloprost)
- *Supplemental oxygen* may be indicated for symptomatic relief
- *Balloon atrial septostomy*: R-L shunt to decompress right heart and increase preload
- *Lung transplantation*: if inadequate response to maximal medical therapy

What are the implications of pulmonary hypertension for the critical care patient?

Admission

- Right HF may require supportive care.
- In PAH, admission to critical care is recommended if: HR > 110/min, systolic BP < 90 mmHg, low UO, and rising lactate not due to comorbidities. RV failure might also be indicated by low $ScvO_2$ (<60%).
- Setting limitations may involve assessment of suitability for transplant.

Prognosis

- Patients under 50 years old with PAH have a 5-year survival rate of 75–80%.
- Pulmonary hypertension requiring ICU care has a poor prognosis and can carry mortality as high as 41%.
- Eisenmenger syndrome may have a better prognosis as RV has been conditioned.
- Intubation frequently causes haemodynamic collapse.
- Those continuing pregnancy to term will be at very high risk of complications (10–20% mortality).
- 50% of those receiving CVVH survive to hospital discharge.

Associations with worse outcome

- Low systemic BP on admission to critical care
- Lower sodium
- Higher creatinine, BNP, CRP

Surgery

- 7% mortality at 30 days in 1 study
- Increased morbidity related to emergency, major, and prolonged surgery
- Regional anaesthesia may result in better outcomes than general anaesthesia.

How is right HF diagnosed?

Right heart dysfunction occurs when a measure of RV function lies outwith the normal range. It may be asymptomatic.

Right HF is present when clinical signs/symptoms of systemic congestion and structural and/or functional abnormalities of the right heart are present:

- Exertional dyspnoea
- Reduced exercise capacity
- Fatigue
- Dizziness
- S3
- *Right-sided decompensation*: JVP distension, hepatomegaly (epigastric fullness/RUQ discomfort), ascites, peripheral oedema

Possible echo findings:

- **RV systolic dysfunction**
  - Tricuspid annular plane systolic excursion (TAPSE) < 17 mm
  - RV fractional area change < 35%
  - RV systolic velocity of the lateral tricuspid annulus < 9.5 cm/s
- **Right-sided pressure/volume overload**
  - TR
  - RV basal end-diastolic diameter > 41 mm
  - RV/LV end-diastolic diameter ratio > 1.0

Rising lactate, low $ScvO_2$ (< 60%), and **anuria** should raise suspicion of imminent right HF. Right heart assessment with a PAC is the gold standard haemodynamic monitor, although its use in the general critical care population has declined following the **PAC-Man** trial.

GUIDELINE   ESC ERS 2015 Pulmonary hypertension

PAC-Man (2005)

- Critically ill patients
- *Intervention*: PAC vs no PAC
- *Primary*: hospital morality – **no difference**
- *Secondary*: LOS ICU/hospital, organ support – no difference
- *10% complication rate*: haematoma (4%), arterial puncture (3%), arrhythmia (3%), PTX, HTX, lost guidewire. No related fatalities.

What supportive care might be involved in the management of the critically unwell patient with right HF?

General
- Reduction in PVR
  - Avoidance of hypoxia, hypercapnia, acidaemia, hypothermia
  - Avoidance of excessive catecholamines, adequate analgesia
  - Reduced Hct
  - Appropriate ventilatory pressures
- Optimisation of fluid balance – **diuretics** vs fluids
- Treatment of trigger (e.g. anaemia, dysrhythmia, infection, comorbidity, thrombus)
- Transfer to a specialist centre
- VA-ECMO – bridge to recovery/transplantation

Cardiovascular drugs
- Maintenance of systemic BP
  - Vasopressors (e.g. **vasopressin** – less pulmonary vasoconstriction than NA)
  - Inopressors (e.g. **adrenaline**)
- Reduction of RV afterload
  - **iNO**
  - Prostacyclin analogues
  - Inodilators (e.g. **milrinone**)
- Improvement of RV function
  - Inotropes (e.g. **dobutamine** preferred for RV, dopamine)
  - Inodilators

(See Chapter 78 Heart Failure)

Can you give some examples of mechanical complications of PAH?

Mechanical complications result from PA dilatation and enlargement:

- PA aneurysm, rupture, dissection
- Compression of left main coronary artery, pulmonary veins, bronchi, recurrent laryngeal nerves

Resources
- Condliffe R, Kiely DG. Critical care management of pulmonary hypertension. BJA Educ. 2017;17(7):228–234.
- Elliot CA, Kiely DG. Pulmonary hypertension. CEACCP. 2006;6(1):17–22.
- Gorter RM, van Veldhuisen DJ, Bauersachs J. Right heart dysfunction and failure in heart failure with pre-served ejection fraction: mechanisms and management. Position statement on behalf of the Heart Failure Association of the European Society of Cardiology. Eur J Heart Fail. 2018;20(1):16–37.
- Kubler P, Gibbs H, Garrahy P. Platypnoea – orthodeoxia syndrome. Heart. 2000;83(2):221–223.

80. AORTIC DISSECTION

What is aortic dissection and when does it occur?

Aortic dissection is the creation of a false lumen between layers of the aortic wall after creation of a defect. The high-pressure blood flow in the defect extends the tear, leading to a variety of clinical effects.

Most commonly, an intimal tear is implicated, occurring at regions of higher stress and pressure fluctuations:

- Predisposing factors relate to BP and ability of the aortic wall to withstand stress/changes.
- Common sites are those subjected to higher mechanical shear force as they are relatively fixed: greater curvature, descending thoracic aorta at the origin of the left SCA.

This condition is more common in males and those aged 50–70 years.

Risk factors are as follows:

- **BP related**
  - Hypertension
  - Stimulant drug use (e.g. cocaine)
  - Pregnancy
  - Deceleration trauma
- **Wall related**
  - Connective tissue disorders (e.g. Marfan, Ehlers-Danlos, Turner syndrome)
  - Vascular disease (e.g. coarctation, Takayasu, syphilis)
  - Aortic aneurysm
  - Iatrogenic defect (e.g. graft anastomosis, cannulation site, cross-clamp)

How is aortic dissection classified?

Classification can be made by chronicity, aetiology (class), or anatomy (type).

Chronicity
- Acute ≤ 2 weeks
- Chronic > 2 weeks

Class
1. Classical aortic dissection
2. Intramural haematoma/haemorrhage
3. Subtle-discrete aortic dissection
4. Plaque rupture/ulceration
5. Traumatic/iatrogenic aortic dissection

KEY POINT

Stanford classification
- A. *Proximal*: involves ascending aorta
- B. *Distal*: distal to origin of left SCA

DeBakey classification
I   Tear in ascending aorta, dissection involves all portions of thoracic aorta (60%)
II Tear in ascending aorta, dissection in ascending only (before origin of innominate artery) (10–15%)
III Tear in descending aorta, almost always involves descending only (25–30%)
   a   Extends to diaphragm
   b   Extends beyond diaphragm

How does classical aortic dissection present?

The presentation may vary but a 2-step process is often involved:

- *Interruption of intima*: severe pain, loss of pulse volume
- *Rupture*: pressure exceeds critical limit
  - Sudden, sharp chest pain, stabbing/tearing/ripping in nature
  - Back/abdominal pain more common in Type B, pain may migrate

Other features
- Tachycardia, hypertension/hypotension, differential/absent extremity pulses, aortic regurgitation
- Pain, anxiety, syncope, stroke

How is diagnosis confirmed?

- High index of clinical suspicion
- *Immediate ECG*: consider acute MI
- *Aortography*: gold standard but not suitable if unstable
- *CT angiography*: more commonly performed, quicker, less invasive
- *TTE/TOE*: image quality may be limited, useful perioperatively, and in unstable patients
- *CXR*: aortic knuckle enlargement, widened mediastinum, cardiomegaly, HTX

A patient is due to be transferred to your unit for emergency surgery: What are your management priorities on arrival?

- Prompt stabilisation and transfer to theatre
- Monitoring/lines
  - Wide bore peripheral venous access
  - Arterial access depending on type of dissection
    - ➤ *A*: **use left side** – avoids innominate artery involvement
    - ➤ *B*: **use right side** – avoids left SCA clamp (femoral line alternatively)
  - CVC and urinary catheter may be better timed after induction of anaesthesia
  - Early intubation and ventilation if unconscious or profoundly unstable
- *BP management*: reduce ventricular force without reducing perfusion
  - Target **systolic BP 110–120 mmHg**
  - Labetalol/esmolol/metoprolol first line (alternatively calcium channel blocker)
  - Sodium nitroprusside/GTN/hydralazine if refractory (vasodilators may cause reflex catecholamine release so should be given second)
- Blood samples including urgent crossmatch, CK, troponin, U&E, FBC, LDH, coagulation
- Analgesia
- Discussion with patient and family as appropriate

How would you manage the patient post-operatively?

- Supportive care
  - Mechanical ventilation until warm, stable, gas exchange adequate, minimal bleeding
  - Ongoing BP control with antihypertensives and good analgesia
  - Analgesia
  - RRT may be required
  - Coagulopathy correction, transfusion
- Further assessment
  - Complete peripheral vascular examination on return/admission from theatre
  - Neurological examination when possible
  - *ECG*: baseline, presence of ischaemia
  - CXR
- Update patient/family

What other management strategies are there for patients with aortic dissection?

Uncomplicated Type B dissections may be managed conservatively (i.e. without surgery). This will still involve rigorous BP control and supportive care. Some may be amenable to IR.

What is the prognosis?

The most common overall causes of mortality are aortic rupture, tamponade, circulatory failure, stroke, and visceral ischaemia.

Approximately 20% of patients with aortic dissection will die before reaching hospital and 50% before reaching a specialist centre. During the first 48 h, mortality increases 1–2% per hour in acute ascending aortic dissection. In those arriving alive to hospital, mortality is approximately 20% at 24 h and 45% at 30 days. The 10-year mortality of treated patients is around 55%.

In-hospital mortality:
- Type A
  - Surgically managed 26%
  - Medically managed 58%
- Type B
  - Surgically managed 31%
  - Medically managed 11%

Resources
- Hebballi R, Swanevelder J. Diagnosis and management of aortic dissection. CEACCP. 2009;9(1):14–18.
- Melvinsdottir IH, Lund SH, Agnarsson BA, et al. The incidence and mortality of acute thoracic aortic dissection: results from a whole nation study. Eur J Cardiothoracic Surg. 2016;50(6):1111–1117.

---

81. AIR LEAK SYNDROME

What is an air leak?

An air leak involves the movement of air from an air-containing cavity to one which is not usually air-containing. Air-containing cavities include the following:

- Tracheobronchial tree
- Sinuses
- GI tract

This can compromise function, usually due to the compression of important structures. It might manifest in several ways:

- PTX
- Pneumopericardium
- Pneumomediastinum
- Pneumoperitoneum
- Pneumocephalus
- Subcutaneous/surgical emphysema
- Gas embolism

Air leak syndrome is characterised by respiratory distress in the setting of an air leak.

How would you classify pneumothoraces?

A PTX is the presence of air in the pleural cavity. The aetiology of a PTX is used in its classification:

- *Spontaneous*
  - *Primary (PSP)*: no lung disease
  - *Secondary (SSP)*: underlying lung disease
    - ➤ *Restrictive*: ARDS, cystic fibrosis, idiopathic pulmonary fibrosis (IPF)
    - ➤ *Obstructive*: asthma, COPD, bronchiolitis
    - ➤ *Other*: bronchopleural fistula, bullous disease, necrotising pneumonia, sarcoidosis, Marfan syndrome, pulmonary haemorrhage, sarcoma, pulmonary contusion, TB, aspergillosis
- *Traumatic*: direct or indirect injury to lung and pleura
- *Iatrogenic*
  - *Barotrauma/volutrauma*: mechanical ventilation, HFOV
  - CVC insertion
  - Surgical intervention
  - Thoracoscopy
  - Laparoscopy
  - Tracheostomy

> **GUIDELINE** BTS 2010 Pneumothorax

What is a bronchopleural fistula?

- A **bronchopleural fistula** is a connection between the pleural space and a major/lobar/segmental bronchus.
- The term **alveolar pleural fistula** is used if the pleural space connects to the lung parenchyma.

How might you determine if an air leak is present?

- Air leak related to PTX is usually demonstrated by the presence of bubbling in the fluid seal column of a chest drain during coughing (increased intrathoracic pressure/gradient).
- In pulmonary surgery, air leak can be investigated by insufflating the lungs whilst bathed in saline and checking for bubbles.
- Air leak may be classified by quantity of leakage/bubbling. A persistent air leak is one which is present for more than 5 days post-operatively.
- Leaks affecting other systems will have specific presentations and may be first detected in the critically unwell patient undergoing CT imaging.

(See Chapter 56 Gas Embolism)

What are the respiratory consequences of a pneumothorax?

- Decrease in lung volume available for gas exchange
- Decreased airflow
- Increased pleural pressure (usually 0–10 cmH$_2$O), increased lung resistance

Chest tube insertion will reverse these effects although the effects of any discomfort will need to be considered.

What is the initial management of ectopic air in patients with a pneumothorax?

Systematic assessment and resuscitation will be required. Oxygen may be indicated to increase reabsorption of ectopic air by denitrogenation – **high-flow oxygen** is recommended in those admitted for observation due to a 4-fold increase in reabsorption and earlier resolution.

Spontaneous PTX:

- If unstable or bilateral – chest drain
- PSP
  - Small, asymptomatic – observation
  - Breathless or size > 2 cm – needle aspiration
    - If remains breathless or size > 2 cm – chest drain
- SSP
  - Breathless or size > 2 cm – chest drain
  - Size 1–2 cm – needle aspiration
    - If size remains > 1 cm – chest drain

Iatrogenic and traumatic pneumothoraces will often require chest drain insertion. In the trauma setting, unilateral/bilateral thoracostomy (or clamshell thoracotomy in extreme circumstances) may be indicated on presentation before chest tube insertion. 'Sucking chest wounds' are a particular concern as tension will result. Open PTX will require the use of a 3-sided occlusive dressing to allow air to escape but not enter.

The requirement for positive pressure ventilation will also influence management. This has the potential to increase air leakage to the pleural space, ultimately resulting in tension. The defect resulting in PTX may heal easily in some cases but any doubt should prompt chest tube insertion. It may be pragmatic and less distressing to do so after induction of anaesthesia and mechanical ventilation if stability allows. (See Chapter 49 Major Trauma)

When would suction be indicated in managing a chest drain?

Suction should not be employed routinely as it risks re-expansion pulmonary oedema amongst other issues. It is occasionally used for persistent air leak ± incomplete re-expansion of the lung.

It is thought that suction will remove air at a higher rate than it crosses the pleural defect, promoting healing by apposition of the pleural layers. Often this is employed after discussion with a respiratory or thoracic surgical team.

High-volume, low-pressure systems are advocated. The converse might cause air stealing, hypoxaemia, and persistence of the air leak. Pressures should be –10 to –20 cmH$_2$O with air flow volume of up to 15–20 l/min.

What are the physiological implications of a significant air leak in the ventilated patient?

- *A*: tube migration, cuff pressure change
- *B*: inability to apply PEEP, loss of V$_T$, persistent collapse, prolonged wean, restriction by subcutaneous emphysema, respiratory failure
- *C*: tension, obstructive shock, dysrhythmias
- *D*: pain, increased sedative requirement
- *E*: increased LOS
- *I*: infection at drain site

How would you manage this patient?

- *Airway*: check device position and cuff pressure
- *Ventilation*: avoid worsening leak
  - Spontaneous mode where possible
  - Lung-protective strategy with minimal MV and PEEP
  - Permissive hypercapnia and hypoxia might be required
  - Consideration of differential lung ventilation
  - ECMO in severe cases
- *Monitoring*
  - Regular CXR (daily)
  - CT imaging to assess defect
  - Consider bronchoscopy

- *Definitive management*
  - Largely conservative
  - Surgery or bronchoscopic repair may be indicated in selected cases
- *Other*: antimicrobials if concomitant infection

When would surgical review be indicated in spontaneous pneumothorax?

- Persistent air leak or failure to re-expand by 3–5 days
- Persistent air leak in SSP at 48 h
- Second ipsilateral PTX
- First contralateral PTX
- Synchronous bilateral spontaneous PTX
- Spontaneous HTX
- Professions at risk (e.g. pilot, diver)
- Pregnancy

Surgery might be required for refractory cases, including thoracoplasty, lung resection/stapling, and pleural abrasion/decortication. Medical or surgical pleurodesis may be indicated to prevent recurrence.

Resources

- Adeyinka A, Pierre L. Air leak. In: StatPearls [Internet]. Treasure Island (FL): StatPEarls Publishing; 2021. Available from: https://www.ncbi.nlm.nih.gov/books/NBK513222/. (Accessed 26 April 2022.)
- Paramasivam E, Bodenham A. Air leaks, pneumothorax, and chest drains. CEACCP. 2008;8(6):204–209.

NEUROSCIENCES

82. SUBARACHNOID HAEMORRHAGE

What is subarachnoid haemorrhage?

Subarachnoid haemorrhage (SAH) is bleeding into the subarachnoid space (the space between the arachnoid and pia mater surrounding the brain) which may result in an acutely life-threatening, multisystem syndrome.

What are risk factors for SAH?

- Hypertension
- Smoking
- Alcohol excess
- Cocaine use
- Family history
- *Genetic*: Ehlers-Danlos syndrome, polycystic kidney disease

What are the causes of SAH?

The bleeding event is often the result of haemodynamic stress (sudden increase in cerebrovascular pressure) ± predisposing condition.

- Traumatic
- Non-traumatic
  - Aneurysm (85%)
    - ➤ Congenital
    - ➤ Acquired
  - Arteriovenous malformation
  - Cerebral venous sinus thrombosis (CVST)
  - Cerebral vasculitis
  - Moyamoya disease

How might SAH present?

- *Headache*: 'thunderclap'/'worst headache ever experienced', occipital, 20% preceding sentinel headache
- *Meningism*: neck pain/stiffness, photophobia, limited neck flexion
- Focal neurology
- Seizure
- *Collapse*: witness account important

- Low GCS
- Cardiac arrhythmia
- Pulmonary oedema

How would you investigate a patient presenting with SAH?

Investigation is time-critical and may have a therapeutic role in addition to diagnostics.

- **CT head** without contrast (highly sensitive at 6 h of headache onset)
- **LP** for xanthochromia
  - Unlikely to help if CT normal ≤6 h symptom onset
  - Consider LP if CT normal >6 h from onset
  - Perform ≥12 h after onset
- **CT angiography**
  - Perform if confirmed diagnosis of SAH or pattern of bleed compatible with aneurysmal rupture
  - Evaluate for underlying vascular anomalies (e.g. aneurysm, arteriovenous malformation)
- **Digital subtraction angiography (DSA)**
  - Useful if CT angiography does not identify cause and aneurysm still suspected
- **MR** imaging ± angiography (as above if DSA contraindicated)

> **GUIDELINE** NICE 2021 SAH (Draft)

What are the most common sites of aneurysmal SAH?

Most aneurysms occur close to bifurcations in the circle of Willis:

- Posterior communicating artery/internal carotid artery take-off
- Anterior communicating artery
- Vertebrobasilar

How can we grade the severity of SAH?

Scoring systems
- *Hunt and Hess*: clinical
- *World Federation of Neurosurgical Societies (WFNS)*: clinical
- *Fisher*: radiological

The WFNS is the most widely used system in contemporary practice. Grades 1–3 are considered 'good' and 4–5 are considered 'poor'.

> **KEY POINT**
>
> WFNS grading of SAH (GCS):
>
> 1. 15
> 2. 13–14, no motor deficit
> 3. 13–14, motor deficit
> 4. **7–12**
> 5. **3–6**

What are 'neuroprotective measures'?

'Neuroprotective measures' are a set of physiologically supportive parameters/measures that are often targeted/instituted with the aim of preventing secondary brain injury.

(See Chapter 83 Traumatic Brain Injury)

How would you manage a patient presenting with SAH?

Management depends on the underlying cause and focuses largely on prevention of complications and secondary brain injury. This will differ slightly depending on whether any culprit lesion has been 'protected'

Table 82.1 Physiological targets in SAH

B	C	D
• P_aO_2 > 11 kPa • S_aO_2 > 95% • P_aCO_2 4.5–5 kPa	• MAP 80–90 mmHg • Systolic BP < 160 mmHg (when aneurysm unprotected)	• Mg^{2+} 0.7–1.0 mmol/l • Glucose 6–10 mmol/l • Temperature 36°C

(i.e. definitively managed). Neuroprotection involves specific physiological targets along with other supportive nuances, as given in Table 82.1:

Other measures
- A
  - Consider intubation and ventilation
- B
  - Head up 30° if ventilated
  - Aim for LPV but this may not be achievable (e.g. neurogenic pulmonary oedema with high ICP)
- C
  - Aim for euvolaemia with crystalloid
  - Vasoactive drugs as required
  - Focused echo helpful
- D
  - Neurosurgical review ± definitive management
  - *Nimodipine*: enteral first line (e.g. 60 mg 4°); if unstable, consider 30 mg 2° or IV
  - Treat hypomagnesaemia, no evidence to support prophylaxis (**MASH-2**)
  - *Analgesia*: may require high dose of opioid
  - CSF drainage/diversion (e.g. EVD) for deterioration due to hydrocephalus
- H
  - Consider liberal transfusion threshold, no definitive guidance (e.g. Hb > 90 g/l, Hct > 30%)
  - Mechanical VTE prophylaxis (pharmacological usually avoided pre-intervention)
  - **SAHaRA** trial to evaluate transfusion threshold, ongoing at time of writing (see Chapter 51 Major Haemorrhage)

STUDY

MASH-2 (2012)

- Aneurysmal SAH
- *Intervention*: $MgSO_4$ 64 mmol/day IV vs placebo
- *Primary*: mRS 4–5 or death at 3 months – **no difference**
- *Secondary*: no symptoms at 3 months – no difference

What are the indications for intubation and ventilation in the context of SAH?

- GCS reduction ≥ 2 points (e.g. cerebral agitation incompatible with plan for imaging)
- GCS < 8 (e.g. obstructive hydrocephalus, extensive injury)
- Seizure control
- Optimisation of oxygenation and ventilation (e.g. failure to meet targets above)

Which definitive interventions might be indicated?

Definitive management (as soon as possible to prevent rebleeding)
- Conservative
- *Coiling*: endovascular occlusion of aneurysm
- *Clipping*: craniotomy with clips across 'stalk' of aneurysm

Anaesthetic review and considerations for emergency theatre will be required if intervention is planned. TXA may be considered if definitive management is not possible ≤24 h hospital admission. Management of non-culprit aneurysms should be considered on an individual basis by the MDT.

STUDY

ULTRA (2021)

- Aneurysmal SAH
- *Intervention*: TXA at diagnosis vs usual care
- *Primary*: mRS 0–3 at 6 months – **no difference**
- *Secondary*: 6-month mortality, serious adverse events, early rebleeding, DCI, thromboembolic events – no difference; mRS 0–2 – **significantly lower**

Do you know of any differences in outcome between coiling and clipping for definitive aneurysmal management?

Endovascular coiling is associated with better short-term outcomes and is less invasive. Intra-arterial vasodilators may be given. However, it is less definitive and may require repeated procedures later in life. Catastrophic bleeding is still a possibility, and anticoagulation is required. The **ISAT** trial found less dependency or death at 1 year with coiling vs clipping, and lower incidence of vasospasm, but a higher rate of rebleeding.

Surgical clipping is useful when anatomical challenges preclude coiling and is a more definitive intervention. However, this is a more invasive early treatment, requiring craniotomy (with associated complications, e.g. infection) and significant anaesthetic considerations.

STUDY

ISAT (2005)

- Aneurysmal SAH
- *Intervention*: endovascular coiling vs neurosurgical clipping
- *Primary*: mRS 3–6 at 12 months – **significantly lower (23.7% vs 30.6%)**, that is coiling resulted in more patients with better outcome
- *Secondary*: late rebleeding – **significantly higher**; seizures – **significantly lower**

How would you manage the ongoing care of this patient?

- C
  - Allow hypertension within first 21 days once protected (unless LV function impaired, myocardial ischaemia, severe valvular disease, other MDT decision)
  - Consider cardiac output monitoring
  - Continue statin if usually prescribed
- D
  - Ongoing analgesia as required
  - Treat seizures aggressively but avoid prophylaxis (worse outcome)
  - Aim to extubate and monitor awake where possible (neurology best indicator)
  - **ICP < 20 mmHg, CPP > 60 mmHg**
  - Repeat non-contrast CT if unexplained neurological deterioration in GCS or subtler signs (e.g. weakness, pronator drift, aphasia, behavioural change)
- Other
  - Feed as indicated
  - Consider reintroduction of any usual anticoagulants and thromboprophylaxis
  - Monitor for and manage complications
  - Rehabilitation and education

STASH (2014)

- Aneurysmal SAH
- *Intervention*: routine simvastatin 40 mg vs placebo for first 21 days
- *Primary*: distribution of mRS scores at 6 months – **no difference**

What are the common complications of SAH and when do they occur?

- Hydrocephalus (20–30%, ≤**72 h**)
- Rebleeding (5–10%, ≤**72 h**)
- Haematoma (30%)
- Cerebral vasospasm (70%, **day 3–10**, resolves by day 21)
- DCI (50%)
- Seizures (1–7%)

What is the difference between vasospasm and DCI?

KEY POINT

- **Cerebral vasospasm** is the narrowing of cerebral blood vessels.
- **DCI** is new neurological deterioration present for >1 h. It may be the clinical manifestation of vasospasm.

Vasospasm is identified radiologically, with the investigation sequence: DSA, MR/CT angiography, TCD. It is a poor prognostic indicator.

Risk factors
- Poor grade
- Age < 50 years
- Hypertension
- Smoking
- Alcohol excess
- Cocaine use

Management of DCI includes the following:

- *Nimodipine*: cerebral vessel vasodilatation, exact mechanism unknown, PO/IV/intra-arterial routes
- *Haemodynamic optimisation*: euvolaemia, individualised BP target, avoidance of anaemia
- *Endovascular intervention*: early coiling, balloon angioplasty, intra-arterial vasodilator infusions

What is 'triple H therapy'?

'Triple H therapy' refers to the strategy of hypervolaemia, hypertension, and haemodilution in the management of DCI. It is no longer recommended, and euvolaemia is preferred.

The rationale for triple H therapy was optimisation of CPP and CBF. Traditional haemodilution aimed for a Hct of 0.3. It has been suggested that volume status does not affect the benefits of induced hypertension, and hypervolaemia may cause significant morbidity. Haemodilution should be avoided.

Resources

- Luoma A, Reddy U. Acute management of aneurysmal subarachnoid haemorrhage. CEACCP. 2013;13(2):52–58.
- Naisbitt J, Ferris P, Claxton A, et al. Northern Care Alliance NHS Group: Sub-Arachnoid Haemorrhage – Guideline for Management of Patients Admitted to Critical Care. November 2019. Available from: https://www. neuroicu.guru/_files/ugd/de5fcc_c7e5ccbb95a749fdbdd9a23f032cc7d7.pdf. (Accessed 25 January 2022.)

83. TRAUMATIC BRAIN INJURY

What is traumatic brain injury?

Traumatic brain injury (TBI) is an insult to the brain which occurs as a result of an external mechanical force.

What do you know about the epidemiology of TBI?

TBI is one of the leading causes of death worldwide and is estimated at affecting 50–60 million people annually. It is the leading cause of disability in patients under 40. Approximately one third of patients presenting with TBI will have polytrauma. Non-accidental injury should be considered in children.

There is a tendency towards a bimodal distribution:

- *Young adults*: road traffic collisions
- *Elderly adults*: falls

What is a primary brain injury?

KEY POINT

A primary brain injury refers to neuronal damage which occurs immediately as a direct result of the initial trauma. It is irreversible.

Mechanisms include the following:

- *Impact*: the head striking an object or vice versa
- *Inertial loading*: the head moves rapidly backwards and forwards or rotates
- *Penetrating*: low- or high-velocity projectiles
- *Blast*: impact from a pressure wave generated by an explosion

What is the pathophysiology of primary TBI?

Deformation of tissues due to compression, tension, and/or shearing forces results in direct neuronal cell damage via local inflammation, vasogenic oedema, cytotoxic oedema, interstitial oedema, and impaired cerebral autoregulation.

Can you describe types of TBI?

Fracture
- *Simple skull fracture*: does not penetrate the dura, may result in EDH or SDH
- *Depressed skull fracture*: more likely to result in dural tears and damage to the underlying parenchyma

Haematoma
- *EDH*: accumulation of blood between the skull and the dura mater, classically associated with temporal bone fractures and tearing of the middle meningeal artery, 'lens shaped'
- *SDH*: accumulation of blood between the dura and arachnoid mater, classically associated with tearing of the bridging veins, crescent-shaped
- *Intraparenchymal haematoma*: commonly caused by a penetrating injury

Other
- *SAH*: accumulation of blood between the arachnoid and pia mater, may occur as primary bleeding from basilar arteries, intracranial vertebral arteries or pial veins, or as secondary extension from intraventricular or intraparenchymal bleeds
- *Intraventricular haemorrhage*: accumulation of blood in the ventricular system, may result in hydrocephalus

- *Contusion*: often caused by coup and contrecoup injuries, commonly frontal/temporal lobes, blossoms over 24–48 h
- *Diffuse axonal injury*: caused by deceleration and rotational forces which cause white matter tract shearing

What is blunt cerebrovascular injury?

Blunt cerebrovascular injury (BCVI) is a non-penetrating injury to the major arteries supplying the brain (carotid ± vertebral arteries). Weakened vessel walls may lead to intimal tearing, thrombus formation, wall haematoma, and lumen occlusion. Pseudoaneurysm may also result. Ischaemic stroke is a major complication, occurring in up to 26% of affected patients.

Incidence may be as high as 9% in patients with severe TBI. Use of the expanded Denver screening tool is recommended, before investigation with CT angiography where appropriate. Management centres on antiplatelet/anticoagulant therapy ± endovascular intervention.

Denver screening criteria (positive if ≥1 present):

- Signs/symptoms
  - Arterial haemorrhage from neck/nose/mouth
  - Cervical bruit (age < 50 years)
  - Expanding cervical haematoma
  - Neurological exam incongruous with head CT findings
  - Stroke on secondary CT
- Risk factors
  - Fractures: Le Fort II/III, mandible, complex skull, basilar skull, occipital condyle, c-spine, or upper rib
  - Severe TBI with GCS < 6
  - C-spine subluxation or ligamentous injury
  - Near hanging with hypoxic brain injury
  - Seat belt abrasion with significant swelling, pain, or altered mental state
  - TBI with thoracic injury
  - Scalp degloving
  - Thoracic vascular injury
  - Blunt cardiac rupture

GUIDELINE Brommeland et al. 2018 BCVI

What is 'secondary brain injury'?

KEY POINT

'Secondary brain injury' refers to neuronal damage due to the sequelae of the primary injury. This occurs hours to days after the primary injury and is the main determinant of outcome.

Causes of secondary brain injury are as follows:

- **Intracranial**
  - Haematoma (e.g. expansion/rebleed)
  - Hydrocephalus
  - Vasospasm/DCI
  - Intracranial infection
  - Seizures
- **Extracranial/systemic**
  - Hypoxia
  - Hyper-/hypocapnia
  - Hypotension

- Hyponatraemia
- Hypo-/hyperglycaemia
- Hyperthermia
- Infection

How can we grade the severity of TBI?

The GCS is the most widely accepted tool for grading the severity of TBI. The individual subscores are of particular importance in prognostication.

KEY POINT

Severity of TBI (GCS):

- *Mild*: 13–15
- *Moderate*: 9–12
- *Severe*: < 8

How would you assess a patient presenting with TBI?

This will be time-critical and should follow trauma resuscitation principles.

History

- *Patient*: age, medical history, allergies, medications including antithrombotic therapy
- *Injury*: mechanism, GCS at the scene, GCS on arrival to hospital, seizure activity, other injuries
- Management thus far

Examination

- Vital signs
- Primary survey
- GCS
- *Pupils*: reactivity, dilation, symmetry
- Focal neurological deficit
- Signs of herniation are as follows:
  - Cranial nerve III palsy
  - Cranial nerve VI palsy
  - Fixed dilated pupils
  - Cushing reflex
  - Diabetes insipidus

How would you investigate this patient?

- *Bedside*: ABG, focused US, ECG
- *Laboratory*: trauma blood panel including coagulation profile, group, and save/cross-match
- *Imaging*: CT – territory determined by nature of presentation (e.g. polytrauma 'pan scan'), X-rays

When would emergency CT imaging be indicated?

CT head imaging should be performed within 1 h with any of the following risk factors:

- GCS < 13 on initial assessment in the emergency department
- GCS < 15 at 2 h
- Suspected open/depressed skull fracture
- *Sign of basal skull fracture*: haemotympanum, 'panda' eyes, CSF leak from ear/nose, Battle's sign
- Post-traumatic seizure
- Focal deficit
- >1 episode of vomiting

A provisional report should be available within 1 h of the scan being performed.

GUIDELINE NHS 2019 CG176 Head injury

(See Chapter 109 Paediatric Trauma)

Which patients should receive ICP monitoring?

Brain Trauma Foundation (BTF) guidelines suggest ICP monitoring in the following:

- Any moderate-to-severe TBI (GCS < 12) who cannot be serially neurologically assessed, for example if sedated
- Any severe TBI (GCS < 8) with an abnormal CT head scan
- Any severe TBI (GCS < 8) with a normal CT head scan if 2 of the following are present:
    - Age > 40 years
    - SBP < 90
    - Abnormal motor posturing

GUIDELINE BTF 2016 TBI

Can you describe the physiological principles used to prevent secondary brain injury?

Maintaining cerebral oxygen supply

- Normoxia
- CPP 60–70 mmHg
- Treat anaemia

Reducing cerebral oxygen demand/rate of consumption (CMRO$_2$)

- Deep sedation
- *NMB*: prevention of coughing/shivering, etc.
- Seizure management
- Normothermia
- Normoglycaemia
- Barbiturate infusion titrated to ICP control/burst suppression

Managing increased ICP

- ICP monitoring
- Blood
    - Increase cerebral venous drainage
        - ➤ Bed tilt or head up to 30°
        - ➤ Head in alignment
        - ➤ *C-spine protection*: remove collar, replace with sandbags at the sides of the head if patient deeply sedated
        - ➤ No taped eyes
        - ➤ Loose tube ties
    - Decrease intracranial blood volume
        - ➤ Low-normal P$_a$CO$_2$
        - ➤ Surgical evacuation of lesion
- Brain
    - *Osmotherapy*: decrease parenchymal swelling
- CSF
    - EVD
- *Decompressive craniectomy*: remove volume/pressure limitation

How would you manage a patient presenting with TBI in the pre-hospital and emergency department setting?

Initial management relies on timely interventions and transfer to a neurosurgical centre. Management of TBI focuses largely on the prevention of secondary injury. Appropriate interventions include the following:

- **Pre-hospital**
  - Management of life-threatening injuries
  - C-spine protection
  - Airway protection
  - *Breathing*: oxygenation; ventilation may include hypocapnia to P_aCO_2 4–4.5 kPa
  - *Circulation*: IV crystalloid fluid resuscitation
  - *Other*: TXA, osmotherapy
- **Emergency Department**
  - Trauma primary survey
  - Transfer to CT once stable enough
  - May require emergency theatre (± prior to CT if unstable polytrauma)
  - Secondary survey
  - Osmotherapy when indicated
  - TXA and major haemorrhage management where relevant
- **Definitive treatment**
  - Determined by lesion
  - Destination theatre/ICU depending on findings
  - Some patients may be appropriate for extubation following CT scan – multifactorial (e.g. intoxication, facial injuries).

(See Chapter 49 Major Trauma and Chapter 50 Complex Injuries)

How would you manage a patient presenting with TBI in the intensive care setting?

Management of TBI focuses largely on the prevention of secondary injury and should follow a tiered approach. Repeat imaging should be considered at each tier. Multimodal monitoring should be considered. Surgical intervention may be required in the form of EVD insertion, evacuation of mass lesions, or decompressive craniectomy.

Tiered therapy
- **Tier 1**
  - Measures to reduce venous congestion (as above)
  - *Ventilation*: SpO_2 > 94%, P_aO_2 > 10 kPa, P_aCO_2 4.5–5 kPa, low PEEP
  - *Induced hypertension*: MAP > 90, SBP > 110, or **CPP 60–70 mmHg**
  - Euvolaemia
  - Deep sedation to RASS −5
  - Normoglycaemia
  - Normothermia
  - NMB infusion
  - Anticonvulsants
  - Treat coagulopathy
  - EVD insertion as indicated
- **Tier 2**
  - P_aCO_2 4–4.5 kPa
  - Osmotherapy
  - Ketamine infusion
- **Tier 3**
  - Barbiturate infusion titrated to ICP control/burst suppression
  - Decompressive craniectomy

Other management priorities
- Consider cardiac output monitoring and echo (myocardial stunning due to catecholamine release)
- *Observe closely for polyuria*: administer DDAVP for diabetes insipidus

- Consider screening for hypopituitarism
- Transfusion thresholds are under evaluation (**HEMOTION**) (see Chapter 51 Major Haemorrhage)

GUIDELINE SIBICC 2019 TBI

What is a good outcome from TBI?

The Glasgow Outcome Scale (GOS) is a global scale of functional outcomes following brain injury. Original classification is as follows:

1 Dead
2 Vegetative state (VS)
3 Severe disability
4 Moderate disability
5 Good recovery

The Extended GOS (GOSE) includes further subcategories. GOSE 1–4 are considered unfavourable and 5–8 favourable.

KEY POINT

GOSE:

1. Dead
2. VS
3. *Lower severe disability (LSD)*: full assistance for ADL
4. *Upper severe disability (USD)*: partial assistance for ADL
5. *Lower moderate disability (LMD)*: independent, unable to resume work or all previous social activities
6. *Upper moderate disability (UMD)*: some disability, partially resume work or previous activities
7. *Lower good recovery (LGR)*: minor physical/mental deficit, affects daily life
8. *Upper good recovery (UGR)*: full recovery or minor symptoms not affecting daily life

(See Chapter 87 Disorders of Consciousness)

Is there a role for decompressive craniectomy in TBI?

Decompressive craniectomy is controversial and is not without significant risk of medical and surgical complications. This operation does still take place occasionally, often as a last resort. Optimising medical management may reduce the need for this invasive intervention.

Several RCTs have examined its role in the management of TBI. Mortality reduction might be offset by significantly higher survival with other 'unfavourable' outcomes (VS/LSD/USD) and reduced survival with UGR.

STUDY

DECRA (2011)

- TBI with refractory intracranial hypertension
- *Intervention*: decompressive craniectomy vs medical therapy
- *Primary*: 6-month GOSE: **dead – no difference, unfavourable score 1–4 – significantly higher (70% vs 42%)**
- *Secondary*: hours of intracranial hypertension, days of MV, ICU LOS – **significantly lower**

STUDY

RESCUEicp (2016)

- TBI with abnormal CT and refractory intracranial hypertension
- *Intervention*: decompressive craniectomy vs medical therapy
- *Primary*: 6-month GOSE: dead – **significantly lower (26.9% vs 48.9%)**; VS, LSD, USD – **significantly higher (8.5% vs 2.1%, 21.9% vs 14.4%, 15.4% vs 8%)**
- *Secondary*: 12-month GOSE similar

Is there a role for steroids in TBI?

Corticosteroids have been linked to worse outcomes and are not recommended in TBI.

STUDY

CRASH (2004)

- Head injury, GCS ≤14
- *Intervention*: early methylprednisolone for 48 h
- *Primary*: 2-week mortality – **higher (21.1% vs 17.9%)** – stopped early
- *Secondary*: 6-week mortality ± severe disability – higher

(The **CRASH-2** and **CRASH-3** trials relate to the use of TXA in major trauma and TBI, respectively.)

(See Chapter 51 Major Haemorrhage)

Is there a role for therapeutic hypothermia in TBI?

Despite its associated reduction in cerebral metabolic oxygen demand, therapeutic hypothermia has not been demonstrated to improve outcomes and carries significant risk of morbidity such as infection. Its use is not recommended (see Chapter 16 Temperature Control).

STUDY

Eurotherm3225 (2015)

- TBI with high ICP refractory to Tier 1 measures
- *Intervention*: therapeutic hypothermia 32–35°C for 48 h until ICP improvement vs standard care
- *Primary*: 6-month GOSE – **trend to poorer outcome (terminated after interim analysis)**
- *Secondary*: 6-month mortality – **significantly higher**; pneumonia in days 1–7 – no difference

STUDY

POLAR (2018)

- Severe TBI
- *Intervention*: cold 0.9% NaCl to target T 35°C vs 36.6–37.5°C
- *Primary*: 6-month favourable GOSE – **no difference**
- *Secondary*: 6-month mortality – no difference, pneumonia – **significantly higher (70.5% vs 57.1%)**, bradycardia – **significantly higher (18.8% vs 4.2%)**

How can we neuroprognosticate in TBI?

This is a difficult task and should be undertaken after a period of stabilisation, accounting for a variety of factors. Consensus opinion of the MDT is required.

Clinical predictors
- Age
- GCS post-resuscitation
- Motor component of GCS post-resuscitation
- Pupillary reactivity to light
- Pupillary size
- Intracranial injury type
- Raised ICP
- Hypoxia
- Hypotension
- Significant comorbidities

Radiological predictors
- Marshall classification of CT head imaging (I–VI including involvement of basal cisterns, midline shift, density of lesions, mass lesion ± evacuation)
- MR head imaging

Research-based predictors
- *Radiological*: MR spectroscopy
- *Electrophysiological*: cEEG, SSEPs
- Biomarkers
  - Serum S100B
  - Neuron-specific enolase (NSE)
  - IL-10
  - *Protein degradation products*: tau, amyloid, glial fibrillary acidic protein

(See Chapter 156 Prognostication)

Resource
- Marshall LF, Marshall SB, Klauber MR, et al. The diagnosis of head injury requires a classification based on computed axial tomography. J Neurotrauma. 1992;9(Suppl1):S287–S292.

---

84. INTRACEREBRAL HAEMORRHAGE

What is ICH?

ICH is bleeding into the brain parenchyma and is a type of stroke.

ICH is responsible for 9–27% of strokes worldwide. Presentation is often with features of abrupt increase in ICP, causing nausea and vomiting, focal deficit, loss of consciousness, or brain stem death.

(See Chapter 85 Ischaemic Stroke)

What are the causes of ICH?

Predisposing factors
- Arterial small-vessel disease
- Arterial large-vessel disease
- Venous disease
- Vascular malformation
- Haemostatic disorders

Precipitants – haemodynamic stress
- Hypertension
- Intracranial hypotension (e.g. post-LP)
- CVST

- Drugs (e.g. cocaine, amphetamines, adrenaline)
- Post-reperfusion (e.g. thrombolysis, endarterectomy)

Specific disease-based causes
- Malignancy
- Amyloidosis
- Haemorrhagic transformation of ischaemic stroke

What are the most common sites of hypertensive ICH?

ICH usually affects deep sites that are as follows:

- Basal ganglia
- Putamen
- Thalamus
- Cerebellum
- Pons

How would you investigate a patient for non-traumatic ICH?

A focused history (± collateral history) and examination for underlying causes are relevant where possible. Medications are of particular importance. Investigation and simultaneous management are time-critical.

- Imaging
  - CT head without contrast
  - *CT angiography*: evaluate any underlying vascular anomalies
  - *MR ± angiography*: role in determining age of haemorrhage
  - *DSA*: diagnostic and therapeutic role
- *Coagulopathy*: FBC, coagulation screen including fibrinogen, viscoelastic testing
- *Hypertension*: consider secondary causes

(See Chapter 73 Hypertension)

How would you manage this patient?

Management depends on the underlying cause and focuses largely on prevention of complications and secondary brain injury. Guidance is inconclusive in several key areas of supportive and definitive management. The majority of care is supportive, in keeping with neuroprotective measures. Transfer to a hyperacute stroke unit (HASU) might be indicated if a patient does not require airway support.

(See Chapter 82 Subarachnoid Haemorrhage)

GUIDELINE   ESO 2014 Spontaneous ICH

GUIDELINE   NICE 2019 NG128 Stroke and TIA

Specific management
- **Intensive BP reduction to 130–140 mmHg < 1 h**, depending on time of presentation:
  - *Indicated within 6 h onset*: if initial systolic BP 150–200 mmHg
  - Consider if presenting after 6 h or if initial systolic BP > 220 mmHg (less strongly recommended)
  - Maintain for **≥7 days**
  - *Contraindications*: underlying structural cause, GCS < 6, early haematoma evacuation planned, massive haematoma with poor prognosis
- **Correction of coagulopathy**
  - Reverse anticoagulant agents (see Chapter 51 Major Haemorrhage)
  - Liaise with haematology
- *Early haematoma evacuation*: not routinely recommended, possible value if GCS 9–12
- VTE prophylaxis with intermittent pneumatic compression (not compression stockings)

- Corticosteroids are not indicated
- BP lowering for secondary prevention recommended

No strong recommendations
- Method of normalising clotting
- Invasive monitoring
- Management of fever
- Prophylactic antiepileptic therapy

STUDY

INTERACT2 (2013)

- Spontaneous ICH
- *Intervention*: intensive BP lowering vs standard treatment
- *Primary*: composite death and dependency at 90 days – **no difference**
- *Secondary*: mRS, mortality – no difference; health-related quality-of-life problems reported – **significantly lower** (except mobility)

STUDY

ATACH-2 (2016)

- Spontaneous ICH
- *Intervention*: BP lowering to 110–139 vs 140–179 mmHg for 24 h
- *Primary*: mRS 4–6 at 3 months – **no difference**
- *Secondary*: haematoma expansion, deterioration, mortality – no difference

---

STUDY

TICH-2 (2018)

- Spontaneous ICH
- *Intervention*: TXA vs placebo
- *Primary*: 90-day mRS – **no difference**
- *Secondary*: 90-day mortality, LOS) – no difference
- *Subgroups*: benefit if SBP < 170 mmHg or baseline haematoma volume 30–60 ml

---

What is the rationale behind intensive BP reduction?

Majority of patients presenting with ICH will display arterial hypertension, with or without a history of raised BP. Appropriate BP targets remain controversial in ICH.

Lowering BP may
- Prevent haematoma enlargement
- Reduce risks of end-organ dysfunction due to hypertension
- Avoid poorer outcomes linked to hypertension in the acute phase of ICH

Counterargument
- Hypotension may predispose to ischaemic damage surrounding the haemorrhage.
- In chronic hypertension, a higher CPP is required to maintain normal CBF; hence, hypotension may lead to impaired CBF.

What is the role of surgical evacuation of haematoma in patients presenting with ICH?

The role of surgical evacuation of haematoma remains controversial in ICH. Minimally invasive surgical techniques are under investigation. Surgery in primary ICH is recommended if hydrocephalus is present.

(See Chapter 85 Ischaemic Stroke)

STUDY

STICH (1998)

- Non-traumatic ICH
- *Intervention*: surgical haematoma evacuation vs medical therapy
- *Primary*: 6-month favourable GOSE – **no difference**
- *Secondary*: 6-month mortality – no difference

STUDY

STICH II (2013)

- Spontaneous ICH ≤1 cm from cortex surface
- *Intervention*: early haematoma evacuation vs initial medical therapy
- *Primary*: 6-month favourable GOSE – **no difference**
- *Secondary*: 6-month mortality – no difference

STUDY

STITCH [Trauma] (2015)

- Traumatic ICH
- *Intervention*: early haematoma evacuation (<12 h) vs conventional management
- *Primary*: 6-month unfavourable GOS – **no difference** (but some reduction) – stopped early due to recruitment difficulties
- *Secondary*: 6-month mortality – **lower**; all additional survivors left with worse functional outcome

Resources

- Fogarty Mack P. Intracranial haemorrhage: therapeutic interventions and anaesthetic management. Br J Anaesth. 2014;113(Suppl2):ii17–ii25.
- Sacco RL, Kasner SE, Broderick JP, et al. An Updated Definition of Stroke for the 21st Century: A Statement for Healthcare Professionals from the American Heart Association/American Stroke Association. Stroke. 2013;44(7):2064–2089.

85. ISCHAEMIC STROKE

What is ischaemic stroke?

> **KEY POINT**
>
> Ischaemic stroke is an episode of neurological dysfunction caused by focal cerebral, spinal, or retinal infarction. It falls within the broader definition of 'stroke'.

Stroke has been defined as 'rapidly developing clinical signs of **focal (or global) disturbance of cerebral function, lasting more than 24 h** or leading to death, with no apparent cause other than that of vascular origin'.

Stroke, ischaemic stroke, and CNS infarction are subtly different concepts. Stroke is defined inconsistently. The following conditions may be considered types of stroke:

- *CNS infarction*: brain, spinal cord, or retinal cell death attributable to ischaemia
- **Ischaemic stroke**
- Silent CNS infarction
- ICH
- Silent cerebral haemorrhage
- SAH
- Stroke caused by SAH
- Stroke caused by cerebral venous thrombosis
- Stroke, not otherwise specified

How might stroke be classified?

> **KEY POINT**
>
> **Bamford Classification**
>
> - Total anterior circulation syndrome (TACS)
> - Partial anterior circulation syndrome (PACS)
> - Lacunar syndrome (LACS)
> - Posterior circulation syndrome (POCS)

TACS – all of the following:
- *Unilateral deficit*: motor/sensory/both – ≥2 of face/arm/leg
- Higher cerebral dysfunction (e.g. dysphasia, dyspraxia, neglect)
- Homonymous hemianopia

PACS – any of the following:
- 2/3 of above criteria
- Pure higher cortical dysfunction
- Pure motor/sensory deficit not as extensive as LACS

LACS:
- Pure motor/sensory deficit – ≥2 of face/arm/leg
- Sensorimotor deficit
- Ataxic hemiparesis
- Dysarthria, clumsy hand syndrome
- Acute onset movement disorder

POCS:
- Isolated hemianopia
- Brain stem signs
- Cerebellar ataxia

What are risk factors for ischaemic stroke?

Risk factors overlap with those for atherosclerosis:

- Hypertension
- Diabetes mellitus
- Smoking
- High BMI
- Dyslipidaemia
- Sickle cell disease
- Pregnancy

What are the common causes of ischaemic stroke?

- Thrombus
- Embolus
- Systemic hypoperfusion

What sites of ischaemic stroke result in the most severe features?

- MCA
- Terminal internal carotid artery
- Basilar artery

How should a patient presenting with suspected ischaemic stroke be investigated?

This will be time-critical, and focus is on ruling out haemorrhagic stroke or a stroke mimic, as well as expediting emergency definitive treatment if indicated. Pre-hospital screening with a validated tool (e.g. FAST) is valuable.

- Exclude hypoglycaemia
- *Rapid diagnosis*: validated tool (e.g. Recognition of Stroke in the Emergency Room [ROSIER])
- *Establish key history*: onset time (or last known to be well), anticoagulants
- *National Institutes of Health Stroke Scale (NIHSS)*: severity assessment
- Imaging
  - Non-enhanced CT
  - CT angiography if thrombectomy indicated
  - ± CT/MR perfusion imaging if thrombectomy indicated >6 h onset
- *Risk factors*: HbA1c, lipid profile, 12-lead ECG, TTE

When is CT imaging indicated in suspected acute stroke?

- Immediate
  - Indications for thrombolysis or thrombectomy
  - Anticoagulants
  - Known bleeding tendency
  - GCS < 13
  - Unexplained progressive/fluctuating symptoms
  - Papilloedema, neck stiffness, or fever
  - Severe headache at onset
- *Within 24 h*: if not meeting above indications

Suspicion of transient ischaemic attack (TIA) does not mandate CT imaging. Carotid imaging should be performed if deemed suitable for carotid endarterectomy. MR might be considered after assessment in a specialist clinic.

What are the key management priorities in ischaemic stroke?

- **Supportive care** as indicated
  - Supplemental O_2 only if hypoxic ($S_aO_2 < 95\%$)
  - Existing evidence does not support cooling in this setting.
- **BP management**
  - Target BP **≤185/110 mmHg** if for IV thrombolysis
  - Otherwise, antihypertensive treatment only if hypertensive emergency: encephalopathy, nephropathy, cardiac failure/MI, aortic dissection, pre-eclampsia/eclampsia
  - Clinical judgement in extreme elevation (≥220/120 mmHg) – European Society of Cardiology (ESC) recommendation, not specified in NICE guideline (see Chapter 73 Hypertension)
- **Definitive management**
  - Aspirin 300 mg loading and daily for 2 weeks (exclude ICH, start within 24 h)
  - IV thrombolysis if indicated **<4.5 h onset** if ICH excluded (e.g. recombinant tissue plasminogen activator, t-PA, alteplase)
  - Intra-arterial thrombectomy
  - *Specialist input*: transfer to HASU if not requiring level 3 support
- **Management of complications**
  - Malignant MCA syndrome
  - Seizures
- **Non-ischaemic aetiology**
  - Treatment-dose anticoagulation for CVST (see Chapter 86 Cerebral Venous Sinus Thrombosis)
  - If ICH, normalise clotting as soon as possible (see Chapter 84 Intracerebral Haemorrhage)

GUIDELINE NICE 2019 NG128 Stroke and TIA

GUIDELINE ESC ESH 2018 Hypertension

STUDY

NINDS (1995)

- Acute ischaemic stroke
- *Intervention*: thrombolysis with t-PA <3 h onset vs usual care
- *Primary*: NIHSS at 24 h – **no difference**
- *Secondary*: favourable Barthel Index, mRS, GOS, NIHSS at 3 months – **significantly higher**

STUDY

IST-3 (2012)

- Acute ischaemic stroke
- *Intervention*: t-PA vs placebo < 6 h
- *Primary*: Oxford Handicap Scale 0–2 at 6 months – **no difference**; did not meet recruitment numbers
- *Secondary*: 7-day mortality – **significantly higher**; 6-month mortality – **significantly lower**

STUDY

EuroHYP-1 (2018)

- Acute ischaemic stroke
- *Intervention*: cooling to target T 34–35°C vs usual care
- *Primary*: mRS at 91 days – **no difference**; stopped early – recruitment difficulty/funding

Which scoring systems are relevant to stroke outcomes?

The NIHSS has been used to quantify stroke severity after its development for the **NINDS** trial, particularly for early use. It includes the following categories which are given an increasing score as features become more severe:

- Level of consciousness
- Response to questions
- Response to commands
- Horizontal extraocular movements
- Visual fields
- Facial palsy
- Motor drift in each limb
- Limb ataxia
- Sensation
- Language/aphasia
- Dysarthria
- Extinction/inattention

The **mRS** is used to measure disability or dependence following stroke and has been extended to use in other causes of brain injury. The Oxford Handicap Scale is similar to the mRS, specifically for patient handicap. The CPC and GOS also relate to brain injury. (See Chapter 83 Traumatic Brain Injury and Chapter 156 Prognostication)

The **Barthel Index for Activities of Daily Living** is used to assess functional independence following stroke and includes feeding, bathing, grooming, dressing, bowel control, bladder control, toilet use, transfers, mobility, and use of stairs.

When is thrombectomy indicated?

KEY POINT

Eligibility for thrombectomy:

- **<6 h symptom onset** and
- Confirmed occlusion of proximal anterior circulation (on CT/MR angiography)

If there is potential to salvage brain tissue demonstrated on CT perfusion or diffusion-weighted MR, it may be offered to patients presenting between 6–24 h onset (including 'wake-up' strokes). Once eligible, thrombectomy should be performed as soon as possible in acute ischaemic stroke. Thrombolysis is given alongside this.

STUDY

DAWN (2018)

- Acute stroke, 6–24 h from onset
- *Intervention*: thrombectomy vs medical care
- *Primary*: utility-weighted mRS at 90 days – **significantly lower**
- *Secondary*: NIHSS decrease, vessel recanalisation – **significantly higher**; infarct volume/change – **significantly lower**

STUDY

DEFUSE 3 (2018)

- Proximal ICA/MCA stroke 6–16 h from onset
- *Intervention*: thrombectomy vs medical care
- *Primary*: mRS at 90 days – **significantly lower**
- *Secondary*: mRS 0–2 at 90 days – **significantly higher**; death at 90 days – no difference

What are the contraindications to IV thrombolysis?

Absolute
- Systolic BP > 185 or diastolic BP > 110 mmHg
- INR > 1.7
- DOAC use within 48 h
- Platelets < 100 × 10⁹/l
- Active internal bleeding
- Arterial puncture at non-compressible site < 7 days
- Intracranial/intraspinal surgery or severe head trauma < 3 months
- Ischaemic stroke < 3 months
- Intracerebral vascular malformations
- Intracranial malignancy
- Previous ICH
- IE

Relative
- Rapidly improving symptoms
- Seizure at onset
- Unruptured intracranial aneurysm
- Pregnancy or post-partum < 14 days
- Major extracranial trauma < 14 days
- Major surgery < 14 days (GI/genitourinary [GU] surgery < 21 days)
- Acute MI < 3 months

GUIDELINE AHA ASA 2019 Early management of stroke

What are potential complications of IV thrombolysis?

- Haemorrhagic transformation
- Other site haemorrhage
- Oral angioedema
- Headache
- Hypertension
- HF
- CS

What is malignant MCA syndrome and is there a role for decompressive craniectomy?

Malignant MCA syndrome is the rapid neurological deterioration due to cerebral oedema following MCA territory ischaemic stroke. Decompressive craniectomy in malignant MCA syndrome remains controversial, and evidence is inconclusive. Mortality reduction has been shown, but functional outcomes in survivors are questionable. It may be considered in some situations.

KEY POINT

Indications for decompressive hemicraniectomy in acute stroke (NICE) are as follows:

- Clinical signs of MCA infarction, NIHSS score > 15
- Decreased level of consciousness, score ≥1 on item 1a on NIHSS
- CT infarct ≥50% MCA territory
  - ± additional infarction of anterior/posterior cerebral artery on same side or
  - Infarct volume > 145 cm³ on diffusion-weighted MRI

STUDY

DESTINY (2007)

- MCA infarction, age 18–60 years
- *Intervention*: decompressive craniectomy vs conservative treatment
- *Primary*: mRS 0–3 at 6 months – **no difference** but non-significant increase (47% vs 27%)
- *Secondary*: 30-day mortality – **significantly lower**

STUDY

DECIMAL (2007)

- MCA infarction, age 18–55 years
- *Intervention*: decompressive craniectomy vs conservative treatment
- *Primary*: mRS ≤3 at 6 months and 12 months – **no difference**; however mRS ≤4 at 12 months **significantly higher (75% vs 22.2%)**
- *Secondary*: 6-month and 12-month mortality – **significantly lower**

STUDY

HAMLET (2009)

- Space-occupying hemispheric infarction
- *Intervention*: decompressive craniectomy vs conservative treatment
- *Primary*: mRS at 12 months – **no difference**
- *Secondary*: mortality – **significantly lower**
- Meta-analysis including **DESTINY** and **DECIMAL** – reduction in poor outcome and case fatality

STUDY

DESTINY II (2011)

- MCA infarction, age ≥61 years
- *Intervention*: decompressive hemicraniectomy < 48 h onset vs conservative treatment
- *Primary*: mRS 0–4 at 6 months – **significantly higher (38% vs 18%)**
- *Secondary*: 12-month mortality – **significantly lower (43% vs 76%)** but no survivors with mRS 0–2

Resources

- Raithatha A, Pratt G, Rash A. Developments in the management of acute ischaemic stroke: implications for anaesthetic and critical care management. CEACCP. 2013;13(3):80–86.
- Sacco RL, Kasner SE, Broderick JP, et al. An updated definition of stroke for the 21st century: a statement for healthcare professionals from the American Heart Association/American Stroke Association. Stroke. 2013;44(7):2064–2089.

86. CEREBRAL VENOUS SINUS THROMBOSIS

What is CVST?

CVST is a rare disorder in which thrombus forms in the cerebral venous system.

It became a more prominent concern following the discovery of vaccine-induced immune thrombocytopaenia and thrombosis (VITT) during the COVID-19 pandemic. Prior to this, the annual incidence was approximately 2–5 cases per million individuals. Younger adults were affected (mean age 35 years) with female predominance.

CVST most commonly affects the **superior sagittal** and **transverse sinuses** (60%), before the **internal jugular** and **cortical veins** (20%). Two thirds of patients will have more than 1 affected sinus.

What is the pathophysiology?

Risk factors include those for other thrombotic disorders, with specific mechanical factors including the following:

- Head trauma
- Neurosurgical procedures
- LP
- Jugular venous catheterisation

CVST then results in the following:

Venous congestion
- Increased hydrostatic pressure upstream of any occlusion
- Variable degree of compensation by anastomotic vessels
- If compensation is overcome, blood-brain barrier disruption can occur
- Fluid extravasation into parenchyma
- Localised oedema

Arterial ischaemia
- If venous pressure greater than arterial pressure
- Haemorrhagic infarction may result
- Perfusion pressure not usually reduced so may have reversible tissue damage

CSF obstruction
- Venous occlusion reduces CSF access to arachnoid granulations
- CSF reabsorption is reduced
- Intracranial hypertension may result
- More common with superior sagittal sinus occlusion

What are the clinical features of CVST?

Patients typically present with **headache** (89%), **seizures** (39%), **paresis** (37%), papilloedema (28%), or altered mental state (22%).

Important characteristics
- *Headache*: new/worsening, diffuse, severe, thunderclap, rapidly progressive over hours
- *Raised ICP*: visual loss on coughing/sneezing/bending, pulsatile tinnitus, papilloedema
- *Focal neurology*: visual disturbance, weakness, speech disturbance

What is VITT?

VITT is a rare syndrome, first described in patients who had received the first dose of a COVID-19 vaccine. It has been found to be more prevalent with some vaccine brands. It resembles HIT clinically. (See Chapter 145 Heparin-Induced Thrombocytopaenia)

VITT is characterised by the following:

- Thrombocytopaenia
- Elevated D-dimer
- Progressive thrombosis (high incidence of CVST)

VITT usually presents 5–28 (median 12) days after vaccination with venous or arterial thrombosis or thromboembolic disease. Approximately 50% will have concomitant ICH and/or SAH.

How would you investigate suspected CVST?

Imaging
- CT cerebral venography – if:
  - Suspected CVST (headache usually > 4 days post vaccine)
  - VITT with extracranial thrombosis
  - VITT with embolic complications within critical care admission
- CT thorax/abdomen/pelvis/limbs
  - Consider if CVST is primary diagnosis to investigate for other complications including PE, portal vein thrombosis, peripheral arterial thrombosis

Bloods in suspected VITT
- *FBC*: platelets < 150×10^9/l
- *Coagulation screen*: low fibrinogen, D-dimer elevation
  - D-dimer > 4000 µg/l or
  - D-dimer 2000–4000 µg/l with high clinical probability
- *Blood film*: confirm true thrombocytopaenia
- *Platelet factor 4 (PF4) antibody assay*: ELISA HIT assay (i.e. not HIT assay by Accustar and Diamend)

These bloods should be repeated daily at first. Haematology should be contacted if a patient presents with acute thrombosis with thrombocytopaenia or isolated thrombocytopaenia in days 5–28 post vaccination.

What are the key management points in CVST?

- Early diagnosis and treatment
- Haematology advice
- Specific treatment
  - **Anticoagulation**
    - When fibrinogen >1.5 g/l and platelets >30×10^9/l
    - Non-heparin (e.g. DOAC, fondaparinux, danaparoid, argatroban)
    - Avoid heparinised saline flushes
  - **Immunosuppression (if caused by VITT)**
    - IVIg 1 g/kg immediately
    - *Steroids if IVIg not available*: methylprednisolone 1 g IV
    - Plasma exchange may be required (monitor for hyponatraemia)
    - Rituximab under consideration in refractory cases
- *Transfusion*: platelets if surgery or major bleeding (target > 50×10^9/l)
- *Tertiary referral*: severe CVST or progression of thrombosis
  - MDT input including haematology, stroke/neurology, neurosurgery, interventional neuroradiology, intensive care medicine
  - *Important features*: potential for intervention, refractory disease, ICH, mass effect, dominant side or bilateral thrombosis, deteriorating GCS
- **Procedures**
  - *IR*: mechanical thrombectomy, intra-sinus thrombolysis, cerebral venous thrombectomy
  - *Decompressive craniectomy*: refractory intracranial hypertension

GUIDELINE ICS 2021 VITT

Resource
- Capecchi M, Abbattista M, Martinelli I. Cerebral venous sinus thrombosis. J Thromb Haemost. 2018;16(10):1918–1931.

What is consciousness?

KEY POINT

Consciousness is a state which requires both wakefulness and awareness.

Wakefulness:
- Eyes open
- Degree of motor arousal
- *Contrast with sleep* (state of eye closure and motor quiescence)

Awareness:
- The ability to have, and the having of, experience of any kind
- *More complex*: physical responses related to environment

What are the main disorders of consciousness caused by sudden onset brain injury?

Disorders of consciousness encompass a continuum of states:

- Normal
- *Confusional state*: confusion, agitation, disorientation
- *Emerged*: reliable and consistent responses (e.g. yes/no, functional object use)
- Minimally conscious state (MCS)
  - *MCS plus*: higher level responses (e.g. following commands, intentional communication)
  - *MCS minus*: lower level behaviours (e.g. visual pursuit, localising motor reactions)
- *Vegetative State (VS)*: reflexive and spontaneous movements only
- Coma

GUIDELINE RCP 2020 PDOC

What are the differences between these disorders and brain stem death?

Wakefulness and awareness can be used to distinguish between these disorders and their differences to brain stem death are important (Table 87.1).

Table 87.1 Differences between disorders of consciousness and brain stem death

	Wakefulness	Awareness	Consciousness	Features
Brain stem death	No	No	No	Irreversible loss of capacity for consciousness and capacity to breathe
Coma	No	No	No	No response to environment or stimulation
VS	Yes	No	No	May open eyes and wake, have basic reflexes, but won't show meaningful responses or interact
MCS	Yes	Yes	Yes	Clear awareness, minimal and inconsistent, may have periods of communicative or interactive behaviour

What is locked in syndrome?

- Upper motor neurone quadriplegia also involving cranial nerves
- Usually results from brain stem pathology
- Clinical impairment of ability to communicate or interact physically
- Not a disorder of consciousness (this is maintained)
- Usually preserves eye movements in 1 or 2 axes, may be able to blink voluntarily
- *Differentials*: myaesthenia gravis, GBS, poliomyelitis, polyneuritis

How is coma classified?

Classification by the presence or absence of lateralising signs, meningism, and brain stem reflexes may aid diagnosis and ongoing management (Figure 87.1).

What are the timescales involved in diagnosing disorders of consciousness?

Brain death may be apparent within hours of injury. Coma usually lasts <2–4 weeks. Prolonged disorder of consciousness (PDOC) can be defined **after 4 weeks**.

MCS

- Continuing (previously 'persistent') MCS >4 weeks
- Chronic MCS plus >9 months (atraumatic), >18 months (TBI)
- Chronic MCS minus >3 months (atraumatic), >12 months (TBI)

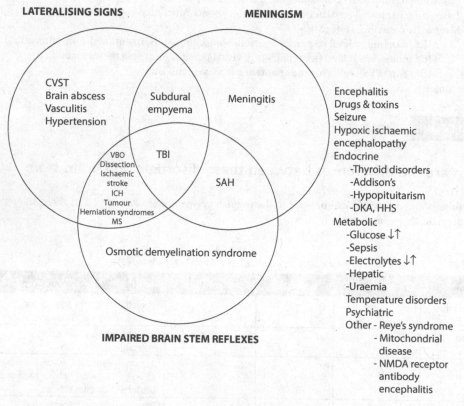

Figure 87.1 Classification of coma by clinical domains affected commonly.

Presentation may vary.

VS
- Continuing VS >4 weeks
- Chronic VS >3 months (atraumatic), >12 months (TBI)

VS or MCS may be diagnosed as 'permanent' after specialist confirmation that there has been no change in trajectory for **6 months**.

How are these disorders diagnosed?

Diagnostic criteria
- Cause established
- Not related to medications
- Reversible causes of loss of awareness treated
- Exclusion of other potentially reversible causes (e.g. primary brain tumour)
- Examinations carried out by trained assessor with experience in PDOC

Assessment
- *Clinical examination*: GCS, Coma Recovery Scale – Revised (CRS-R)
- *Imaging*: CT, MR
- *Functional*: EEG, functional MR limited to research

What is the prognosis in PDOC?

- Patients with PDOC may survive several years.
- The longer someone is in a PDOC, the less likely they are to regain consciousness.
- Most patients never recover consciousness (isolated reports exist).
- Those who do recover consciousness often have severe disability from brain injury.

(See Chapter 156 Prognostication)

How are patients with PDOC managed in the longer term?

- Clinically assisted nutrition and hydration (CANH)
- Pressure area relief
- Physiotherapy to prevent joint and muscle stiffness
- Washing
- Bladder and bowel management
- Oral hygiene measures
- Offering opportunities for meaningful activity
- Sensory stimulation to attempt to increase responsiveness

Affected patients are usually fully dependent on nursing care from family and/or external services and require specialised accommodation. A palliative care team might be involved.

If there is almost no chance of recovery, an MDT decision might be made to withdraw CANH. This may involve referral to court.

GUIDELINE BMA & RCP 2018 CANH

Resource
- Patel S, Hirsch N. Coma. CEACCP. 2014;14(5):220–223.

88.   STATUS EPILEPTICUS

Define convulsive status epilepticus.

> **KEY POINT**
>
> Convulsive status epilepticus:
>
> - Prolonged convulsive seizure >5 min or
> - Convulsive seizures (>1) occurring one after the other with incomplete recovery between them

Definitions regarding ongoing seizure activity vary but examples include the following:

- *Refractory status epilepticus*: failure to respond to first-line therapies at 60–90 min (e.g. adequately dosed benzodiazepine and second antiepileptic drug)
- *Super-refractory status epilepticus*: present for 24 h

What is epilepsy?

- *Epilepsy*: neurological disorder characterised by recurrent epileptic seizures
- *Epileptic seizure*: transient signs and/or symptoms resulting from a primary change to electrical activity in the brain

Why is status epilepticus a concern?

- Can cause sudden death
- Significant neuronal injury occurs within minutes of onset
- Morbidity related to rapidity of seizure control

Major complications

- Airway obstruction
- Aspiration
- Hypoxic ischaemic injury (multisystem)
- Pulmonary oedema
- Dysrhythmias
- Lasting neurological dysfunction
- Cerebrovascular accident
- Rhabdomyolysis
- Trauma

Mortality (e.g. at hospital discharge)

- *Convulsive*: 9–21%
- *Non-convulsive*: 18–52%
- *Refractory*: 23–61%

How does a generalised seizure affect the autonomic nervous system?

Sympathetic predominance is most common, but ictal changes may also include its inhibition or parasympathetic activation.

Parasympathetic

- Bradypnoea
- Bradycardia
- Hypotension
- Miosis
- Increased salivation, gastric acid secretion, peristalsis

Sympathetic
- Tachypnoea
- Tachycardia
- Hypertension
- Mydriasis
- Diaphoresis

What are the specific management principles in status epilepticus?

The overall goal is to prevent secondary injury by reducing CMR and optimising CPP.

Principles
- Airway protection
- Rapid termination of seizure activity with antiepileptic drugs – practice may vary locally (Figure 88.1)
- Treating the underlying cause of decompensation
- Diagnosis of any underlying disorder
- Treating complications

Specific therapies
- *Eclampsia*: magnesium sulphate, delivery
- *Toxicity*: antidotes as indicated (see Chapter 32 Poisoning Overview)
    - *Cholinergic syndrome*: atropine, pralidoxime
    - *Sodium channel blockers*: sodium bicarbonate, intralipid
- *Infection*: antibiotics, antivirals, consider steroids
- *Alcohol withdrawal or impaired nutrition*: glucose, thiamine

GUIDELINE NICE 2021 CG137 Epilepsies

What investigations might you consider alongside your initial management?

- *Collateral history*: precipitants, psychosocial factors, lifestyle, trauma
- *Bloods*: FBC, U&E, glucose, Mg^{2+}, TFT, serum antiepileptic drug levels, metabolic panel, other (e.g. ADAMTS13)

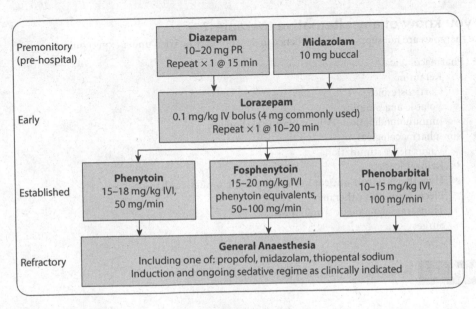

Premonitory (pre-hospital)	**Diazepam** 10–20 mg PR Repeat × 1 @ 15 min	**Midazolam** 10 mg buccal

Early	**Lorazepam** 0.1 mg/kg IV bolus (4 mg commonly used) Repeat × 1 @ 10–20 min

Established	**Phenytoin** 15–18 mg/kg IVI, 50 mg/min	**Fosphenytoin** 15–20 mg/kg IVI phenytoin equivalents, 50–100 mg/min	**Phenobarbital** 10–15 mg/kg IVI, 100 mg/min

Refractory	**General Anaesthesia** Including one of: propofol, midazolam, thiopental sodium Induction and ongoing sedative regime as clinically indicated

Figure 88.1 Adult status epilepticus treatment algorithm.

- Urine/serum βhCG
- Toxicology
- *CT*: if acute neurological lesion or illness suspected
- cEEG
- LP

What are the pharmacological recommendations in children?

- *5 min*: midazolam (0.5 mg/kg buccal) or lorazepam if IV access (0.1 mg/kg)
- *15 min*: lorazepam IV
- *25 min*: phenytoin (20 mg/kg IV infusion, 20 min) or phenobarbital (20 mg/kg IVI, 5 min)
- *45 min*: general anaesthesia using thiopental sodium (4 mg/kg)

What is your strategy for sedating a patient with refractory status epilepticus in the critical care unit?

Sedative infusions with antiepileptic properties are prioritised in addition to background maintenance antiepileptic therapy. Opioid infusions should be avoided as they lower the seizure threshold.

Recommencing usual medications is important, and adjustments to polypharmacy with intermittently dosed agents may need to be guided by a neurologist. Transfer to a specialist centre may be indicated.

Continuous infusions
- Midazolam
- Propofol
- Thiopental
- Pentobarbital

Intermittent anti-epileptic drugs (AED)
- *Benzodiazepines*: diazepam, lorazepam, midazolam
- Fosphenytoin, phenytoin
- Levetiracetam
- Valproate sodium
- Phenobarbital
- Topiramate
- Lacosamide
- Clobazam

Do you know of any alternative therapies?

Some therapies are not supported by evidence to date but may be tried under expert guidance:

- Pharmacological
  - Ketamine
  - Corticosteroids
  - Volatile anaesthetics
  - Immunomodulation (IVIg or plasma exchange)
- Non-pharmacological
  - Vagus nerve stimulation
  - Ketogenic diet
  - Hypothermia (role unclear in status epilepticus post-cardiac arrest)
  - Electroconvulsive therapy
  - Transcranial magnetic stimulation
  - Surgery

GUIDELINE Neurocritical Care Society 2012 Status epilepticus

HYBERNATUS (2016)

- Convulsive status epilepticus
- *Intervention*: target T 32–34°C for 24 h vs no target
- *Primary*: GOS 5 – **no difference**
- *Secondary*: mortality, seizure duration, LOS – no difference; progression in EEG-confirmed status epilepticus – **significantly lower**

When would you wake the patient up?

NICE guidance advocates **12–24 h anaesthesia** after the last clinical or electrographic seizure in status epilepticus. The Neurocritical Care Society recommends 24–48 h electrographic control in refractory status epilepticus. Infusions should be withdrawn slowly with cEEG monitoring.

What is non-convulsive status epilepticus?

KEY POINT

Non-convulsive status epilepticus is defined as status seizure activity on EEG without clinical findings associated with generalised convulsive status epilepticus.

There are 2 main phenotypes: the 'wandering confused' and the 'acutely ill patient with severely impaired mental status' (may have subtle motor movements).

Features

- *Negative symptoms*: anorexia, aphasia/mutism, amnesia, catatonia, coma, confusion, lethargy, staring
- *Positive symptoms*: agitation/aggression, automatisms, blinking, crying, delirium, delusions, echolalia, facial twitching, laughter, nausea/vomiting, nystagmus/eye deviation, perseveration, psychosis, tremulousness

89.   MENINGITIS

What is meningitis?

- *Meningitis*: pathological diagnosis of inflammation of the meninges
- *Meningoencephalitis*: inflammation of meninges and adjoining brain parenchyma
- *Meningococcal sepsis*: sepsis ± characteristic petechial/purpuric rash and hypoperfusion (*N. meningitidis* in blood/CSF/skin)
- *Invasive meningococcal disease*: invasion of normally sterile site by *N. meningitidis*

What are the causes of meningitis?

Infectious
- Bacterial
  - *Pneumococcal (Streptococcus pneumoniae)*: over 50s
  - *Meningococcal (N. meningitidis)*: adolescents, young adults

- *Listeria monocytogenes*: over 60s, rare
- *Haemophilus influenzae* type B
- *Escherichia coli*
- *Mycobacterium tuberculosis*
- Lyme disease (*Borrelia burgdorferi*)
- *Viral*: HSV-1, **HSV-2** (20–40 years), VZV, mumps, HIV, influenza, enteroviruses, tick-borne viruses
- *Fungal*: Cryptococcus (particularly with HIV, CD4 < 100 μl^{-1}), histoplasmosis
- *Parasitic*: malaria, schistosomiasis, trypanosomiasis

Non-infectious
- Malignancy
- *Inflammatory*: vasculitidies, SLE, sarcoid
- *Medication-related*: antibiotics, NSAIDs, IVIg

A cause is not identified in the majority of cases.

What are risk factors for meningitis?

- Incomplete vaccination history
- *Immunocompromise*: HIV, transplant
- Splenectomy (encapsulated bacterial infection)
- Systemic autoimmune disease
- Malignancy
- Animal contact
- Travel

How might meningitis present?

- Classical triad
  - **Fever**
  - **Meningism** (headache, neck stiffness, photophobia)
  - **Altered mental state**
- Neurological
  - Headache
  - Seizures
  - Cranial nerve abnormalities
  - Hydrocephalus
  - CVST
- Systemic
  - Rash
  - Meningococcal features
  - Sepsis and septic shock
  - Multi-organ dysfunction
  - DIC
  - Waterhouse-Friderichsen syndrome (haemorrhage into adrenal glands)

What is the significance of meningococcal disease?

Meningococcal bacteria (*N. meningitidis*) may result in meningococcal meningitis, meningococcal septi-caemia, or a combination of the two. There are several groups of bacteria: A, B, C, W, and X. These are often present in the nose and throat.

Meningococcal meningitis is associated with a high risk of neurological sequelae. Meningococcal sepsis may present in extremis with multi-organ dysfunction, DIC, and gangrene.

Risk factors for fatal outcome in meningococcal disease are as follows:

- Rapidly progressing rash
- Coma
- Hypotension and shock
- Lactate > 4 mmol/l

- Low/normal peripheral WCC
- Low acute phase reactants
- Low platelets
- Coagulopathy
- Absence of meningitis

GUIDELINE   Joint Specialist Societies 2016 Meningitis

How would you manage a critically unwell patient with suspected meningitis?

Stabilisation and investigation may occur concomitantly. GCS should be documented.

Management priorities
- **Supportive care** as indicated
  - May require intubation and ventilation (e.g. low GCS, severe agitation)
  - Euvolaemia, MAP ≥65 mmHg, NA first-line vasopressor
  - If suspected high ICP, measures to maintain CPP
  - Seizure management
  - CSF drainage if raised ICP
- **LP within 1 h** if safe to do so
  - Neuroimaging first only if clinically indicated (e.g. CT without contrast)
  - Delay if respiratory/cardiovascular compromise, severe sepsis, rapidly evolving rash, coagulopathy, infection at site of LP
- **Sepsis management** as per usual guidance (see Chapter 26 Sepsis)
  - *Blood cultures*: within 1 h
  - *Antimicrobials*: liaise with microbiology
- **Corticosteroids**
  - **Dexamethasone 10 mg 6°** on admission (start before, with, or up to 12 h after first dose of antibiotics)
- **Infection prevention and control**
  - Respiratory isolation and barrier nursing until diagnosis excluded or received 24 h treatment
  - Droplet precautions until received 24 h antibiotics
- **Neurosurgical opinion** may be indicated (e.g. if empyema)

When would CT imaging be required prior to LP?

CT may be indicated prior to LP to exclude cerebral oedema and mass effect which may predispose to herniation in cases with:

- Focal neurological signs
- Papilloedema
- Continuous or uncontrolled seizures
- GCS ≤ 12

When should LP be performed in patients on anticoagulants or with coagulopathy?

- *Warfarin*: when INR ≤1.4
- *Clopidogrel*: 7 days post cessation unless DDAVP/platelets given, guided by haematology
- *DOACs*: guided by haematology
- Platelets ≥40 × 10⁹/l, not rapidly falling

Which specific investigations might be helpful?

Investigations should also consider a diagnosis of encephalitis. Those recommended in all cases are listed in bold:

- Laboratory
  - **FBC, U&E, LFT, clotting, glucose, lactate, PCT**

- *Blood*: HIV screen, **meningococcal PCR, pneumococcal PCR**
- *Urine*: pneumococcal antigen
- *Nose and throat swab*: **meningococcal culture**
- Other investigations for infections as suspected
- Radiological
  - *CT head*: exclude differentials, complications (e.g. subdural empyema, hydrocephalus), may be normal
  - *MR head*: first-line imaging but often impractical, may be normal
  - *MR venogram*: complications (e.g. CVST)
- LP
  - **Opening pressure**
  - *Cell count*: **differential**
  - *Biochemistry*: **protein, glucose (and concurrent plasma glucose), lactate**
  - **MC+S**
  - *PCR*: **pneumococci, meningococci**
  - *Viral PCR*: HSV, VZV, other
  - *TB*: Ziehl-Neelsen stain, TB culture
  - *Cryptococcus*: India ink stain, cryptococcal antigen
  - Autoimmune encephalitis panel (see Chapter 90 Encephalitis)
  - Oligoclonal bands
  - Cytology
  - Additional sample for storage
  - If HSV PCR negative a second LP may be performed after 3–7 days

Gram stain

- *Gram-positive diplococci*: *S. pneumoniae* likely
- *Gram-negative diplococci*: *N. meningitidis* likely
- *Gram-positive bacilli*: *Listeria monocytogenes*
- Gram-negative rods (e.g. extended-spectrum beta-lactamase-producing organism [ESBL])

How would you manage antimicrobials in suspected meningitis?

Antimicrobials should be given as soon as possible, ideally **within 1 h** and after blood cultures and LP. Encephalitis should be considered and covered empirically (see Chapter 90 Encephalitis).

Empirical cover

- Ceftriaxone 2 g 12 hourly IV or cefotaxime 2 g 6 hourly
  - Chloramphenicol 25 mg/kg 6 hourly IV if anaphylaxis to penicillins/cephalosporins
- Amoxicillin 2 g 4 hourly IV (add if age ≥60 y)
  - Co-trimoxazole 10–20 mg/kg second line
- Vancomycin 15–20 mg/kg 12 hourly or rifampicin 600 mg 12 hourly (add if suspect penicillin-resistant pneumococci)
- Aciclovir 10 mg/kg 8 hourly for 14 days (foscarnet second line for herpes viruses)
- Other as indicated (e.g. antiretrovirals, anti-TB, antimalarial)

Course length

- *Pneumococcal*: 10 days (14 if not recovered or resistance)
- *Meningococcal*: 5 days
- *Listeria monocytogenes*: 21 days
- *H. influenzae*: 10 days
- *Enterobacteriaceae*: 21 days
- No pathogen identified, recovered: 10 days

Post-exposure prophylaxis may be indicated for others:

- Staff with transient close contact only if exposed to aerosols/secretions from respiratory tract
- Prolonged close contacts in household-type setting in preceding week before onset of illness
- For example, ciprofloxacin 500 mg single dose

What is the role of steroids in bacterial meningitis?

Corticosteroids have potential anti-inflammatory effects and are indicated in the prevention of neurological complications of meningitis, supported by a Cochrane review in 2015 (Brouwer et al.).

Corticosteroids should be given **before or with the** first **dose of antibiotics, ideally within 4 h**. They should not be started >12 h after starting antibiotics. Dexamethasone 10 mg IV 6 hourly is recommended and should be continued for 4 days in probable/confirmed **pneumococcal** disease.

STUDY

Brouwer et al. (2015)

- Cochrane review of corticosteroids for acute bacterial meningitis
- *Any hearing loss, severe hearing loss, neurological sequelae*: **significantly lower (RR 0.74, 0.67, 0.83)**
- *S. pneumoniae*: mortality – **significantly lower (RR 0.84, 29.9% vs 36.0%)**
- *N. meningitidis* or *H. influenzae*: mortality – no difference
- *H. influenzae in children*: severe hearing loss – **significantly lower (RR 0.84, 4% vs 12%)**

Are steroids used in paediatric cases?

Corticosteroids are recommended in bacterial meningitis in children aged 3 months or older based on LP findings as follows:

- Frankly purulent CSF
- CSF WCC > 1000 × 10^6/l
- CSF WCC elevated with protein >1 g/l
- Bacteria on gram stain

Dexamethasone is recommended at 0.15 mg/kg (maximum 10 mg) 6 hourly for 4 days. Steroids are recommended against in children <3 months old and in meningococcal sepsis unless indicated for refractory shock. If TB is suspected, steroid therapy may be harmful without appropriate anti-tuberculous therapy.

GUIDELINE NICE 2015 CG102 Paediatric meningitis

---

90. ENCEPHALITIS

What is encephalitis?

Encephalitis is inflammation of the brain parenchyma associated with neurological dysfunction.

What are the causes of encephalitis?

Infectious
- Viral
  - HSV-1 or 2 (most common)
  - *Other herpes viruses*: VZV, HHV6, HHV-7, EBV, CMV
  - Measles
  - Rubella
  - Influenza A
  - *Arboviruses*: Japanese encephalitis, West Nile virus (WNV)
  - *Zoonoses*: rabies

- Bacterial
  - Listeria
  - Mycoplasma
  - TB
  - Neuroborreliosis (Lyme disease)
  - Leptospirosis
  - Brucellosis
  - Neurosyphilis
- *Fungal*: Cryptococcus
- *Protozoal*: malaria, toxoplasmosis
- *Prion*: CJD

Post-infectious

- *Autoimmune*: ADEM

Non-infectious (autoimmune)

- Anti-NMDA receptor
- Anti-VGKC (most common autoimmune cause in adults)
- *Paraneoplastic limbic encephalitis*: small cell lung cancer, thymoma, breast, ovarian, testicular
- Non-paraneoplastic limbic encephalitis

As with meningitis, a cause is often not identified.

How might encephalitis present?

- **Neurological**
  - Altered mental state
  - Seizures
  - Headache
  - Cranial nerve abnormalities
  - Speech disorders
  - Movement disorders
  - Coexistent meningism
- **Psychiatric**
  - Altered behaviour
  - Altered personality
- **Systemic**
  - Fever
  - *Skin signs*: vesicles, rashes, bites

How would you diagnose encephalitis?

KEY POINT

Major criteria for diagnosis of encephalitis (required):

- **Altered mental status ≥24 h** with no alternative cause identified

Minor criteria (2 – possible, ≥**3** – probable/confirmed):

- Temperature ≥ 38°C ≤ 72 h before/after presentation
- *Seizures*: generalised/partial, not fully attributable to pre-existing disorder
- New focal neurology
- CSF WCC ≥ 5 × 10^6/l
- Abnormal brain parenchyma on imaging suggestive of encephalitis (new/acute)
- EEG abnormality consistent (not attributable to another cause)

GUIDELINE International Encephalitis Consortium 2013 Encephalitis

Which investigations would support the diagnosis?

- *LP*: as for meningitis (see Chapter 89 Meningitis); specific additions are as follows:
  - HSV-1/2, VZV, enterovirus PCR
  - Cryptococcal antigen and/or India ink staining
  - Oligoclonal bands and IgG Index
  - VDRL
- Serum
  - HIV serology
  - Treponemal testing
  - *Paired antibody testing*: acute sample and in convalescence 10–14 days later
- Imaging
  - **MR** first line (CT if not): HSV encephalitis commonly affects the limbic system with hyperintensity of frontal/temporal areas on T2/FLAIR.
  - CXR
- *Neurophysiology*: EEG
  - Non-convulsive status epilepticus
  - *HSV*: lateralised periodic discharges or spikes in temporal regions
  - *Anti-NMDA receptor encephalitis*: delta brush pattern
- Testing for extra CNS involvement (e.g. skin biopsy, BAL, endobronchial biopsy, throat swab, stool culture, investigation of malignancy)
- Brain biopsy
  - Gold standard, highly invasive, rarely performed premortem
  - May be indicated in extreme circumstance of rapid deterioration without a diagnosis

What would an autoimmune panel include?
Antibodies to the following:

- VGKC
- GAD
- AMPA receptor
- GABA$_b$ receptor
- mGluR5
- Hu
- CV2/CRMP5
- Ma2
- Amphiphysin

Which other investigations might be indicated depending on specific circumstances in the history?

- Host immunocompromise
  - CMV, HHV-6, HIV PCR; *T. gondii* serology and/or PCR; TB, fungal, WNV tests
- Geographic
  - *Africa*: malaria, trypanosomiasis, dengue
  - *Asia*: Japanese encephalitis, dengue, malaria, Nipah virus testing
  - *Australia*: Murray Valley encephalitis virus, Kunjin virus, Australian bat lyssavirus
  - *Europe*: tick-borne encephalitis, Toscana virus
  - *Central/South America*: dengue, malaria, WNV, Venezuelan equine encephalitis
  - *North America*: WNV, Powassan, La Crosse, eastern equine encephalitis
- Season/exposure
  - *Summer*: arbovirus, tick-borne disease
  - *Cat*: Bartonella antibody, ophthalmological evaluation
  - *Animal bite/bat exposure*: rabies
  - *Swimming in warm freshwater/sinus irrigation*: Naegleria fowleri

Which causes would be suggested by specific signs?

- *Psychosis/movement disorder*: anti-NMDA, rabies, malignancy, CJD
- *Limbic*: autoimmune limbic encephalitis, HHV-6/7, malignancy
- *Respiratory*: *Mycoplasma pneumoniae*, respiratory viruses
- *Acute flaccid paralysis*: arbovirus, rabies
- *Parkinsonism*: arbovirus, toxoplasmosis
- *Nonhealing skin lesions*: *Balamuthia mandrillaris*, *Acanthamoeba*

How would you manage encephalitis?

Management is in keeping with principles used in suspected meningitis, and antimicrobial cover is often required for both diseases until gram stain and culture results are known. IV acyclovir is life-saving and significantly reduces mortality. (See Chapter 89 Meningitis)

Autoimmune encephalitis
- Steroids, IVIg, plasma exchange
- Rituximab, cyclophosphamide
- Treat underlying malignancy

Resources

- Chaudhuri A, Kennedy PGE. Diagnosis and treatment of viral encephalitis. Postgrad Med J. 2002; 78(924):575–583.
- Kennedy PGE. Viral encephalitis: causes, differential diagnosis, and management. J Neurol Neurosurg Psychiatry. 2004;75(Suppl1):i10–i15.

---

91.   TETANUS AND BOTULISM

What is tetanus?

Tetanus is a disease caused by the bacterium *Clostridium tetani* (Gram-positive anaerobe). It is preventable but causes 20 cases per year in the UK. Diagnosis is clinical, but positive cultures may be seen.

What is the pathophysiology of tetanus?

- Incubation period 1–2 weeks (<5 days heralds severe disease)
- Tetanospasmin (toxin) released into the systemic circulation
- Irreversible binding to neuromuscular junction
- Retrograde travel to spinal cord
- Cleaves synaptobrevin membrane protein
- Prevents inhibitory neurotransmitter (GABA) release
- Stimulation of motor neurons predominates
- Results in spasm and autonomic instability
- Recovery requires growth of new nerve terminals

C. tetani spores are found in the environment, particularly soil, faeces, and dust. Contaminated wounds are often implicated, including illicit IV/IM/subcutaneous drug use.

When might a patient with tetanus require critical care?

The clinical features of tetanus result from muscular spasm and autonomic instability or 'storms'. Risus sardonicus and opisthotonus might be seen. Tetanus can range from mild to very severe (as per the Ablett classification).

Higher level supportive care may be indicated with the following life-threatening features as follows:

- *A*: trismus, laryngospasm, hypersalivation
- *B*: respiratory muscle rigidity, apnoeic spells

- *C*: autonomic instability with labile BP and HR
- *F*: rhabdomyolysis, AKI
- *H*: thromboembolism including PE

Other important effects include significant musculoskeletal injury, dysphagia, and pain.

What are the key management principles in tetanus?

Primary prevention through the national vaccination schedule has had the most significant effect on outcomes.

- **Minimising toxin exposure** (e.g. wound washout, debridement)
- **Bacterial eradication** (e.g. metronidazole)
- **Neutralising unbound toxin** with human tetanus immunoglobulin (HTIg)
- **Investigation of differential diagnoses** (e.g. hypocalcaemia, meningitis, SAH, strychnine)
- **Supportive care**
  - *Spasm/rigidity*: benzodiazepines, opioids, other sedative agents, NMB if refractory (atracurium or vecuronium first line)
  - *Autonomic instability*: sedation (opioids, clonidine), magnesium
  - *VTE*: appropriate prophylaxis
- **Notifiable disease** under Public Health (Control of Disease) Act 1984 and Health Protection (Notification) Regulations 2010

A long stay is expected, requiring multidisciplinary involvement, particularly:

- Nutritional support
- Psychological support
- *Prevention of respiratory complications*: physiotherapy, mouth care, suction

What is the prognosis of tetanus?

- Most patients will require 4–6 weeks of supportive care.
- 10% mortality in developed world (20% in severe cases)
- >50% mortality in developing countries
- Higher mortality with increasing age and absence of vaccination

What is botulism?

Botulism is a rare disease caused by exposure to botulinum toxin. In suitable conditions, this is produced by *Clostridium botulinum* (another Gram-positive anaerobe found in soil and dust). Serological types A–G exist but A, B, and E are responsible for most human cases.

Botulism encompasses the following:

- *Food-borne botulism*: ingested pre-formed toxin
- *Wound botulism*: bacterial growth and toxin production
- *Intestinal colonisation botulism*: bacterial growth and toxin production
- *Deliberate release of botulinum toxin*: bioterrorism
- *Accidental botulism*: therapeutic botulinum toxin for spasm/contracture or cosmesis
- *Inhalational botulism*: during toxin purification

What is the pathophysiology of botulism?

- Onset 2–8 h post ingestion, peak at 48 h
- Botulinum toxin binds to cells
- Cleaves SNARE proteins (docking protein usually allowing vesicles of ACh to fuse with presynaptic membrane)
- ACh not released into synaptic cleft
- Flaccid paralysis and anticholinergic features result
- Recovery requires growth of new nerve terminals

Anaerobic food manufacture (e.g. tins, fermentation) has been responsible for food-borne outbreaks. Intestinal colonisation is more common in infants.

What are the main clinical features of botulism?

Botulism can vary from mild to severe disease, with death possible within 24 h. It causes a syndrome of **afebrile, descending, symmetrical, flaccid paralysis**.

Specific features include the following:

- *A*: loss of muscle tone and airway integrity, neck weakness
- *B*: type 2 respiratory failure
- *C*: postural hypotension
- *D*: diplopia, blurred vision, photophobia, ptosis, mydriasis/miosis, nystagmus, sore throat, dysphagia, dysarthria, dysphonia
- *E*: ileus, abdominal pain
- *F*: urinary incontinence/retention

What are the differential diagnoses of botulism?

- GBS
- Poliomyelitis
- Myaesthenia gravis
- LEMS
- Tick bite
- Viral encephalitis

What are the main priorities in critical care management?

- *Supportive care*
  - Consider semi-elective intubation and mechanical ventilation (similar to with GBS).
  - Tracheostomy often required
- *Confirm diagnosis with early toxin bioassay*: faeces, vomitus, serum, tissue, pus
- *Source control*: wound debridement, washout, antibiotics where applicable
- *Specialist input*: infectious diseases, microbiology
- *Administration of trivalent antitoxin*: after clinical diagnosis, repeat after 24 h if no improvement (ideally skin test first, available through duty doctor at Health Protection Agency)
- Investigation of differential diagnoses
- Multidisciplinary involvement as above for long-stay patient
- Notifiable disease (as above)

Antibiotics are not indicated routinely but may be appropriate in some cases (e.g. wound botulism).

Immunisation is less valuable in botulism (compared to tetanus) due to the rarity of disease, scarcity of toxoid, and potential elimination of benefit from therapeutic uses of botulinum toxin. Pentavalent toxoid has been given to laboratory workers and the military in the United States.

What is the prognosis of botulism?

- Several months of supportive care may be required.
- Ventilatory muscle strength usually normal by 1 year but exercise capacity reduced.
- 7–10% mortality (doubled over 60 years of age)
- Type A mortality higher

Resources

- Taylor AM. Tetanus. CEACCP. 2006;6(3):101–104.
- Wenham T, Cohen A. Botulism. CEACCP. 2008;8(1):21–25.

92. GUILLAIN-BARRÉ SYNDROME

What is Guillain-Barré syndrome?

Guillain-Barré syndrome (GBS) is an **acute polyneuropathy**, which typically occurs as an **autoimmune** response following a respiratory or GI infection.

There is typically a bimodal distribution, occurring more commonly in younger adults (<40 years) and the elderly (>60 years), with a male preponderance.

What are the causes of GBS?

The majority of cases occur within 1 month of a respiratory or GI infection. Common pathogens include the following:

- *Campylobacter jejuni*
- *M. pneumoniae*
- CMV
- EBV

Other causes are as follows:

- *Infection*: HIV, hepatitis A–E, VZV, Zika virus
- *Drugs*: vaccinations (e.g. influenza, rabies), penicillins
- *Systemic disease*: SLE, sarcoid, lymphoma

What is the pathophysiology of GBS?

The precise mechanism is unclear. It is thought to involve an autoimmune pathway whereby an immune activation event leads to autoantibody production. Subtypes result from different immune activation events, with the most common being acute inflammatory demyelinating polyradiculopathy (AIDP).

KEY POINT

Subtypes of GBS:

- *AIDP*: targets myelin sheath, Schwann-cell components
- *Acute motor axonal neuropathy (AMAN)*: targets axonal membrane
- *Acute motor sensory axonal neuropathy (AMSAN)*

GBS triggered by *C. jejuni*:

- Serological antibody response against GM1 and GD1a gangliosides
- Associated with AMAN

How would you diagnose GBS?

GBS should be suspected in cases of rapidly progressive bilateral limb weakness and/or sensory deficits, hypo/areflexia, facial/bulbar palsy, and ophthalmoplegia and ataxia.

KEY POINT

Diagnosis of GBS by NINDS criteria:

- Progressive bilateral weakness of arms and legs
- Absent/decreased tendon reflexes in affected limbs

Other supportive features are as follows:

- Progressive phase lasting days to 4 weeks (usually <2 weeks)
- Symmetry
- Mild sensory features
- Cranial nerve involvement, especially VII
- Autonomic dysfunction
- Muscular/radicular back/limb pain
- CSF protein high
- Electrophysiology demonstrating motor/sensorimotor neuropathy

Consider other cause if:

- Asymmetry
- Bladder/bowel dysfunction at onset/persistent
- Limited weakness
- Fever
- Nadir < 24 h, progression > 4 weeks
- Sharp sensory level
- Hyper-reflexia/clonus
- Extensor plantars
- Abdominal pain
- Altered consciousness
- CSF mononuclear/polymorphonuclear cells high (>50 × 10^6/l)

Which symptom patterns exist?

- **Classic sensorimotor** (30–85%)
- **Pure motor** (5–70%)
- *Miller Fisher syndrome*: **ophthalmoplegia, areflexia, ataxia** (5–25%), 15% overlap with classical
- *Paraparetic (5–10%)*: paresis restricted to legs

More rarely
- Pharyngeal-cervical-brachial
- Bilateral facial palsy with paraesthesias
- Bickerstaff brain stem encephalitis
- Pure sensory

Which differential diagnoses are relevant?

- *CNS*: brain stem inflammation (e.g. sarcoid, Sjögren, neuromyelitis optica), spinal cord inflammation (e.g. sarcoid, Sjögren, transverse myelitis), brain stem/cord compression, brain stem stroke, vitamin deficiency
- *Anterior horn cells*: acute flaccid myelitis (e.g. polio, enterovirus, WNV, Japanese encephalitis, rabies)
- *Nerve roots*: compression, leptomeningeal malignancy, infection (e.g. Lyme, CMV, HIV, EBV, VZV)
- *Peripheral*: CIDP, metabolic/electrolytes, vitamin deficiency, toxins, CIP, neuralgic amyotrophy, vasculitis, infection (e.g. diphtheria, HIV)
- *Neuromuscular junction*: myaesthenia gravis, LEMS, neurotoxins, organophosphates
- *Muscle*: metabolic/electrolytes, myositis, rhabdomyolysis, toxic myopathy, mitochondrial
- *Other*: functional/conversion disorder

How would you investigate a patient suspected to have GBS?

Investigations may be helpful to assess complications, differential diagnoses or determine GBS subtypes. Diagnosis remains clinical, and negative antibody results may not rule out GBS.

- **Serum**
  - FBC, U&E, glucose, LFT
  - Anti-ganglioside GM1 and GD1a antibodies (axonal)
  - Anti-GQ1b (Miller Fisher)

- **CSF**
  - *Typically*: elevated protein, normal cell count (albumino-cytological dissociation) from day 5 to 7
  - Oligoclonal bands may be present
- **Electrophysiology**
  - 'Sural sparing' pattern, may be normal, most pronounced at 2 weeks from onset
  - Sensorimotor polyradiculoneuropathy/polyneuropathy:
    - ➤ Reduced conduction velocities
    - ➤ Reduced sensory and motor evoked amplitudes
    - ➤ Abnormal temporal dispersion
    - ➤ Partial motor conduction blocks
- *Imaging*: rule out high cervical lesion, may be required prior to LP (see Chapter 89 Meningitis)
- *PFT*: progression of respiratory insufficiency
- **Infection screening**

How is GBS managed?

- Treat underlying cause
- Immunomodulation
  - *IVIg*: 0.4 g/kg for 5 days
  - *Plasma exchange*: 200–250 ml plasma/kg, 5 sessions
  - Corticosteroids not found to be beneficial in several RCTs, may have negative effect

Indications for immunomodulation are as follows:

- Inability to walk >10 m independently
- Rapid progression of weakness
- Severe autonomic/bulbar features
- Respiratory insufficiency

When would you admit a patient with GBS to critical care?

Indications for critical care admission are as follows:

- Rapid progression of weakness
- Severe autonomic/swallowing dysfunction
- Evolving respiratory distress
- Erasmus GBS Respiratory Insufficiency Score (EGRIS) > 4

Twenty-two per cent of GBS patients require mechanical ventilation within a week of admission. Focus is on early identification of those at risk of respiratory failure.

The **EGRIS** prognostic tool can be used to calculate probability of requiring ventilation within 1 week of assessment. The following criteria are assessed at hospital admission:

- Days since onset of weakness
- Facial and/or bulbar weakness
- MRC sum score

Signs of imminent respiratory insufficiency are as follows:

- Breathlessness at rest or during talking
- Accessory respiratory muscle use
- Increased RR or HR
- Abnormal ABG or S_pO_2
- **Inability to count to 15 in a single breath**
- **Vital capacity < 15–20 ml/kg or < 1 l**

What are the ongoing management priorities in critical care?

- Definitive management if not started already (as above)
- Rule out differential diagnoses

- Other care is largely supportive and may be required for months
  - Airway protection for bulbar weakness, secretion management (likely to require tracheostomy)
  - *Ventilatory support*: LPV, VAP prevention
  - Cardiovascular support for hypotension/hypertension, arrhythmias
  - Multimodal analgesia
  - Nutritional support
  - Bowel management
  - Urinary catheter
  - Thromboprophylaxis
  - Skin/pressure care
  - Rehabilitation and psychological support

Which important complications are you aware of?

- *A/B*: aspiration, choking
- *C*: arrhythmias, haemodynamic instability
- *D*: pain, allodynia, delirium, depression, corneal ulceration, compression neuropathy
- *F*: urinary retention, hyponatraemia
- *G*: constipation, malnutrition
- *I*: nosocomial infection
- *Other*: pressure sores, contractures, ossifications

Resources

- Leonhard SE, Mandarakas MR, Gondim FAA, et al. Diagnosis and management of Guillain-Barré syndrome in ten steps. Nat Rev Neurol. 2019;15(11):671–683.
- Richards KJC, Cohen AT. Guillain-Barré syndrome. BJA CEPD Reviews. 2003;3(2):46–49.
- Willison HJ, Jacobs BC, van Doorn PA. Guillain-Barré syndrome. Lancet. 2016;388(10045):717–727.

What is myaesthenia gravis?

Myaesthenia gravis is a chronic autoimmune neuromuscular disease, which results in skeletal muscle weakness. It is characterised by **fatiguability** (i.e. it is worsened by activity and improved by rest).

Myaesthenia gravis has a bimodal distribution, affecting younger females (<40 years) and older males (>60 years) more. Neonates may be affected by transfer of maternal autoantibodies.

What is the pathophysiology of myaesthenia gravis?

Normal neuromuscular physiology
- ACh released into synaptic cleft in response to nerve impulse
- ACh binds to postsynaptic nicotinic AChRs in motor end plate
- Action potential triggered, resulting in muscle contraction
- Acetylcholinesterase usually present in synaptic cleft and postsynaptic folds breaks down ACh

Myaesthenia gravis
- Auto-antibodies produced are as follows:
  - Postsynaptic nicotinic AChR (80%)
  - Postsynaptic muscle-specific kinase (MuSK) (10%)
  - Seronegative disease (10%)
- Block attachment of ACh
- Increase rate of degradation of receptors
- Complement induced damage to neuromuscular junction
- Skeletal muscle is affected. The AChRs of smooth and cardiac muscle have a different antigenicity.

Associated with
- Thymus pathology (75%)
  - Hyperplasia (85%)
  - Thymoma (15%)
- *Other autoimmune disease*: hypothyroidism, SLE, RA

What are the clinical features?

- Weakness and fatiguability of skeletal muscles
- Worsening later in the day
- Ocular weakness on presentation (10% don't progress from this)
- Craniocaudal progression
- *Neuromuscular breathlessness*: orthopnoea resolves rapidly on sitting up, 'diaphragmatic paradox'

How is myaesthenia gravis classified?

Osserman's classification
1 **Ocular myaesthenia** (confined to ocular muscles)
2 **Generalised** myaesthenia gravis
  a) mild
  b) moderate
3 **Severe generalised**
4 **Myaesthenic crisis with respiratory failure**

Classification by aetiology
1 Acquired autoimmune
2 Transient neonatal
3 Drug induced
4 Congenital myaesthenic syndromes

How would you investigate a patient presenting with myaesthenia gravis?

Diagnosis may be made clinically with a strong history. Confirmation is useful to support this prior to long-term treatment.

- **Diagnostic**
  - Serum AChR antibodies, anti-MuSK antibodies
  - *Neurophysiological*: repetitive nerve stimulation, single-fibre EMG
  - Edrophonium (Tensilon) test
    - ➤ *Acetylcholinesterase inhibitor*: ACh accumulates in the neuromuscular junction with more available to receptors, transiently reducing muscle weakness and fatiguability
    - ➤ *Rarely performed*: may precipitate cholinergic crisis
- **Thymus evaluation**
  - Anti-striated muscle antibody
  - CXR, CT, MR
- **Respiratory function**
  - ABG
  - Peak expiratory flow rate (PEFR)
  - FVC

What is a myaesthenic crisis?

Myaesthenic crisis is worsening of myaesthenic weakness of the respiratory muscles, requiring intubation or NIV.

Decompensation may be precipitated by infection, early effects of steroid therapy, or inadequate treatment. In pregnancy, a third of patients will improve, a third will deteriorate, and a third will not experience a change. Severe bulbar weakness often accompanies respiratory muscle weakness or may be predominant, resulting in upper airway obstruction or aspiration.

What is a cholinergic crisis and when might it present?

Cholinergic crisis is a syndrome of overstimulation of nicotinic and muscarinic receptors at the neuromuscular junction. It is usually secondary to the inactivation or inhibition of acetylcholinesterase.

- **Muscarinic toxicity** ('SLUDGE' syndrome)
  - *Visual*: miosis, blurred vision
  - *Respiratory*: bronchoconstriction
  - *Cardiovascular*: bradycardia
  - *GI*: nausea, vomiting, diarrhoea
  - *GU*: urinary urgency and frequency
  - *Secretory*: increased respiratory and GI secretions
- **Nicotinic toxicity**
  - *Muscular*: weakness, fasciculation, flaccid paralysis
  - *Cardiovascular*: tachycardia

Scenarios

- Patients with myaesthenia gravis on treatment with high-dose acetylcholinesterase inhibitors
- Patients after general anaesthesia who receive high-dose acetylcholinesterase inhibitors to reverse the effects of neuromuscular blocking agents
- Exposure to organophosphates

Management is supportive. Atropine may be used for its muscarinic effect and oximes for nicotinic effects.

(See Chapter 32 Poisoning Overview)

Which drugs may exacerbate myaesthenia gravis?

Some medications are relatively contraindicated as they exacerbate the condition. Some might be avoided due to their effects on respiratory function (e.g. opioids).

KEY POINT

Medications exacerbating myaesthenia are as follows:

- *Antibiotics*: aminoglycosides, fluoroquinolones, macrolides
- *Cardiovascular*: beta-blockers, procainamide, magnesium, statins
- Other
  - Botulinum toxin
  - Chloroquine, hydroxychloroquine
  - Desferrioxamine
  - Penicillamine
  - Immune checkpoint inhibitors (ICI)
  - Iodinated contrast agents
  - Quinine
  - Telithromycin

GUIDELINE Neurology 2020 Myasthenia gravis

How would you manage the myaesthenic patient in critical care?

The critically unwell patient will require supportive care with the following priorities:

- Airway/ventilatory support
- Treatment of precipitant (e.g. infection)
- Prompt disease control with **IVIg or plasmapheresis**
- Anticholinesterase therapy (e.g. pyridostigmine enterally)
- Neurologist input

Non-emergency treatment strategy is as follows:

- *First line*: **acetylcholinesterase inhibitors** (also known as **anticholinesterases**)
  - *Pyridostigmine*: onset 30 min, peak 2 h, half-life 4 h
- *Addition of immune-directed treatment*: corticosteroids or thymectomy initially
- *Long term*: steroid-sparing strategy (e.g. other immunosuppressant, plasmapheresis, thymectomy)
  - Azathioprine
  - Cyclosporin

Resource

- Thanvi BR, Lo TCN. Update on myasthenia gravis. Postgrad Med J. 2004;80(950):690–700.

---

94. OTHER NEUROMUSCULAR DISORDERS

Which neuromuscular disorders are you aware of?

Hereditary

- Pre-junctional
  - *Peripheral neuropathies*: Charcot-Marie-Tooth, Friedrich's ataxia
- Postjunctional
  - *Dystrophicas*: Duchenne, Becker's
  - *Myotonias*: myotonic dystrophy, myotonia congenita, hyper-/hypokalaemic periodic paralysis
  - Metabolic/mitochondrial disorders

Acquired

- Pre-junctional
  - Motor neurone disease (MND)
  - MS
  - GBS
  - Peripheral neuropathies (e.g. diabetes mellitus)
- Junctional
  - Myaesthenia gravis
  - LEMS
- Postjunctional
  - Inflammatory myopathies
  - CIP/myopathy

When might affected patients present to critical care?

- **Respiratory complications** (commonest cause of death in this group)
  - Recurrent aspiration due to bulbar muscle weakness
  - Respiratory muscle weakness
  - OSA
  - Spinal deformity
- **Cardiac complications**
  - Cardiomyopathy
  - Arrhythmias
- **Post-operative management**
  - Respiratory insufficiency possible despite attempts to avoid
- **Unrelated condition** (e.g. sepsis)

Why are the hereditary neuromuscular disorders relevant to critical care?

Respiratory failure is common due to muscular weakness. Some hereditary neuromuscular disorders are life-limiting and may be rapidly progressive. A thorough consideration of the underlying functional status, likely progression (with specialist input), and cardiac and respiratory complications should be made.

Patients may have had involvement with paediatric critical care services, and those with certain conditions are increasingly surviving to adulthood. They may have struggled with the transition from paediatric to adult services, and family members may have been heavily involved in decision-making around medical care previously. It is not unusual for families to have already had discussions about treatment limitations and futility in extremis.

An awareness of key features and likely disease progression is essential in considering which therapies may or may not benefit these patients. Temporary organ support may often be appropriate. Multidisciplinary input is recommended where time allows.

Can you outline the features of a hereditary neuromuscular disorder?

Friedrich's ataxia
- **Autosomal recessive** ataxia
- Risk of aspiration from upper motoneurone involvement
- Diaphragmatic weakness
- Progressive myocardial degeneration occurs resulting in cardiac failure

Duchenne muscular dystrophy
- Most common childhood muscular dystrophy (1:3500), **X-linked recessive**
- *Lack of dystrophin*: protein anchoring myocytes to extracellular matrix
- Progressive wasting and weakness, proximal predominance
- Scoliosis, contractures, restrictive lung function, cardiomyopathy (50% DCM by teens)
- *Fatal by second or third decade*: cardiorespiratory failure

Becker's muscular dystrophy
- **X-linked recessive**, less common
- Partial absence of dystrophin protein, milder than Duchenne, presents in teens
- DCM, arrhythmias also manifest
- Increased risk of blood loss due to smooth muscle and platelet dysfunction
- Cardiorespiratory failure possible by third or fourth decade but life expectancy may be normal

Myotonic dystrophy
- **Autosomal dominant**, chromosome 19, 'anticipation' with presentation earlier in subsequent generations
- Abnormal sodium/chloride channels, hyperexcitability of myocytes
- *Characterised by myotonia*: sustained muscle contraction, inability to relax
- Myotonia precipitated by hypothermia, shivering, mechanical/electrical stimulation
- *Myotonia treatment*: treat cause, Na+ channel blockade (e.g. phenytoin, local anaesthetics)
- Cardiomyopathy may progress to require permanent pacemaker

Myotonia congenita
- **Autosomal dominant**, chromosome 17, dysfunctional chloride channel
- Widespread muscle hypertrophy, more severe contractures, myotonic features
- Dysphagia, cardiomyopathy

Mitochondrial myopathies
- Disorders of mitochondrial dysfunction in tissues with high metabolic demand
- Variable manifestation, may present from neonatal period to adulthood
- Some may cause mild weakness; others severe, progressive features early in life
- For example MELAS (mitochondrial encephalopathy, lactic acidosis, and stroke-like episodes)

What pharmacological considerations should be made when treating these patients?

- *All*: avoid volatile agents, depolarising NMB (MH, rhabdomyolysis, hyperkalaemia)
- *All*: lower doses of NMB (risk of prolonged block)
- *Autonomic dysfunction*: lower doses of cardiovascular drugs (increased sensitivity of receptors)
- *Friedrich's ataxia*: avoid negative inotropy
- *Myotonias*: avoid depolarising NMB, anticholinesterases (prolonged contractures)

What is LEMS?

LEMS is an autoimmune condition in which antibodies are produced against calcium channels in the presynaptic membrane, preventing calcium release into the synaptic cleft. It is characterised by **proximal weakness, hyporeflexia**, and **autonomic dysfunction**.

LEMS may be paraneoplastic (usually small cell lung cancer) or associated with other autoimmune disorders. Repetitive nerve stimulation results in an improvement in symptoms, in contrast to the fatiguability of myaesthenia gravis. Management follows similar principles as well as managing any underlying malignancy.

(See Chapter 93 Myaesthenia Gravis)

When might patients with MS require critical care input?

Multiple sclerosis (MS) is an immune-mediated condition of neuronal demyelination. Features and progression are variable, and several clinical subtypes exist. The most common indication for admission to critical care is respiratory insufficiency.

Indications

- *Respiratory failure*: infection most commonly
- Circulatory failure
- Impaired consciousness
- Status epilepticus
- Other infection
- Plasma exchange

What do you know about MND in the context of invasive ventilation?

Motor neurone disease (MND) is a progressive neuromuscular disorder that most commonly causes death through respiratory failure (diaphragmatic, intercostal, and accessory muscle weakness). Bulbar weakness and inadequate cough increase the risk of pulmonary aspiration.

Respiratory failure is usually anticipated after diagnosis and appropriate advanced care planning instituted. NIV may be used in the community to provide symptomatic relief and improve life expectancy. Some patients will undergo tracheostomy.

Acute respiratory failure may present a challenge to the admitting intensivist. Patients may be undiagnosed or not yet have had significant discussions. Occasionally, patients with MND will be invasively ventilated. Acute invasive ventilation is unlikely to lead to independence from the ventilator. Ideally, discussions and decisions about the risks and benefits of such treatment should take place outwith the acute setting.

Resources

- Bradley MD, Orrell RW, Clarke J, et al. Outcome of ventilatory support for acute respiratory failure in motor neurone disease. J Neurol Neurosurg Psychiatry. 2002;72(6):752–756.
- Karamyan A, Dünser MW, Wiebe DJ. Critical illness in patients with multiple sclerosis: a matched case-control study. PLoS One. 2016;11:e0155795.
- Marsh S, Pittard A. Neuromuscular disorders and anaesthesia. Part 2: specific neuromuscular disorders. CEACCP. 2011;11(4):119–123.
- Marsh S, Ross N, Pittard A. Neuromuscular disorders and anaesthesia. Part 1: generic anaesthetic management. CEACCP. 2011;11(4):115–118.
- Ragoonanan V, Russell W. Anaesthesia for children with neuromuscular disease. CEACCP. 2010;10(5):143–147.

95.   SPINAL CORD INJURY

What is a spinal cord injury?

A spinal cord injury is damage to the spinal cord and/or surrounding structures, which may be temporary or permanent. Injury can occur at any level of the spinal cord and may be incomplete or complete.

What are the causes of spinal cord injury?

Causes can be divided into the following:

- Traumatic
  - Falls
  - Road traffic collisions
  - Sports injuries
  - *Violence*: hanging, gunshot/stab wounds
- Non-traumatic
  - Degenerative disease
  - Abscess
  - Tumour
  - Congenital

What is the difference between spinal shock and neurogenic shock?

> **KEY POINT**
>
> - *Spinal shock*: depression or loss of spinal reflex activity below the level of the lesion
> - *Neurogenic shock*: distributive shock, may be caused by spinal cord injury disrupting sympathetic pathways, resulting in the following:
>   - Decreased SVR (hypotension)
>   - Unopposed parasympathetic activity (bradycardia)

What is the clinical significance of the level of injury in a complete spinal cord injury?

- Lesions >T6 will cause neurogenic shock and autonomic dysreflexia, requiring haemodynamic support.
- Patients with lesions >C5 will be quadriplegic.

Respiratory implications depending on level of injury are as follows:

- *C1–C2*: fully dependent on mechanical ventilation (apnoeic and unable to cough, diaphragmatic palsy)
- *C3–C5*: likely to require early mechanical ventilation, may require long-term support (partial phrenic/diaphragmatic involvement)
- *>T8*: likely to require early ventilation for secretion management, may require long-term support (inspiratory intercostal muscles lost)
- *<T8*: may require short-term support (lower expiratory and abdominal muscles lost)

What are the management priorities for patients presenting with a spinal cord injury?

- *Trauma principles*: time-critical, multidisciplinary (see Chapter 49 Major Trauma)
  - *Spinal precautions*: C-spine immobilisation, log roll
  - Documentation of focal deficit
- **Cardiovascular support** for neurogenic shock

- **Prevention of secondary injury**
  - Cord ischaemia extends in both directions
  - Ascending level of injury may manifest within first 72 h
- **Timely transfer** to specialist centre

Medications that have been considered for prevention of secondary spinal cord injury include methylprednisolone, nimodipine, and naloxone. They are not recommended by current guidance. The role of corticosteroids is controversial. They were thought to be beneficial due to reduction in the level of injury with early treatment. However, increased mortality and rates of sepsis are associated with their use.

GUIDELINE NICE 2016 NG41 Spinal injury

STUDY

NASCIS 2 (1990)

- Acute spinal cord injury
- *Intervention*: methylprednisolone or naloxone vs placebo
- *Primary*: neurologic change score – **significantly higher** with methylprednisolone <8 h; naloxone – no difference

How would you immobilise the spine initially?

- Spinal bed
- Remove collar and blocks
- Unstable C-spine
  - Sand bags either side of head, deep sedation
  - Specialised collar (e.g. Aspen, Miami J, Philadelphia)
- Unstable thoracic/lumbar spine
  - *Whole-bed tilt*: 30° reverse Trendelenburg position
  - Log roll for turns (e.g. back examination, cleaning)

Would you continue to immobilise the cervical spine of a patient with polytrauma and no obvious abnormality on neck imaging?

- Will depend on local policy
- Some healthcare providers will clear the C-spine radiologically based on high sensitivity of investigations.
- Others will not support C-spine clearance until the patient can be cleared clinically or by MDT input.

What might ongoing critical care involve?

- *A*: early intubation to optimise oxygenation and ventilation
- *B*: low-pressure suction (avoid vagal response), bronchodilators may be required due to autonomic instability
- *C*: vasopressors, chronotropic support (e.g. atropine, dobutamine, pacing)
- *D*: analgesia, secondary/tertiary survey, thorough clinical examination
- *E*: normothermia
- Surgery may be indicated in the subacute phase
- Other supportive care (e.g. thromboprophylaxis, gut protection, VAP prevention, skincare, rehabilitation)

What is autonomic dysreflexia?

Autonomic dysreflexia is a complication that occurs in patients with a spinal cord injury level of **T6 and above**. Stimulation below the level of the lesion results in sympathetic stimulation and peripheral vasoconstriction. A reflex parasympathetic response is triggered above the level of the lesion, but this does not transmit below the level of the lesion.

Common stimuli
- Urinary bladder distension
- Rectal distension
- Acute abdominal pathology
- Pain
- Pressure ulcers
- Tight clothing

Signs and symptoms
- Hypertension, bradycardia, arrhythmias
- Headache, blurred vision, agitation, change in GCS
- Profuse sweating

Which features of incomplete spinal cord injury are you aware of?

Incomplete cord injury syndromes
- Anterior cord syndrome
- Posterior cord syndrome
- Central cord syndrome
- Brown-Séquard syndrome
- Cauda equina syndrome
- Conus medullaris syndrome

Cauda equina and conus medullaris syndromes arise from injury at these levels. They involve loss of bladder and bowel reflexes and lower limb weakness. Conus medullaris syndrome may spare the sacral segments (Figure 95.1).

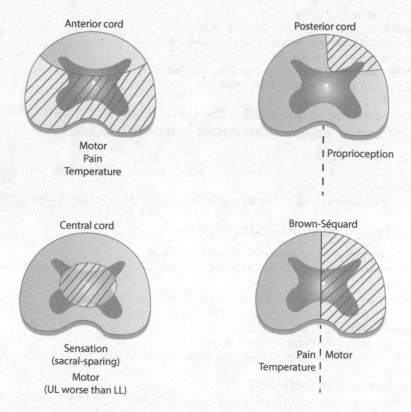

Figure 95.1 Incomplete spinal cord injury syndromes.

Deficits below the level of injury are listed, with unilateral defects indicated by separation in the midline.

How is the severity of a spinal cord injury graded?

Spinal cord injuries are graded in severity according to the **American Spinal Injury Association (ASIA) Scale**.

> **KEY POINT**
>
> ASIA Scale
>
> A. *Complete spinal cord injury*: complete motor and sensory loss
> B. *Incomplete injury*: complete motor loss
> C. *Incomplete injury*: some movement, less than half of muscle groups can oppose gravity
> D. *Incomplete injury*: some movement, more than half of muscle groups can oppose gravity
> E. *Normal*

Resource

- Bonner S, Smith C. Initial management of acute spinal cord injury. CEACCP. 2013;13(6):224–231.

96. THE POST-OP MAJOR SPINAL PATIENT

Can you name some conditions requiring major spinal surgery?

- Trauma
- Deformity (e.g. kyphoscoliosis)
- Myelopathy

Examples of operations are as follows:

- Posterior lumbar interbody fusion
- Anterior cervical decompression and fusion
- Spinal reconstructive surgery

What are the main challenges presented in these patient groups?

- Difficult airway management
- Ventilatory compromise
- Demographic with degenerative scoliosis often frail
- Acute on chronic pain management
- Occasionally congenital muscular or rheumatological disease
- Mental health diagnoses common in younger demographic with deformity
- Metastatic neoplastic disease
- Immobilisation and deconditioning

What are the main physiological challenges presented by the surgery?

- Prone positioning
- Commonly associated with massive haemorrhage
- Lengthy procedures
- Spinal cord monitoring may be required
- May require use of double-lumen tube and one-lung ventilation

Which intraoperative details might be relevant on admission to critical care?

- Duration of surgery
- Difficulty with intubation, technique used, use of throat pack

- Airway device particularly if remains intubated (e.g. flexible armoured tube)
- Blood loss, transfusion, cell salvage use, TXA
- Positioning (e.g. eye checks if prone)
- Pressure sores noted
- Concern over evoked potentials, use of 'wake-up test'

How might analgesia be managed post-operatively for scoliosis correction?

Corrective surgery for scoliosis has the potential to be significantly painful, often on a background of chronic pain management.

Opioids are the mainstay of acute pain management, but a **multimodal approach** is often used to reduce this requirement.

Simple analgesia
- Regular paracetamol
- Gabapentin, pregabalin
- Tramadol
- *NSAIDs avoided*: concerns about coagulopathy leading to haematoma and cord compression

Regional
- Epidural infusion
- Paravertebral catheter infusion
- Intercostal blocks (shorter acting)

Infusions
- Opioid infusion vs PCA
- Ketamine (1–2 mg/kg/24 h)
- *Lidocaine used in some centres*: controversy surrounding safety

Which significant and specific early complications might arise in critical care and how would you recognise and manage them?

Major blood loss, infection, and post-operative respiratory complications are common. PTX is possible. More specific complications include the following:

Airway compromise (supraglottic oedema, anterior neck haematoma, neurological deficit)
- Patients may need to remain intubated and ventilated post-operatively in critical care.
- Consideration of staged extubation once leak around tube confirmed
- If extubated, may become symptomatic up to 36 h post-operatively:
  - Neck swelling, stridor, hoarseness, voice change, tracheal tug, respiratory distress, agitation, reaching for throat
  - May cause carotid sinus compression with hypotension and bradycardia
  - May be a difficult airway if/when reintubation required

- Management algorithm suggested includes the following:
  - Administering high-flow oxygen ± CPAP
  - Senior anaesthetic and surgical review
  - Surgeon to consider removing clips or cutting sutures
  - If oxygenation adequate, transfer to theatre
  - If not, for immediate surgical cricothyroidotomy by anaesthetist

Spinal cord compromise (haematoma, oedema, CSF leak, nerve transection, ischaemia)
- Approximately 1% of deformity correction surgeries will be complicated by paralysis.
- Lower limb neurological observations should be monitored.
- Urinary or faecal incontinence should be considered (complicated by catheterisation).
- Concern should trigger immediate surgical review.

Abdominal organ ischaemia (liver, pancreas)
- Reports of cardiovascular instability and MODS with lactic acidosis 2 h into surgery
- Unexplained metabolic acidosis may present.

- Liver enzymes and platelets should be investigated.
- Prevention and recognition intraoperatively is key.
- Measures to reduce IAP may help.

Post-operative visual loss (central retinal artery occlusion, ischaemic optic atrophy)

- Procedure often >6 h long
- Early assessment of vision post-op is advocated
- If any suspected visual compromise, ophthalmological opinion recommended
- *Perfusion should be optimised*: Hb, BP, oxygenation
- Acetazolamide not shown to be beneficial
- *Prevention key*: careful positioning, monitoring of eyes throughout surgery

CSF leak (dural tear)

- May manifest with headache and wound leakage post-operatively
- *May require further operation*: surgical review prudent

Resource

- Nowicki RWA. Anaesthesia for major spinal surgery. CEACCP. 2014;14(4):147–152.

OBSTETRICS

97. THE PREGNANT CRITICAL CARE PATIENT

Why is the optimal management of pregnant critical care patients important?

There are 2.4 critical care admissions per 1000 maternities. ICNARC data suggest that 83% of peripartum admissions occur in the postnatal period with the most common causes of admission being haemorrhage, infection, and pre-eclampsia.

Respiratory failure has been the most common cause of admission in the antepartum group since before the COVID-19 pandemic. The **INTERCOVID** study found that 8.4% pregnant patients with COVID-19 required ICU admission during March–October 2020. UK Obstetric Surveillance System (UKOSS) data revealed that 9% women required critical care admission and 0.6% received ECMO.

Management may be affected by the following:

- Physiological changes during pregnancy
- *Pregnancy-specific conditions*: pre-eclampsia, MOH, PPCM, amniotic fluid embolism (AFE)
- *Presence of fetus*: viability depends on gestational age and assessment of development (US and Doppler analysis)
- Clinicians' level of familiarity

Transfer to specialist maternal critical care centre is recommended if anticipating ventilation >48 h. Plans and equipment should be available immediately for performing a perimortem caesarean section in the event of maternal cardiac arrest.

> **GUIDELINE**   FICM ICS 2022 GPICS 2.1

> **GUIDELINE**   RCoA 2018 Enhanced maternal care

INTERCOVID (2021)

- COVID-19 in pregnancy (laboratory, radiological, or symptomatic diagnosis)
- 8.4% admitted to critical care
- Higher risk of pre-eclampsia/eclampsia (RR 1.76), severe infections (3.38), ICU admission (5.04), maternal mortality (22.3), preterm birth (1.59), medically indicated preterm birth (1.97), Severe Neonatal Morbidity Index (2.66), Severe Perinatal Morbidity and Mortality Index (2.14)
- *Fever and SOB*: higher risk of severe maternal complications (2.56) and neonatal complications (2.56)
- *Asymptomatic*: higher risk of maternal morbidity (1.24) and pre-eclampsia (1.63)

How might the airway differ in this population and how would you adapt your intubation technique?

- **Increased airway oedema during pregnancy and labour** leading to potentially more difficult laryngoscopy and intubation (1:30–1:100 difficult, 1:224–1:390 failed).
  - *Optimise positioning*: ramping, head up.
  - Pre-oxygenate to $F_{ET}O_2 \geq 0.9$.
  - Have short-handled laryngoscopy blade and videolarygnoscope available.
  - *May require smaller tracheal tube*: common practice to 'downsize' (e.g. 7.0 mm internal diameter first line).
  - Consideration of decision to wake/proceed is complex in the setting of delivery.
  - Refer to specific Obstetric Anaesthetists' Association (OAA) and DAS guideline for failed intubation.
- **Increased risk of aspiration**
  - Ideally give sodium citrate 30 ml and omeprazole prior to RSI.

OAA DAS 2015 Airway

What cardiorespiratory adaptations need to be considered in the management of obstetric patients?

Respiratory
- *Rapid desaturation during apnoea*: reduced FRC due to pregnant uterus and increased O_2 consumption
  - Adequate pre-oxygenation essential.
  - HFNO during intubation may be helpful.
- Fetal oxygenation
  - Maintain $P_aO_2 > 9$ kPa.
- Lower maternal baseline P_aCO_2 (4.3 kPa) (progesterone-induced hyperventilation)
  - Aim for lower P_aCO_2 (4.0–4.5 kPa) when ventilated.
  - Effects of permissive hypercapnia not well known, may lead to fetal acidaemia.
  - Hyperventilation may reduce uterine blood flow.
- Aspiration risk
  - NIV has been used but may exacerbate gastric hyperinflation.
- Prone positioning is challenging in the third trimester.

Cardiovascular
- Aortocaval compression from the gravid uterus can occur when in supine position.
  - *Lateral displacement of uterus required*: left tilt 15–30° or manual displacement during maternal collapse/arrest

- Expanded fluid volume and reduced oncotic pressure near term
  - Caution with fluid
- Deleterious effects of some medications
  - NA is the vasopressor of choice.
  - Vasopressin is uterotonic.
  - Modified RSI with rapid-onset opioid as co-induction agent in hypertensive disease

Which other systemic adaptations are relevant?

CNS
- Risk of ICH in pre-eclamptic patient undergoing laryngoscopy
  - Ensure BP well-controlled prior to induction
- Psychological vulnerability

Haematological
- Physiological anaemia as plasma volume increases faster than red blood cell production
- WCC count higher in pregnancy, confounding diagnosis (e.g. of infection)
- Increased clotting factors and fibrinogen
  - *Increased risk of VTE*: need appropriate prophylaxis until 6 weeks post-partum
  - Caution with anticoagulation around time of delivery (i.e. if neuraxial anaesthesia required)

GI
- *Nutritional requirements not fully understood*: population excluded from major trials
  - Involve dietitians early
- *ALP is released from the placenta*: higher levels in pregnancy

Renal
- *Increased GFR*: lower baseline serum creatinine and urea
- *Uraemia concerning for fetal well-being*: consider RRT if 17–20 mmol/l persistently

Can you give some examples of pathological conditions that might be concerning in this population?

- *B*: worsening asthma (note decompensation threshold P_aCO_2 4.0 kPa), PE
- *C*: haemorrhage, pre-eclampsia, sepsis, PPCM, myocarditis, HCM, ARVC, ventricular failure, increasing prevalence of ischaemic heart disease (IHD), AFE
- *D*: eclampsia, local anaesthetic systemic toxicity, PTSD, postnatal depression, in pre-eclampsia – ICH, PRES, reversible cerebral vasoconstriction syndrome, venous sinus thrombosis
- *F*: water intoxication and severe hyponatraemia, lupus nephritis may present
- *G*: acute fatty liver of pregnancy, starvation ketoacidosis, HELLP
- *H*: VTE, DIC

How would you consider the fetus in your critical care management?

- **Monitoring**
  - Liaise with obstetric and midwifery teams.
  - For example twice-daily cardiotocography (CTG) or intermittent auscultation/Doppler until in labour.
- **Delivery**
  - Timing decided by MDT on case-by-case basis
  - Consider delivery to benefit mother if intractable hypoxia or hypercarbia.
  - Mode guided by obstetric indication and maternal condition
  - Lung maturation with corticosteroids may be required between 24 and 34 weeks.
  - Separation of neonate from mother should be minimised facilitate skin-to-skin and breastfeeding if possible.
- **Resuscitation**
  - Specialised equipment should be available in the critical care unit.

- Teratogenicity
  - Pharmacological considerations should be made where possible.
  - Imaging risks require balance with necessity.

What is your approach to imaging studies in the pregnant patient?

A balance of clinical indication and risk of ionising radiation should be considered. Most risks relate to fetal exposure, particularly between 10 and 17/40, although there are some notable risks to the mother above usual considerations. The mother should be involved in decision-making where possible.

Mother

- *CT might be required*: VTE, blunt trauma, acute intracranial event.
- Considerations in suspected PE:
  - CTPA associated with higher risk of maternal breast cancer.
    - ➢ Up to 20 mGy radiation may be required (20–100 × dose for V/Q).
    - ➢ 10 mGy to breast increases lifetime risk by 13.6% above background risk.
  - V/Q may have slightly increased risk of childhood cancer for fetus.
  - V/Q may be difficult to perform if significant oxygen requirement, must be awake.

Fetus

- Ionising radiation
  - No increased risk with radiation under background levels (<5 rad or 50 mGy)
  - Risk of microcephaly and developmental delay from 10/40, maximal at 10–17/40, lower at 18–27/40
- Contrast media
  - Largely safe
  - Paramagnetic agents for MR only when absolutely necessary (e.g. gadolinium – specific risks)
- Radioisotopes
  - Higher exposure earlier in pregnancy
  - *Except iodine*: increasing effect on fetal thyroid with gestational age, avoid iodinated agents
  - *V/Q scan*: technetium macroaggregated albumin (perfusion) and inhaled xenon (ventilation) used
- MR
  - Safe (historically avoided in first trimester)
- US
  - Concern about thermal and mechanical effects (focused point-of-care study safe)

What are the pharmacological concerns when treating pregnant patients?

- **Teratogenicity** particularly concerning in first trimester
  - For example ACE-I, ARB, lithium, warfarin
  - *Antibiotics*: tetracyclines, trimethoprim (penicillins, macrolides, cephalosporins safe)
  - Antiepileptics: most, will require balance of risk
- **Analgesics**
  - Paracetamol is safe.
  - NSAIDs cause closure of ductus arteriosus (avoid after 30/40).
  - Unpredictable codeine metabolism (avoid breastfeeding, consider dihydrocodeine with caution)
  - Opioids are linked to neonatal respiratory depression and withdrawal after prolonged usage – minimise.
- **Sedatives**
  - *Depressant effect on fetus at delivery*: minimise exposure where possible
  - Neonatal withdrawal possible (e.g. midazolam)
  - Dexmedetomidine and clonidine safety profile unknown

Resources

- Banerjee A, Cantellow S. Maternal critical care: part I. BJA Educ. 2021;21(4):140–147.
- Banerjee A, Cantellow S. Maternal critical care: part II. BJA Educ. 2021;21:164–171.
- Chambers D, Huang C, Matthews G. Basic Physiology for Anaesthetists. 2nd ed. Cambridge: Cambridge University Press; 2019.

- Eskandar OS, Eckford SD, Watkinson. Review: Safety of diagnostic imaging in pregnancy. Part 1: X-ray, nuclear medicine investigations, computed tomography and contrast media. Obstet Gynecol. 2010;12(2):71–78.
- Ray JG, Vermeulen M, Bharatha A, et al. Association between MRI exposure during pregnancy and fetal and childhood outcomes. JAMA. 2016;316(9):952–961.
- Royal College of Obstetricians & Gynaecologists. Thromboembolic Disease in Pregnancy and the Puerperium: Acute Management: Green-top Guideline No. 37b. April 2015. Available from: https://www.rcog.org.uk/globalassets/documents/guidelines/gtg-37b.pdf. (Accessed 23 January 2022.)
- The Newcastle upon Tyne Hospitals NHS Foundation Trust. Teratogenic Drugs. 2021. Available from: https://www.newcastle-hospitals.nhs.uk/services/clinical-genetics/information-for-healthcare-professionals/preconception-counselling/teratogenic-drugs/. (Accessed 23 January 2022.)
- Vousden N, Bunch K, Morris E, et al. The incidence, characteristics and outcomes of pregnant women hospitalized with symptomatic and asymptomatic SARS-CoV-2 infection in the UK from March to September 2020: A national cohort study using the UK Obstetric Surveillance System (UKOSS). PLoS One. 2021;16(5):e0251123.

98. HYPERTENSIVE DISORDERS OF PREGNANCY

What is the significance of hypertensive disease in pregnancy?

Hypertensive disorders in pregnancy affect 8–10% of all pregnant women and are associated with increased maternal and fetal mortality and morbidity.

What is gestational hypertension and how is it usually managed?

> **KEY POINT**
>
> Gestational hypertension is a new diagnosis of hypertension **after 20/40 gestation** without features of pre-eclampsia.

- **BP 140/90–159/109 mmHg** (ideally on 2 occasions >4 h apart)
  - Pharmacological treatment given to target BP ≤135/85 mmHg
  - *Agents used*: labetalol, nifedipine, methyldopa – dependent on pre-existing treatment, side effects, risk, and patient preference
  - *Investigations*: FBC, LFT, U&E, urinalysis
  - Placental growth factor (PlGF)-based testing if suspicion of pre-eclampsia
- *Severe*: **BP ≥ 160/110 mmHg**
  - As above but admit to hospital
  - Measure BP every 15–30 min until BP < 160/110 mmHg then 4× daily

Hypertension diagnosed in the first 20 weeks of gestation falls within the definition of chronic hypertension.

- Medication is likely to need to be reviewed and safer alternative offered.
- Thiazide diuretics, ACEI, and ARB are associated with increased risk of congenital abnormalities.

GUIDELINE NICE 2019 NG133 Hypertension in pregnancy

What are the diagnostic criteria for pre-eclampsia?

KEY POINT

Pre-eclampsia:

- **Systolic BP ≥140 mmHg or diastolic BP ≥90 mmHg**, plus
- *Proteinuria*: urinary PCR ≥30 mg/mmol, ACR ≥8 mg/mmol, or
- ≥1 of the following:
  - *AKI*: creatinine ≥90 µmol/L
  - *Liver involvement*: ALT > 70 IU/l or 2 × upper limit of normal
  - Neurological complications (e.g. eclampsia, severe headaches)
  - *Haematological complications*: platelets < 150 × 10⁹/l, DIC, haemolysis, or HELLP syndrome
  - Uteroplacental dysfunction (e.g. fetal growth restriction or abnormal umbilical artery Doppler waveform analysis)

Severe pre-eclampsia is defined by the presence of any of the following:

- *A/B*: pulmonary oedema
- *C*: systolic BP ≥ 160 or diastolic BP ≥ 110 mmHg
- *D*: visual disturbance (flashing lights, blurring), severe headache
- *F*: renal insufficiency (×2 creatinine)
- *G*: ALT > 70 IU/l or 2 × upper limit of normal, liver tenderness
- *H*: platelets < 100 × 10⁹/l
- HELLP syndrome

Other indicative features are as follows:

- *Significant oedema*: sudden swelling of face, hands, or feet
- Ongoing/recurring severe headaches
- Epigastric pain
- Nausea and vomiting

What is the pathophysiology of pre-eclampsia?

- Impaired trophoblastic cell invasion
- Reduced spiral artery development
- Placental hypoxaemia
- Placenta releases cytokines and inflammatory factors into maternal circulation.
- *Decrease in proangiogenic factors*: vascular endothelial growth factor (VEGF), PlGF
- *Increase in anti-angiogenic factors*: soluble FMS-like tyrosine kinase 1 (sFlt1), soluble endoglin (sEng), asymmetric dimethyl arginine (ADMA)
- Increased vascular tone and permeability, activation of coagulation cascade
- Resultant organ dysfunction

What are the most common risk factors?

- Previous pre-eclampsia
- Chronic hypertension
- Raised BMI
- Diabetes mellitus prior to pregnancy
- Antiphospholipid syndrome, SLE
- Assisted reproduction
- Primiparity
- Advanced maternal age > 40 years
- Family history
- Multiple pregnancy
- Chronic kidney disease

Do you know of any risk prediction models that are used for pre-eclampsia?

PRediction of complications in Early-onset Pre-eclampsia (PREP-S) and Pre-eclampsia Integrated Estimate of RiSk (fullPIERS) are validated risk prediction models for severe disease that are recommended by NICE to guide decision-making.

What does management involve?

- Initially managed by obstetric team
- *HDU level care common*: IV antihypertensives, magnesium infusion, continuous arterial pressure monitoring
- *Addressing underlying cause (i.e. delivery)*: disease process will not improve until delivery of placenta
    - Timing dependent on gestation and severity of disease
    - If over 37/40, delivery usually expedited to next 24–48 h
    - If planned preterm birth, offer antenatal corticosteroids and magnesium

- *Management of hypertension – example regimes*:
    - Enteral
        - Labetalol (200 mg 12 hourly, increased to max 2.4 g/day)
        - Nifedipine (10 mg, repeat dose after 30 min)
    - IV
        - Labetalol (20 mg over 2 min, up to 80 mg, then infusion)
        - Hydralazine (5–10 mg over 2 min, further 10 mg after 20 min if required, then infusion)
- *Seizure management*: **magnesium sulphate**
    - Indicated in eclamptic seizure or evidence of severe pre-eclampsia
    - 4 g MgSO$_4$ over 5–15 min
    - 1 g/h MgSO$_4$ infusion until 24 h post-delivery or last seizure (whichever is later)
    - Further 2–4 g bolus if recurrent seizures
    - Monitoring including tendon reflexes essential
    - Caution with dose in patients with renal impairment
- Treat magnesium toxicity with calcium gluconate
    - Avoid benzodiazepines, phenytoin, other antiepileptics in women with eclampsia
- **Fluid status**
    - Monitor UO
    - Restrict input to 80 ml/h (balance with adequate output)
- Thromboprophylaxis

STUDY

Magpie (2002)

- Women with pre-eclampsia
- *Intervention*: magnesium sulphate vs placebo
- *Primary*: eclampsia – **significantly lower**, death of baby – **no difference**

What are the complications of pre-eclampsia?

Fetal
- Fetal demise
- Preterm birth
- Neonatal ICU admission

Maternal
- Eclamptic seizures
- Fluid overload, pulmonary oedema
- Cardiomyopathy, HF

- AKI
- Liver dysfunction, hepatic rupture
- Coagulopathy including DIC
- ICH and stroke
- Visual loss
- Post-partum haemorrhage (PPH)

When would you consider admission for higher levels of care?

A minimum of high-dependency (level 2) care is indicated in severe pre-eclampsia with any of the following:

- *C*: initial stabilisation of severe hypertension, IV antihypertensives, cardiac failure, haemorrhage
- *D*: eclampsia, abnormal neurology
- *F*: hyperkalaemia, severe oliguria
- *G*: HELLP syndrome
- *H*: coagulation support

Level 3 care might be indicated in severe pre-eclampsia if:

- Requiring mechanical ventilation
- Additional vasopressor or other cardiovascular support required
- Acid-base or severe electrolyte abnormalities present
- RRT may be indicated

Which disease-specific considerations will be required in critical care?

- Increased risk of **airway problems**
  - Generalised airway and subglottic oedema
    - ➤ Smaller-sized tube should be available.
    - ➤ *Caution with extubation*: leak test
- Increased risk of **pulmonary oedema**
  - Restrictive fluid balance
  - Likely to require higher airway pressures and PEEP.
  - May have reduced response to furosemide.
  - GTN infusion may be required.
- Risk of **cerebrovascular haemorrhage** with increased SBP during laryngoscopy
  - Pre-empt and actively manage with short-acting IV opioids (e.g. alfentanil) ± antihypertensives.
  - Aim to maintain BP at pre-induction values.
  - Avoid swings in BP.
- *Coagulopathy*: cautious removal of epidural if used
- Magnesium increases the duration of action of muscle relaxants.

Post-partum

- Hypertension can persist for 6–8 weeks post-delivery.
- Women have increased risk of cardiovascular disease, stroke, diabetes, CKD, and VTE in later life.

What is the difference between HELLP syndrome and acute fatty liver of pregnancy?

HELLP syndrome and acute fatty liver of pregnancy (AFLP) are 2 similar disorders of acute liver dysfunction in pregnancy. Delivery is the key to preventing both conditions from progressing.

HELLP syndrome

- Severe form of pre-eclampsia (4–20% patients)
- Often preceded by 'hepatic angina' (right upper quadrant pain)
- Diagnosis based on spectrum of platelet count, ALT/AST, LDH
- Low-grade haemolysis, platelet dysfunction more significant, 20% develop DIC

- *Rare complications*: hepatic haematoma or rupture, shock, <1% mortality
- IR/surgery may be required after early imaging

AFLP

- Rare, may be a variant of pre-eclampsia, can also deteriorate post-partum
- 60% require ICU admission, mortality < 2%, perinatal mortality 20–50%
- Often follows several week history of nausea, vomiting, malaise
- May develop fulminant hepatic failure but platelet function more stable than in HELLP
- *Diagnosed using Swansea criteria (≥6 of)*: vomiting, abdominal pain, polydipsia/polyuria, encephalopathy, elevated bilirubin, hypoglycaemia, hyperuricaemia, leukocytosis, ascites/echogenic liver on US, elevated transaminases, elevated ammonia, AKI, coagulopathy, microvesicular steatosis on liver biopsy

(See Chapter 135 Acute Liver Failure)

Resources

- Goddard J, Wee MYK, Vinayakarao L. Update on hypertensive disorders in pregnancy. BJA Educ. 2020;20(12): 411–416.
- Griffiths S, Nicholson C. Anaesthetic implications for liver disease in pregnancy. BJA Educ. 2016;16(1):21–25.

---

99. MAJOR OBSTETRIC HAEMORRHAGE

What is the significance of obstetric haemorrhage?

Haemorrhage remains one of the leading causes of maternal morbidity and mortality both in the developed and developing world. The latest Mothers and Babies: Reducing Risk through Audits and Confidential Enquiries across the UK (MBRRACE-UK) report found that 9% of perinatal deaths were due to haemorrhage. Internationally, this increases to up to 50%.

What types of obstetric haemorrhage are you aware of?

KEY POINT

- *Antepartum haemorrhage (APH)*: bleeding from/in genital tract **from 24/40 until delivery**
- *PPH*:
    - *Primary PPH*: loss of **≥500 ml blood within the first 24 h** after delivery
    - *Secondary PPH*: bleeding occurring between **24 h and 12 weeks** after delivery

When grading severity, the size of the patient is relevant in terms of percentage blood loss. Volume criteria are also described as follows:

- *APH*: usually considered massive if >**1000 ml**
- *PPH*:
    - *Minor*: 500–1000 ml
    - Major
        - Moderate 1000–2000 ml
        - Severe > 2000 ml

GUIDELINE   RCOG 2016 PPH

What are the most common causes of major obstetric haemorrhage?

APH causes MOH less commonly than PPH does, but it can also be catastrophic.

APH

- *Placental abruption*: abnormal separation of the placenta from the uterus
- *Placenta praevia*: low-lying placental implantation close to/over the uterine os
- *Placenta accreta*: villi attach to myometrium instead of decidua
  - *Placenta increta*: villi penetrate myometrium
  - *Placenta percreta*: villi attach to uterine serosa or adjacent organs
- *Vasa praevia*: fetal vessels traverse the uterine os
- *Uterine rupture*: increased risk following previous caesarean section, short duration since last caesarean section, and artificial induction of labour

PPH

- *Tone*: atony post-delivery
  - Multiparity
  - Multiple pregnancy
  - Prolonged labour
  - Polyhydramnios
  - Placenta praevia
  - Previous PPH from atony
  - Increased maternal age
  - Chorioamnionitis
- *Trauma*: to the perineum, vagina, or uterus/abdomen during delivery
  - Increased risk with large neonate
- *Tissue*: retained placenta
- *Thrombotic*
  - Bleeding disorder
  - Anticoagulants
  - DIC (e.g. secondary to placental abruption or AFE)

How would you recognise MOH?

- *Visual estimation of blood loss*: notoriously inaccurate, clinical signs and symptoms should be used.
- *Gravimetric estimation*: weighing of swabs/absorbent pads
- *Volumetric estimation*: suction containers, etc.

What are the specific treatment priorities in MOH?

- Prompt resuscitation with simultaneous interventions by multiple team members
- Multidisciplinary involvement including obstetricians, paediatricians, and midwifery
- Left-lateral uterine displacement if antepartum
- Consider other causes of shock (e.g. sepsis)
- *Address underlying cause*: may require immediate transfer to theatre

Management of bleeding

- Wide-bore IV access
- *Send bloods*: cross-match if not done previously, FBC, coagulation screen including fibrinogen
- Activate major haemorrhage protocol (may involve specific obstetric protocol)
- Blood product administration may be guided by point of care testing (e.g. VHA – TEG®, ROTEM®) and may include the following:
  - FFP empiric dose 12–15 ml/kg
  - Cryoprecipitate/fibrinogen concentrate
- TXA 1 g IV
- Warmed crystalloid if blood not immediately available
- Cell salvage in theatre to minimise other transfusion requirement
  - Second suction circuit for amniotic fluid
  - Leukodepletion filters not recommended routinely

- Liaise with haematology for ongoing advice regarding transfusion
- Uterotonics and surgical intervention

Other supportive care
- Normothermia
- Arterial, central venous access
- Cardiac output monitoring

Transfusion goals
- Hct > 0.3
- Platelets > 75 × 10⁹/l
- Fibrinogen > 2 g/l
- Ionised calcium > 1.0 mmol/l
- Temperature > 36°C

STUDY

WOMAN (2017)

- PPH
- *Intervention*: TXA 1 g IV over 10 min vs placebo
- *Primary*: composite of 42-day all-cause mortality/hysterectomy – **no difference**
- *Secondary*: death due to bleeding – **significantly lower**; thromboembolism – no difference

(See Chapter 51 Major Haemorrhage)

How would you address the underlying cause of bleeding?

Atony
- *Stimulation of contraction*: uterine massage and bimanual compression
- Uterotonics
  - Syntocinon (synthetic oxytocin)
    - ➤ 5 IU IV slow bolus, can repeat, IV infusion 10 IU/h
    - ➤ Causes hypotension, tachycardia
    - ➤ Also given prophylactically in third stage of labour
  - Ergometrine (ergot alkaloid)
    - ➤ 500 µg IM – avoid in hypertensive/cardiac disease
  - Carboprost (Hemabate®) (prostaglandin F2α)
    - ➤ 250 µg IM – repeat every 15 min (max 2 mg)
    - ➤ Caution in asthmatic patients (may induce bronchospasm)
    - ➤ Avoid in pulmonary hypertension (increases PAP)
  - Misoprostol (synthetic prostaglandin analogue)
    - ➤ 1 mg PR
- Surgical intervention
  - *Intrauterine balloon tamponade*: Bakri balloon
  - *Uterine compression suture*: brace suture
  - *IR*: uterine artery embolisation
  - Ligation of pelvic vessels
  - Hysterectomy

Other causes
- *Tissue*: removal of any retained placenta, require manual removal in theatre
- *Trauma*: surgical repair
- *Thrombus*: actively treat coagulopathy

What are the additional considerations after MOH?

- High-dependency care on delivery suite or transfer to critical care
- May require period of cardiovascular support or ventilation depending on severity
- Close monitoring of fluid balance
- Antibiotic prophylaxis from theatre may need to be repeated if blood loss >1500 ml
- Thromboprophylaxis as soon as bleeding settled and coagulation normalised

Resources

- Knight M, Bunch K, Tuffnell D, et al. Saving Lives, Improving Mothers' Care – Lessons learned to inform maternity care from the UK and Ireland Confidential Enquiries into Maternal Deaths and Morbidity 2017–19. November 2021. Available from: https://www.npeu.ox.ac.uk/assets/downloads/mbrrace-uk/reports/maternal-report-2021/MBRRACE-UK_Maternal_Report_2021_-_FINAL_-_WEB_VERSION.pdf. (Accessed 23 January 2022.)
- Plaat F, Shonfeld A. Major obstetric haemorrhage. BJA Educ. 2015;15(4):190–193.

100.   MATERNAL SEPSIS

What is puerperal sepsis and what is its significance?

Many definitions exist surrounding sepsis in pregnant patients, differing in their inclusion of sepsis due to genital tract infection (vs other site) and timing (puerperium vs throughout pregnancy).

> **KEY POINT**
>
> The WHO describes **maternal sepsis** as 'a life-threatening condition defined as organ dysfunction resulting from infection during pregnancy, childbirth, post-abortion, or postpartum period'.

Sepsis is the leading cause of maternal morbidity and mortality worldwide. MBRRACE-UK identified that approximately 11% (23/217) of maternal deaths in the puerperal period were due to sepsis. Signs and symptoms of sepsis can often go unrecognised and may be attributed to the haemodynamic changes associated with labour pain or blood loss.

Maternal sepsis care bundles have been developed to improve early recognition. Diagnosis usually involves the use of specific maternity early warning scores such as the Modified Early Obstetric Warning System (MEOWS).

What are the most common causes?

Direct (genital tract or wound infection)
- Group A *Streptococcus*
- *Chorioamnionitis*: *E. coli*

Indirect
- Influenza (A, B – including H_1N_1)
- *UTI*: pyelonephritis
- Pneumonia
- TB
- Disseminated herpes simplex
- Meningitis
- COVID-19

What are the main risk factors?

- **In pregnancy**
  - *Intervention*: amniocentesis, cervical suture
  - Premature rupture of membranes (especially in preterm group)
  - Intrauterine fetal death
- **During labour**
  - Prolonged labour
  - Vaginal trauma
- **Surgical**
  - Episiotomy
  - Caesarean section
  - Retained products
- **Non-obstetric**
  - *Maternal comorbidities*: diabetes, anaemia, obesity
  - Immunosuppression
  - History of group B *Streptococcus* infection
  - Black or other minority ethnic group
  - Maternal age > 35 years
  - Group A *Streptococcus* infection in close contacts

Which physical adaptations in pregnancy might make detection difficult?

- Baseline tachycardia
- Further increases in HR associated with pain of labour
- State of relative vasodilatation
- Increased plasma volume
- Increased WCC during labour
- Other complications associated with pregnancy and delivery (e.g. pre-eclampsia, MOH)

What are the management priorities in maternal sepsis?

Prevention is ideal during the following:

- *Appropriate vaccinations*: influenza, COVID-19
- Active treatment of premature rupture of membranes
- Prophylactic antibiotics at time of surgical intervention

Timely recognition is the key to effective management in established sepsis. Management principles follow those recommended for other causes, with specific adaptations. (See Chapter 26 Sepsis)

- General
  - Early involvement of senior MDT staff is important.
  - Cultures should include a high vaginal swab.
  - Monitor for coagulopathy.
- Cardiovascular support
  - Left-lateral uterine displacement is important after 20/40 gestation until delivery.
  - Fluid management may be tricky with pre-eclampsia or underlying cardiac disease.
  - Oxytocin infusion may cause/exacerbate hyponatraemia.
  - Bedside echo is helpful.
- **Surgical source control**
  - Debridement of wound infection
  - Evacuation of retained products
  - Delivery of fetus in chorioamnionitis
  - Percutaneous drainage of abscesses
  - Stenting for obstructive pyelonephritis

GUIDELINE NICE 2019 NG121 Existing conditions or complications

RCOG 2012 Bacterial sepsis

SSC 2021 Sepsis

When might intensivists be involved with patients with maternal sepsis?

- Airway protection
- *Respiratory failure*: pulmonary oedema, ARDS
- Persistent hypotension requiring vasopressor therapy
- Severe AKI potentially requiring RRT
- Decreased conscious level
- Multi-organ dysfunction
- Uncorrected acidosis

NICE recommend senior intensivist input if any of:

- Altered consciousness
- $F_1O_2 \geq 0.4$ to maintain $S_pO_2 > 92\%$
- Systolic BP < 90 mmHg
- UO < 0.5 ml/kg/h (despite fluid resuscitation)
- Tympanic temperature < 36°C

When would delivery of the fetus be considered with sepsis?

This should be an MDT decision including the wishes of the woman if possible. Considerations are as follows:

- Source
- Severity
- Gestational age
- Fetal wellbeing
- Stage and progress of labour
- Parity
- Response to treatment

What are your concerns if this patient requires general anaesthesia?

- As per general obstetric considerations (see Chapter 97 The Pregnant Critical Care Patient)
- Desaturation may be even more problematic due to higher oxygen demand.
- *Haemodynamic compromise a significant risk* (increased vasoplegia)
- Increased risk of PPH, especially if source is chorioamnionitis

How would you adapt your management for COVID-19 pneumonitis?

- Self-proning is challenging in later stages of pregnancy but advised if possible.
- Corticosteroids
  - Indicated if oxygen requirement
  - Prednisolone 40 mg OD for 10 days or until discharge
  - Regular blood glucose monitoring (e.g. 6°)

(See Chapter 124 COVID-19)

Resources

- Burlinson CEG, Sirounis D, Walley KR, et al. Sepsis in pregnancy and the puerperium. Int J Obstet Anesth. 2018;36:96–107.
- Knight M, Bunch K, Tuffnell D, et al. Saving Lives, Improving Mothers' Care – Lessons learned to inform maternity care from the UK and Ireland Confidential Enquiries into Maternal Deaths and Morbidity 2017–2019. November 2021. Available from: https://www.npeu.ox.ac.uk/assets/downloads/mbrrace-uk/reports/maternal-report-2021/MBRRACE-UK_Maternal_Report_2021_-_FINAL_-_WEB_VERSION.pdf. (Accessed 23 January 2022.)

101. AMNIOTIC FLUID EMBOLISM

Why is amniotic fluid embolism a concern?

AFE continues to cause severe morbidity and mortality to mother and baby. Its incidence is approximately 1.7 per 100000 maternities, with a case fatality rate of 19%. The potential for permanent neurological injury is significant.

It often presents as sudden, unexplained, profound maternal collapse. Due to its rarity and difficulty to diagnose, there remain large gaps in evidence. Most cases are thought to occur during labour, but it may also present during caesarean section and the immediate period following vaginal delivery.

What are the clinical features of AFE?

- Fetal distress
- *Maternal*
    - *B*: pulmonary oedema, ARDS, hypoxia
    - *C*: cardiovascular collapse/hypotension, cardiorespiratory arrest, uterine atony
    - *D*: seizures
    - *H*: consumptive coagulopathy, DIC

How is AFE diagnosed?

Diagnosis must be made clinically due to the emergent nature of the condition but can only be confirmed on histological analysis (e.g. post-mortem presence of fetal squames in maternal lung tissue).

> **KEY POINT**
>
> UKOSS criteria for AFE diagnosis:
>
> - Acute hypotension/cardiac arrest
> - Acute hypoxia and coagulopathy or severe haemorrhage in the absence of any other potential explanation for observed signs and symptoms

Differentials which should be excluded:

- *Anaphylaxis*: send serum tryptase
- Eclampsia
- PE
- Sepsis
- MI
- Local anaesthetic systemic toxicity
- Concealed major haemorrhage

What are the risk factors?

There are many suggested risk factors but none of which justify any prospective alteration of standard obstetric practice to reduce risk of AFE:

- Maternal
    - **Age > 35 years**
    - Ethnic minority
    - Eclampsia
- Fetal
    - **Multiple pregnancy**
    - Polyhydramnios
    - Male fetus

- Obstetric
  - **Induction of labour**
  - **Placenta praevia**
  - Evidence of hyperstimulation
  - Oxytocin augmentation
  - Placental abruption
  - Assisted delivery (forceps/vacuum)
  - Caesarean section
  - Uterine rupture
  - Cervical trauma

What is the pathophysiology of AFE?

It is thought that exposure of the maternal circulation to certain substances causes immune activation with an anaphylactoid response. These include substances within amniotic fluid (e.g. fetal squamous cells, trophoblasts, fetal gut mucin, bile-stained meconium, prothrombotic substances) or fetal antigens.

KEY POINT

There are 2 phases in AFE as follows:

1. Initial entry of amniotic fluid into the circulation causes **pulmonary hypertension** secondary to vascular occlusion either by debris or vasoconstriction. This leads to RV failure, microvascular damage, and hypotension.
2. **LV failure** develops, and endothelial activation leads to capillary leakage and DIC.

Discuss the management of these patients.

- General
  - Supportive care
  - Senior staff present early
  - Emergent delivery of fetus/perimortem caesarean section
- Respiratory
  - Early intubation
  - F_IO_2 1.0
- Cardiovascular support
  - Vasopressors likely to be required
  - Echo helpful
  - Early aggressive haemorrhage management
  - Recombinant factor VII only if not corrected by massive blood component replacement
  - Early aggressive treatment of coagulopathy
- Ongoing care
  - Intensive care normally required for survivors.
  - May require ECMO, mechanical circulatory support, RRT

GUIDELINE   RCOG 2019 Maternal collapse

Resources

- Fitzpatrick KE, Tuffnell D, Kurinczuk JJ, et al. Incidence, risk factors, management and outcomes of amniotic-fluid embolism: a population-based cohort and nested case-control study. BJOG. 2016;123(1):100–109.
- Metodiev Y, Ramasamy P, Tuffnell D. Amniotic fluid embolism. BJA Educ. 2018;18(8):234–238.

102. OBSTETRIC CARDIAC ARREST

What is the significance of obstetric cardiac arrest in the UK?

Obstetric cardiac arrest is that occurring during pregnancy and **up to 6 weeks post-partum**.

Obstetric cardiac arrest is rare, with an incidence of around 1 in 36000 maternities (1:16000 including post-partum data). Maternal survival rates of over 50% have been reported; 25% of cases are related to anaesthesia, but this subgroup has a high survival rate.

Management should follow standard resuscitation principles with a few extra considerations. Perimortem caesarean section is indicated after 20 weeks' gestation to improve maternal and fetal outcome by relieving aortocaval compression, therefore improving venous return. The fetus acts as an end organ with limited autoregulatory mechanisms to maintain perfusion in extremis. It is unlikely that the fetus will have a good outcome if the mother's cardiac output is not prioritised.

GUIDELINE RCOG 2019 Maternal collapse

What are the causes of cardiac arrest specific to obstetric patients?

- Hypoxia
  - **Pulmonary embolus**
  - Failed intubation/aspiration
  - HF
  - Anaphylaxis
  - *Eclampsia/pre-eclampsia*: pulmonary oedema, seizure
- Hypovolaemia
  - *Haemorrhage*: MOH, splenic/hepatic artery rupture, aneurysm rupture
  - **Sepsis**
  - Anaphylaxis
  - High regional anaesthesia
- *Hypo-/hyperkalaemia*: consider other imbalance – magnesium, sodium, glucose, calcium
- *Hypothermia*: unlikely in inpatient setting
- Tamponade
  - Trauma
  - Aortic dissection
- 'Thrombosis'
  - **AFE**
  - Air embolus
  - PE
  - MI
- Toxins
  - Local anaesthetic systemic toxicity
  - Opioids (e.g. remifentanil PCA for labour)
  - Illicit drugs
  - Self-harm
  - Magnesium
- *Tension PTX*: unlikely but exacerbated by N_2O

- Other
  - Intracranial haemorrhage
  - PPCM

What are the priorities during an obstetric cardiac arrest?

- *Calling appropriate team members*: anaesthetists, obstetricians, neonatologists if ≥20/40
- *Relieving aortocaval compression*: manual displacement of uterus
- Effective CPR
- **Early intubation**
- Consideration of causes specific to obstetrics
- **Timely perimortem caesarean section**
  - Avoid moving patient
  - Within 5 min of cardiac arrest
  - Midline vertical or suprapubic transverse incision
  - Non-obstetrician may be required to perform this
- **Consideration of E-CPR** if prolonged, depending on availability

Which specific pharmacological treatments should be considered in the obstetric setting?

- *Eclampsia*: magnesium 4 g IV bolus
- *Magnesium toxicity*: 10 ml 10% calcium chloride/gluconate
- *PE*: thrombolysis (e.g. alteplase)
- *Local anaesthetic toxicity*: 20% lipid emulsion (1.5 ml/kg bolus then 15 ml/kg/h infusion)
- *Haemorrhage*: TXA 1 g, uterotonics (see Chapter 99 Major Obstetric Haemorrhage)

How would you perform spinal immobilisation in major trauma?

The spine should be protected with a spinal board before applying 15–30° left tilt. If no spinal board is available, manual displacement of the uterus should be performed.

Resources

- Beckett VA, Knight M, Sharpe P. The CAPS Study: incidence, management and outcomes of cardiac arrest in pregnancy in the UK: a prospective, descriptive study. BJOG. 2017;124(9):1374–1381.
- Resuscitation Council UK and Obstetric Anaesthetists' Association. Obstetric Cardiac Arrest quick reference guide. Available from: https://www.oaa-anaes.ac.uk/assets/_managed/cms/files/Clinical%20Guidelines/Obstetric%20Cardiac%20Arrest%20QRH%20OAA%20V1%201.pdf. (Accessed 23 January 2022.)

PAEDIATRICS

103. BRONCHIOLITIS

What is bronchiolitis?

Bronchiolitis is an infection of the respiratory tract, characterised by a high secretion load, typically presenting in children under 2 years old. It is most common in the winter months in infants (particularly aged between 3 and 6 months).

How is bronchiolitis diagnosed?

Bronchiolitis is a clinical diagnosis and may be supported by microbiology. Typical features include coryza, cough, wheeze, and fine crepitations, with varying degrees of respiratory failure. Fever (<39°C) and poor feeding are common. Symptoms may last several weeks.

KEY POINT

Bronchiolitis diagnostic criteria:

- Coryzal prodrome 1–3 days
- Persistent cough
- Either of:
  - Tachypnoea and/or chest recession
  - Wheeze and/or crackles on chest auscultation

GUIDELINE   NICE 2021 NG9 Bronchiolitis

Which important differential diagnoses should be considered?

- *Pneumonia*: particularly if temperature >39°C or persistently focal crackles
- *Early-onset asthma*: absence of crackles, episodic wheeze, atopy
- Viral-induced wheeze

What are the causes?

Causative pathogens include the following:

- **RSV** (80%)
- Metapneumovirus
- Influenza

- Parainfluenza
- Adenovirus
- Rhinovirus
- Boca virus
- *Mycoplasma*

What constitutes severe disease?

Severe
- $F_IO_2 > 0.5$ to maintain $S_pO_2 > 95\%$
- Severe intercostal recession
- Tachypnoea
- Tachycardia
- Frequent apnoeas (>2/h)

Life-threatening
- $S_pO_2 < 88\%$ despite high-flow oxygen or CPAP
- Respiratory acidosis
- Episodes of desaturation
- Apnoeas requiring bag mask ventilation or increased frequency with desaturation
- Exhaustion, grunting, marked recession

Which factors are associated with a worse outcome?

- Chronic lung disease
- Congenital cardiac disease
- Prematurity
- Immunodeficiency
- Adenovirus as causative pathogen
- Presentation at less than 6 weeks of age

Outline the initial therapeutic principles in severe disease

There are no specific treatments and therapy is supportive:

- *Airway*: ensure nose not blocked by superficial secretion clearance
- *Respiratory*:
    - Humidified, high-flow oxygen
    - Nasal CPAP or BiPAP as titrated to capillary blood gas and clinical features
    - Gastric decompression may be required
- **Hydration**
- **Treat secondary bacterial infection**

Which therapies are recommended against routinely?

- Antibiotics
- Hypertonic saline
- Nebulised adrenaline
- Salbutamol
- Montelukast
- Ipratropium bromide
- Corticosteroids

Caffeine and aminophylline have been tried for prevention of apnoeas (with limited evidence).

When might invasive ventilation be required?

- Severe disease not responding to initial therapy, or deteriorating.
- Intubation and invasive ventilation may be required in presence of life-threatening features, significant respiratory acidosis, or hypoxia despite NIV.
- 3–5% of infants with bronchiolitis will require intensive care admission.

What would ongoing management in the ICU involve?

- LPV
- Appropriate tube positioning as directed by CXR
- Secretion management
- Change to nasal tube if prolonged intubation anticipated
- Appropriate feeding regime
- Supporting parents or carers

Can you list some common problems encountered in these patients in the ICU?

- Secondary bacterial infection
- Mucous plugging
- Bronchospasm and gas trapping
- Bradycardic episodes
- Hyponatraemia

Resource

- Shetty N, Phatak R. Guidelines for Management of Severe and Life-threatening Bronchiolitis. Version 2. North West & North Wales Paediatric Transport Service. June 2016. Available from: https://www.nwts.nhs.uk/_file/NMlaVTfxoy_306198.pdf. (Accessed 05 January 2022.)

---

104. CONGENITAL HEART DISEASE

What types of congenital heart disease do you know of?

Congenital heart disease is one of the commonest birth defects, affecting up to 8:1000 babies in the UK. Risk factors include chromosomal conditions (e.g. Down syndrome) and maternal infection, medications, smoking, alcohol consumption, and diabetes.

Examples (Figure 104.1)
- *Septal defects*: atrial, ventricular
- Patent ductus arteriosus
- Coarctation of the aorta
- Pulmonary stenosis
- Transposition of the great arteries
- *Tetralogy of Fallot*: ventricular septal defect, pulmonary stenosis, overriding aorta, RV hypertrophy
- Aortic stenosis
- Ebstein's anomaly
- Hypoplastic left heart syndrome
- Tricuspid atresia
- Total/partial anomalous pulmonary venous connection/drainage (TAPVD)
- Truncus arteriosus

What is meant by 'duct-dependent' congenital heart disease?

'Duct-dependent' disease refers to pathological configurations that are reliant on a patent ductus arteriosus in order to maintain end-organ perfusion. Most of the above conditions may have significant duct-dependency.

Typical presentation is with cyanosis unresponsive to increased F_IO_2. Femoral pulses may be poor or absent and saturations different in pre-/post-ductal sites.

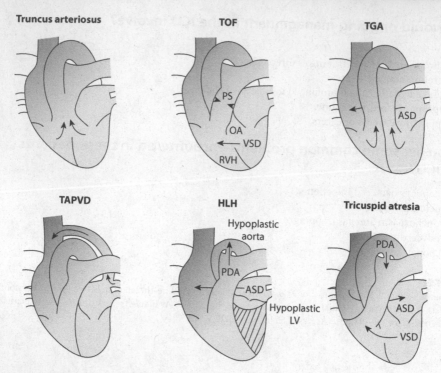

Figure 104.1 Congenital heart disease.

ToF, tetralogy of Fallot; PS, pulmonary stenosis; OA, overriding aorta; VSD, ventricular septal defect; RVH, right ventricular hypertrophy; TGA, transposition of the great arteries; ASD, atrial septal defect; TAPVD, total anomalous pulmonary venous drainage; HLH, hypoplastic left heart; PDA, patent ductus arteriosus.

How might a child with congenital heart disease present to hospital?

- Cardiorespiratory arrest
- Respiratory tract infection
- Dysrhythmia
- HF symptoms
- Cyanosis
- Protein-losing enteropathy
- Haemoptysis
- Drug side effects
- IE
- Complications of corrective surgery

What is the Fontan circulation?

This is the name of a circuit formed during repair of certain cardiac malformations with a single functional ventricle (e.g. tricuspid/pulmonary atresia, hypoplastic left heart syndrome). This would otherwise cause arterial desaturation and chronic volume overload, usually leading to death by the fourth decade.

It requires a multi-stage procedure (Figure 104.2), with these main steps:

- *4–12 months*: cavopulmonary connection or bidirectional shunt created, permitting increased blood flow to the lungs
- *1–5 years*: completion of Fontan circuit – IVC connected to PA

How might a child present with congenital heart disease to the intensivist?

Malformations requiring intensive care management are often those resulting in severe cyanosis or HF early in life. Some less severe defects may become apparent during other intensive care management (e.g. sudden desaturation during ventilation or failure to wean). Many affected children are surviving into

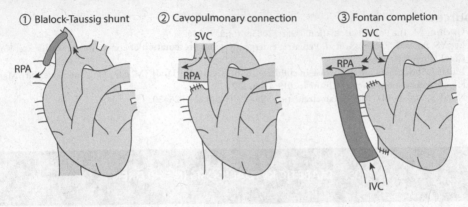

① Blalock-Taussig shunt   **② Cavopulmonary connection**   **③ Fontan completion**

Figure 104.2   Formation of the Fontan circulation.

RPA, right pulmonary artery; SVC, superior vena cava.

adulthood and could present to adult intensive care. Presentation to obstetric services later in life might involve an extremely high-risk puerperium.

Severe cyanosis
- Usually respiratory, congenital heart disease an important differential
- Murmur may not be present
- *Differentials*: transposition of the great vessels, pulmonary atresia/stenosis, Ebstein's anomaly, obstructed TAPVD, persistent pulmonary hypertension of the newborn

Cardiac failure
- Obstruction to the left side of the heart (e.g. aortic stenosis, coarctation, hypoplastic left heart)
- May present as the ductus arteriosus closes and collateral flow is lost
- Cold, pale, weak peripheral pulses, deteriorating rapidly
- Progressive hepatomegaly, pulmonary oedema, cardiomegaly, severe metabolic acidosis
- *Differentials*: sustained SVT, myocarditis, sepsis, metabolic disorders

What are the main management principles in these patients?
- *Reduce oxygen demand*: invasive ventilation may be required
- Treat respiratory disease
- Correct acidosis
- Avoid high PVR (e.g. high ventilatory pressures, hypercarbia, hypoxaemia, certain drugs)
- Consider iNO in pulmonary hypertension
- Consider keeping ductus arteriosus open with prostaglandins
- Inotropes for cardiac dysfunction
- *Discussion with specialist paediatric cardiac centre*: may require transfer ± ECMO, surgery

What is the significance of congenital heart disease to adult critical care?
Survival of patients with congenital heart disease has increased significantly in recent decades. Around 85% survive to adult life, with so-called 'adult congenital heart disease' (ACHD), which is stratified by complexity. It is possible that such patients will present to adult critical care services acutely unwell or perioperatively and an awareness of appropriate management is important.

Examples of management considerations are as follows:

- ACHD passport carried by patient
- Specialist input from regional ACHD centre
- Cardiac catheterisation might be helpful
- Transfer if appropriate (e.g. moderate to high-risk conditions)

GUIDELINE   ACC AHA 2008 ACHD

Resources

- Gwelling M. The Fontan circulation. Heart. 2005;91(6):839–846.
- Lee YS, Baek JS, Kwon BS, et al. Pediatric emergency room presentation of congenital heart disease. Korean Circ J. 2010;40(1):36–41.
- Millar J, Shock and cardiac disease in children. In: Berstein AD, Handy JM, eds., Oh's Intensive Care Manual, 8th ed. Amsterdam: Elsevier LImited; 2019: 1308–1321.
- Nayak S, Booker PD. The Fontan circulation. CEACCP. 2008;8(1):26–30.

105. DIABETIC KETOACIDOSIS IN CHILDREN

How is DKA diagnosed in children?

KEY POINT

Paediatric DKA:

- HCO_3^- < 15 mmol/l or pH < 7.30
- and ketones > 3.0 mmol/l

Severity is determined by venous pH or serum bicarbonate as follows:

- *Mild*: pH 7.20–7.29 or HCO_3^- 10–15 mmol/l
- *Moderate*: pH 7.10–7.19 or HCO_3^- 5–10 mmol/l
- *Severe*: pH < 7.10 or HCO_3^- < 5 mmol/l

How does the presentation and management of DKA differ in children?

- First presentation of diabetes more likely
- More susceptible to cerebral oedema hence difficulty in adequate fluid resuscitation
- Blood glucose will fall more readily with rehydration. Avoid insulin until 1–2 h initial therapy trialled (dose 0.05–1 units/kg/h)
- VTE thromboprophylaxis in those >16 years, indwelling lines minimised
- *Abdominal pain common*: differentials include liver swelling, gastritis, urinary retention, ileus, acute appendicitis

GUIDELINE   BSPED 2021 Children and young people with DKA

(See Chapter 149 Diabetes Emergencies)

What are the main causes of mortality in this population?

- **Cerebral oedema**
- Hypokalaemia
- Aspiration pneumonia
- Inadequate resuscitation

How should fluid therapy be managed in paediatric DKA?

Shock

- Bolus 10 ml/kg crystalloid over 15 min (0.9% NaCl currently recommend)
- Further 10 ml/kg boluses to restore adequate circulation up to a total of 40 ml/kg
- Inotropes or vasopressors may be required subsequently.

Stable
- If not shocked, consider 10 ml/kg 0.9% NaCl over 60 min.
- Replacement of deficit over 48 h
- Maintenance fluid as indicated (Holliday-Segar formula).
- Potassium supplementation (20 mmol per 500 ml fluid until glucose < 14 mmol/l)
- Monitor corrected sodium levels.
- Avoid IV sodium bicarbonate unless life-threatening hyperkalaemia or impaired myocardial contractility in the context of severe acidosis.

> **KEY POINT**
>
> Holliday-Segar formula for 24-h fluid requirement
>
> Sum of:
>
> - 100 ml/kg/day for first 10 kg body weight
> - 50 ml/kg/day for second 10 kg
> - 20 ml/kg/day for each additional kg

What signs might indicate that cerebral oedema is developing?

Early
- Headache
- Agitation or irritability
- Bradycardia
- Hypertension

Late
- Decreased level of consciousness
- Abnormal breathing pattern
- Oculomotor palsies
- Abnormal posturing
- Pupillary abnormalities

What might initial therapy for cerebral oedema include?

- Hypertonic saline (2.5–5 ml/kg of 3%) or mannitol (0.5–1 g/kg) over 15 min
- Repeated after 30 min if no improvement
- Consideration of intubation and ventilation
- CT head to exclude other diagnosis (e.g. thrombosis, haemorrhage, infarction) once treated

106. NEONATAL LIFE SUPPORT

What are the risk factors for requiring stabilisation or resuscitation at birth?

Antepartum
- Fetal
  - Intrauterine growth restriction
  - <37/40 gestation
  - Multiple pregnancy

- Congenital abnormality
- Oligo-/polyhydramnios
- Maternal
  - Infection
  - Gestational diabetes
  - Pregnancy-induced hypertension
  - Pre-eclampsia
  - High BMI
  - Short stature
  - Preterm lack of antenatal steroids

Intrapartum

- Evidence of fetal compromise
- Meconium
- Breech vaginal delivery
- Forceps/vacuum delivery
- Bleeding
- Caesarean section before 39/40
- Emergency caesarean section
- General anaesthesia

Can you describe the main steps in the newborn life support algorithm?

First 60 s

- Delay cord clamping if possible, dry the neonate unless <32/40, maintain normothermia
- Assess colour, tone, breathing, HR
- Open airway, consider CPAP if preterm
- **5 rescue breaths** (PEEP 5–6 cmH$_2$O if possible)

Ongoing

- Reassess
  - If no HR improvement, look for chest movement
  - If no chest movement, use 2-person airway control ± other manoeuvres
- **Repeat 5 breaths**
- **Ventilate for 30 s** if HR remains < 60 min^{-1}
- **Start chest compressions at 3:1** if HR < 60 min^{-1} (increase F$_I$O$_2$ to 1.0)
- Reassess every 30 s, consider venous access and drugs

The algorithm also emphasises the need to maintain temperature, consider help, titrate oxygen as guided by oximetry, as well as updating the parents and debriefing the team.

> **GUIDELINE** Resuscitation Council UK 2021 Newborn resuscitation

How is oxygen therapy managed in neonatal life support?

Starting F$_I$O$_2$:

- *Term/preterm ≥32/40*: **air**
- *28–31/40*: **0.21–0.3**
- *<28/40*: **0.3**

Target pre-ductal oxygen saturation above 25th centile for healthy term infants initially:

- *2 min*: 65%
- *5 min*: 85%
- *10 min*: 90%

Ongoing oxygenation:

- If no increase in heart rate or saturations despite effective ventilation, increase F_IO_2
- Check F_IO_2 and S_aO_2 frequently every 30 s, titrate to effect (avoid $S_aO_2 > 95\%$)

How are chest compressions performed in the neonate?

- Increase F_IO_2 to 1.0
- 3:1 compressions to breaths (15 cycles per 30 s)
- Hand encircling technique, thumbs over lower half of sternum
- Aim 1/3 depth of chest, adequate recoil

What vascular access might be used?

- Umbilical venous access first line
- IO access
- Peripheral access is likely to be difficult and inadequate for vasopressors

What drugs are used in neonatal life support?

- If bradycardic despite adequate airway, ventilation, and chest compressions, drugs may be considered:
  - Adrenaline IV/IO 20 µg/kg (intra-tracheal 100 µg/kg if necessary)
  - Repeat every 3–5 min if no response to CPR
- Glucose IV/IO 250 mg/kg (2.5 ml/kg 10% dextrose)
- Crystalloid/blood 10 ml/kg
- Sodium bicarbonate if refractory intracardiac acidosis IV/IO 1–2 mmol/kg (2–4 ml/kg 4.2%)

The Resuscitation Council UK dosing of IV adrenaline differs subtly to that mentioned in the most recent Advanced Paediatric Life Support (APLS) manual (10 µg/kg, followed by 10–30 µg/kg if unsuccessful).

APLS advocates continuation of 10% glucose infusion 100 ml/kg/day to prevent rebound hypoglycaemia as risks of hyperglycaemia are thought to be less significant in this population.

What is the role of therapeutic hypothermia in neonatal life support?

If there is clinical and/or biochemical evidence of significant risk of moderate/severe hypoxic ischaemic encephalopathy, consider inducing hypothermia.

A temperature of 33–34°C is targeted only where justified with supporting evidence. This is likely to be harmful in other circumstances. This differs to management in adult patients. (See Chapter 16 Temperature Control)

Why might there be a poor response to resuscitation?

- Oesophageal intubation
- Intubation of right main bronchus
- PTX
- Hypovolaemia
- Equipment failure
- Congenital heart disease

When should neonatal resuscitation be withheld or discontinued?

An undetectable heart rate for > 10 min after delivery should prompt review: clinical factors (e.g. dysmorphism, effectiveness of resuscitation, clinical team views about continuing).

Discontinuation should be discussed if there has been no response after **20 min,** and reversible causes have been excluded. Partial response complicates matters, and further navigation in the neonatal/paediatric ICU may be more appropriate.

Withholding resuscitation usually involves discussion with parents about evidence surrounding outcomes:

- Resuscitation is usually deemed inappropriate if > 90% predicted neonatal mortality and unacceptably high morbidity in survivors.

- If discussion has not taken place, resuscitation is usually started.
- Resuscitation is usually indicated if >50% survival rate and acceptable morbidity.
- If survival < 50%, high morbidity and anticipated burden for the child is high, seek parental wishes. These are usually supported.

Resource

- Samuels M, Wieteska S. (Eds.) Advanced Paediatric Life Support: A Practical Approach to Emergencies, 6th ed. Chichester: John Wiley & Sons; 2016.

107. PAEDIATRIC RESUSCITATION

What are the challenges of paediatric resuscitation?

- Anatomical and physiological differences
- Equipment and dosing very specific to size/age
- May not yet have presented with conditions (e.g. diabetes mellitus)
- Conditions relatively unique to paediatrics (e.g. uncorrected significant cardiac malformation)
- Variable autonomy and capacity, still developing
- Potential for longer-term implications of therapies and complications (e.g. radiation-related)
- Emotive for healthcare providers

What is your approach to managing bradycardia in children?

- Treat hypoxia and shock
- If signs of vagal overactivity give atropine (20 µg/kg)
- Otherwise give adrenaline (10 µg/kg)
- Following this, adrenaline infusion or pacing should be considered

GUIDELINE Resuscitation Council UK 2021 PALS

What is your approach to management of tachycardia with circulatory compromise?

- **Narrow complex**
  - Sinus tachycardia (infant < 220 min⁻¹, child < 180 min⁻¹, gradual onset)
    - ➢ *Treat cause*: pain, anxiety, exercise
    - ➢ *Identify precipitant*: hypovolaemia, sepsis, anaemia, cardiovascular/respiratory failure
  - SVT (infant > 200 min-1, child > 180 min⁻¹, abrupt onset)
    - ➢ Synchronised DCCV 1 J/kg, 2–4 J/kg subsequently
    - ➢ Adenosine (<1 year 150 µg/kg max 2 doses; neonate 500 µg/kg; infant 1–11 years 100 µg/kg max 12 mg; 12–17 years 3 mg, 6 mg, 12 mg)
- **Broad complex**
  - VT
    - ➢ Synchronised DCCV (start 2 J/kg then 4 J/kg subsequently)
    - ➢ Amiodarone before third shock (5 mg/kg IV infusion 20 min)

(Note: APLS and Resuscitation Council UK guidance differs in the normal range values for heart rate and the use of adenosine in shock/non-shocked states.)

How would you approach a paediatric cardiac arrest?

Follow algorithm as per 2021 guidelines:

- Recognise and call for help

- 5 rescue breaths
- CPR at 15:2 in 2-min cycles
- *Non-shockable*: adrenaline 10 µg/kg immediately
- *Shockable*: 1 × 4 J/kg DC shock
  - Adrenaline after 3 shocks (10 µg/kg), give every 3–5 min
  - Amiodarone after third and fifth shocks (both doses 5 mg/kg)
- If definitive airway, ventilate at following rates:
  - Infant 25 min^{-1}
  - 1–8 years 20 min^{-1}
  - 8–12 years 15 min^{-1}
  - 12+ 10–12 min^{-1}

When is ECLS indicated?

IHCA
- Presumed reversible cause
- Where conventional resuscitation doesn't lead to ROSC promptly
- In an appropriate context to rapidly initiate ECLS

Out-of-hospital hypothermic cardiac arrest may be suitable for E-CPR where cannulation is possible pre-hospitally.

Resource
- Samuels M, Wieteska S. (Eds.) Advanced Paediatric Life Support: A Practical Approach to Emergencies, 6th ed. Chichester: John Wiley & Sons; 2016.

---

108. PAEDIATRIC SEPSIS

How is sepsis defined in the paediatric population?
The 2016 Sepsis-3 definition of sepsis applies more to the adult population. Formal revisions in paediatrics are yet to be made, and the 2005 definition remains in use for severe sepsis.

> **KEY POINT**
>
> **Paediatric sepsis** can be defined as per Sepsis-3 as a life-threatening organ dysfunction caused by a dysregulated host response to infection.
>
> **Severe sepsis (paediatric)**
> - ≥2 SIRS criteria
> - Confirmed or suspected invasive infection
> - Cardiovascular dysfunction, ARDS, or ≥2 other organ system dysfunctions
>
> **Septic shock (paediatric)**
> - Severe infection
> - Leading to cardiovascular dysfunction (hypotension, need for vasoactive medication, or impaired perfusion)

GUIDELINE   SSC 2020 Sepsis in children

(See Chapter 26 Sepsis)

What are the paediatric SIRS criteria?

Paediatric SIRS criteria are in keeping with those used previously in definitions in the adult population, with subtle differences including the use of age-appropriate observations. Heart rate criteria rely on the absence of external stimulus, chronic drugs, painful stimuli, and vagal stimulus.

Paediatric SIRS is defined by the presence of ≥2 of the 4 criteria (one must be abnormal temperature or WCC) (Table 108.1).

How are paediatric organ dysfunctions defined?

For each system, the presence of any of the main criteria listed will define organ dysfunction:

- **Respiratory**
  - P/F < 300 in absence of cyanotic heart disease or pre-existing lung disease
  - P_aCO_2 > 20 mmHg over baseline
  - Need for non-elective invasive or non-invasive mechanical ventilation
- **Cardiovascular** (despite isotonic IV bolus ≥40 ml/kg in 1 h)
  - Hypotension > 5th percentile for age **or** systolic BP < 2 SD below normal for age
  - Need for vasoactive drug (dopamine > 5 µg/kg/min or any dose of other)
  - ≥2 of the following:
    - ➤ *Unexplained metabolic acidosis*: base deficit > 5.0 mEq/l
    - ➤ Increased arterial lactate > 2 × upper limit normal
    - ➤ UO < 0.5 ml/kg/h
    - ➤ CR > 5 s
    - ➤ Core-to-peripheral temperature gap > 3°C
- **Neurological**
  - GCS ≤11
  - Acute change in mental status with GCS decrease ≥3 from abnormal baseline
- **Renal**
  - Creatinine ≥2 × upper limit normal for age
  - 2 × baseline creatinine
- **Hepatic**
  - Bilirubin ≥4 mg/dl
  - ALT 2 × upper limit normal for age
- **Haematological**
  - Platelets < 80 × 10⁹/l
  - 50% drop in platelet count from highest in last 3 days (chronic haematology/oncology patients)
  - INR > 2

Table 108.1 Paediatric SIRS criteria

Criterion		0–1 week	1 week–1 month	1 month–1 year	2–5 years	6–12 years	13–17 years
Temperature (°C)		>38.5, < 36					
WCC (× 10⁹/l)		>34	>19.5, < 5	>17.5, < 5	>15.5, < 6	>13.5, < 4.5	>11, < 4.5
		>10% immature neutrophils					
HR (min⁻¹)	>2 SD above normal	>180			>140	>130	>110
	Unexplained persistent elevation for 0.5–4 h						
	<10th percentile	<100	<100	<90			
	Unexplained persistent depression for 0.5 h						
RR (min⁻¹)	>2 SD above normal	>50	>40	>34	>22	>18	>14
	Mechanical ventilation for acute process unrelated to underlying neuromuscular disease/GA						

What are the other important differentials of neonatal collapse?

Neonates may not present with a typical picture. Other than sepsis, neonatal collapse may also be due to other groups of disorders, predominantly:

- **Cardiac** (second most common after sepsis)
- **Trauma** (including non-accidental injury)
- **Metabolic**
- **Surgical**

How are antimicrobials managed in paediatric sepsis?

Current guidance includes the following:

- *Septic shock*: start antimicrobials as soon as possible, < 1 h of recognition
- *Organ dysfunction*: start antimicrobials as soon as possible after evaluation, < 3 h recognition
- Empiric broad-spectrum therapy to cover all likely pathogens
- Narrow cover once culture result known
- Daily assessment for de-escalation

What other resuscitative measures are suggested?

- Source control as soon as possible
- Balanced crystalloid bolus **40–60 ml/kg in 10 ml/kg challenges** during first hour if septic shock or organ dysfunction
    - Avoid fluid bolus in absence of hypotension
- Adrenaline or NA suggested rather than dopamine as has been used previously
    - Add vasopressin if high dose
- IV hydrocortisone in refractory haemodynamic instability
- High PEEP in sepsis-induced paediatric ARDS
- iNO only as a rescue therapy in refractory hypoxaemia
- Transfusion threshold Hb 70 g/l

Which therapies should not be used?

- Colloids
- Routine use of levothyroxine in sick euthyroid state
- Prokinetics for feed intolerance
- Trace elements and vitamins
- Routine IVIg unless specific indication
- Prophylactic platelet or plasma transfusion in non-bleeding state with coagulation abnormalities

When might extracorporeal support be indicated?

- *RRT*: fluid overload unresponsive to fluid restriction and diuresis
- *VV-ECMO*: sepsis-induced paediatric ARDS with refractory hypoxaemia
- *VA-ECMO*: refractory septic shock
- Plasma exchange is not recommended

Resource

- Goldstein B, Giroir B, Randolph A, et al. International pediatric sepsis consensus conference: Definitions for sepsis and organ dysfunction in pediatrics. Pediatric Crit Care Med. 2005;6(1):2–8.

109. PAEDIATRIC TRAUMA

Can you describe the epidemiology of paediatric trauma?

- Incidence higher in males than females
- Type of injury related to stage of development
- 2–6 × mortality from injury in social class V (attributed to overcrowding, poor housing, fewer safety-related adaptations)
- More common in families with mental illness, substance abuse, marital discord, moving home

What are the commonest injuries causing death in paediatrics?

- Motor vehicle collisions
- Drownings
- Burns
- Falls from height
- Poisonings

Name some types of injury prevention.

- *Primary*: speed limits, cycle lanes, fireguards, child-resistant medication closures
- *Secondary*: fitted seatbelts, bicycle helmets
- *Tertiary*: application of cold water to burns, pressure to laceration, CPR training

Are there any special considerations to injury patterns in children?

The physiology of children can vary significantly depending on age, and some differences may mitigate or exacerbate injury effects.

Chest

- Relatively elastic tissue so rib fractures sign of high energy transfer, serious injury may occur without fracture
- High incidence of pulmonary contusion

Abdomen

- Blunt injury, commonly due to road collisions
- Thin wall, less protective
- Liver and spleen low and more anterior, more exposed
- Bladder intra-abdominal so more exposed

Head

- Most commonly due to road traffic collisions
- Most common single cause of trauma death
- Fontanelle/sutures relevant to ICP under 12–18 months of age (may have significant bleed and Hb drop) before overt neurological change
- Prone to cerebral oedema

Spine/limbs

- Extremity injury is common but unlikely to be life-threatening in polytrauma and should not distract from main life-threatening injuries.
- Pelvic fractures are relatively uncommon.
- Closed femoral fractures may cause 20% circulating volume loss.
- Significant spinal cord damage can occur without fracture.
- *Spinal imaging*: plain film before MR, avoidance of CT due to susceptibility to radiation
- If GCS < 13, whole spine and head CT are indicated

Which presentations might alert you to physical non-accidental injury?

Physical abuse may present with the following:

- *Head injuries*: fractures, SDH, signs of raised ICP
- *Fractures*: long bones (possibly multiple, different stages of healing), spine, ribs
- Ruptured abdominal viscus
- *Burns and scalds*: glove and stocking, imprints
- Cold injury
- Poisoning
- Suffocation
- *Bruising*: non-mobile infant, non-exposed areas, imprints

It is important to also consider signs of neglect, emotional abuse, and sexual abuse.

What approach would you take to managing the seriously injured child?

- Similar principles apply to the management of the adult trauma patient (see Chapter 49 Major Trauma)
- *Primary survey*: <C>A+CBCDE
  - Catastrophic external haemorrhage control is paramount and may be managed with direct pressure, haemostatic dressings, or tourniquet in the first instance. TXA should be given as soon as possible.
- *Secondary survey*: head, face, neck, chest, abdomen, pelvis, spine/back, extremities
- *Continuing stabilisation*: respiration, circulation, nervous system, metabolism, host defence
- Consideration of non-accidental injury and safeguarding issues

What are the doses of resuscitative agents in paediatric haemorrhage?

KEY POINT

- *TXA*: 15 mg/kg
- *Packed red cells/FFP*: 5 ml/kg
- *Crystalloid*: 10 ml/kg
- After 20 ml/kg blood products:
  - 10–15 ml/kg platelets
  - 0.1 ml/kg 10% calcium chloride
- *Cryoprecipitate*:10 ml/kg
- Activated factor VII (NovoSeven®) after 2 cycles

What transfusion targets will you aim for?

Transfusion targets should be used second line to restoration of circulating volume and cessation of bleeding.

KEY POINT

- Platelets > 50 × 10^9/l
- Fibrinogen > 1 g/dl
- Ionised calcium > 1 mmol/l
- Hb 80–120 g/l

How would you determine a child's conscious level?

Children aged <4 years require the modified Children's GCS:

Eye opening
4   Spontaneous
3   Verbal

2 Pain
1 No response to pain

Best motor response
6 Spontaneous or obeys command
5 Localises or withdraws to touch
4 Withdraws from pain
3 Abnormal flexion to pain (decorticate)
2 Abnormal extension to pain (decerebrate)
1 No response to pain

Best verbal response*
5 Alert; babbles, coos words to usual ability
4 Less than usual words, spontaneous irritable cry
3 Cries only to pain
2 Moans to pain
1 No response to pain

*Pre-verbal patients should be assessed with a 'grimace' response as follows:

5 Spontaneous normal facial/oromotor activity
4 Less than usual spontaneous ability or only response to touch stimuli
3 Vigorous grimace to pain
2 Mild grimace to pain
1 No response to pain

When would an emergency (<1 h) CT scan be indicated in a child with a head injury?

KEY POINT

CT head criteria in children
One of the following:

- Suspected non-accidental injury
- Seizure and no history of epilepsy
- Initial departmental GCS < 14 or < 15 under 1 year
- 2-h GCS < 15
- Suspected open/depressed fracture/tense fontanelle
- Suspected basal skull fracture
- Focal neurology
- <1 year with bruise/swelling/laceration > 5 cm on the head

Two of the following:

- Loss of consciousness > 5 min
- Abnormal drowsiness
- 3 × discreet vomiting episodes
- Dangerous mechanism
- Amnesia > 5 min (retro/anterograde)

(See Chapter 49 Major Trauma, Chapter 53 Drowning, Chapter 54 Burns, and Chapter 55 Electrical Injury)

Resource
- Samuels M, Wieteska S. (Eds.) Advanced Paediatric Life Support: A Practical Approach to Emergencies, 6th ed. Chichester: John Wiley & Sons; 2016.

110. PIMS-TS

Can you name some inflammatory syndromes that present in children?

- Kawasaki disease
- TSS
- Sepsis
- Macrophage activation syndrome (MAS)
- Haemophagocytic lymphohistiocytosis (HLH)
- Paediatric multisystem inflammatory syndrome temporally associated with SARS-CoV-2 (PIMS-TS)

(See Chapter 144 Haemophagocytic Lymphohistiocytosis)

When might you diagnose PIMS-TS?

PIMS-TS emerged during the COVID-19 pandemic (2020).

The Royal College of Paediatrics and Child Health (RCPCH) case definition for PIMS-TS is as follows:

- Child presenting with persistent fever, inflammation, evidence of organ dysfunction, with additional features
- Exclusion of other microbial cause, TSSs, other infective myocarditis

SARS-CoV-2 PCR testing may be positive or negative. Inflammation is indicated by neutrophilia, elevated CRP, and lymphopaenia. The main differential is Kawasaki disease, and it may be difficult to distinguish between the 2 conditions.

GUIDELINE RCPCH 2020 PIMS-TS

What clinical features might you see?

All will have the following:

- **Persistent fever > 38.5°C**
- **Oxygen requirement**
- **Hypotension**

Other features are as follows:

- A/B
  - Mucus membrane changes
  - Neck swelling
  - Respiratory symptoms
  - Cough
  - Sore throat
  - Lymphadenopathy
- C
  - Syncope
- D
  - Confusion
  - Headache
  - Conjunctivitis
- E
  - Abdominal pain
  - Diarrhoea
  - Vomiting
  - Rash
  - Swollen hands and feet

What investigation findings might you expect?

Laboratory (all)
- High fibrinogen, CRP, D-dimer, ferritin, neutrophils
- Low albumin, lymphocytes
- Absence of other causative organisms on blood culture/PCR

Sometimes
- High IL-10, IL-6
- High CK, LDH, triglycerides, transaminitis, troponin
- Thrombocytopaenia
- Proteinuria
- AKI
- Anaemia
- Coagulopathy

Imaging
- *CXR*: patchy infiltrates, effusion
- *Echo*: myocarditis, valvulitis, effusion, coronary artery dilatation
- *Abdominal US*: colitis, ileitis, lymphadenopathy, ascites, hepatosplenomegaly

Other recommended initial investigations are as follows: blood film, glucose, blood gas with lactate, pro-BNP, vitamin D, and amylase.

What microbiological tests should you request?

- Urine, blood, stool, throat swab MC+S
- *Nasopharyngeal aspirate/throat swab PCR*: respiratory panel, SARS-CoV-2
- *Blood PCR*: pneumococcal, meningococcal, group A *Streptococcus*, *Staph. aureus*, EBV, CMV, adenovirus, enterovirus, SARS-CoV-2
- *Stool PCR*: SARS-CoV-2, viral screen
- SARS-CoV-2 serology
- Anti-streptolysin titre (ASOT)
- Enterotoxin, staph toxins

What management principles apply to children with PIMS-TS?

- Treat as suspected COVID-19, use appropriate PPE.
- Evaluate degree of cardiac dysfunction.
- Suspect multisystem involvement.
- Empirical antibiotics are usually indicated on presentation.
- Early involvement of critical care services, infectious diseases, immunology, rheumatology
- Anticoagulation may be required.
- Immunomodulation on discussion with MDT
- Consider IVIg if Kawasaki disease or TSS criteria fulfilled.
- Consideration for recruitment into research studies

What critical care involvement may be required?

The commonest presentation in the critically ill is with shock, and 60% of patients require mechanical ventilation, often for cardiovascular indications. Respiratory failure is uncommon.

Critical care support often involves vasopressors, central venous access, ± inotropes for cardiac dysfunction. ECLS may be indicated rarely. RRT is uncommon.

What is the prognosis of PIMS-TS?

Most patients survive, with an average LOS in paediatric ICU of approximately 3–4 days.

Resources

- Paediatric Intensive Care Society. Paediatric Inflammatory Multi-system Syndrome – temporally associated with SARS-CoV (PIMS-TS): Critical care guidance. May 2020. Available from: https://pccsociety.uk/wp-content/uploads/2020/05/PIMS-TS-Critical-Care-Clinical-Guidance-v4.pdf. (Accessed 06 January 2022.)
- Penner J, Abdel-Mannan O, Grant K, et al. Six-month multidisciplinary follow-up and outcomes of patients with paediatric inflammatory multisystem syndrome (PIMS-TS) at a UK tertiary paediatric hospital: a retrospective cohort study. Lancet Child Adolesc Health. 2021;5(7):473–482.

111. TOXIC SHOCK SYNDROME

What is toxic shock syndrome?

TSS is an acute inflammatory multisystem disorder mediated by exotoxin release from severe Gram-positive infections. It is characterised by early shock, rash, desquamation, and fever.

What causes TSS?

- *Strep. pyogenes* (group A)
  - Burns
  - Necrotising fasciitis
- *Staph. aureus*
  - Menstrual products
  - Nasal packing
  - Intrauterine devices
  - *Soft tissue infection*: burns, surgical wounds, post-partum
  - Pneumonia

How might this condition present?

- Fever, flu-like symptoms
- Tissue swelling, erythema, rash
- Flu-like symptoms
- Circulatory compromise and multi-organ dysfunction
- Myocarditis
- Severe pain in extremity
- Abdominal pain and tenderness
- Endophthalmitis
- Hypothermia

Which investigations may aid diagnosis and management?

General

- Blood cultures (positive in 60% *Strep.* and < 5% *Staph.*)
- MC+S pleural fluid, peritoneal fluid, tissue, throat swab, CSF
- FBC, U&E, LFT, albumin, calcium, lactate, CK, coagulation profile
- *Urinalysis*: haemoglobinuria
- *CXR*: ARDS

Specific

- *Serology*: Rocky Mountain spotted fever (a rickettsia), leptospirosis, measles
- Acute and convalescent staphylococcal antibody
- Streptococcal exotoxin subtypes

How is toxic shock diagnosed?

Streptococcal TSS

- *Probable*: **clinical case definition** in absence of another identified aetiology + isolation of group A *Streptococcus* from nonsterile site
- *Confirmed*: as above but from normally sterile site (blood, CSF, joint, pleural, pericardial)

Clinical case definition for streptococcal TSS is as follows:

- Hypotension (SBP ≤90 mmHg or 5th centile if age < 16 years)
- *Multi-organ involvement (≥2 systems)*:
  - *Renal*: creatinine ≥177 μmol/l or ≥2 × upper limit normal or baseline
  - *Haematologic*: platelets ≤100 × 10⁹/l
  - *Liver*: ALT, AST, or bilirubin ≥2 × upper limit normal or baseline
  - ARDS
  - Generalised erythematous macular rash that may desquamate
  - Soft-tissue necrosis including necrotising fasciitis or myositis, or gangrene

Non-streptococcal TSS

- *Probable*: laboratory criteria + ≥4 **clinical criteria**
- *Confirmed*: laboratory criteria + 5 clinical criteria (including desquamation)

Laboratory criteria

- Negative blood/CSF cultures (except blood culture for *Staph. aureus*)
- Negative serology for Rocky Mountain spotted fever, leptospirosis, measles

Clinical criteria

- Temperature ≥38.9°C
- *Rash*: diffuse macular erythroderma
- *Desquamation*: 1–2 weeks after rash onset
- *Hypotension*: as above
- Multisystem involvement (≥3 organ systems)
  - *GI*: vomiting/diarrhoea
  - *Muscular*: severe myalgia or CK twice upper limit of normal
  - *Mucous membrane*: oropharyngeal/conjunctival/vaginal hyperaemia
  - *Renal*: urea/creatinine twice upper limit of normal or urinary sediment with pyuria without UTI
  - *Liver*: as above
  - *Haematologic*: as above
  - *CNS*: altered level of consciousness without focal signs (when fever and hypotension absent)

How is TSS managed?

Specific
- **Source control**
  - *Antimicrobials*: broad-spectrum (e.g. beta-lactam) plus antitoxin (e.g. clindamycin, linezolid)
  - May require immediate debridement
- **IVIg** in streptococcal TSS
- *Possible in future*: hyperbaric oxygen, anti-TNF, pentoxifylline

Supportive care
- Supportive therapy including high fluid requirement
- Corticosteroids as indicated
- Wound care
- Notification of public health services

Primary prevention is best:

- Handwashing
- Hygiene measures
- Avoidance of extended tampon use
- Isolation until 24 h post start of antibiotic course in *Strep.* throat

What is the mortality in TSS?

- *Streptococcal*: 30–85%
- *Staphylococcal*: 5% non-menstrual, 1.8% menstrual

Resources

- Centers for Disease Control and Prevention. Streptococcal Toxic Shock Syndrome. 2022. Available from: https://www.cdc.gov/groupastrep/diseases-hcp/Streptococcal-Toxic-Shock-Syndrome.html. (Accessed 06 January 2022.)
- Centers for Disease Control and Prevention. Toxic Shock Syndrome (Other Than Streptococcal) (TSS) 2011 Case Definition. 2021. Available from: https://ndc.services.cdc.gov/case-definitions/toxic-shock-syndrome-2011/. (Accessed 04 March 2022.)

MICROBIOLOGY

112. ANTIMICROBIAL STEWARDSHIP

What are the mechanisms of antimicrobial resistance?

Pathogens may be intrinsically resistant, or resistance may be induced or evolve. Broad-spectrum agent use is relevant to the development of resistance. Infection with resistant organisms is associated with poor outcome if not treated appropriately (e.g. in VAP).

> **KEY POINT**
>
> Mechanisms of resistance are as follows:
>
> - *Inactivation*: enzyme production (e.g. beta-lactamase – beta-lactam antibiotics)
> - *Target site modification*: structural changes to bacterial components (e.g. ribosomal proteins – macrolides)
> - *Decreased cell wall permeability*: structural changes to cell wall/channels/transporters (e.g. porins in pseudomonas – imipenem)
> - *Active expulsion*: modification of efflux pumps (e.g. enterobacter – tetracyclines)
> - *Metabolic*: development of alternative pathway or target (e.g. peptidoglycan production in MRSA – flucloxacillin [methicillin])

Which resistant organisms are you aware of and which agents might be effective against them?

- *MRSA*: vancomycin, teicoplanin
- *Clostridium difficile*: vancomycin, metronidazole, fidaxomicin (complications may require surgery)
- *Vancomycin-resistant Enterococcus (VRE)*: linezolid, tigecycline
- *ESBL (e.g. E. coli, K. pneumoniae)*: carbapenems
- *Carbapenemase-producing Enterobacteriaceae (CPE)*: carbapenems (an increasing problem in many units)
- *Pseudomonas*: aminoglycoside, piperacillin-tazobactam, quinolones, carbapenems
- *Other gram negatives (e.g. Acinetobacter spp., Stenotrophomonas maltophilia)*: carbapenems, gentamicin; quinolones

Increasingly resistant bacteria can be remembered with the 'ESCAPE' acronym:

- *Enterococcus faecium* (VRE)
- *S. aureus* (MRSA)

- *C. difficile*
- *Acinetobacter baumannii*
- *P. aeruginosa*
- *Enterobacteriaceae* (e.g. *K. pneumoniae, E. coli*)

(See Chapter 137 Diarrhoea)

What do you understand by the term 'antimicrobial stewardship' in critical care?

Antimicrobial stewardship is the practice of linking infection control measures with judicious antibiotic management. The aim is to optimise drug choice, timing, dose, and duration in order to eradicate infection whilst reducing the negative effects of antimicrobials:

- Nosocomial infection
- Toxicity
- Resistant organisms
- Associated costs

Antimicrobial stewardship programmes should be overseen by a MDT involving clinicians, clinical pharmacists, and clinical microbiologists/infection specialists.

What strategies might be used in antibiotic stewardship?

- *Prospective audit and feedback*: antimicrobial ward round recommended
- *Formulary restriction*: by clinical area, speciality, seniority (e.g. if broad spectrum)
- *Evidence-based guidelines*: including local patterns
- *Antibiotic optimisation*: de-escalation, short courses, enteral conversion if possible
- *Antibiotic cycling*: planned withdrawal for scheduled period, 'antibiotic holiday'
- *Restrictive antibiotic strategies*: avoiding prescription without significant evidence
- *Dose optimisation*: avoidance of subtherapeutic doses
- *Education and training*: mandatory training, awareness, pharmacist guidance
- *Information technology and computer-assisted support*: safety alerts, decision tools
- *Microbiology laboratories*: systems facilitating culture, identifying sensitivity/resistance
- *Leadership and teamwork*: coordination by hospital management board

Biomarker evaluation is underway and may be helpful in future. PCT is a precursor of calcitonin that is produced in the thyroid C cells. Infection triggers its release. Clinical trials have focused on the role of serum PCT testing in clinical practice recently, and evaluation is ongoing. So far, it has been found to reduce antibiotic duration (used in de-escalation) but with no change in mortality.

Which factors might impact bactericidal activity of antibiotics?

- *Minimum inhibitory concentration (MIC)*: concentration of antimicrobial required to completely inhibit visible growth of a target organism (in vitro)
- *Time-dependent killing*: bactericidal when concentration above MIC consistently (e.g. penicillins, cephalosporins, carbapenems)
- *Concentration-dependent killing*: bactericidal when peak concentration at infection site above a certain level is achieved (e.g. aminoglycosides, metronidazole)
- *Area under curve (AUC)/MIC*: both concentration- and time-dependent killing effects (e.g. quinolones, macrolides, glycopeptides)

What is SDD?

SDD is a strategy in which oral, enteral, and systemic antimicrobials are used to decontaminate the GI tract. It is based on the theory that most infections in ICU arise from endogenous bacterial colonisation.

SDD has been shown to reduce overall mortality by 6% and the odds ratio of lower airway infections. It is not practised commonly in the UK. Evidence is limited, and there are concerns about antimicrobial resistance (although not demonstrated).

Resources

- Inweregbu K, Dave J, Pittard A. Nosocomial infections. CEACCP. 2005;5(1):14–17.
- Johnson I, Banks V. Antibiotic stewardship in critical care. BJA Educ. 2017;17(4):111–116.
- Varley AJ, Williams H, Fletcher S. Antibiotic resistance in the intensive care unit. CEACCP. 2009;9(4):114–118.

---

113.   BACTERIAL INFECTION

How common is fever in critical care patients?

Fever is common and will affect most patients during a critical care stay. It may be difficult to distinguish between infectious and non-infectious sources. Data depend on threshold temperature and population studied:

General critical care population
- One study found infection responsible for 73% pyrexia episodes
  - Pneumonia responsible for 70% of these
- Another found 44% incidence of fever (≥38.3°C)
  - Highest in patients with trauma/neurological disease
  - Cultures positive in 17% fever and 31% high-fever episodes
  - Cultures more likely to be positive in medical population

Post-operative admission
- 26% patients affected by fever
- 46% fevers due to infection, more likely if present at time of admission in emergency
- *Elective surgery*: early fever < 72 h likely to be non-infectious

Acute neurological conditions
- Incidence of fever 23–51%
- Highest amongst patients with TBI/SAH, lowest in acute ischaemic stroke
- Infection more common in TBI, central fever more likely in SAH
- *SAH*: fever < 72 h of admission likely to be non-infectious

(See Chapter 59 Malignant Hyperthermia)

Which sources of infection might be relevant in critical care?

Bacteraemia, pneumonia, and UTI are typically considered in a 'septic screen'. However, many other systems could be responsible for infection. All relevant potential sources should be considered. A detailed history (or collateral), focused examination, and appropriate investigation should be involved. Pathogens may be bacterial, viral, fungal, or parasitic.

Notable sources
- *A*: dental abscess, mucosal lesions, sinusitis, tonsillitis
- *B*: tracheitis, pneumonia, empyema, TB
- *C*: IE
- *D*: meningitis, encephalitis, cerebral abscess, botulism, tetanus
- *E*: cellulitis, necrotising fasciitis, otitis media, lymphangitis, Lyme disease, septic arthritis, pressure sores
- *F*: UTI, pyelonephritis
- *G*: cholecystitis, cholangitis, intra-abdominal abscess, diverticulitis, appendicitis, peritonitis, perforated viscus/GI tract, gastroenteritis
- *GU*: pelvic inflammatory disease, prostatitis, epididymo-orchitis, sexually transmitted infections

What specific features might your history cover when investigating a pyrexia of unknown origin?

In addition to usual components of history taking such as systems review and functional status, the following are particularly relevant to patients with pyrexia:

- *Presentation*: time course, detailed symptomatology, recent issues (e.g. back pain)
- *Fever*: onset, duration, severity, course, exacerbating/relieving factors, rigors
- *Symptoms*: weight loss, night sweats, skin lesions, systems review
- *Vaccination*: national, specific diseases, occupational requirements
- *Contact*: unwell close contacts, occupations, living situation
- *Activities*: travel abroad, country of origin, hobbies, animal contact, drug misuse, alcohol, smoking
- *Relevant diseases*: HIV, sickle cell disease, immunocompromise, malignancy, malnutrition, autoimmune conditions, previous infectious diseases
- *GU*: pain, lesions, menstruation, contraception, pregnancy, miscarriage, sexual transmission (may be history of abuse)
- *Surgical*: splenectomy, prostheses, recent operations

Which factors are important when considering how to manage a suspected bacterial infection in critical care?

- *Suspected source*: broad or narrow spectrum, required tissue penetration, institutionalisation
- *Toxin production*
- *Type of cover*: empirical treatment, culture positive, prophylaxis
- *Route*: note poor enteral absorption, high IV fluid volumes, bioavailability
- *Existing culture results*: screening (e.g. CPE, MRSA), previous infections
- *Severity of illness*: refractory septic shock vs pyrexia in stable patient
- *Comorbidity*: renal/liver dysfunction, allergies, concomitant medications, susceptibility to specific side effects
- *Extra-corporeal circuits*: CVVH, ECMO
- *Local antimicrobial guidelines*: formulary, local resistance patterns, hospital policy
- *Microbiology review*: daily input recommended

(See Chapter 26 Sepsis and Chapter 112 Antimicrobial Stewardship)

How would you prescribe an antibiotic?

Antibiotic prescribing should follow the principles of antimicrobial stewardship according to local policy. Of note, course length should be specified where known or estimated. The indication should be recorded appropriately, including for empirical courses. Drug interactions should be anticipated and managed appropriately (e.g. withholding statin in the presence of clarithromycin).

When would you consider stopping an antibiotic?

Course lengths are usually individualised in critical care and may be unpredictable. An antibiotic course would usually cover a typical time frame for a specific infection.

Clinical improvement or stabilisation would also be expected, for example:

- Improvement in gas exchange
- Resolving pyrexia
- Reduced secretion volume
- Resolution in CXR infiltrates

Prolonged course lengths (weeks onwards) might be anticipated in patients with certain conditions. Examples are as follows:

- CNS infection
- IE
- Osteomyelitis
- Abscess, empyema

Biomarkers may be useful in future. (See Chapter 112 Antimicrobial Stewardship)

Which antibiotics are most commonly associated with anaphylaxis?

Although surgical prophylaxis and treatment may involve different spectra of diseases and antibiotics to the critical care population, the NAP 6 report shared some insight into the risk of anaphylaxis with different therapies.

Perioperative anaphylaxis was caused by antibiotics in 46% of cases; 89% of these were due to co-amoxiclav or teicoplanin. The most prevalent antibiotics were co-amoxiclav, teicoplanin, and cefuroxime. Elective orthopaedic patients were most likely to be affected due to high usage of teicoplanin. Hypotension was the most common first clinical feature (42%).

Antibiotic anaphylaxis rate per 100000 administrations (4:100000 overall) is as follows:

- *16.4*: **teicoplanin**
- *8.7*: **co-amoxiclav**
- *5.7*: vancomycin
- *3.5*: piperacillin-tazobactam
- *0.94*: cefuroxime
- *0.94*: flucloxacillin
- *0.49*: gentamicin
- *0.37*: metronidazole

(See Chapter 42 Anaphylaxis)

A patient's GP record indicates that they have an allergy to penicillin. There is a previous cephalexin prescription. Is it safe to prescribe ceftriaxone?

The nature of the reaction is important when considering an allergy history. It would be prudent to find out more information about the penicillin allergy if possible. Attribution of penicillin allergy was discovered to be unfounded in >90% cases of teicoplanin anaphylaxis in the NAP 6 study, and the risks of alternative choices must be considered. Emphasis has been placed on improving allergy history taking. It would be reasonable to extrapolate this to patients admitted to critical care, where collateral history may be more significant.

Beta-lactam cross-reactivity is worth considering. Cross-reactivity with penicillins was more significant with first-generation cephalosporins such as cephalexin. Cefuroxime is a third-generation cephalosporin; this class is thought to demonstrate negligible cross-reactivity. Carbapenem cross-reactivity is thought to be less than 1%.

Prior exposure to an antibiotic (e.g. cephalexin in this example) does not mean that it will be tolerated in future. In fact, it may have acted as a sensitising event for future reactions. Patients with penicillin allergy may also lose sensitivity and tolerate it later in life.

In summary, further information is needed, but cross-reactivity is unlikely. There is no reassurance that a primary allergy to cephalexin or ceftriaxone will not occur.

Resources

- Campagna JD, Bond MC, Schabelman E, et al. The use of cephalosporins in penicillin-allergic patients: a literature review. J Emerg Med. 2012;42(5):612–620.
- Harper NJN, Cook TM, Garcez T, et al. Anaesthesia, surgery, and life-threatening allergic reactions: management and outcomes in the 6th National Audit Project (NAP6). Br J Anaesth. 2018;121(1):172–188.
- Maker HJ, Stroup CM, Huang V, et al. Antibiotic hypersensitivity mechanisms. Pharmacy (Basel) 2019;7(3):122.
- Niven DJ, Laupland HB. Pyrexia: aetiology in the ICU. Crit Care. 2016;20:247.
- Varley AJ, Jumoke S, Absalom AR. Principles of antibiotic therapy. CEACCP. 2009;9(6):184–188.

Can you name some viruses (or their diseases) that might be relevant to critical care?

Common

- *Orthomyxoviridae*: **Influenza A/B/C**
- *Coronaviridae*: **SARS-CoV (SARS), SARS-CoV-2 (COVID-19), Middle East respiratory syndrome (MERS)-CoV**
- *Herpesviridae*: **HSV1, HSV2, VZV, CMV, EBV**

Other

- *Paramyxoviridae*: RSV, measles, mumps, parainfluenza
- *Caliciviridae*: norovirus
- *Picornaviridae*: poliovirus, HAV, rhinovirus
- *Flaviviridae*: dengue fever, yellow fever, HCV
- *Bunyaviridae*: hantavirus
- *Rhabdoviridae*: rabies
- *Filoviridae*: Ebola, Marburg
- *Arenaviridae*: Lassa
- *Hepadnaviridae*: HBV
- *Poxviridae*: smallpox

How can human viruses be classified?

Viruses consist of DNA or RNA surrounded by a protein-based capsid, termed a nucleocapsid in combination. Nucleocapsids can be helical, icosahedral, or complex in shape. Some have lipid bilayer forming an outer envelope (or 'naked' without this).

Viruses may be classified by type of genetic material and structure, for example:

RNA

- Icosahedral
  - *Naked*: picornavirus, calicivirus, reovirus, togavirus
  - *Enveloped*: togavirus, flavivirus
- *Helical, enveloped*: coronavirus, bunyavirus, orthomyxovirus, paramyxovirus, rhabdovirus, filovirus, arenavirus
- *Complex*: retroviruses

DNA

- Icosahedral
  - *Naked*: parvovirus, papovavirus, adenoviruses
  - *Enveloped*: herpesviruses, hepadnavirus
- *Complex*: poxviruses

How might viral diseases present to critical care?

Viral disease may be relevant due to the severity of presentation.

Influenza (Type A) and **RSV** bronchiolitis cause an increase in demand for respiratory support over the winter in the UK. COVID-19 (SARS-CoV-2) resulted in global demand for critical care services for severe acute respiratory failure. SARS and MERS carry a high mortality but are less transmissible. Croup is viral in origin. (See Chapter 124 COVID-19 and Chapter 103 Bronchiolitis)

Mumps virus replicates in the upper respiratory tract and lymph nodes and may cause meningitis or encephalitis, pancreatitis, myocarditis, thyroiditis, hepatitis, or nephritis. Measles may also cause multisystem disease after the prodrome, resulting in pneumonia, myocarditis, or encephalitis.

EBV may cause infectious mononucleosis: fever, pharyngitis, headache, malaise, lethargy. Lymphadenopathy and splenomegaly may occur, and it may cause malignancy. Rarer effects include meningitis, encephalitis, haemolysis, and splenic rupture.

Rarer but significant viral infections include **viral haemorrhagic fevers**: Ebola, Marburg, Lassa, hantavirus, Crimean-Congo, Rift Valley, severe dengue, and yellow fever. These all carry a high mortality and are characterised by fever, haemorrhagic events, leukopaenia, thrombocytopaenia, liver toxicity, and renal impairment. Travel history is important.

Immunocompromised patients are also at risk of developing overwhelming viral disease through what would usually be mild infections. Notably, herpesviruses, and CMV may be reactivated in critical illness in otherwise immunocompetent patients.

Which usually mild viral infections may have severe complications in the immunocompromised?

- *Adenovirus*: hepatitis, encephalitis, pneumonia, life-threatening diarrhoea, and haemorrhagic cystitis
- *HSV*: pneumonia, hepatitis, colitis, encephalitis
- *VZV*: congenital varicella syndrome, neonatal chickenpox, pneumonia, encephalitis
- *CMV*: disseminated infection, retinitis, pneumonia

What is the significance of HSV encephalitis in immunocompromised?

HSV encephalitis may present with pyrexia, altered mental state, temporal lobe symptoms (personality/behavioural change), psychiatric symptoms, seizures, and focal neurology. CSF is usually clear with lymphocytosis, normal/slightly elevated protein, and normal glucose ratio. Mortality is 6 times higher in the immunocompromised. (See Chapter 90 Encephalitis)

How might CMV infection manifest?

- *Asymptomatic infection*: common in immunocompetent, 80% adults have antibodies
- *Placental transfer*: severe fetal brain damage or other neurology, occurs in 40% with primary infection in pregnancy
- *Infectious mononucleosis*: similar to EBV
- Reactivation in immunocompromised patient

How might viral disease be investigated?

Other than taking a full history and examining the patient, viral investigations may include the following:

- Influenza, parainfluenza, RSV, COVID-19, adenoviruses
  - *PCR*: throat/pharyngeal swabs, nasopharyngeal/tracheal aspirate, BAL
  - *PCR*: conjunctival swab (adenovirus)
- Mumps, measles
  - *Reverse transcriptase PCR*: buccal swab, saliva, CSF, urine
  - *Serology*: IgM, IgG
- HIV
  - Antibodies, p24 antigen
- HSV1, VZV
  - *PCR*: blood, CSF, lower respiratory tract, vesicle fluid
- CMV
  - *CMV-PCR and histology*: blood, lower respiratory tract, CSF, tissue specimen
  - *Serology*: IgM, IgG
- EBV
  - Peripheral blood film
  - *Serology*: IgG, IgM
  - *PCR*: blood

What specific pharmacological therapies might be used in common viral diseases?

- *Influenza*: neuraminidase inhibitors – oseltamivir, zanamivir
- *Adenovirus*: cidofovir
- *HSV1*: aciclovir
- *VZV*: aciclovir
- *EBV*: corticosteroids (if significant neurology, haemolysis, thrombocytopaenia)
- *SARS-CoV-2*: remdesivir, molnupiravir (See Chapter 124 COVID-19)

Some therapies are usually reserved for the immunocompromised or pregnant women:

- *Measles*: IVIg
- *VZV prophylaxis*: VZIg, valaciclovir
- *CMV*: ganciclovir, foscarnet
- *RSV, parainfluenza, human metapneumovirus*: aerosolised ribavirin

Consideration should be made of suspending immunosuppressive medications in significant infection.

What are standard precautions?

Standard or universal precautions are used for all patients regardless of infection status

- Hand hygiene
- Use of PPE
- Respiratory hygiene/cough etiquette
- Sharps safety
- Safe injection practices
- Sterile instruments and devices
- Clean and disinfected environmental surfaces

Other precautions may be required when standard precautions cannot prevent transmission alone: transmission-based precautions. Appropriate patient placement and limiting transport/movement of patients are essential. Cleaning and disinfection of rooms should be prioritised.

Which types of transmission-based precautions are there?

Contact precautions: pathogen transmitted by direct/indirect contact

- Single-patient room (alternatives such as cohorting may be required)
- Wear gown, gloves for contact with patient or potentially contaminated environment

Droplet precautions: pathogen spread through close respiratory/mucous membrane contact with respiratory secretions

- *Source control*: patient to wear mask
- Single-patient room ideally
- Spatial separation of ≥3 ft, drawing curtain between beds
- *PPE*: face mask for close contact, don upon entry to room

Airborne precautions: pathogen infectious over long distances when suspended in air

- *Source control*: patient to wear mask
- PPE
  - Mask or respirator depending on disease-specific recommendations, donned prior to room entry
  - *Respiratory protection programme*: education, fit-testing, seal checks
- Airborne infection isolation room
  - Monitored negative pressure relative to surrounding area
  - Specified number of air exchanges per hour
  - Air exhausted outdoors or recirculated through high-efficiency particulate absorbing (HEPA) filter

- Non-immune staff to avoid vaccine-preventable airborne disease
- Immunise susceptible persons as soon as possible after unprotected contact

Which workplace precautions are required for specific pathogens?

- *Standard universal precautions*: HIV, CMV, EBV
- *Contact precautions*: HSV1
- *Contact and droplet precautions*: influenza, parainfluenza, human metapneumovirus, adenoviruses
- *Contact, droplet, airborne precautions*: measles, SARS-CoV, MERS-CoV, VZV, SARS-CoV-2
- *Non-immune staff exclusion*: mumps, measles, VZV, smallpox
- Specific Occupational Health recommendations may be required (e.g. shielding in pregnancy).

GUIDELINE NHS 2022 Infection prevention and control

What are the 'high-consequence infectious diseases' (HCIDs)?

KEY POINT

A HCID is an acute infectious disease which is characterised by the following:

- High case-fatality rate
- Absence of effective prophylaxis or treatment
- Difficulty in recognition and rapid detection
- Ability to spread in the community and healthcare settings
- Requirement for an enhanced response

The majority of HCIDs are viral in origin. They are classified into contact and airborne groups according to mode of transmission as follows:

Contact HCID
- Argentine haemorrhagic fever (Junin virus)
- Bolivian haemorrhagic fever (Machupo virus)
- Crimean-Congo haemorrhagic fever
- Ebola virus disease
- Lassa fever
- Lujo virus disease
- Marburg virus disease
- Severe fever with thrombocytopaenia syndrome

Airborne HCID
- Andes virus infection (hantavirus)
- Avian influenza A H7N9, H5N1, H5N6, H7N7
- MERS
- Mpox (formerly 'monkeypox')
- Nipah virus infection
- Pneumonic plague (*Yersinia pestis*)
- SARS

COVID-19 was removed from the UK HCID list in March 2020.

GUIDELINE PHE 2022 HCID

How would you manage a patient with suspected viral haemorrhagic fever in critical care?

- *Specialist input*: close liaison with the infectious diseases team
- Supportive care as required
- *Isolation*: appropriate precautions (includes aerosols)
- *Diagnosis*: high index of suspicion in sick traveller from endemic area, PCR
- *Malaria cover*: send malaria thick blood films, empirical antimalarials
- *Specific treatment*: early IV ribavirin (discontinue if filoviral/flaviviral infection)
- *Notification*: local infection control, national authorities (may trigger public health investigation)
- May require transfer to national centre

Resources

- CDC. Infection Control. Part III: Precautions to Prevent Transmission of Infectious Agents. 2019. Available from: https://www.cdc.gov/infectioncontrol/guidelines/isolation/precautions.html. (Accessed 24 November 2021.)
- Geisbert TW, Jahrling PB. Exotic emerging viral diseases: progress and challenges. Nat Med. 2004;10:S110–S121.
- Johnstone C, Hall A, Hart IJ. Common viral illnesses in intensive care: presentation, diagnosis, and management. CEACCP. 2014;14(5):213–219.

115. FUNGAL INFECTION

What challenges do fungal infections in critical care patients present?

- High mortality
- Difficult distinction between infection and colonisation
- Insidious onset and non-specific signs requiring high index of suspicion
- Effects also due to direct saprophytic destruction of tissues (e.g. GI perforation)
- Significant side effects of therapeutic agents make treatment challenging.
- Patients affected have not typically endured a straightforward critical care stay.

What types of human fungal infection are you aware of?

The following groups of fungi are notable in critical care:

- Moulds: **Aspergillus**, *Zygomycetes*
- Yeasts: **Candida**, *Cryptococcus*
- Dimorphic: *Blastomyces, Histoplasma, Coccidioides*

What are the risk factors for fungal infection?

- Admission to ICU
- Immunocompromise
- *Respiratory compromise*: suppurative (cystic fibrosis, bronchiectasis), COPD, mechanical ventilation
- *Invasive procedures*: CVC, PN, urethral catheterisation, PD, prostheses
- *Other*: broad-spectrum antibiotics, contamination of sterile sites by gut bacteria (peritonitis, oesophageal perforation), IV drug misuse

What do you know about invasive candidiasis?

Candida albicans is the most common cause of fungal infection in the critically ill in the UK. *Candida* infection is usually secondary to superficial colonisation on the skin or mucous membranes. Mortality associated with candidaemia is up to 40% and higher with non-albicans species.

Invasive candidiasis is a disease caused by candidaemia resulting in haematogenous spread to end organs (e.g. heart, liver, spleen, brain, and eyes). IE and endophthalmitis are most commonly reported.

Affected indwelling lines should be removed if possible, particularly with positive *Candida parapsilosis* culture. Ophthalmology review is indicated, and echo should be performed to look for seeding/disseminated infection. Assessment for endovascular involvement is important with persistently positive blood cultures despite treatment and may require surgery.

Fluconazole is the first-line antifungal agent, followed by an echinocandin (**anidulafungin**) or amphotericin as per Trust guidelines.

How can *Aspergillus* affect the body?

- Saprophytic infection
  - **Invasive pulmonary aspergillosis**
  - Chronic necrotising pulmonary aspergillosis
  - Chronic cavitatory aspergillosis
  - *Tracheobronchial aspergillosis*
  - *Aspergillus bronchitis*
  - Extrapulmonary aspergillosis (e.g. sinus/cerebral spread)
- Other
  - Allergic bronchopulmonary aspergillosis
  - Allergic sinusitis
  - Aspergilloma
- Complications
  - Sepsis related
  - Angio-invasion (e.g. massive haemoptysis)
  - *Dissemination*: abscesses in other organs

Can you describe some features of other fungal infections?

Pneumocystis pneumonia
- Gradually progressive dyspnoea
- Dry cough
- Desaturation on exertion
- Low-grade fever
- *Air leaks*: pneumatocoeles, PTX, pneumomediastinum

Cryptococcus neoformans/gattii
- *Pulmonary cryptococcosis*: infiltrative pneumonia, effusions, hilar lymphadenopathy, nodules, collapse
- *Meningoencephalitis*: slow progression, cranial nerve signs, cryptococcomas, raised ICP (hydrocephalus due to CSF 'sludging')

Zygomycosis (e.g. mucormycosis)
- Angio-invasion
- Disseminated infection
- Extensive tissue necrosis
- Rhinocerebral form in patients with DKA

Self-limiting pneumonia (or haematogenous spread in immunocompromised)
- *Histoplasma capsulatum*: cavitating pulmonary disease, similar to TB
- *Blastomyces dermatitidis*: granulomatous skin ulcers
- *Paracoccidioides brasiliensis*: erosion and destruction of palate and orpharynx
- *Coccidioides immitis*

How might suspected fungal disease be investigated?

Serum assay for **1,3-beta-D-glucan** can be helpful in most fungal infections (alongside MC+S of any relevant body fluids/tissue/sputum/pus). False positives may occur with the use of immunoglobulin or albumin, therapies involving cellulose membranes or filters (e.g. haemodialysis, blood product filtration, gauze), and potentially some antimicrobials.

Invasive candidiasis
- Blood culture
- Serum mannan, anti-mannan
- Whole-blood PCR
- Fundoscopy: cotton-wool ball changes within retina (candidal choroidoretinitis)

Aspergillosis
- Serum/BAL galactomannan
- Whole-blood PCR
- *CT chest*: air crescent formations, halo sign, pleural wedges of consolidation
- *Histology*: confirm diagnosis with septae, branching hypae invading lung tissue

Pneumocystis jirovecii
- Sputum/BAL immunofluorescence, PCR
- CXR
- CT chest

Other
- *Cryptococcus*: lumbar puncture, antigen test, CXR
- *Zygomycosis*: whole-blood PCR, tissue scrapings/skin biopsies
- *Histoplasmosis*: antigen radioimmunoassay, blood/marrow culture, blood smear
- *Blastomycosis*: urine antigen assay
- *Paracoccidioidomycosis*: antigen complement fixation text, tissue granuloma biopsy
- *Coccidioidomycosis*: coccidioidin skin test, serum latex agglutination test, serum/CSF complement fixation test, MC+S joint fluid, lumbar puncture

Which antifungal agents are indicated in invasive aspergillosis?
First-line therapy in invasive aspergillosis is usually **voriconazole ± amphotericin** (AmBisome®), a polyene.

What are the most significant side effects of commonly used antifungal agents?

- *Fluconazole/voriconazole**: liver dysfunction, QTc prolongation, cytochrome P450 inhibition
- *Anidulafungin*: liver dysfunction
- *Amphotericin*: nephrotoxicity, anaphylactoid reaction, electrolyte disturbance, marrow suppression

When else might antifungal agents be indicated?
Prophylaxis may be given against invasive fungal infections in certain groups:

- Neutropaenia
- Immunosuppression following solid organ transplant
- HIV with low CD4 count
- ALF
- GI perforation

Pneumocystis jirovecii pneumonia (PJP) prophylaxis is usually co-trimoxazole.

High-risk patients may be given empirical cover for sepsis with antifungal therapy, usually with broad spectrum (e.g. anidulafungin).

Resources
- Beed M, Sherman R. Fungal infections and critically ill adults. CEACCP. 2014;14(6):262–267.
- Marty FM, Lowry CM, Lempitski SJ, et al. Reactivity of (1→3)-β-D-glucan assay with commonly used intravenous antimicrobials. Antmicrob Agents Chemother. 2006;50(10):3450–3453.

---

* Voriconazole requires monitoring to ensure levels are in the therapeutic range.

116. NOSOCOMIAL INFECTION

How would you define a nosocomial infection?

> **KEY POINT**
>
> Healthcare-associated infection occurring within
>
> - 48 h of hospital admission,
> - 3 days of discharge, or
> - 30 days of an operation.

Why are nosocomial infections significant?

- *Common*: 20% ICU patients, 10% hospital admissions
- Preventable in a third of cases
- *Increased morbidity and mortality*: 5000 extra deaths per year
- Increased LOS in hospital (× 2.5)

Which factors predispose to nosocomial infections?

- **Patient**
  - Advanced age
  - Malnutrition
  - Alcohol excess
  - Heavy smoking
  - Chronic lung disease
  - Diabetes
- **Disease**
  - Surgery
  - Trauma
  - Burns
- **Treatment**
  - *Invasive procedures*: tracheal intubation, CVC, RRT, drains, NG tube, tracheostomy, urinary catheter
  - Transfusion
  - Recent antimicrobials
  - Immunosuppression
  - Stress ulcer prophylaxis
  - Recumbent position
  - PN
  - Increased LOS

Can you give some examples of nosocomial infections and common causative pathogens in critical care?

- Blood stream infection (BSI)/central line-associated BSI (CLABSI)
- Pneumonia
- UTI/catheter-associated UTI (CAUTI)
- SSI

Pathogens

- Coagulase-negative *staphylococci*: BSI, CLABSI, SSI
- *Staph. aureus*: pneumonia, SSI, BSI, CLABSI

- *P. aeruginosa*: pneumonia, UTI
- *Enterococci* spp.: SSI, UTI
- *Enterobacter* spp.: pneumonia
- *E. coli*: UTI, CAUTI, SSI
- *C. albicans*: UTI, CLABSI
- *K. pneumoniae*: pneumonia

(See Chapter 25 Ventilator-Associated Pneumonia)

What are catheter-related BSI (CRBSI) and CLABSI?

KEY POINT

CRBSI

- BSI attributed to intravascular catheter by
- quantitative culture of catheter tip, or
- differences in growth between catheter/peripheral blood cultures

CLABSI

- Laboratory-confirmed BSI, in
- patient with indwelling central line ≤48 h prior to BSI development,
- unrelated to infection at another site

CLABSI is a surveillance definition, whereas CRBSI is more clinical and may not be proven. In the case of tunnelled lines, the distinction between **exit site infection** (<2 cm) vs **tunnel infection** (extending beyond 2 cm from exit site) is significant to management.

Indwelling catheters become colonised within hours of insertion. Threshold levels of organisms are likely to be relevant to the likelihood of developing infection. This is increased further by the presence of adherent thrombus, which may become infected and cause severe disease.

Infection might be suggested by signs at the insertion site, bacteraemia, resolution after removal, and positive paired blood cultures. Risk factors also include frequent accessing of the device and use for PN administration. Risk in femoral > internal jugular > subclavian catheters.

Typical organisms
- *37%*: **Coagulase-negative *Staphylococcus***
- *22%*: ***Staph. aureus***
- *12%*: enteric Gram-negative *Bacilli*
- *9%*: yeasts (e.g. *Candida* spp.)
- *5%*: *Pseudomonas*
- *5%*: *Enterococci* and *Streptococci*
- *9%*: other

How should line infections be prevented and managed?

Prevention
- **Evaluate need for indwelling devices** daily and remove if clinically appropriate
- **Catheter type**
  - ➢ Minimise lumen number for what is required
  - ➢ PN through dedicated line or lumen
  - ➢ Implantable or tunnelled line if long term (>30 days)
  - ➢ Consider antimicrobial impregnated catheter if high risk (chlorhexidine/silver, minocycline/rifampicin)
- **Site**
  - ➢ Balance of risk against mechanical risk of insertion
  - ➢ Subclavian route recommended unless contraindicated (although in practice likely to be less commonly performed)

- **ANTT**
  - ➢ Optimum technique during insertion with sterile gown, gloves, drapes
  - ➢ Disinfection of site with alcohol/chlorhexidine or alcohol/iodine, allow to dry
- **Care**
  - ➢ Disinfect external surfaces and ports before use (with above solutions)
  - ➢ Use sterile gauze or transparent dressing over insertion site
  - ➢ Flush containing anticoagulant
- **Replacement**
  - ➢ Avoid routine replacement of central lines
  - ➢ Guidewire exchange acceptable in malfunction if no evidence of infection

Management

- Ideally, **catheter removal** if infection suspected
- 'Precious' lines
  - ➢ May be appropriate to leave and treat medically
  - ➢ Guidewire exchange followed by complete replacement at other site if microbiology proves line is the source of sepsis
  - ➢ *Indications for removal rather than salvage*: persistent symptoms, septic shock, metastatic infection, persistently positive blood cultures, difficult to clear organisms, or recurrence
- **Antimicrobials** based on culture
  - ➢ 1 week once catheter removed
  - ➢ 2 weeks if *Staph. aureus* or fungal
  - ➢ Longer if deep-seated ± surgery
  - ➢ Empirical therapy should include MRSA and Gram-negative cover

The subject of 'line changes' is contentious in critical care, particularly in the context of catheters older than 7 days in a patient with fever. Around 80% catheters removed on the basis of fever and/or leukocytosis alone are sterile.

Which other strategies might prevent nosocomial infection?

Reduction in modifiable risk factors may help to reduce the incidence of nosocomial infection.

Other important strategies are as follows:

- *Hand hygiene*: poor hand hygiene responsible for 40% infections transmitted in hospitals
- Appropriate use of PPE and isolation precautions
- Management of indwelling devices (e.g. CVC as above)
- Ventilator care bundle
- Antimicrobial stewardship

(See Chapter 112 Antimicrobial Stewardship and Chapter 25 Ventilator-Associated Pneumonia)

What is the role of infection surveillance in the critical care unit?

The critical care environment has great potential to give rise to resistant organisms. Surveillance can help to identify emerging outbreaks and causative factors.

Multiple patients with similar infections at one time could indicate a problem with water-borne pathogens (e.g. *P. aeruginosa*, *Stenotrophomonas* spp.). The infection prevention/control team should be involved, and water testing might be necessary. Some units are moving towards 'water-free' care.

Active surveillance cultures have been introduced in many hospitals (e.g. CPE, MRSA, SARS-CoV-2 screening on admission). Financial penalties are also attached to some healthcare-associated infections (e.g. MRSA bacteraemia).

Resources
- Fletcher S. Catheter-related bloodstream infection. CEACCP. 2005;5(2):49–51.
- Haddadin Y, Annamaraju P, Regunath H. Central Line Associated Blood Stream Infections. 2022. Available from: https://www.ncbi.nlm.nih.gov/books/NBK430891/. (Accessed 14 February 2022.)
- Hopman J, Tostmann A, Wertheim H, et al. Reduced rate of intensive care unit acquired gram-negative bacilli after removal of sinks and introduction of 'water-free' patient care. Antimirob Resist Infect Control. 2017;6:59.
- Inweregbu K, Dave J, Pittard A. Nosocomial infections. CEACCP. 2005;5(1):14–17.

What is HIV?

Human immunodeficiency virus (HIV) is a **retrovirus** which causes illness characterised by destruction of the CD4 cells in the immune system.

Two forms of HIV virus exist: HIV-1 (more common worldwide) and HIV-2. Viral RNA is transcribed into DNA by viral reverse transcriptase enzyme. This DNA is then incorporated into the host cell's genome, preferentially in CD4+ T cells.

The HIV pandemic came to light in the 1980s, and advances in understanding and therapeutic options have resulted in a near normal life expectancy from what used to be a rapidly progressive, fatal disease. There are approximately 100000 people living with HIV in the UK, and the undiagnosed prevalence is around 0.016%. Cases are emerging of patients 'cured' of HIV with sustained remission through bone marrow transplant from donors with rare genetic mutations.

Occasional presentations to critical care still occur, and an awareness of optimal management is the key to maximising good outcomes in these patients.

How are HIV and acquired immunodeficiency syndrome (AIDS) diagnosed?

HIV infection is diagnosed based on specific laboratory testing but is undetectable immediately after exposure. Multi-test algorithms may be used, or a positive result may be diagnostic from specific serological tests (e.g. HIV-1 p24 antigen test). Antigen testing may be positive from day 18 and antibodies from 3 months. HIV is classified by the CDC into 5 stages by CD4+ cell count preferentially before percentage criteria (Table 117.1).

AIDS is Stage 3 HIV infection, characterised by **CD4+ count < 200 × 10⁶/l (or < 14%)** or immune dysfunction resulting in specific 'AIDS-defining' **opportunistic illnesses** (OIs):

- **Bacterial**
  - *Mycobacteria*: TB, avium complex*, other*
  - Recurrent pneumonia (≥2 episodes in 12 months)
  - Recurrent salmonella septicaemia
- **Fungal**
  - *P. carinii* (PJP)
  - *Candidiasis*: oesophageal, lower respiratory tract
  - *Cryptococcosis*: extrapulmonary (e.g. meningoencephalitis)
  - Histoplasmosis*
  - Coccidioidomycosis*
  - *Talaromycosis*: disseminated
- **Viral**
  - *CMV*: retinitis, other (except liver, spleen, glands)

Table 117.1   HIV classification (adult ranges given)

Stage	Description	CD4+ count (× 10⁶/l)	CD4+ cells (%)
0	Early HIV infection	Negative/indeterminate	
1	Acute HIV infection	≥500	≥26
2	Chronic HIV infection	200–499	14–25
3	AIDS	<200 or OI	<14
U	Unknown	e.g. missing information	

---

* Disseminated/extrapulmonary disease.

- *HSV*: ulcers > 1 month, bronchitis, pneumonitis
- *JC*: PML
- **Parasitic**
  - *Toxoplasmosis*: cerebral
  - *Cryptosporidiosis*: diarrhoea > 1 month
  - Isosporiasis > 1 month
  - Atypical disseminated leishmaniasis
  - *Reactivation of American trypanosomiasis*: meningoencephalitis, myocarditis
- *Neoplastic*: cervical cancer, non-Hodgkin lymphoma (NHL), Kaposi's sarcoma

When might patients with HIV present to critical care?

As with any condition, patients may present with a complication of the disease, significant side effects from treatment (e.g. toxicity causing 5% HIV-related admissions), or pathology not directly related to AIDS (70% admissions).

Bacterial sepsis and **exacerbated comorbidities** are now the leading causes of admission to ICU. **Respiratory and CNS failure** account for the majority of admissions (Table 117.2).

Severe OIs tend to occur in patients with previously unknown HIV or restricted access to antiretroviral therapy, and there may be >1 concurrent OI on presentation. The commonest presentations are as follows:

- Acute respiratory failure (40–60%)
- Bacterial sepsis (10–20%)
- Impaired consciousness (10–20%)

Organ support usage in all HIV seropositive individuals admitted to critical care is as follows:

- Invasive ventilation (40–50%)
- Vasopressors (15–30%)
- RRT for AKI (8–15%)

Table 117.2   Critical illness due to respiratory/CNS failure in patients with HIV

	Respiratory	Neurological
All stages	Bacterial pneumonia TB	Bacterial meningitis (*S. pneumoniae*)
Stage 3 (AIDS)	**PJP** Kaposi sarcoma CMV Toxoplasmosis MAC Nocardiosis Aspergillosis Rhodococcosis Histoplasmosis Cryptococcosis	**Toxoplasmosis** **TB** **Cryptococcosis** CMV Nocardiosis Aspergillosis PML HIV encephalitis NHL Neurosyphilis
Other	COPD Bronchiectasis Lung cancer Pulmonary hypertension Pulmonary fibrosis HF	Stroke Epilepsy Non-infectious encephalitis Bacterial brain abscess
Indirect	Interstitial pneumonitis Drug toxicity Asthma PE	Sepsis Endocarditis Hypoxia Metabolic disorder Drug toxicity/overdose Malignancy Thrombotic microangiopathy

Other presentations are as follows:

- Post-operative care
- GI
  - *Bleeding*: infectious ulceration, Kaposi's sarcoma, lymphoma, thrombocytopaenia (also indirectly: peptic ulceration, varices, gastritis)
  - *Bowel perforation*: CMV enteritis, Kaposi's sarcoma, lymphoma, mycobacterial infection
  - AIDS cholangiopathy
  - Pancreatitis
- AKI
  - Glomerulonephritis
  - CCF
- Cardiovascular
  - Sepsis

Can you list some significant side effects of antiretroviral medications?

> **KEY POINT**
>
> ART classification:
>
> - *NRTI (nucleoside/nucleotide reverse transcriptase inhibitors)*: abacavir, lamivudine, zidovudine, tenofovir, emtricitabine
> - *NNRTI (non-NRTI)*: efavirenz, etravirine, nevirapine, rilpivirine
> - *Integrase inhibitors*: raltegravir, dolutegravir
> - *Protease inhibitors*: atazanavir, darunavir, fosamprenavir, lopinavir, tipranavir
> - *Fusion inhibitors*: enfuvirtide
> - *CCR5 inhibitors*: maraviroc

Most antiretrovirals can cause hepatitis. Other significant severe toxicities include the following:

- *Lactic acidosis*: zidovudine, didanosine
- *Pancreatitis*: didanosine
- *AKI*: tenofovir, nevarapine
- *TEN*: tenofovir, nevirapine
- *Rhabdomyolysis*: raltegravir
- *Neutropaenia*: emtricitabine, nevirapine

What is immune reconstitution inflammatory syndrome (IRIS)?

IRIS describes a collection of inflammatory disorders associated with paradoxical worsening of pre-existing infectious processes following antiretroviral initiation. It may occur up to months after initiation.

Presentations
- Worsening of a treated condition
- Unmasking of undiagnosed OI

Effects
- Acute respiratory failure (e.g. worsening *Pneumocystis* pneumonia)
- Severe systemic inflammatory response (including HLH)
- Neurological deterioration (e.g. lesion enlargement causing raised ICP, seizures)

How would you manage antiretroviral therapy in a critical care patient known or suspected to have HIV?

Management principles differ according to whether or not patients are already established on medication at admission; 70% HIV-infected patients admitted to ICU are receiving long-term antiretroviral therapy.

Antiretroviral initiation involves weighing the benefits of HIV suppression against the potential for toxicity and IRIS in the acute setting, which requires individualisation. Liaison with infectious disease (specifically HIV) specialists is common practice. One proposed strategy:

- **Existing therapy**
  - Continue where possible
  - *Adapt dosing according to risk of toxicity*: organ failure, interactions
  - May require alternative route if GI absorption affected
- **De novo**
  - *Immediate*: severe acute OI, HIV encephalitis, PML
  - *<2 weeks*: other OI (e.g. *Pneumocystis*, extra-CNS TB)
  - *Delayed (>4 weeks, disease control)*: CNS TB, cryptococcosis
  - *Late (after ICU discharge)*: non-HIV-related admission, CD4+ > 200 × 10^6/l

Can you describe how you would diagnose and manage one of the common severe opportunistic infections?

The most common OIs in the ICU are PJP, TB, and cerebral toxoplasmosis.

PJP
- Diagnosis
  - *BAL*: *P. jirovecii* cystic/trophic forms on staining/immunofluorescence (90% sensitivity, 100% specificity)
  - *PCR*: high sensitivity, poor specificity (colonisation in 70% patients)
  - *Beta-D-glucan*: 92% sensitivity, poor specificity (80%)
  - *High-resolution CT*: reticular infiltrates, intra-parenchymal cysts, ground-glass opacities, alveolar consolidation sparing peripheries, absence of effusion or lymphadenopathy
- Management
  - Sulfamethoxazole + trimethoprim
  - *Second line*: pentamidine
  - Corticosteroids if P$_a$O$_2$ < 9 kPa (reduced invasive ventilation and in-hospital mortality)
  - Early NIV beneficial

TB
- Diagnosis
  - *All samples*: acid-fast bacilli (AFB), MC+S, PCR for *Mycobacterium tuberculosis*
  - *Meningitis*: CSF lymphocytic pleocytosis, low glucose, high protein
  - *Disseminated*: blood cultures
  - *Other*: tissue biopsy, adenosine deaminase (serositis/meningitis)
  - *Imaging*: usual patterns unless AIDS (e.g. miliary pneumonia, no cavitation)
- Management
  - *Intensive phase (2 months)*: isoniazid + rifampicin/rifabutin + pyrazinamide + ethambutol
  - *Continuation phase (6–9 months)*: isoniazid + rifampicin/rifabutin
  - Liaise with infectious diseases specialist particularly with multidrug resistance
  - *CNS*: dexamethasone (2–4 weeks, 8–10 week taper)
  - *Pericardial*: prednisolone (6 weeks)

Cerebral toxoplasmosis
- *Presentation*: altered mental state, motor deficit, seizures
- Diagnosis
  - IgG serology
  - *CSF/blood*: PCR *T. gondii* (sensitivity ≤ 50%, specificity > 95%)
  - *MR*: multifocal ring-enhanced lesions (± haemorrhagic) in cortex or basal ganglia, mass effect (oedema), rarely solitary lesion or diffuse encephalitis
- Management
  - Pyrimethamine once
  - Then pyrimethamine + sulphadiazine + leucovorin (>6 weeks)
  - *Second line*: pyrimethamine + clindamycin, or sulphamethoxazole + trimethoprim
  - Corticosteroids if mass effect

What is the prognosis?

Prognosis of HIV itself is good in patients with access to appropriate resources and good compliance with medications. Social and logistical issues and deprivation complicate disease control for many patients.

In-hospital mortality has reduced from 80% to 20–40% and now largely depends on indirect factors (e.g. age, comorbidity, extent of organ dysfunction) rather than HIV-related factors (CD4 count, viral load, AIDS-related admission, and prior antiretroviral use). ART initiation/maintenance in ICU might be associated with improved outcome.

When would HIV testing be indicated in critical care patients?

Any presentation with **AIDS-defining OI** should prompt testing. Other **indicator conditions** are relevant in the context of critical care presentation. A thorough social history is indicated.

Risk factors

- Men who have sex with men, and their female sexual partners
- Black African ethnicity
- People who inject drugs
- Sex workers
- Prisoners
- Transgender women
- People from countries with high HIV seroprevalence, and their sexual partners

British HIV Association (BHIVA) guidelines recommend testing in the following people:

- Increased risk of exposure
- Sexual partners of diagnosed individual
- Users of services where users have associated risk (e.g. sexual health clinics)
- Healthcare users in areas with high prevalence (e.g. at emergency departments)
- HIV indicator conditions (undiagnosed prevalence > 1:1000)

Notable indicator conditions

- *B*: CAP, invasive pneumococcal disease, unexplained oral candidiasis
- *D*: peripheral neuropathy, GBS
- *E*: unexplained fever
- *F*: unexplained chronic renal impairment
- *G*: unexplained weight loss, unexplained chronic diarrhoea
- *H*: malignant lymphoma, unexplained leukocytopaenia/thrombocytopaenia > 4 weeks
- *I*: VZV, HAV, HBV, HCV, candidaemia, sexually transmitted infection

Contaminated sharps injury is also an indication for testing but is controversial in the context of a donor patient lacking capacity.

GUIDELINE   BHIVA 2020 HIV Testing

Resources

- Barbier F, Mer M, Szychowiak P, et al. Management of HIV-infected patients in the intensive care unit. Intensive Care Med. 2020;46(2):329–342.
- Centers for Disease Control and Prevention. Terms, Definitions, and Calculations Used in CDC HIV Surveillance Publications. 2022. Available from: https://www.cdc.gov/hiv/statistics/surveillance/terms.html. (Accessed 24 January 2022.)
- Prout J, Agarwal B. Anaesthesia and critical care for patients with HIV infection. CEACCP. 2005;5(5):153–156.

What is malaria?

Malaria is a life-threatening tropical infection, the most common to present in the UK. It is caused by a protozoa transmitted via mosquitos. In the UK, it is seen in travellers returning from endemic areas, and compliance with chemoprophylaxis is often poor.

Around 10% malaria in the UK is considered severe, and mortality is 1% amongst all cases of *falciparum* malaria.

The major indications for critical care are cerebral involvement, renal failure, respiratory failure, and coexisting infection.

What is the causative agent?

Malaria is caused by protozoa which are carried and transmitted by anopheles mosquito. *Plasmodium falciparum* is the causative agent in nearly all serious illness. Other types are *P. vivax, P. ovale, P. malariae,* and *P. knowlesi* – rarely related to serious illness.

What are the risk factors for malaria?

- *Travel to endemic areas*: Africa, Asia, Latin America
- Mosquito bites
- Poor compliance with chemoprophylaxis

What is the pathophysiology of malaria?

The malaria life cycle relies on 2 hosts: the anopheles mosquito and humans. Human disease is caused by the asexual phases involving schizonts, trophozoites, and merozoites.

> **KEY POINT**
>
> Stages of malaria
>
> 1. **Human liver stage**
>   - Human bitten by mosquito
>   - Parasites travel to the liver and invades cells
>   - They mature into **schizonts** which rupture hepatocytes
>   - **Merozoites** are released into the bloodstream
> 2. **Human blood stage**
>   - Merozoites infect erythrocytes
>   - These multiply into **trophozoites** and onto **schizonts**
>   - Erythrocyte rupture releases further merozoites back into the bloodstream
>   - *Some differentiate into gametocytes*: can be taken up by a mosquito following another bite
> 3. **Mosquito stage**
>   - Gameocytes in the mosquito undergo sexual reproduction and produce eggs
>   - These release **sporozoites** which travel to mosquito salvia
>   - Human inoculation restarts the human liver stage

How is malaria diagnosed?

Malaria is notoriously non-specific. Therefore, a high index of clinical suspicion, careful history taking, and investigations must be used together:

- History
  - Travel to endemic area
  - Mosquito bites
  - Presents 12–14 days after inoculation (can be up to 3 months after return)
- *Clinical signs*: fever, altered mental state, seizures, jaundice, splenomegaly, nonspecific illness

- Investigations
  - *Blood film*: **thick and thin blood film microscopy**
    - ➢ *Thick film*: identifies organism and species for diagnosis
    - ➢ *Thin film*: quantifies parasitaemia to assess severity
  - *Rapid diagnostic tests (often finger-prick samples)*: simple tests will pick up presence of malaria, used more often outwith healthcare facilities to diagnose and treat
  - *Other*: FFBC, U&E, LFT, coagulation profile – aid assessment of severity and complications

How would you define severe malaria?

WHO guidelines have set out criteria to define severe malaria. Those at risk of poor outcomes include elderly patients, pregnant patients, and those with AIDS.

KEY POINT

Severe *P. falciparum* malaria (in adults) include the following:

- *B*: pulmonary oedema (CT/CXR, S_pO_2 < 92% on air, RR > 30 min^{-1})
- *C*: shock (CR ≥3 s, temperature gradient on leg, SBP < 80 mmHg in adults)
- *D*: GCS < 11, seizures (>2 in 24 h), prostration (unable to sit/stand independently), glucose < 2.2 mmol/l
- *F*: creatinine > 265 µmol/l or urea > 20 mmol/l
- *G*: bilirubin > 50 µmol/l
- *H*: Hb < 70 g/l or Hct < 20% with parasite count > 10000 µl^{-1}, significant bleeding (e.g. gums, venepuncture sites, GI)
- *I*: parasitaemia > 10%
- *Acidaemia*: BE < −8, HCO_3^- < 15 mmol/l, lactate > 5 mmol/l

---

GUIDELINE   WHO 2021 Malaria

What pharmacological treatments are available?

Parenteral treatment is recommended with **parasitaemia > 2%** or **jaundice**, regardless of other features of severe disease. All patients with evidence of severe disease should receive high-dose parenteral antimalarial treatment.

Antimalarials
- **Artesunate**
  - Now the preferred treatment option, newer treatment
  - Shown to have mortality benefit
  - Reduces parasite counts faster than quinine
  - 2.4 mg/kg IV 12° for 3 doses then once daily
  - *Issues with availability*: start quinine if not immediately available
- **Quinine**
  - Mainstay of treatment for many years, readily available
  - *Side effects*: arrhythmias (long QT), hypoglycaemia, cinchonism
  - 20 mg/kg loading (up to 1400 mg), then 10 mg/kg 8°

How would you manage the complications of malaria?

Management of complications requires early administration of IV antimalarial drugs; otherwise, it is primarily supportive treatment. All cases should be discussed with specialist units and consider transfer.

ARDS
- Usual ARDS evidence-based management
- Neutral fluid balance (consider evidence of overload and AKI)
- *Case by case management in those with concomitant cerebral malaria*: ARDS vs neuroprotective measures
- High risk of superadded bacterial pneumonia

Cerebral malaria (GCS < 11 or seizures)
- Rule out or treat hypoglycaemia (due to malaria or quinine)
- *Seizures*: antiepileptics
- *Cerebral oedema*: supportive care
- No benefit shown from other treatments including corticosteroids, mannitol, NAC, aspirin

AKI
- *Supportive*: fluid balance, electrolyte correction, RRT if required
- Good prognosis, most recover renal function

Anaemia and DIC
- *Anaemia (haemolysis and removal of infected red blood cells by the spleen)*: restrictive transfusion
- *Coagulopathy (platelet consumption, DIC)*: liaise with haematology, transfusion as indicated

Resources
- Centers for Disease Control and Prevention. Malaria. 2022. Available from: https://www.cdc.gov/parasites/malaria/index.html. (Accessed 24 January 2022.)
- Marks M, Gupta-Wright A, Doherty JF, et al. Managing malaria in the intensive care unit. Br J Anaesth. 2014;113(6):910–921.
- Whitty CJM. Chapter 292: Diagnosis and management of malaria in the ICU. In: Webb A, Angus D, Finfer S, et al. (Eds.) Oxford Textbook of Critical Care, 2nd ed. Oxford: Oxford University Press; 2016. Available from: https://oxfordmedicine.com/view/10.1093/med/9780199600830.001.0001/med-9780199600830-chapter-292. (Accessed 24 January 2022.)

---

119. OTHER RARE INFECTIONS

What is the relevance of vaccination in the UK to critical care?
Vaccination programmes have reduced the incidence of certain viral and bacterial illnesses in the UK. However, uptake is not universal, particularly after misinformation was spread about the MMR vaccine in the 1990s. It is possible that patients will present with such diseases occasionally. An awareness of their features is important. Outbreaks have been seen in certain environments (e.g. meningitis at universities).

Vaccination effectiveness may be affected by anaesthesia, and some vaccines may have significant side effects (see Chapter 86 Cerebral Venous Sinus Thrombosis).

The UK National Vaccination Schedule covers the following conditions (in order):

- Diphtheria
- Hepatitis B
- Haemophilus influenzae type B
- Polio
- Tetanus
- Pertussis
- Rotavirus
- Meningitis B
- Pneumococcus
- Measles
- Mumps
- Rubella
- Influenza
- Meningitis A, C, W, Y
- Human papilloma virus (age 12–13)
- *Shingles (Herpes zoster)*: VZV (age ≥ 70)

Table 119.1   Examples of significant infections covered by the childhood vaccination schedule

	Presentation	Complications
Diphtheria (*Corynebacterium diphtheria*)	Sore throat, fever, headache	Airway obstruction by pseudomembrane presence or dislodgement, endocarditis
Poliomyelitis (poliovirus)	Asymptomatic or flu-like illness	Meningitis (1:25), paralysis (1:200)
Whooping cough (*Bordetella pertussis*)	Coryza, fever, coughing fits, vomiting	Exhaustion, apnoeas
Measles	Cough, coryza, conjunctivitis, fever, Koplik spots, rash	Otitis media, croup, pneumonia, diarrhoea, hepatitis, myocarditis, pancreatitis, appendicitis, encephalitis, subacute sclerosing panencephalitis
Mumps	Parotitis, epididymo-orchitis	Myocarditis, meningitis, pancreatitis, oophoritis, arthritis, encephalitis, sensorineural deafness
Rubella	Mild fever, maculopapular rash, occipital lymphadenopathy	Arthritis, thrombocytopaenia, encephalitis, (in utero infection: deafness, blindness, heart defects in baby)

What are the features of some conditions for which routine childhood vaccination exists?

Diphtheria, poliomyelitis, and whooping cough are examples of conditions which may have severe complications (Table 119.1).

(See Chapter 89 Meningitis and Chapter 91 Tetanus and Botulism)

What are the significant complications of varicella infection?

VZV usually causes mild fever and a maculopapular, vesicular rash which starts centrally and leads to scab formation. The incubation period is 10–21 days. The infectious period starts 2 days before rash becomes apparent and lasts until all lesions have dried and crusted.

Notable complications
- Secondary bacterial infection (common)
- Arthritis
- Pneumonitis
- Myocarditis
- Encephalitis
- Facial nerve palsy
- Thrombosis
- DIC
- Purpura fulminans

What do you know about dengue virus?

Dengue virus is transmitted by the *Aedes aegypti* and *Aedes albopictus* mosquitoes. Incubation is 4–7 days, and presentation is commonly with fever, severe headache, generalised muscle, and bone pains ('breakbone fever').

Some patients develop severe disease at defervescence, **dengue haemorrhagic fever**:

- **Acute vascular permeability syndrome**
  - Hypoproteinaemia
  - *Hypovolaemia*: elevated Hct
  - *Effusions*: pleural, ascites
  - Dengue shock syndrome
- **Abnormal haemostasis**
  - Haemorrhage
  - Thrombocytopaenia

Dengue shock syndrome is managed supportively with balanced fluid resuscitation, avoiding overload but maintaining cardiovascular stability and renal function. Reabsorption usually begins after 48–72 h. Steroids and top-up platelet transfusion without bleeding do not improve outcome.

How might tick-borne illnesses present?

Most present with non-specific flu-like illness: fever, myalgia, headache, malaise, and GI upset. Lyme disease is most common but does not often result in critical illness. Splenectomy might predispose to these conditions.

- *Anaplasmosis*: confusion, neck stiffness, ARDS, rhabdomyolysis, AKI, myocarditis, pancreatitis, DIC, HLH
- *Babesiosis*: intravascular haemolysis, AIHA, altered mental state, ARDS, HF, splenic rupture, AKI, DIC
- *Ehrlichiosis*: rash, meningoencephalitis, ARDS, multi-organ failure (including liver/AKI), HLH
- *Rocky Mountain spotted fever*: rash, nondependent oedema, GI upset, meningoencephalitis, cerebral oedema, gangrene, multi-organ failure

Which other tropical diseases might cause meningoencephalitis?

Viral

- Enteroviruses
- Nipah virus
- HSV
- Rift Valley fever
- Japanese encephalitis
- WNV
- Venezuelan equine encephalitis

Other

- Chagas disease
- African trypanosomiasis (*Trypanosoma brucei gambiense/rhodesiense*)
- Leptospirosis

What do you know about leptospirosis?

Leptospirosis is a zoonotic illness caused by *Leptospira* spirochetes. Carriers include animals including **rodents**, cattle, dogs, and pigs. Spirochetes are excreted in animals' **urine**, and transmission to humans may occur through direct inoculation with infected tissue/fluids or mucosal contact with contaminated substances (e.g. water, soil).

Incubation takes 5–14 days typically. Features range from asymptomatic infection, to flu-like illness, to multi-organ dysfunction (around 40% mortality in MODS). It is diagnosed based on typical features, history of exposure, and evidence of organ involvement. Confirmation is with positive culture, PCR, or microscopic agglutination test.

Complications
- Systemic vasculitis
- Renal dysfunction
- Liver dysfunction
- Intra-alveolar haemorrhage
- Myocarditis
- Meningoencephalitis
- Uveitis

Definitive management includes antimicrobials (e.g. doxycycline if mild, IV penicillins/cephalosporins in more severe disease) alongside supportive care, specialist input, and consideration of transfer to a tertiary centre.

What is toxoplasmosis?

Toxoplasmosis is a protozoal infection caused by *T. gondii*. It may result from food-borne (uncooked meats), congenital, or zoonotic transmission, with **infected cats** implicated through faecal contamination. Ingestion of oocytes results in human infection.

Presentation is with flu-like symptoms. Retinochoroiditis may cause blindness. Other features include lymphadenopathy, seizures, and myocarditis. Immunocompromised patients are particularly at risk of severe disease which may be prevented by prophylaxis with co-trimoxazole.

Treatment may involve the folic acid antagonist, **pyrimethamine**, alongside **sulphonamide** and **leucovorin** (folinic acid). Other options include clindamycin, spiramycin (unlicenced use in pregnancy), and atovaquone.

What is the causative organism in cat scratch disease?

Cat scratch disease is a bacterial infection caused by *Bartonella henselae*. This is transmitted when an infected cat contaminates an open wound, through saliva or scratches. It often presents with tender lymphadenopathy and flu-like illness. Severe complications include meningoencephalitis, seizures, and endocarditis.

Can you describe the features of other rarer infections that might require organ support in critical care?

Rarer infections might require specific organ support (Table 119.2).

(See Chapter 39 Environmental Poisons and Chapter 137 Diarrhoea)

Table 119.2   Rarer infections requiring critical care

	Presentation	Complications
Amoebiasis (*Entamoeba histolytica*)	Dysentery, crampy abdominal pain, bloody diarrhoea	Abscess (liver), stricture, haemorrhage, UC, peritonitis, amoeboma
Brucellosis (*Brucellae*)	Pyrexia, fatigue, headache, myalgia	Endocarditis (aortic more common than mitral), CCF, CS
Chagas disease (*Trypanosoma cruzi*)	Chagoma, lymphadenopathy, hepatosplenomegaly	Myocarditis, DCM, conduction block, meningoencephalitis, autonomic destruction causing megacolon, megaoesophagus
Hydatid disease (*Echinococcus granulosus*)	Cysts in liver, lungs (20%)	Spread to other organs (eye, brain, peritoneal, splenic, bone), cyst rupture, hypersensitivity to hydatid antigens entering circulation including anaphylaxis
Noma	Infectious oral gangrene – periodontitis, ulcerative stomatitis	Gangrene, bone necrosis, complete trismus, death
Rabies (lyssavirus)	Bite with incubation period of weeks to months; initially flu-like illness, generalised weakness	Delirium, abnormal behaviour, hydrophobia, insomnia (almost always fatal once symptomatic)
Schistosomiasis (*Schistosoma*)	Fever, myalgia, rash, malaise, dry cough, nausea, vomiting, diarrhoea	Haematuria, bladder perforation/fibrosis/calcification, hepatic fibrosis, oesophageal varices, pulmonary spread causing pulmonary hypertension, cor pulmonale
Syphilis (*Treponema pallidum*)	Primary – chancre	Secondary – rash, lymphadenopathy, condyloma lata, meningism, alopecia, laryngitis, hepatitis, nephrotic syndrome, bone pain, uveitis Tertiary – aortitis, aortic incompetence, angina, aortic aneurysm, neurosyphilis (paresis, tabes dorsalis, meningitis, meningovascular syphilis)
Typhoid (*Salmonella enterica*)	Headache, fever, cough, abdominal pain, altered bowel habit	Intestinal perforation, GI bleeding
Yellow fever	Flu-like illness, fatigue, fever, nausea, vomiting	High fever, jaundice, haemorrhage, shock, multi-organ failure (30–60% mortality if severe disease)

Which tropical conditions might require surgical intervention?

- *Typhoid*: laparotomy, repair of perforation
- *Hydatid disease*: percutaneous cyst aspiration, surgical resection of complications
- *Amoebiasis*: laparotomy, repair of perforation/intussusception, aspiration of abscess
- *Lymphatic filariasis*: hydrocelectomy
- *Brucellosis*: valve surgery

Resources

- Bashford T, Howell V. Tropical medicine and anaesthesia; part 1. BJA Educ. 2018;18(2):35–40.
- Bashford T, Howell V. Tropical medicine and anaesthesia; part 2. BJA Educ. 2018;18(3):75–81.
- Bhatia N, Barber N. Dilemmas in the preoperative assessment of children. CEACCP. 2011;11(6):214–218.
- Centers for Disease Control and Prevention. Available from: https://www.cdc.gov. (Accessed 24 January 2022.)
- Epidemiology Unit, Ministry of Health. National Guidelines on Management of Leptospirosis. 2016, Sri Lanka. Available from: https://www.epid.gov.lk/web/images/pdf/Publication/leptospirosis/lepto_national_guidelines. pdf. (Accessed 05 April 2022.)
- Farkas J. Internet Book of Critical Care: Tick-borne Illnesses. July 2021. Available from: https://emcrit.org/ibcc/ tick/#presentation:_signs_&_symptoms. (Accessed 24 January 2022.)
- Oswal S, Lyons G. Syphilis in pregnancy. CEACCP. 2008;8(6):240–227.
- Webb A, Angus D, Finger S, et al. (Eds.) Oxford Textbook of Critical Care, 2nd ed. Oxford: Oxford University Press; 2016.

MEDICINE

What is asthma and why is it significant?

Asthma is a common disease of often reversible airway obstruction characterised by mucus hypersecretion, smooth muscle contraction, and airway inflammation.

- In the UK, 5.4 million people are currently being treated for asthma.
- On average, 3 people die from asthma in the UK every day.

Diagnosis is based upon typical symptoms (e.g. recurrent cough, wheeze, dyspnoea, chest tightness, and history of atopy) with a corroborated history of wheeze witnessed by a healthcare professional, and ideally with variable PEFR recordings. Fractional exhaled nitric oxide, **FeNO, ≥40 ppb** is diagnostic in stable patients.

Spirometry revealing reversible obstruction **>12%** in response to inhaled bronchodilators increases the likelihood of asthma. Normal spirometry in an asymptomatic patient does not rule out the diagnosis.

What are the risk factors for exacerbations?

Adults
- *Greatly increased risk*: history of previous exacerbations
- *Moderately increased*: poor control, inappropriate/excessive short-acting beta-2 agonist (SABA) use
- *Slightly increased*: older age, female sex, obesity, smoking, depression, reduced lung function

Children
- *Greatly increased*: history of previous attacks, persistent symptoms
- *Moderately increased*: suboptimal drug regimen, atopy, low-income family, vitamin D deficiency
- *Slightly increased*: younger age, tobacco smoke exposure, obesity, low parental education

How is asthma managed pharmacologically in the community?

Step-wise approach
- SABA
- *Regular preventer*: low-dose inhaled corticosteroid
- *Initial add-on*: inhaled long-acting beta agonist (LABA)
- *Additional controller*: increase inhaled corticosteroid dose or add leukotriene receptor antagonist (LTRA)
- *Specialist therapies:* monoclonal antibodies, oral steroids

Table 120.1   Severity of acute asthma exacerbations

Moderate	Severe	Life-threatening	Near-fatal

• Increasing symptoms
• PEFR > 50–75% best/predicted
• No severe features
	• PEFR 33–50%
	• RR ≥25 min^{-1}
	• HR ≥110 min^{-1}
	• Inability to complete sentences in one breath
		33–92-CHEST:
		  • PEFR < 33%
		  • S_pO_2 < 92%
		  • C: cyanosis
		  • H: hypotension
		  • E: exhaustion
		  • S: silent chest
		  • T: (tachy)arrhythmia
		  • Poor respiratory effort
		ABG:
		  • Normal P_aCO_2 (4.6–6.0 kPa)
		  • Severe hypoxia (P_aO_2 < 8 kPa irrespective of F_iO_2)
		  • Low pH (or high H$^+$)
			• Raised P_aCO_2
			• Requiring mechanical ventilation with raised pressures

How is the severity of exacerbations graded?

The British Thoracic Society (BTS) and Scottish Intercollegiate Guidelines Network (SIGN) have extensive guidelines outlining the management of asthma (Table 120.1).

GUIDELINE   BTS SIGN 2019 Asthma

How is acute asthma managed initially?

- *Assessment*: clinical features, PEFR (determine severity)
- *Oxygenation*: S_pO_2 94–98%, if <92% perform ABG
- *Investigation*: CXR only indicated if other diagnosis considered (e.g. pneumonia, PTX)
- Treat bronchospasm
  - *High-dose nebulised beta-2 agonists*: salbutamol 5 mg (IV infusion only if inhaled route impossible)
  - *Corticosteroids*: prednisolone PO 40–50 mg daily (hydrocortisone 100 mg 6° if not absorbing)
  - Add nebulised ipratropium bromide 500 µg 4–6 hourly if poor response to beta-2 agonists
  - Consider magnesium sulphate 1.2–2 g IV over 20 min if poor response to nebulisers
  - Aminophylline infusion may be used but not proven to be effective
  - Continue long-term medications where suitable pending specialist review
- Consider ventilatory support

STUDY

3Mg (2013)

- Severe acute asthma
- *Intervention*: IV vs nebulised MgSO$_4$ vs placebo
- *Primary*: hospital admission rate, breathlessness – **no difference**
- *Secondary*: mortality, respiratory support, hospital LOS, HDU/ICU admission, change in PEFR/physiological variables – no difference
- Note exclusion of life-threatening/near-fatal asthma

When should a patient with acute asthma be referred to critical care for assessment?

Patients should be referred if requiring ventilatory support or failing to respond to therapy.

Indications for intubation and ventilation in suitable patients are as follows:

- Absolute
    - Coma
    - Respiratory/cardiac arrest
    - Severe refractory hypoxaemia
- Relative
    - Adverse trajectory
    - Fatigue, somnolence
    - Cardiovascular compromise
    - PTX

What are the concerns surrounding RSI in patients with decompensated asthma?

RSI for the critically unwell asthmatic patient is one of the most high-risk inductions in anaesthesia.

Haemodynamic collapse and cardiac arrest may result from several factors:

- Switch from high intrinsically produced **negative intrathoracic pressure** to high positive pressure
- Reduced **venous return** from high ventilatory pressure against poorly compliant lung
- Absolute **hypovolaemia** from high respiratory effort
- Loss of high **sympathetic tone** with anaesthesia

These may be mitigated by pre-oxygenation, fluid preloading, minimising hand ventilation, and maintaining sympathetic tone (e.g. use of ketamine for induction, early vasopressors).

Which adjunctive therapies may be used on critical care?

There is little RCT evidence to support the use of additional therapies in asthma, but they may be used to break persistent bronchospasm:

- **Aminophylline** IV loading dose, followed by infusion
- **Ketamine** infusion
- **Adrenaline** infusion
- *Volatile anaesthetic agents*: **isoflurane, sevoflurane** (with anaesthetic machine or in-circuit device, e.g. AnaConDa®, Sedana Medical)

Additionally, medications increasing the likelihood of bronchospasm can be swapped for more favourable alternatives (e.g. cisatracurium or pancuronium instead of atracurium, different opioid profiles).

How would you ventilate a patient with near-fatal asthma?

The use of NIV is controversial in mild-moderate exacerbations. It is contraindicated in life-threatening asthma outside critical care but may be considered as a ceiling of care. The usefulness of heliox is limited by F_IO_2 restriction.

Ventilator settings

- **Low RR** (e.g. 12–14 min^{-1})
- **Prolonged expiratory phase** (e.g. I:E 1:4)

- **Minimal PEEP**
- Consideration of manual decompression
- *Lung-protective strategy*: permissive hypercapnia (pH > 7.2)
- *Choice of mode important for patient-ventilator interaction*: extrinsic PEEP, trigger sensitivities

Other

- Minimise NMB and deep sedation.
- VV-ECMO may be required.
- VAP prevention
- Respiratory physician input

Resource

- Stanley D, Tunnicliffe W. Management of life-threatening asthma in adults. CEACCP. 2008;8(3):95–99.

121. BRONCHIECTASIS

What is bronchiectasis?

Bronchiectasis is a radiologically diagnosed pulmonary disease characterised by chronic inflammation, persistent production of mucopurulent sputum, and recurrent infection.

Which common organisms might be responsible for exacerbations?

- *Pseudomonas aeruginosa*
- *S. pneumoniae*
- *Haemophilus influenzae*
- *Moraxella catarrhalis*
- *Staph. aureus*
- *Coliforms: Klebsiella, Enterobacter*

What is the pathophysiology of bronchiectasis?

Pathophysiology is complex and is thought to involve a vicious cycle of multiple processes. Causative conditions may affect different parts of the cycle as follows:

- *Respiratory insult causes inflammation*: infection (e.g. pneumonia, measles, TB), aspiration
- *Impaired bronchial drainage*: obstruction by tumour, foreign body, lymph nodes
- *Impaired mucociliary clearance*: cystic fibrosis, primary ciliary dyskinesia (Kartagener's, Young's syndromes)
- Mucus hypersecretion
- Further impairment of mucociliary clearance
- Microbial colonisation ± infection
- Widening of airways

Which other conditions are associated with bronchiectasis?

- COPD
- Alpha-1 antitrypsin deficiency
- Asthma
- Inflammatory bowel disease (IBD)
- Rheumatoid arthritis
- *Other connective tissue diseases*: Sjogren's, Marfan's, systemic sclerosis, SLE, ankylosing spondylitis
- *Chronic systemic infection*: HIV, human T-lymphotropic virus (HTLV)-1
- Chronic rhinosinusitis

Causative conditions

- Cystic fibrosis
- Allergic bronchopulmonary aspergillosis
- Primary antibody deficiency syndromes

How is it diagnosed?

Diagnosis is confirmed by demonstration of **bronchial dilatation on CT**:

- Bronchoarterial ratio > 1 (signet ring sign)
- Lack of tapering
- Airway visibility within 1 cm of pleural surface or touching mediastinal pleura

Further investigations include baseline CXR and those directed at aetiology:

- *Full history*: particularly for associated diseases
- FBC
- *Sputum culture*: routine (when well), during exacerbation, mycobacterial
- PFT
- *Specialist*: IgE to *Aspergillus fumigatus*, serum IgG/IgA/IgM, antibodies to *S. pneumoniae*, test for cystic fibrosis ± primary ciliary dyskinesia

When is bronchiectasis 'severe'?

Severity can be determined using scoring systems (e.g. Bronchiectasis Severity Index, FACED). Important features include age, BMI, FEV_1, exacerbations, admissions, MRC breathlessness score, colonisation, radiological severity. *P. aeruginosa* colonisation carries a higher risk of bronchiectasis-related complications.

Complications

- Chronic respiratory failure
- Haemoptysis
- Chest pain
- Vascular disease
- Pulmonary hypertension
- *Other*: depression, anxiety, nutritional deficiency, fatigue

How is bronchiectasis managed?

Bronchiectasis is managed in a stepwise approach depending on frequency of exacerbations with existing therapies. The following interventions may be involved:

- Treat underlying cause
- Airway clearance techniques ± pulmonary rehabilitation
- *Prompt antibiotic treatment of exacerbations*: direct at known culture results
- Annual influenza immunisation
- Mucoactive treatment
- Long-term antibiotics: inhaled antipseudomonal (colistin/gentamicin) or oral macrolide
- Regular IV antibiotics every 2–3 months

There is no role for routine inhaled/oral steroids, phosphodiesterase-4 inhibitors, methylxanthines, LTRA, CXCR2 antagonists, neutrophil elastase inhibitors, or statins. Bronchodilators and steroids may be used if indicated for concomitant disease (e.g. COPD, asthma).

Double lung transplantation may be considered in those under 65 years old with FEV_1 <30% and clinical instability or rapid progression despite optimal medical management. Earlier transplantation may be appropriate if massive haemoptysis, pulmonary hypertension, ICU admissions, or respiratory failure is notable.

GUIDELINE BTS 2019 Bronchiectasis

What challenges might bronchiectasis present to the intensivist?

- *Assessment of premorbid function*: comorbidity common
- *Ventilation*: variable compliance, gas trapping, mucus plugging, poor absorption of inhaled agents
- *Nutrition*: poor baseline common
- *Complications*: pulmonary haemorrhage, pulmonary hypertension
- *Microbiology*: colonisation, resistant organisms

What do you know about cystic fibrosis?

Cystic fibrosis is a multisystem autosomal recessive disorder characterised by impaired clearance of secretions, resulting in obstruction of various organ systems.

It is usually diagnosed by neonatal screening for the defective cystic fibrosis transmembrane conductance regulator (CFTR) gene (F508del and other mutations) which affects chloride ion channels and secretion consistency. It is the most common genetic disease in the UK occurring in 1:2500 live births. The disease is progressive with death occurring due to lung disease and liver cirrhosis most commonly. Median age at death had been around 30–35 years but is improving with newer disease modulators.

Multisystem effects

- *A*: viscous secretions
- *B*: bronchiectasis
- *F*: CKD, renal stones
- *G*: malnutrition, abdominal pain, diabetes, liver disease, bowel obstruction, musculoskeletal disorders, in-/subfertility
- *I*: colonisation (*P. aeruginosa, Staph. aureus, H. influenzae, Stenotrophomonas maltophilia, Burkholderia cepacia, Aspergillus*)

How is cystic fibrosis managed?

- *Minimise pulmonary infection*: chest physiotherapy, mucolytics (DNA-ase nebuliser, inhaled hypertonic saline), antibiotics
- *Optimise nutritional status*: may require supplementation (150% non-CF requirement), high fat, exogenous insulin
- *Slow disease progression*: anti-inflammatories, gene therapy (nebulised plasmid DNA)
- *Symptomatic management*: home oxygen, NIV, CPAP
- *Psychological input*: transplantation, end-of-life care, adherence to treatment

CFTR modulators are a new group of precision medicines that have been shown to improve outcomes such as quality of life and FEV_1 in those with specific genetic mutations:

- *Kalydeco® (ivacaftor)*: rarer mutations
- *Symkevi® (ivacaftor + tezacaftor)*: F508del mutation
- *Orkambi® (ivacaftor + lumacaftor)*: homozygotes for F508del mutation
- *Kaftrio® (tezacaftor, ivacaftor, elexacaftor)*: F508del mutation

Transplantation may be indicated in severe disease and could involve simultaneous/combination transplants such as lung-liver or heart-lung.

STUDY

Middleton et al. (2019)

- Cystic fibrosis, heterozygous Phe508del CFTR mutation, age ≥12 years
- *Intervention*: elexacaftor-tezacaftor-ivacaftor vs placebo
- *Primary*: absolute change in % predicted FEV_1 at 4 weeks – **significantly higher**
- *Secondary*: exacerbations, sweat chloride concentration – **significantly lower**; quality of life – **significantly higher**

Resource

- Fitzgerald M, Ryan D. Cystic fibrosis and anaesthesia. CEACCP. 2011;11(6):204–209.

122. COMMUNITY-ACQUIRED PNEUMONIA

What is community-acquired pneumonia?

Community-acquired pneumonia (CAP) is an acute infection of the pulmonary parenchyma with symptoms occurring in the community or **within 48 h** of hospital admission. Diagnosis requires significant findings on chest examination (crackles, altered breath sounds) or infiltrates on chest imaging.

Severity is assessed clinically and can be assisted using scoring systems. Severe CAP is often a multisystem disorder with a requirement for critical care support. Causes may be bacterial, viral, or fungal. The most common cause is *S. pneumoniae*.

CAP is common with an annual incidence of 6–10/1000 adults in Europe. Severe CAP is associated with high mortality rates with a CURB-65 score of 3–5 associated with a mortality >15%.

(See Chapter 115 Fungal Infection and Chapter 124 COVID-19)

How would you stratify risk in CAP?

Several risk prediction tools exist and may be indicated to alert senior team members to review, confirm severity, and enact a management plan. The most commonly used is the CURB-65 score (CRB65 when urea is unavailable); 1 point is given for each feature present.

> **KEY POINT**
>
> CURB-65 score:
>
> - **C**onfusion (abbreviated Mental Test Score ≤8, or new disorientation in person/place/time)
> - Blood **u**rea > 7 mmol/l
> - **R**R ≥ 30 min⁻¹
> - **B**P (diastolic ≤ 60 or systolic < 90 mmHg)
> - Age ≥ **65** years

Significance of total score is as follows:

- *0–1*: low risk (<3% mortality) – consider treatment in the community
- *2*: intermediate risk (3–15% mortality) – hospital treatment probably required
- *3–5*: high risk (>15% mortality) – hospital treatment required, consider HDU/ICU

A proposed score to assess the risk of requiring Invasive ventilation or vasoactive support is 'SMART-COP'. It considers 8 variables with a score of ≥3 identifying 92% of patients requiring ICU admission. This requires further validation.

> **GUIDELINE** NICE 2019 NG138 CAP

How is CAP investigated?

- *Bloods*: ABG, U&E, FBC, LFT, CRP
- Sputum culture (preferably a deep cough sample)
- Blood cultures
- *Chest imaging*: CXR, lung US, CT
- Urine for legionella and pneumococcal antigen
- *Pleural fluid aspiration*: culture, biochemistry (may determine indication for drainage)
- PCR respiratory pathogens (e.g. COVID-19, influenza, RSV, Mycoplasma, Chlamydophilia)
- HIV test

How is CAP treated?

- **Supportive care**
  - NIV not routinely recommended
  - Concomitant management of sepsis if present as per usual guidelines
- **Close collaboration with respiratory specialists**
- **Antimicrobial therapy**
  - Local policy may be based on CURB-65
  - Duration 7–10 days (longer if resistant organism or *Staph. aureus* bacteraemia)
  - May require notification of Health Protection Unit (e.g. *Legionella*), involvement of microbiology
- **Treatment of concomitant viral infection** (see Chapter 124 COVID-19)
- **Management of complications**
  - *Parapneumonic effusion*: early thoracocentesis
  - *Empyema (or pH < 7.2)*: early pleural drainage

What do you know about the role of NIV/CPAP in this context?

Evidence is limited, but some observations have been made:

- NIV
  - Systematic reviews have shown no clear benefit in non-COPD population
  - Some data suggest reduced need for intubation but no effect on mortality
- CPAP
  - An RCT of 213 patients showed no reduction in intubation or improved outcome
  - CPAP appeared to delay intubation with adverse consequences

The use of NIV or CPAP is not recommended routinely in CAP. Any trial of non-invasive respiratory support for this indication should be conducted in a critical care area where a rapid transition to intubation can be facilitated if appropriate. HFNO has not been shown to reduce intubation rates in a study of mostly pneumonia patients (**FLORALI**).

GUIDELINE BTS 2009 CAP

STUDY

Delclaux et al. (2000)

- Acute hypoxaemic, non-hypercapnic, respiratory insufficiency
- *Intervention*: addition of CPAP vs conventional oxygen therapy
- *Primary*: rate of tracheal intubation – **no difference**
- *Secondary*: ICU LOS, hospital mortality – no difference; respiratory indices (subjective response to treatment, P/F ratio) – significantly improved at 1 h then no difference; adverse events – **significantly higher**

STUDY

FLORALI (2015)

- Acute hypoxaemic respiratory failure
- *Intervention*: HFNO vs NIV vs facemask oxygen
- *Primary*: rate of tracheal intubation – **no difference**
- *Secondary (e.g. LOS, complications)*: no difference, 90-day mortality – **significantly lower** with high flow, discomfort at 1 h – **significantly lower** with high flow

What is 'PVL' pneumonia?

Panton-Valentine leukocidin-producing (PVL) *Staph. aureus* is a rare cause of severe community-acquired pneumonia associated with lung cavitation and multi-organ dysfunction. Leukocidin toxin may be suppressed using linezolid, clindamycin, or rifampicin (also covering MRSA strains).

Clinical features

- *Prodromal illness*: diarrhoea, 'flu-like' illness, necrotising soft tissue infection
- High fever
- Haemoptysis
- Profound hypotension
- Skin pustules

Is there any specific treatment for viral pneumonia?

Supportive care is the key, but some specific therapies exist:

- *Influenza*: neuraminidase inhibitors (e.g. oseltamivir 75 mg PO BD up to 10 days, zanamivir IV)
- *COVID-19*: dexamethasone if dependent on supplemental O_2 ± other therapies (see Chapter 124 COVID-19)
- *RSV*: ribavirin sometimes used in immunocompromised patients

(See Chapter 114 Viral Infection)

Why is influenza significant to critical care?

Influenza is a single-stranded RNA orthomyxovirus spread by respiratory droplets. Subtypes are named according to variations in the **haemagglutinin** (H number) and **neuraminidase** (N number) proteins on the viral envelope.

It causes a mild, self-limiting illness in many but may result in severe, life-threatening infection in a minority of patients. Prior to the 2020 COVID-19 pandemic, influenza outbreaks were the most common and problematic viral lung infection. Influenza has also been responsible for pandemic disease, most recently in 2009 with the '**A(H1N1)pdm09**' strain. Types B and C usually cause milder disease and more local outbreaks.

Influenza should be suspected in presentation with pneumonia, exacerbations of respiratory disease, sepsis, myocarditis, acute neurological disorders, or rhabdomyolysis.

At-risk groups for complicated disease are as follows:

- *Chronic disease*: neurological, hepatic, renal, pulmonary, cardiovascular
- *Immunosuppression*: diabetes mellitus, hyposplenism, pregnancy, immunosuppressive medications (e.g. for solid organ transplant, haematopoietic stem cell transplant)
- Age > 65 years
- BMI ≥ 40 kg/m²

Primary influenza virus pneumonia is difficult to distinguish clinically from other viral or bacterial pneumonia, so rapid PCR testing is recommended in all suspected infections. Management is supportive, with consideration of preventing further transmission. Neuraminidase inhibitors should be commenced on clinical suspicion within 48 h of symptom onset to reduce the duration of symptoms (see Chapter 124 COVID-19).

GUIDELINE PHE 2019 Influenza

Resource

- Morgan AJ, Glossop AJ. Severe community-acquired pneumonia. BJA Educ. 2016;16(5):167–172.

What is COPD?

> **KEY POINT**
>
> COPD is
>
> - a common, preventable, and treatable disease, characterised by
> - persistent respiratory symptoms and
> - variable airflow limitation
> - due to airway and/or alveolar abnormalities
> - caused by significant exposure to noxious particles or gases

COPD encompasses emphysema and chronic bronchitis and may involve exacerbations of illness.

An **exacerbation** is an acute, sustained worsening of symptoms beyond normal day-to-day variations. Common symptoms include worsening breathlessness, cough, increased sputum production, and change in sputum colour.

> **GUIDELINE**   GOLD 2017 COPD

What are the risk factors for developing COPD?

- *Smoking*: more than 80% patients have a significant tobacco smoking history
- Industrial exposure
- Recurrent infection
- Airway hyperreactivity and chronic inflammatory response
- Air pollution
- Genetic (alpha-1 antitrypsin deficiency)

Risk factors for exacerbations are as follows:

- Smoking/passive smoke exposure
- Infection
- Air pollution
- Lack of physical activity
- *Seasonal*: winter/spring

What is the pathophysiology of COPD?

- Small airway inflammation and parenchymal destruction affect proximal and peripheral airways, lung parenchyma, and vasculature.
- Airway obstruction with poor reversibility occurs.
- Airway remodelling, increased goblet cells and mucous production, and changes in PVR result.
- Leads to clinical picture of airway obstruction, pulmonary hypertension, dynamic hyperinflation, respiratory muscle dysfunction (secondary to diaphragm flattening), and V/Q mismatch.

How is the severity of COPD assessed?

Diagnosis should be suspected clinically and supported by spirometry. Suggestive features in combination with risk factors (current or previous smoking history) are as follows:

- Exertional breathlessness
- Chronic cough

- Regular sputum production
- Frequent 'winter' bronchitis
- Wheeze

Spirometry showing **FEV_1/FVC ratio < 0.7** is supportive of a diagnosis of COPD. Severity should then be assessed with a multimodal approach, including the Global Initiative for Chronic Obstructive Lung Disease (GOLD) guide values for severity. Other systems for grading of airflow obstruction include those from NICE, American Thoracic Society (ATS), and European Respiratory Society (ERS). Breathlessness should be graded using the MRC Dyspnoea Scale.

NICE recommends against using the BODE Index for COPD survival as its indices are not routinely available in primary care and it is not suitable for acute exacerbations.

Other investigations should centre around ruling out differentials (e.g. BNP – HF) and assessing complications (e.g. CT, echo for pulmonary hypertension).

KEY POINT

GOLD Stage (% predicted FEV_1):

1. Mild ≥ 80
2. Moderate ≥ 50, < 80
3. Severe ≥ 30, < 50
4. Very severe < 30

KEY POINT

MRC Dyspnoea Scale:

1. Only on strenuous exercise
2. On hurrying or walking up a slight hill
3. Slower than contemporaries on level ground or stopping for breath at own pace
4. Stopping for breath after walking 100 m or a few minutes on level ground
5. On dressing/undressing, too breathless to leave the house

GUIDELINE   NICE 2018 NG115 COPD

Which factors might affect severity?

- Frailty
- Severity and frequency of exacerbations
- Smoking status
- Chronic hypoxia and cor pulmonale
- Low BMI
- Hospital admissions
- *Symptom burden*: consider the COPD Assessment Test (CAT) score
- Exercise capacity (6MWT or recent cardiopulmonary exercise test)
- TLCO
- Whether the person meets criteria for long-term oxygen therapy (LTOT) or NIV
- Multimorbidity

How is COPD managed pharmacologically in the community?

Smoking cessation is prioritised, and **non-pharmacological management** should be targeted in addition to relevant **vaccinations** before pharmacological management:

- *Initial*: short-acting bronchodilator
- *No asthmatic features*: LABA + long-acting muscarinic antagonist (LAMA)

- *Asthmatic features*: LABA + inhaled corticosteroid
- *Next*: LAMA + LABA + inhaled corticosteroid
- Other
  - Long-term oral corticosteroids when unable to wean following exacerbation
  - *Theophyllines*: after trial of bronchodilators or if unable to tolerate inhalers
  - *Chronic productive cough*: oral mucolytics (e.g. carbocysteine)

When is LTOT recommended?

LTOT improves outcomes and might be appropriate in **very severe airflow obstruction (<30%)**, cyanosis, polycythaemia, peripheral oedema, raised JVP, and $S_pO_2 < 92\%$ on air. After optimal medical management, 2 ABGs taken at least 3 weeks apart are required for assessment. There should not be a significant rise in P_aCO_2 (i.e. ≤1 kPa) when on oxygen.

Criteria for LTOT in stable COPD are as follows:

- $P_aO_2 < 7.3$ kPa
- P_aO_2 7.3–8 kPa if any of:
  - Secondary polycythaemia
  - Peripheral oedema
  - Pulmonary hypertension

How would you assess a patient with a suspected exacerbation of COPD?

- *History*: sputum change, sepsis, functional status, comorbid disease
- *Consideration of differentials/complications*: pneumonia, PTX, high BMI, HF, PE
- *Investigations*
  - *ABG, bloods*: FBC, U&E, inflammatory markers
  - CXR
  - *ECG*: exclude comorbidities
  - *Theophylline level*: if taking at home
  - *Sputum MC+S*: if purulent
  - *Blood cultures*: if pyrexial
  - *TTE*: HF, pulmonary hypertension
  - FEV_1 not recommended in acute setting

What are the management priorities?

- **Controlled oxygenation**
  - Venturi mask
  - Individualised target S_aO_2
- **Bronchospasm**
  - Short-acting bronchodilators
  - Oral corticosteroids (30 mg prednisolone 5 days)
  - *Aminophylline*: if inadequate response to nebulised bronchodilators, monitor levels
- **Ventilatory support**
  - NIV
  - Invasive ventilation
  - *Respiratory stimulants (e.g. doxapram)*: only if NIV unavailable/inappropriate
- **Respiratory physiotherapy**
- **Treatment of concomitant infection**
- **Smoking cessation advice**
- **Respiratory team input**
- **Pulmonary rehabilitation** may be appropriate when recovered

What are the indications for NIV?

Following failure of optimal medical therapy NIV should be initiated when:

- pH 7.25–7.35 (H+ 45–56 nmol/l)
- P_aCO_2 > 6.5 kPa
- RR > 23

Severe acidosis alone doesn't preclude a trial of NIV in an appropriately staffed and experienced area. The use of NIV should not delay escalation to invasive ventilation when this is appropriate. A decision surrounding tracheal intubation should be made before commencing NIV in any patient.

NIV has been used successfully to wean from invasive ventilation and may be appropriate where conventional strategies fail.

NIV is not indicated in the presence of impaired consciousness, severe hypoxaemia, or copious respiratory secretions (e.g. concomitant bronchiectasis). Absolute contraindications include recent facial surgery/trauma, fixed upper airway obstruction, and vomiting.

GUIDELINE BTS/ICS 2016 Acute hypercapnic respiratory failure

What are some indications for referral to ICU?

- Impending respiratory arrest
- NIV failing to augment chest wall movement or reduce P_aCO_2
- Inability to maintain S_aO_2 > 85–88% on NIV
- Need for IV sedation or adverse feature indicating the need for closer monitoring and/or possible difficult intubation
- To facilitate appropriate decision-making about potential NIV failure

What ventilatory strategies can be employed during invasive ventilation in COPD?

- Mandatory ventilation should be continued until airway resistance falls.
- Spontaneous breathing as soon as possible
- *Reduction of dynamic hyperinflation with IMV:*
  - Prolonged expiratory time (I:E ratio 1:3 or longer)
  - Low RR 10–15 min^{-1}
  - Permissive hypercapnia with pH 7.2–7.25
- Extrinsic PEEP < 12 cmH_2O
- Carbonic anhydrase inhibitors for metabolic alkalosis
  - Not recommended routinely (no evidence of benefit, significant side effects)
  - Short courses have been used during weaning stage (can normalise severe metabolic alkalosis, thought to reduce risk of apnoea)

STUDY

DIABOLO (2016)

- Critically ill patients with COPD and metabolic alkalosis
- *Intervention*: acetazolamide for up to 28 days vs placebo
- *Primary*: duration of invasive ventilation – **no difference**
- *Secondary*: duration of invasive ventilation, numbers of SBTs, VAP – no difference, serum bicarbonate – **significantly lower**, days with metabolic alkalosis – **significantly lower**

What is the role of extracorporeal therapies in COPD?

Candidacy for further invasive treatment is likely to be problematic. Clear benefit has yet to be demonstrated, and risk of adverse events is high.

ECCO$_2$R might be indicated in COPD for the following:

- Severe hypercapnic acidosis (pH < 7.15) despite optimal mandatory ventilation
- LPV where hypercapnia contraindicated (e.g. coexistent brain injury – although any bleed may preclude circuit anticoagulation)

(See Chapter 9 ECMO and ECCO$_2$R)

---

124.   COVID-19

Why are the coronaviruses relevant to critical care?

Coronavirus strains usually cause common cold symptoms but several are responsible for severe respiratory disease as follows:

- SARS-CoV
  - SARS epidemic 2002–2003
  - 10% mortality
  - Around 8000 cases reported
- MERS-CoV
  - MERS described 2012 onwards
  - 35% mortality
  - Several thousand cases reported (around 2000 in first 6 years)
- SARS-CoV-2
  - COVID-19 pandemic 2020 onwards (ongoing at time of writing)
  - 0.1 to >25% case fatality ratio, variable by country
  - 15–30% develop severe ARDS (prevaccination)
  - *Globally*: >600 million cases, >6 million deaths
  - *UK*: >20 million cases, >170,000 deaths

GUIDELINE   NICE 2022 NG191 COVID-19

(See Chapter 122 Community-Acquired Pneumonia and Chapter 114 Viral Infection)

What is the pathophysiology of COVID-19?

SARS-CoV-2 is an enveloped RNA betacoronavirus which causes COVID-19. It is characterised by 4 structural proteins related to infectivity and replication as follows:

- *Spike (S)*: protrudes from membrane, tip is crown-shaped
  - Binds to angiotensin-converting enzyme 2 (ACE2) receptor (point of entry to host)
  - Thought to be major contributor to immunogenic response (target of most vaccines)
- *Membrane (M)*: important in viral pathogenesis
- *Envelope (E)*: role in viral replication and infectivity
- *Nucleocapsid (N)*: regulation of viral RNA replication, transcription, and synthesis

The ACE2 receptor is abundant in the lower respiratory tract, hence COVID-19's predominance for respiratory symptoms. Following respiratory infection, rapid replication causes high levels of IL and other inflammatory substances. A microangiopathic angiopathy follows. The magnitude of immune response may dictate the clinical syndrome experienced by the patient, ranging from mild/asymptomatic disease to florid multi-organ dysfunction.

What do you know about SARS-CoV-2 variants?

Different variants have been identified, with differing characteristics (Table 124.1).

Variants of interest (VOI) have genetic changes predicted/known to affect characteristics such as transmissibility, severity, immune escape, or diagnostic/therapeutic escape. These have usually caused significant community transmission or multiple clusters in multiple countries with increasing relative prevalence (or other suggestion of emerging risk to global public health).

Variants under monitoring (VUM) also exist whereby the above criteria are not fulfilled, along with **formerly monitored variants** – those that have become insignificant.

What are the non-respiratory features of COVID-19?

- Taste/olfactory disorders (53% with early strains)
- *Cardiovascular*: myocardial injury, myocarditis, myopericarditis, arrhythmias, HF
- *Neurological*: ICH, ischaemic stroke, dizziness, headache, altered mental state, GBS, acute necrotising encephalopathy
- *Ocular (32%)*: conjunctival hyperaemia, chemosis, lacrimation
- Diarrhoea (2–40%)
- VTE
- Skin changes
- PIMS-TS in children

What are the specific management priorities for patients with severe COVID-19 pneumonitis?

- Infection prevention and control (See Chapter 114 Viral Infection)
- *Holistic assessment*: discussion of treatment expectations and care goals
- Manage comorbidities/differentials
- Non-pharmacological therapies (e.g. changing body positioning – conscious proning) (see Chapter 8 Proning)
- Pharmacological
  - **Dexamethasone** if oxygen-dependent

Table 124.1 Early SARS-CoV-2 variants

WHO label	Lineage	First documentation	Features
Alpha	B.1.1.7	UK, September 2020	
Beta	B.1.351	South Africa, May 2020	
Gamma	P.1	Brazil, November 2020	
Delta	B.1.617.2	India, October 2020	Highly transmissible, disease more severe
Omicron	B.1.1.529	Multiple countries, November 2021	More transmissible, disease less severe

- Specific therapies as indicated
- *Anxiolysis*: trial of benzodiazepine recommended
- *Thromboprophylaxis*: unclear whether increased dosing of value
- *Antibiotics*: only if appropriate for co-infection
- Non-invasive respiratory support
  - When above optimised
  - *CPAP*: consider if F_IO_2 requirement ≥0.4 and invasive ventilation not immediately needed, or as ceiling of treatment
  - *HFNO*: indicated for breaks from CPAP, weaning from CPAP, humidification
- Invasive ventilation
  - Lung-protective strategy
  - Often prolonged, approximately 20% require tracheostomy
- *VV-ECMO*: poorer outcomes when compared to other indications, candidacy limited

What is the evidence behind steroid use in the management of COVID-19 pneumonitis?

The **RECOVERY** and **REMAP-CAP** trials studied a variety of different treatments as adaptive RCTs (and are ongoing at the time of writing). Results from the corticosteroid arms supported the use of dexamethasone in patients receiving oxygen. A 10-day course length is recommended and alternative corticosteroids (e.g. hydrocortisone, prednisolone) may be used.

STUDY

REMAP-CAP (2020) Corticosteroid

- Severe COVID-19
- *Intervention*: hydrocortisone 50 mg IV 6° 7 days (up to 28 days whilst in shock) vs standard care
- *Primary*: 21-day respiratory/cardiovascular support-free days – **no difference, probability of superiority – 93% (80% in shock)**
- *Secondary*: for example in-hospital mortality probability of superiority 54% (62%)

STUDY

RECOVERY (2021) Dexamethasone

- Hospitalised SARS-CoV-2 infection
- *Intervention*: dexamethasone 6 mg OD 10 days vs usual care
- *Primary*: 28-day mortality – **significantly lower (21.6% vs 24.6%)**
- *Secondary*:
  - *28-day mortality subgroups*: MV – **significantly lower (29% vs 40.7%)**, supplemental O_2 – **significantly lower (21.5% vs 25%)**, no respiratory support – no difference
  - *Other*: hospital LOS – **significantly lower** (12 vs 13 days), composite IMV and death – **significantly lower**, use of MV – **significantly lower**

Which specific therapies have been considered and used in the management of COVID-19 pneumonitis?

In addition to corticosteroids, the most significant results so far have been seen with IL-6 inhibitors, antivirals, monoclonal antibodies, and baricitinib (Table 124.2).

- **IL-6 inhibitors,** such as tocilizumab and sarilumab, have shown modest benefit in terms of time to organ support-free days and avoidance of invasive ventilation.
- **Antivirals** may be of benefit. Remdesivir may improve time to hospital discharge, but a mortality benefit has not been demonstrated yet. The combination of nirmatrelvir and ritonavir has been shown to reduce risk of progression to severe disease in unvaccinated patients.

Table 124.2 Specific pharmacological therapies for COVID-19

Class	Drug	Dose	Indications	Contraindications
IL-6 inhibitors	**Tocilizumab**	8 mg/kg IV infusion (max 800 mg)	CRP > 75 mg/l ≤ 48 hours advanced respiratory support if required Receiving/completed steroid	Other infection that may be worsened
	Sarilumab	400 mg IV infusion	Second line to tocilizumab	
JAK inhibitors	**Baricitinib**	4 mg daily (10 days)	Receiving/completed steroid	Other infection that might be worsened Age < 2 years
Antivirals	Remdesivir	200 mg IV day 1, 100 mg day 2 onwards (5 days if F_iO_2 > 0.21; 3 days otherwise)	Within 7 days symptom onset High risk of severe illness	Age < 12 years Weight < 40 kg Advanced respiratory support
	Molnupiravir (Lagevrio®)	800 mg 12 O (5 days)	Mild to moderate disease At risk of severe illness Within 5 days symptom onset	Pregnancy Age < 18 years Weight < 40 kg
	Nirmatrelvir/ ritonavir (Paxlovid®)	300/100 mg 12 O (5 days)	High risk of severe illness Within 5 days symptom onset	Weight < 40 kg
nMABs	Casirivimab/ imdevimab (Ronapreve®)	2.4 g IV infusion	Seronegative Susceptible variant	Omicron variant Age < 12 years
	Sotrovimab (Xevudy®)	500 mg IV infusion	Symptomatic Risk of severe illness Within 5 days symptom onset	

Note: All drugs described are indicated when there is a supplemental O_2 requirement, except those in grey, which require there to be no supplemental O_2 requirement. The most strongly recommended therapies are highlighted in **bold**.

- **Neutralising monoclonal antibodies (nMABs)** bind to the spike protein and prevent entry into the host cell and subsequent replication. Casirivimab/imdevimab reduces the relative risk of mortality by 20% in appropriate patients. However, it is less effective against the Omicron variant. It is important to determine if patients are seronegative/seropositive by investigating for serum **anti-spike (anti-S) antibody**, which is directed against SARS-Cov-2 spike protein, also known as 'spike protein antibody'.
- The **Janus kinase (JAK) inhibitor**, baricitinib, acts specifically on the JAK1 and JAK2 enzymes involved in mediation of signalling for some cytokines thought to be implicated in COVID-19. Mortality, hospital LOS, and severity of disease were shown to be reduced across several trials.

There is an ever-growing list of other therapies that are being, or have been, monitored for significant effects against COVID-19. Examples include the following: ACE-I, acetylcysteine, imatinib, and mesenchymal stem cell therapy.

STUDY

REMAP-CAP (2021) IL-6

- Critically ill COVID-19
- *Intervention*: tocilizumab vs sarilumab vs standard care
- *Primary*: organ support-free days up to day 21 – **probability of superiority 99.9% and 99.5%**, hospital mortality – **significantly lower (28% vs 22.2% vs 35.8%)**
- *Secondary*: 90-day survival, respiratory support-free days, cardiovascular support-free days – **significantly higher**; progression to IMV, ECMO, or death – **significantly lower**

STUDY

STUDY

RECOVERY (2022) Casirivimab/Imdevimab

- Hospitalised COVID-19
- *Intervention*: Casirivimab/imdevimab (REGEN-COV®, USA)
- *Primary*: (seronegative) 28-day mortality – **significantly lower if seronegative (24% vs 30%)**
- *Secondary*: (seronegative) progression to NIV/IMV – **significantly lower**, discharged alive from hospital at 28 days – **significantly higher**
- No difference in above when including seropositive patients

STUDY

RECOVERY (2022) Baricitinib

- Hospitalised COVID-19
- *Intervention*: Baricitinib vs usual care
- *Primary*: 28-day mortality – 13% proportional reduction in mortality (12% vs 14%), 20% reduction in updated meta-analysis

Which therapies are recommended against?

- Azithromycin
- Inhaled budesonide
- Colchicine
- Doxycycline
- Ivermectin

What is the role of vitamin D supplementation in COVID-19?

Vitamin D supplementation is encouraged to maintain bone and muscle health for all people aged > 4 years between October and early March in the UK due to the lack of sunlight and limitations of dietary supplementation. It is not recommended solely to prevent or treat COVID-19 at present.

GUIDELINE NICE 2020 NG187 COVID-19 Vitamin D

What is COVID-19-associated pulmonary aspergillosis ('CAPA')?

CAPA may occur in the critically ill with or alongside COVID-19. Risk may increase with age and chronic lung disease. Multimodal testing should include BAL if possible. Antifungal treatment may be indicated and should be coordinated by a MDT.

How might you detect COVID-19-related myocardial injury initially?

NICE recommend the following tests and typical results:

- High-sensitivity troponin I or T (elevation, particularly increasing over time)
- N-terminal pro B-type natriuretic peptide > 400 ng/l
- ECG (evolving ischaemia)

What measures might reduce the risk of infection towards staff during airway procedures?

There has been much debate about how SARS-CoV-2 is thought to be spread and what constitutes an 'aerosol-generating procedure' (AGP). These factors have significant implications in terms of infection prevention and control and service delivery.

Adaptations to tracheal intubation suggested early in the pandemic included the following:

- *Aerosol precautions*: including PPE, appropriately ventilated room
- Setting up for highest chance of intubation on first attempt (e.g. staff with greatest airway experience/expertise)
- Preparing equipment as much as possible prior to procedure to minimise disconnections (e.g. closed-circuit suction attached to catheter mount)
- Minimising ventilation during apnoeic time
- Inflation of cuff prior to starting ventilation
- Minimising touching contaminated equipment, appropriate disposal (transfer of fomites)
- Allowing appropriate air turnover time before entering room after AGP

> **GUIDELINE** ICS 2020 COVID-19 Airway

How about tracheostomy insertion?

Tracheostomy procedure has also been considered. Ideally, it should be performed when the patient is SARS-CoV-2 negative. However, this may not occur within a realistic time frame. Ventilation is likely to be required during the procedure, but ventilatory pressures/frequency should be reduced or suspended where possible. Again, experienced operators – both 'procedural' and at the 'top end' – are recommended.

> **GUIDELINE** NTSP 2020 COVID-19 Tracheostomy

How do the COVID-19 vaccinations work?

Vaccination has been proven to be effective in preventing COVID-19. Available types are as follows:

- *mRNA*: Pfizer BioNTech (Comirnaty), Moderna (Spikevax)
- *Adenovirus (ChAdOx) vector*: AstraZeneca (Vaxzevria), Covishield
- *Adenovirus based*: Janssen, Sputnik, CanSinoBIO
- *Whole inactivated coronavirus*: Sinopharm, Sinovac, Covaxin
- *Recombinant spike protein with novel adjuvant*: Novavax

mRNA vaccines (e.g. Pfizer BioNTech, Moderna) contain the genetic sequence for the spike protein, wrapped in a lipid envelope. Vaccine mRNA is absorbed by host cells which then translate this to produce spike proteins. An immune response is generated.

Adenovirus (ChAdOx) vector vaccines use weakened adenovirus as a carrier to deliver the genetic sequence of the spike protein to host cells. It cannot replicate so cannot cause disease. The body destroys the adenovirus once the sequence has been delivered. Spike protein production again produces an immune response.

Can you describe any ethical challenges that arose during the COVID-19 pandemic?

- *Resource prioritisation for COVID-19*: PPE, beds, oxygen, staffing
- *Working outside of specialty*: redeployment of staff
- *Vulnerability of staff*: shielding, occupational exposure, and subsequent illness/death
- Service pressure managing non-COVID-19 caseload (e.g. cancer waiting lists, elective surgery)
- Managing patients who had previously declined vaccination
- *Vaccination of staff*: whether mandatory or not
- *Vaccination of children and pregnant women*: limitations to research trials
- *Face-to-face vs remote contact*: professional, visiting restrictions, and effect on families' well-being

> **GUIDELINE** RCP 2021 Ethical dimensions of COVID-19

Resources

- Attaway AH, Scheraga RG, Bhimraj A, et al. Severe COVID-19 pneumonia: pathogenesis and clinical management. BMJ. 2021;372:n436.
- Dandachi D, Rodriguez-Barradas. Viral pneumonia: etiologies and treatment. J Investig Med 2018;66(6):957–965.
- Johnstone C, Hall A, Hart IJ. Common viral illnesses in intensive care: presentation, diagnosis, and management. CEACCP. 2014;14(5):213–219.
- National Institute for Health and Care Excellence. Treatments Being Monitored by RAPID C-19. Available from: https://www.nice.org.uk/covid-19/rapid-c-19-treatments-currently-monitored. (Accessed 31 August 2022.)
- UK Health Security Agency. COVID-19 Vaccination Programme: Information for Healthcare Practitioners. February 2022. Available from: https://assets.publishing.service.gov.uk/government/uploads/system/uploads/attachment_data/file/1052112/COVID-19_vaccine_Information_for_healthcare_practitioners_250122__2_.pdf. (Accessed 07 February 2022.)
- Vetter P, Vu DL, L'Huillier AG, et al. Clinical Features of COVID-19. BMJ 2020;369:m1470.
- World Health Organization. Estimating Mortality from COVID-19: Scientific Brief. August 2020. Available from: https://www.who.int/news-room/commentaries/detail/estimating-mortality-from-covid-19. (Accessed 07 February 2022.)
- World Health Organization. Tracking SARS-CoV-2 Variants. February 2022. Available from: https://www.who.int/en/activities/tracking-SARS-CoV-2-variants/. (Accessed 07 February 2022.)

125. PLEURAL EFFUSION

What is a pleural effusion?

A pleural effusion is a non-physiological collection of fluid in the pleural space (between the visceral and parietal pleura).

Normal pleural fluid comprises approximately 0.1–0.2 ml/kg and is alkaline (pH 7.62) with a low protein content (<1.5 g/dl). The pleural space may hold as much as 4–5 l.

What types of pleural effusions are there?

Pleural effusions can be classified by site, as unilateral or bilateral, or by composition as transudate or exudate. Other fluids may accumulate in rarer circumstances (Table 125.1).

- **Transudates** have a low protein content due to hydrostatic pressure resulting in filtration. They occur largely due to organ failures or fluid accumulation.
- **Exudates** contain more protein and result from leakage across membranes as a result of inflammatory conditions.

Table 125.1 Causes of pleural effusions

Transudates	Exudates	Other
• **LV failure** • **Cirrhosis with ascites** • Hypoalbuminaemia • Nephrotic syndrome • PD • Mitral stenosis • Hypothyroidism • Constrictive pericarditis • Meig's syndrome (benign ovarian tumour with ascites and pleural effusion)	• **Parapneumonic** • **Malignancy** • **TB** • PE • Pancreatitis • MI • Autoimmune pleuritis • Asbestos • CABG • Yellow nail syndrome (and other lymphatic disorders) • Sarcoidosis • *Drug reaction*: methotrexate, amiodarone, phenytoin, B-blockers, nitrofurantoin • Fungal infection • Ovarian hyperstimulation syndrome	• Chylothorax (lymph from thoracic duct defect) • Urinothorax (GU tract obstruction/injury with extravasation of urine) • GI contents (Boerhaave syndrome) • Cholothorax/bilothorax (biliary fistula) • Pyothorax (pus) • Catamenial HTX (thoracic endometriosis syndrome)

How would you investigate a pleural effusion?

A thorough history, examination, and CXR should be performed in the initial workup. Investigation and subsequent management depend on the degree of respiratory compromise caused and whether the effusion is suspicious in nature. Unilateral effusions are more likely to require investigation.

Bilateral effusion likely to be transudate should not be aspirated unless atypical or failing to respond to therapy. If management of the likely cause is ineffective, referral should be made to a chest physician. In the context of sepsis or pneumonia, diagnostic pleural tap should be carried out.

Pleural aspiration may be performed for the following:

- Cytology (60% sensitivity in malignant cause)
- Protein
- LDH
- pH
- MC+S

Pleural fluid pH < 7.30 may occur in malignancy, infection, connective tissue diseases, TB, and oesophageal rupture.

Pleural fluid appearance may be helpful for the following:

- *Putrid odour*: anaerobic empyema
- *Food particles*: oesophageal rupture
- *Bile staining*: cholothorax/bilothorax
- *Milky*: chylothorax, pseudochylothorax
- *'Anchovy sauce'*: ruptured amoebic abscess

Additional pleural fluid tests as indicated:

- *Glucose*: may be useful in rheumatoid
- AFB, TB culture
- *Triglycerides, cholesterol*: chylothorax
- *Amylase*: pancreatitis-related
- *Hct*: HTX

CT is indicated in undiagnosed exudative effusion, ideally before complete drainage as image quality is better. Further investigation might include percutaneous pleural biopsy or thoracoscopy. Bronchoscopy is only indicated if haemoptysis or obstruction is suggested in this context.

> **GUIDELINE** BTS 2010 Pleural disease

What are Light's criteria?

Crude distinction between transudative and exudative effusion can be made by the pleural fluid protein content (transudate < 30 g/l, exudate > 30 g/l). Light's criteria are recommended as more accurate, particularly when serum protein/albumin are outwith the normal range.

> **KEY POINT**
>
> Light's criteria for exudative pleural effusion – 1 or more of the following:
>
> - Pleural/serum protein > 0.5
> - Pleural/serum LDH > 0.6
> - Pleural LDH > ⅔ upper limit of normal serum LDH

What causes chylothorax?

- *Trauma*: chest injury, thoracic surgery (e.g. oesophagectomy)
- *Malignancy*: lymphoma, metastasis
- *Other*: LAM, TB, cirrhosis, obstruction of central veins, chyloascites

- Idiopathic (10%)
- *Pseudochylothorax*: TB, RA

When is pleural drainage indicated?

General
- Respiration compromised
- HTX

Infection
- pH < 7.20
- Frankly turbid/cloudy fluid
- Presence of organisms on Gram stain and/or culture of pleural fluid
- Loculated pleural collection

Considerations
- Volume drained should be limited to 1.5 l in the immediate setting (or <500 ml/h due to the risk of re-expansion pulmonary oedema.
- *No consensus on ideal tube size*: effective drainage must be balanced against discomfort.
- Drain removal can be considered when exudate has drained completely, or when transudate is insignificant (50–100 ml in 24 h).

Resource
- Paramasivam E, Bodenham A. Pleural fluid collections in critically ill patients. CEACCP. 2007;7(1):10–14.

---

126. PULMONARY EMBOLISM

What is the significance of PE?

PE is a form of VTE – third most common acute cardiovascular syndrome behind MI and stroke. It may be fatal or result in significant morbidity, with around 34% deaths occurring within hours of the event. PE may be preventable by addressing modifiable risk factors.

Do you know of any risk factors?

Many risk factors for PE have been identified (Table 126.1).

(See Chapter 141 Bleeding and Clotting Disorders)

Table 126.1   Risk factors for PE

Strong	Moderate	Weak
• Lower limb fracture • Spinal cord injury • Hip/knee replacement • Major trauma • Previous VTE • Spinal cord injury • Hospitalisation for HF/AF (last 3/12)	• Arthroscopic knee surgery • Autoimmune disease • Thrombophilia • Post-partum • Malignancy • Transfusion • Superficial vein thrombosis • Oral contraceptive pill • CVC • Infection • IBD • CCF • Stroke • In vitro fertilisation	• Bed rest >3 days • Immobility due to sitting • Laparoscopy • Obesity • Arterial hypertension • Pregnancy • Varicose veins • Diabetes mellitus • Increasing age

Table 126.2 ESC classification of PE

High risk	Intermediate risk		Low risk
Cardiovascular instability: • Syncope, • Sustained hypotension (systolic BP < 90 mmHg 15 min), or • Cardiac arrest	• PESI III–IV, sPESI ≥1, ≥1 Hestia criterion, or • RV dysfunction on TTE/CTPA		Stable, other factors negative
	Intermediate-high: • Troponin +ve	Intermediate-low: • Troponin –ve	

Table 126.3 AHA classification of PE

Massive	Submassive	Low risk
• Sustained hypotension (systolic BP < 90 mmHg 15 min or requiring inotropes), and • Not due to another cause (e.g. arrhythmia, hypovolaemia, sepsis, LV dysfunction, pulselessness, persistent profound bradycardia	Absence of sustained hypotension, and either: • RV dysfunction (echo, CT, BNP, ECG), or • Myocardial necrosis (elevated troponin)	Absence of clinical markers of massive/submassive PE

How would you classify PE?

Several classifications exist. The ESC/ERS classification is currently in use in the UK (Table 126.2). Reference might be made to terms used in the American Heart Association (AHA) classification (Table 126.3).

GUIDELINE ESC/ERS 2019 PE

How would you investigate a PE?

Diagnosis should be based on clinical suspicion, followed by confirmation with appropriate investigations. Validated prediction rules may be of value.

- *TTE*: first line in the unstable patient
- If RV dysfunction, perform **CTPA** if immediately available and feasible
  - *Positive*: treat as high risk
  - *Negative*: search for other causes of shock/instability
  - If CTPA not possible, treat as high risk
- *No RV dysfunction*: search for other causes

In a stable patient, clinical probability would be assessed using clinical judgement or a prediction rule, before consideration of CTPA (high probability) or D-dimer (low/intermediate probability). D-dimer can be used to rule out PE, but a positive result should prompt CTPA.

Can you describe some scoring systems that are used in PE?

Diagnostic scores involve point allocation of variable weighting for known risk factors and clinical findings. The Wells' criteria include a judgement-based question of whether PE is the most likely diagnosis or equally likely to other diagnoses.

- **Revised Geneva rule**
  - *Three-level score*: low (0–1), intermediate (2–4), high (≥5) risk
  - *Two-level score*: PE unlikely (0–2), PE likely (≥3)
- **Wells rule**
  - *Three-tier model*: low (0–1), moderate (2–6), high (>6) risk
  - *Two-tier model*: PE unlikely (≤4), PE likely (≥5)
- **PE rule-out criteria (PERC)**
  - Gestalt estimation of low risk + all criteria negative 'rules out' PE (probability < 2%)
  - Used in Emergency Department setting to avoid over-investigation
- **Hestia criteria**: used in stable patients to determine suitability for outpatient management

The **PE Severity Index (PESI)** is the most extensively validated system in assessment of overall mortality risk and early outcome. Points are allocated to the criteria of age, sex, cancer, chronic HF, COPD, HR, systolic BP, RR, temperature, altered mental status, and S_aO_2. Simplified PESI (S-PESI) has fewer criteria and can be used to facilitate discharge decisions (but is less accurate). Risk stratification according to 30-day mortality is as follows:

PESI Class by points (mortality in brackets):

i. ≤65 very low (0–1.6%)
ii. 66–85 low (1.7–3.5%)
iii. 86–105 moderate (3.2–7.1%)
iv. 106–125 high (4.0–11.4%)
v. >125 very high (10.0–24.5%)

What ECG signs might you see in severe PE?

A normal ECG is the most common finding in PE, but sinus tachycardia is the most common abnormality.

Features of RV strain are as follows:

- T inversion in V1–4
- QR pattern in V1
- S1Q3T3
- Incomplete or complete RBBB

What are the principles of management in the critically unwell patient with PE?

- *Reperfusion*
  - Thrombolysis
    - ➢ Indicated in **high-risk PE**
    - ➢ Alteplase 10 mg over 1–2 min, then 90 mg IV infusion over 2 h (max 1.5 mg/kg if under 65 kg)
  - Percutaneous catheter-directed treatment
  - *Surgical embolectomy/endarterectomy if thrombolysis fails/contraindicated*: requires cardiopulmonary bypass at specialist centre
- *Anticoagulation*: heparin-based (unfractionated initially)
- *Supportive care*
  - Target S_aO_2 ≥90%
  - *Noradrenaline*: RV inotropy, systemic BP, positive ventricular interactions, coronary perfusion gradient restoration
  - *Dobutamine*: RV inotropy, filling pressure reduction
  - ECLS (e.g. VA-ECMO) may be of benefit if surgical embolectomy performed
- *Multidisciplinary involvement*: respiratory medicine, IR, cardiothoracic surgery
- *Prevention of recurrence*
  - Anticoagulation
  - Vena cava interruption (e.g. IVC filter)

(See Chapter 79 Pulmonary Hypertension)

What do you know about thrombolysis in more stable patients with PE?

- Decision-making is tricky and most contentious in intermediate-high-risk PE.
- High risk of potentially life-threatening bleeding complications vs expected benefits
- Routine full-dose systemic thrombolysis in intermediate- or low-risk PE is not recommended.
- **Rescue thrombolysis** is recommended only if there is haemodynamic deterioration despite anticoagulation.
- The role of half-dose thrombolysis is unclear and as yet unsupported.

STUDY

MOPETT (2013)

- Moderate PE
- *Intervention*: addition of low-dose thrombolysis vs anticoagulation alone
- *Primary*: pulmonary hypertension on echo at 28 months – **significantly lower**
- *Secondary*: composite pulmonary hypertension and recurrent PE at 28 months – **significantly lower**; recurrent PE, mortality, bleeding – no difference.

STUDY

PEITHO (2014)

- Intermediate-risk PE
- *Intervention*: addition of tenecteplase vs heparin alone
- *Primary*: 7-day composite death and haemodynamic decompensation – **significantly lower**
- *Secondary*: haemodynamic decompensation – **significantly lower**, major haemorrhagic stroke – **significantly higher**, major extracranial bleeding – **significantly higher**, 7-day and 30-day mortality – no difference

Resources

- Jaff MR, McMurty MS, Archer SL, et al. Management of massive and submassive pulmonary embolism, iliofemoral deep vein thrombosis, and chronic thromboembolic pulmonary hypertension: a scientific statement from the American Heart Association. Circulation. 2011;123(16):1788–1830.
- Kline JA, Courtney DM, Kabrhel C, et al. Prospective multicenter evaluation of the pulmonary embolism rule-out criteria. J Thromb Haemost. 2008;6(5):772–780.

127. RESTRICTIVE LUNG DISEASE

What is restrictive lung disease?

Restrictive lung diseases are disorders of compliance, encompassing those which impair lung volume, with potential to develop into type II respiratory failure.

Causes may be pulmonary or extrapulmonary and can be classified according to aetiology:

- **Extrapulmonary**
  - *Respiratory centre (reduced respiratory drive)*: trauma, drugs (e.g. opioids)
  - *Neuronal*: poliomyelitis, GBS, diaphragmatic palsy, MND
  - *Neuromuscular junction*: MG
  - *Muscle*: muscular dystrophy
  - *Thoracic wall*: obesity, kyphoscoliosis, eschar, rib fractures
  - *Pleural*: effusion, PTX, plaques, mesothelioma
- **Pulmonary**
  - ILD
  - ARDS
  - TB
  - *Surgical*: lobectomy, pneumonectomy

What types of ILD are there?

There are over 300 different conditions that would qualify as ILDs, previously known as diffuse parenchymal lung diseases. Only 1 in 3 has a known cause.

- **Known aetiology**
  - Pneumoconioses (e.g. asbestosis, silicosis)
  - Extrinsic allergic alveolitis (EAA) (hypersensitivity pneumonitis) (e.g. farmer's lung, pigeon breeder's lung)
  - Iatrogenic (e.g. drugs*, radiation)
  - Post-infectious
- **Unknown aetiology**
  - Sarcoidosis
  - **Idiopathic interstitial pneumonias**
  - Related to connective tissue diseases and collagen-vascular diseases (includes rheumatoid arthritis and progressive systemic sclerosis)
  - Lymphangioleiomyomatosis (LAM)

What is the significance of LAM?

LAM is very rare but usually affects women of childbearing age. It can present with PTX or respiratory distress and is often fatal without lung transplantation. Associated features include renal angiomyolipomas, lymphangioleiomyomas, chylothorax, and lymph node involvement. Lung cysts are found on CT.

How are the idiopathic interstitial pneumonias classified?

The ATS and ERS classify idiopathic interstitial pneumonias as follows:

- Major idiopathic interstitial pneumonias
  - *IPF*: idiopathic pulmonary fibrosis
  - *NSIP*: idiopathic nonspecific interstitial pneumonia
  - *RB-ILD*: respiratory bronchiolitis-ILD
  - *DIP*: desquamative interstitial pneumonia
  - *COP*: cryptogenic organising pneumonia
  - *AIP*: acute interstitial pneumonia
- Rare idiopathic interstitial pneumonias
  - Idiopathic lymphoid interstitial pneumonia
  - Idiopathic pleuroparenchymal fibroelastosis
- Unclassifiable idiopathic interstitial pneumonias

They can also be classified by clinical behaviour as follows:

- *Reversible, self-limited*: RB-ILD
- *Reversible, risk of progression*: NSIP, DIP, COP
- *Stable with residual disease*: NSIP
- *Progressive, irreversible, potential for stabilisation*: NSIP
- *Progressive, irreversible despite therapy*: IPF, NSIP

What do you know about AIP?

AIP is characterised by progressive hypoxaemia and carries a high mortality (50%) with no proven treatment. Survivors have a good long-term prognosis, similar to that of ARDS. Some may experience recurrences or chronic progressive disease. On CT, early disease is exudative, before distortion of bronchovascular bundles and development of traction bronchiectasis.

What do you know about sarcoidosis?

Sarcoidosis is the second most common ILD and is characterised by granuloma formation in the lungs but may spread to other organs: skin, lymph nodes, liver, heart, and brain.

The classical finding on CXR is bilateral hilar lymphadenopathy, with more progressive disease exhibiting a reticulonodular pattern. Staging is based on CXR findings.

---

* Amiodarone, bleomycin, methotrexate, and nitrofurantoin are common causes of drug-induced ILD.

It has a high rate of spontaneous remission (55–90% stage I disease). Progressive disease is managed using prednisolone at treatment dose for several weeks, before low-dose maintenance for up to 2 years. Other immunosuppressants have a role if corticosteroids are not effective or tolerated (methotrexate first line). Lung transplantation may be indicated in end-stage disease.

How is severity of IPF determined?

Severity is difficult to determine and no set criteria apply. Concurrent disease is common (e.g. emphysema in 40%). Judgement may be made based on a combination of exercise tolerance, CXR, PFT, high-resolution CT, and multidisciplinary review over time.

What is the prognosis of ILD?

5-year survival
- *IPF*: 20%
- *Lymphoid interstitial pneumonia*: 60%
- *Cellular NSIP*: 80%
- *EAA*: 82%
- *Sarcoidosis*: 90%
- COP ~100%

Intubation and ventilation
- IPF ~ 100% short-term mortality even if discharged from ICU

What are the management priorities in ILD outwith the critical care environment?

- Known aetiology
  - Prevention
  - Cessation of exposure
- Unknown aetiology
  - *Antifibrotic therapies*: pirfenidone, nintedanib
  - *Anti-pulmonary hypertensives*: endothelin-1 antagonists (e.g. bosentan), phosphodiesterase-5 inhibitors (e.g. sildenafil)
  - *Anti-inflammatory drugs (not in IPF)*: corticosteroids, others including cyclophosphamide, methotrexate, biologics
- Advanced ILD
  - *Oxygen*: symptomatic relief only (no effect on survival)
  - *Rehabilitation*: quality of life
  - Pulmonary hypertension: referral to specialist centre if disproportionate or severe (PASP > 50 mmHg)
  - Lung transplantation where appropriate
  - Palliative care

GUIDELINE BTS 2008 ILD

When is lung transplantation indicated in IPF?

Patients with IPF or fibrotic NSIP may be suitable for transplantation if TLCO < 40% predicted or progressive (FVC decline ≥10%). Candidates are usually otherwise physiologically and psychologically robust and <65 years of age.

How would you approach the referral of a patient to critical care with ILD and acute respiratory failure?

This should trigger an individualised assessment with the input of respiratory physicians. Underlying diagnosis is crucial. The most common diagnoses are AIP, acute exacerbation of IPF, and fulminant COP.

Seek information
- **Nature of presentation**
  - Exacerbation of ILD

- Initial presentation of rapidly progressive ILD
- Other pathology with ILD as a comorbidity
- **Important considerations**
  - *Aetiology*: reversibility, response to treatment, accuracy of diagnosis
  - *Severity of disease*: usual therapy (specifically use of home oxygen)
  - Behaviour prior to acute deterioration (particularly progression despite treatment)
  - *Complications*: pulmonary hypertension, cor pulmonale
  - Functional status
  - *Investigation results*: PFT, exercise tolerance, echo, BAL, transbronchial/surgical lung biopsy
  - *Specialist opinion*: clinic review, expected prognosis
  - Involvement of palliative care team

Management of acute respiratory failure due to ILD is as follows:

- *Respiratory support*: if potentially reversible pending further investigation
  - Intubation and ventilation often not appropriate in IPF due to high associated mortality
  - BTS guidance advocates that the decision for NIV but not IMV should be made jointly by a respiratory physician and an intensivist, ideally not at the point of immediate requirement of this support.
  - Mechanical ventilation is increasingly an absolute contraindication to lung transplantation due to high risk of pneumonia from colonisation and deconditioning (×3 post-transplant mortality at 1 year).

- **Investigation**
  - If nature of ILD defined and distinction made between disease progression and infection (treat as appropriate)
  - Otherwise, consider BAL, transbronchial biopsy (± surgical biopsy).
- **Corticosteroids**
  - In rapidly progressive ILD with respiratory failure (once any concomitant infection controlled)
  - Pulsed IV methylprednisolone
- **Cyclophosphamide**
  - Second line in above
  - First line in suspected vasculitis
- *Palliation*: if irreversible (majority of patients)

Resources

- European Respiratory Society. European Lung White Book: Interstitial Lung Diseases. 2022. Available from: https://www.erswhitebook.org/chapters/interstitial-lung-diseases/. (Accessed 31 August 2022.)
- Johnson SR, Cordier JF, Lazor R. European Respiratory Society guidelines for the diagnosis and management of lymphangioleiomyomatosis. Eur Respir J. 2010;35(1):14–26.
- Travis WD, Costabel U, Hansell DM, et al. An Official American Thoracic Society/European Respiratory Society Statement: Update of the International Multidisciplinary Classification of the Idiopathic Interstitial Pneumonias. Am J Respir Crit Care Med. 2013;188(6):733–748.

128. SLEEP BREATHING DISORDERS

What is sleep-disordered breathing?

Sleep-disordered breathing encompasses several conditions characterised by hypoventilation during sleep:

- *Snoring*: intermittent, partial airway obstruction without sleep disturbance
- *OSA*: intermittent full airway obstruction, irrespective of daytime symptoms
- *Obstructive sleep apnoea syndrome (OSAS)*: OSA with daytime symptoms, also known as obstructive sleep apnoea/hypopnoea syndrome (OSAHS)

- *Central sleep apnoea (CSA)*: periodic cessation of breathing without airway obstruction
- *OHS*: breathing reduced throughout sleep, with/without upper airway narrowing/obstruction

What else do you know about OSAS?

OSAS is common and can result in daytime somnolence, cognitive impairment, hypertension, and cardiovascular morbidity. Untreated disease increases the rate of road traffic collisions and work-related and domestic accidents.

It results from pharyngeal obstruction and is most commonly caused by obesity. Other contributory factors are as follows: male, smoking, alcohol use, muscle-relaxant medication, supine posture, reduced nasal patency, and anatomical variations.

KEY POINT

- *Obstructive apnoea*: cessation of airflow despite continued breathing efforts ≥10 s
- *Hypopnoea*: 30–50% reduction in thoraco-abdominal movement from baseline for ≥10 s (with 3% desaturation or an arousal)

KEY POINT

Severity can be measured by the Apnoea/Hypopnoea Index (AHI):

- *Mild*: 5-15 events per hour of sleep
- *Moderate*: 15–30
- *Severe*: >30

Overnight polysomnography may be used in diagnosis, involving the following: nasal/oral airflow, thoraco-abdominal movement, snoring, EEG, electro-oculogram, EMG, and oxygen saturation.

Management might include the following:

- *Lifestyle measures*: weight loss, alcohol reduction, smoking cessation
- Nocturnal CPAP
- Mandibular repositioning device
- *Surgery*: tonsillectomy, upper airway surgery (e.g. in craniofacial abnormality), bariatric, hypoglossal nerve stimulation

What is the main physiological difference between OSAS and OHS?

The key difference is the hypercapnia when awake in OHS, whereas P_aCO_2 is normal in awake patients with OSAS. NIV may be used in preference to CPAP, and supplemental oxygen may often be required.

KEY POINT

OHS is defined by the following:

- BMI > 30 kg/m²
- Type II respiratory failure (P_aCO_2 > 6.5 kPa)
- Sleep-disordered breathing

When other causes of type II respiratory failure have been excluded.

Resource

- European Respiratory Society. European Lung White Book: Sleep breathing disorders. 2022. Available from: https://www.erswhitebook.org/chapters/sleep-breathing-disorders/. (Accessed 31 August 2022.)

What is TB?

TB is an airborne disease caused by *Mycobacterium tuberculosis*, manifesting as a spectrum of illness from respiratory symptoms to multisystem disease.

What are the clinical features of TB?

The most common presenting features of TB are cough and haemoptysis.

Other characteristic features are as follows:

- Fever
- Weight loss
- Night sweats

Multisystem involvement is possible, and presentation may arise from other organs.

When might patients with TB be admitted to critical care?

Common causes of admission directly related to TB are as follows:

- **Respiratory failure due to pulmonary TB** (1.5% of hospitalised pulmonary TB)
  - 72% have concomitant bacterial pneumonia, COPD, or malignancy
  - 20% also have extrapulmonary TB
  - Often have significant comorbidities (e.g. HIV infection)
- **Miliary TB**
  - Haematological dissemination to multiple organs
  - Immunosuppression contributory
  - 80% develop multi-organ dysfunction
  - May cause adrenal insufficiency
- *CNS TB*: meningitis, tuberculomas (1% TB cases)
  - 6–18% ICU admissions from TB
  - Hydrocephalus common (77%)
  - *Hyponatraemia problematic*: SIADH and cerebral salt-wasting syndrome (CSWS) contributory

Other indications are as follows:

- **TB-related**
  - *CS*: pericardial effusion
  - *Massive haemoptysis*: Rasmussen aneurysm (dilatation of PA branch adjacent to tuberculoma)
  - *DIC*: miliary TB
  - *Pituitary apoplexy*: cerebral TB
  - *Airway obstruction*: laryngeal/retropharyngeal TB
- **Treatment-related**
  - *Renal failure*: rifampicin
  - *Liver failure*: rifampicin, isoniazid
- **Unrelated**
  - *Post-operative*: known TB undergoing other surgery (e.g. thoracic)
  - Concurrent disease in patient with known TB

What are the challenges of managing TB in critical care?

- Microbiological samples may be difficult to obtain, prolonged culture time
- Administration of effective anti-TB treatment (poor absorption, organ dysfunction)
- Paradoxical reactions, side effects
- Inability to monitor for ocular toxicity with ethambutol
- Managing infectivity

- Maintaining compliance with treatment as patients recover
- Emergence of multidrug-resistant TB

How is TB diagnosed?

Positive culture is ideal. Diagnosis may be made if clinical features, radiology, and microbiological samples are in keeping with TB. Presence of AFB may facilitate diagnosis in this context whilst culture is pending.

Workup should follow the following sequence, progressing if each stage is inconclusive:

- *Sputum*: AFB (or PCR)
- *Bronchoscopy or induced sputum if stable enough*: AFB (or PCR)
- *Seek evidence at other sites*: lymph nodes, pleural effusion, CSF
- Decision based on overall clinical picture (including radiology, interferon gamma release assay)

Microbiological culture
- Suspected patients should have ≥2 sputum specimens sent for MC+S.
- Culture takes 2–4 weeks (up to 12 weeks in some cases).
- Initial staining (auramine/Ziehl-Neelsen) is useful for AFB.
- High sensitivity of samples from bronchoscopy (87%) or tracheal aspirates (88%)
- Biopsy may be indicated for histology.

Extrapulmonary samples
- Blood cultures for mycobacteria (disseminated TB)
- CSF characteristics (TB meningitis)
- TB PCR
- Interferon gamma release assays/nucleic acid amplification tests

Radiology
- *CXR*: upper lobe disease, nodules, cavities
- *CT*: centrilobular nodules, 'tree in bud' pattern, mediastinal lymphadenopathy, miliary shadowing

What are the main anti-TB drugs and important side effects?

- *R*: **rifampicin*** – hepatotoxicity, AKI
- *H*: **isoniazid*** – hepatotoxicity
- *Z*: **pyrazinamide**
- *E*: **ethambutol** – optic nerve toxicity
- Fluoroquinolones* (e.g. moxifloxacin)
- Aminoglycosides* (e.g. streptomycin, amikacin)
- Cycloserine
- Prothionamide

What specific management priorities are relevant to TB in critical care?

- **Multidisciplinary input**
  - For example microbiology, infectious diseases, respiratory, neurology, neurosurgery
- **Infection control measures**
  - *Aerosol precautions*: isolation, PPE
  - Ensuring compliance as patients recover
  - *Rarely*: involuntary isolation (ethically complex)
- **Anti-TB treatment**
  - *Non-multidrug-resistant*: R+H 6–9 months (12 if CNS)
  - Parenteral therapy may be commenced initially.
- **Treatment of co-infection**
  - *HIV*: may require antiretroviral therapy
  - *Bacterial infection*: may require additional antimicrobial cover

---

* Parenteral preparations available.

- **Management of complications**
  - Corticosteroids for meningitis, pericardial effusion, some cases of advanced pulmonary disease
  - *Hyponatraemia*: depends on cause, may be multifactorial
  - *Hydrocephalus*: EVD, third ventriculostomy
  - *Paradoxical reaction/immune reconstitution syndrome possible (median onset at 26 days from treatment)*: may respond to corticosteroids, thalidomide, montelukast
    - ➢ Recurrent fever
    - ➢ Lymph node inflammation
    - ➢ Airway obstruction
    - ➢ Splenic rupture
    - ➢ Worsening neurology

What is the prognosis of TB requiring critical care?

- *Mechanical ventilation for active TB*: 69% in-hospital mortality
- *CNS TB requiring ICU admission*: 65% 1-year mortality

Resources

- Bashford T, Howell V. Tropical medicine and anaesthesia 1. BJA Educ. 2018;18(2):35–40.
- Hagan G, Nathani N. Clinical review: tuberculosis on the intensive care unit. Crit Care. 2013;17:240.
- World Health Organization Regional Office for Europe. Tuberculosis, Ethics and Human Rights: Report of a Regional Workshop. October 2013. Available from: https://www.euro.who.int/__data/assets/pdf_file/0004/242941/Tuberculosis,-ethics-and-human-rights.pdf. (Accessed 09 February 2022.)

---

130.   ACUTE KIDNEY INJURY

What is 'AKI'?

AKI is a rapid deterioration in kidney function and may be caused by multiple pathological processes. The prevalence of AKI requiring RRT in the ICU is around 5–6%, with a hospital mortality of 60%.

It can be defined using the KDIGO criteria, which stage AKI based on changes in creatinine and/or UO. Requirement for acute RRT qualifies the patient for stage 3 automatically. RIFLE criteria were used prior to KDIGO. Automated detection may have a significant impact on recognition of AKI.

Table 130.1   Comparison of KDIGO and RIFLE criteria for AKI

	KDIGO Serum creatinine (mmol/l)		Both	RIFLE		
	Absolute	Change from baseline	UO (ml/kg/h)		Serum creatinine change from baseline	eGFR reduction (%)
1	≥26.5 rise in 48 h	× 1.5–1.9	<0.5 for 6–12 h	**Risk**	× 1.5–1.9	>25
2		× 2.0–2.9	<0.5 for ≥12 h	**Injury**	× 2.0–2.9	>50
3	≥353.6 or RRT or (if <18 years) eGFR < 35%	× 3.0	<0.3 for ≥24 h or Anuria for ≥12 h	**Failure**	× 3.0 or >354 with acute rise >44 mmol/l	>75
				Loss	Persistent AKI – complete loss of kidney function >4 weeks	
				End-stage	>3 months	

What are the causes of reduced renal function?

Prerenal
- *Hypoperfusion*: hypovolaemia, reduced cardiac output, increased vascular resistance

Intrinsic
- *Tubular*: ischaemia, nephrotoxins, endogenous toxins (e.g. myoglobin, uric acid)
- *Glomerular*: glomerulonephritis*
- *Interstitial*: infection, medications
- *Vascular*
  - *Large vessel*: renal artery stenosis, renal vein thrombosis
  - *Small vessel*: vasculitis, hypertension emergency, emboli, thrombotic microangiopathy (TMA)

Postrenal
- *Extra-renal obstruction*: prostatic hypertrophy, catheter blockage, malignancy
- *Intra-renal obstruction*: nephrolithiasis, 'clot retention', papillary necrosis

When does AKI become CKD?

> **KEY POINT**
>
> Duration of renal dysfunction is as follows:
>
> - Persistent AKI > 48 h
> - Acute kidney disease (AKD) > 7 days
> - CKD > 90 days

What are the limitations of the KDIGO criteria?

- Creatinine is unreliable:
  - Baseline values are often not known.
  - Variation in muscle mass and turnover between patients may lead to falsely low or high values.
  - Altered by some drugs independently of renal function
  - Unreliable in sepsis, liver disease, neuromuscular disorders
  - Measurement is affected by volume status.
- No differentiation between patients with normal baseline renal function vs CKD
- No indication of underlying aetiology
- Not validated in pregnancy (GFR physiologically increased, diagnosis may be delayed)
- UO is unreliable as oliguria may be an appropriate physiological response (e.g. stress, hypovolaemia).

Do you know of any biomarkers for AKI?

Serum creatinine reflects GFR. An alternative is the biomarker, **cystatin C**, which is a small cysteine protease inhibitor produced by nucleated cells. Its levels are not dependent on muscle mass, so it is being used increasingly in renal clearance calculations at extremes of body weight and in paediatrics.

Newer biomarkers are under evaluation to detect kidney damage, although these are not used clinically at the moment. Examples are as follows:

- *Tubular stress*: TIMP-2
- *Tubular damage*: urinary or plasma NGAL, urinary KIM-1

---

* There are many causes of acute and chronic glomerulonephritis, often classified in terms of histopathological appearance. Rapidly progressive glomerulonephritis is characterised by a 50% drop in function within 3 months – causes include anti-GBM disease, SLE, IgA, Henoch-Schönlein purpura (HSP), and ANCA-associated vasculitis (AAV).

- *Inflammation*: urinary ILs (e.g. IL-18)
- *Nephrocheck®*: product of urine TIMP-2 and IGFBP-7, used in the United States to detect risk of AKI

What are the causes of AKI?

Exposure to **causative** factors:

- Sepsis
- Critical illness
- Circulatory shock
- Burns
- Trauma
- Cardiac surgery (especially with cardiopulmonary bypass)
- Major non-cardiac surgery
- Nephrotoxic drugs
- Radiocontrast agents
- Poisonous plants and animals
- *Immune complex deposition*: SLE, glomerulonephritis
- *Formation of microvascular thrombi*: TMA, pre-eclampsia

Factors increasing **susceptibility** are as follows:

- Dehydration or volume depletion
- Advanced age
- Female sex
- CKD
- Chronic diseases (heart, lung, liver)
- Diabetes mellitus
- Cancer
- Anaemia

What might your 'AKI screen' include?

All

- *Bloods*: FBC, blood film, U&E, bicarbonate, glucose, bone profile, VBG, coagulation screen, LDH, CRP
- Urine dip
- *Imaging*: renal US

Case dependent

- *Cultures*: blood, sputum, urine, wound, etc.
- *Viral*: HBV, HCV, HIV serology
- *Immune*: autoantibodies (e.g. ANCA, ANA, anti-GBM), C3, C4
- *Myeloma*: serum/urine electrophoresis, urine Bence-Jones protein, serum-free light chains
- *Rhabdomyolysis*: CK, myoglobin
- *Post-streptococcal glomerulonephritis*: ASOT, throat swab
- *Rarer infections*: leptospirosis, hantavirus PCR

What are the main causes of AKI in the critical care population?

Most AKI will involve multiple aetiologies. In order of incidence:

- Septic shock
- Major surgery
- Cardiogenic shock
- Hypovolaemia
- Drug-related

Name some important nephrotoxins used commonly in critical care.

- *Antibiotics*: aminoglycosides, glycopeptides (e.g. vancomycin)
- *Antifungals*: amphotericin B

- *Antivirals*: aciclovir, ganciclovir
- Mannitol
- Large volumes of 0.9% NaCl

(See Chapter 32 Poisoning Overview)

Would you give IV radiological contrast to a patient at risk of AKI?

Contrast-induced nephropathy is a decline in renal function seen in the days following contrast administration.

It is not felt to be as high a threat as previously thought. There is no robust evidence to support an association between contrast dye and significant adverse outcome, whilst there are clear benefits of using contrast to accurately visualise pathology.

Most critically unwell patients should receive contrast when indicated, except perhaps those with very severe AKI. Consideration should be made to patients' likelihood to receive RRT in this cohort.

What are the important management principles in AKI?

Early recognition is the key as there is no specific treatment. Thromboprophylaxis dosing should be adjusted as indicated to avoid harm. Care is aimed at optimising renal function and preserving any further decline:

- **Maintain adequate volume status** (may include fluid resuscitation or restriction)
- **Correct electrolytes**
- **Minimise tubular toxins**
- **Treat any glomerular disease**
- **Relieve postrenal obstruction**

Is there any role for early commencement of RRT in stage 3 AKI?

No mortality benefit has been shown by commencing RRT early. Conversely, not all patients with severe AKI will require RRT, and it is not without morbidity (e.g. risks of line insertion, anticoagulation). It may be that early initiation carries greater risk of continued dependence on RRT and possible RRT-related kidney injury.

Indications to start RRT are often described as follows:

- *A*: acidosis – significant metabolic acidosis
- *E*: electrolytes – refractory hyperkalaemia
- *I*: intoxication – clearance of toxins including drugs and alcohols
- *O*: overload – fluid overload causing compromise
- *U*: uraemia – compromise (e.g. pericarditis or encephalopathy, around 30 mmol/l)

KDIGO recommend commencing RRT emergently in life-threatening changes in fluid, electrolyte, and acid-base balance. Other indications might include temperature management or removal of inflammatory mediators in sepsis (controversial). The broader clinical context should be considered.

In cases of AKI, a stage-based approach following KDIGO guidelines should be employed. There is no evidence to support pre-emptive RRT, but its consideration is recommended in Stage 2 or 3 AKI.

GUIDELINE KDIGO 2012 AKI

STUDY

STARRT-AKI (2020)

- Critically ill patients with severe AKI
- *Intervention*: accelerated RRT (<12 h of meeting criteria) vs standard care (classical indications or AKI > 72 h)
- *Primary*: 90-day mortality – **no difference**
- *Secondary*: composite of death/dependence, MAKE, sustained reduction in kidney function, death in ICU at 28/7, hospital LOS – no difference; RRT dependence at 90 days – **significantly higher (10.4% vs 6%)**.
- Higher incidence of adverse events in the accelerated strategy group

AKIKI (2016)

- Critically ill patients with stage 3 AKI
- *Intervention*: early RRT < 6 h vs delayed RRT (conventional criteria, e.g. hyperkalaemia)
- *Primary*: 60-day mortality – **no difference**
- *Secondary*: 8-day mortality, ICU LOS, hospital LOS, RRT dependency – no difference; number receiving RRT – **significantly higher**; CRBSI – **significantly higher**

ELAIN (2016)

- Severe AKI
- *Intervention*: early (within 8 h of stage 2 AKI) vs delayed initiation (within 12 h of stage 3) of RRT
- *Primary*: 90-day mortality – **significantly lower (39.3% vs 54.7%)**
- *Secondary*: duration of RRT, hospital LOS – **significantly lower**; recovery of renal function by day 90 – **significantly higher**; requirement for RRT after day 90, organ dysfunction, ICU LOS – **no difference**
- Single centre, predominantly surgical population

What is the role of sodium bicarbonate infusion in severe AKI with acidaemia?

Sodium bicarbonate has not been shown to improve outcomes such as mortality or LOS on ICU. However, the amount and duration of RRT might be reduced with its use, with potential to minimise associated complications and morbidity.

BICAR-ICU (2018)

- Critically ill patients with severe metabolic acidosis (pH ≤ 7.20)
- *Intervention*: 4.25% sodium bicarbonate infusion vs none
- *Primary*: composite 28-day mortality and ≥1 organ failure at 7 days – **no difference**
- *Secondary*: RRT use – **significantly lower**, RRT-free days – **significantly lower**, time to RRT – **significantly higher**, ICU LOS – no difference

How would you define renal recovery?

The KDIGO definition of renal recovery is the absence of diagnostic criteria for AKI.

RRT might be stopped when treatment limitations are reviewed or native kidney function return, or if a complication arises (e.g. circuit clotting) in more borderline cases, with a view to balance risks against probability of recovery.

Cessation of RRT should be considered when UO > 400 ml/24 h without diuretic use, or >2300 ml/day with diuretics. Creatinine clearance >20 ml/min can also be considered, as used in the **ATN** and **ELAIN** trials. (See Chapter 20 Renal Replacement Therapy)

When should a renal referral be made from critical care?

Indications for specialist renal review include the following:

- Unknown aetiology of AKI
- Suspected glomerular or vasculitic disease
- Renal transplant
- Ongoing requirement for RRT

What is the prognosis in terms of renal function for those with AKI who require RRT on critical care?

- 40% survival to hospital discharge
  - Additional 10% mortality per year following discharge (study period of 8 years)
- In survivors to hospital discharge, at 1 year
  - 48% complete renal recovery (peak at 90 days)
  - 33% incomplete recovery
  - 19% dialysis dependent (28% at 3 years)
- *MAKE*: death, incomplete renal recovery, ESRF on RRT
  - 83% at hospital discharge
  - 94% at 3 years

Resources

- De Corte W, Dhondt A, Vanholder R, et al. Long-term outcome in ICU patients with acute kidney injury treated with renal replacement therapy: a prospective cohort study. Crit Care. 2016;20(1):256.
- Uchino S, Kellum JA, Bellomo R, et al. Acute renal failure in critically ill patients: a multinational, multicenter study. JAMA. 2005;294(7):813–818.

---

131. CHRONIC KIDNEY DISEASE

How is CKD diagnosed?

CKD is diagnosed when an abnormality of kidney structure and/or function has been present for >3 months, with implications for health. Causes are largely as for AKI. (See Chapter 130 Acute Kidney Injury)

KEY POINT

Diagnostic Criteria for CKD

Estimated glomerular filtration rate (eGFR) <60 for >3 months plus one of:

- ACR ≥3 mg/mmol (≥30 mg/g)
- Urinary sediment abnormalities
- Electrolyte and other abnormalities due to tubular disorders
- Abnormalities detected by histology
- Structural abnormalities detected by imaging
- History of renal transplant

GUIDELINE KDIGO 2012 CKD

How is CKD classified?

CKD may also be classified as GFR category or albuminuria category as follows.

> **KEY POINT**
>
> GFR category (ml/min/1.73 m²)
>
> 1. ≥90
> 2. 60–89
> 3. 30–59
>   a. 45–59
>   b. 30–44
> 4. 15–29
> 5. <15
>
> *Albuminuria categories*: albumin excretion rate (mg/24 h), ACR (mg/mmol)
>
> 1. <30, <3
> 2. 30–300, 3–30
> 3. >300, >30

What does the management of CKD involve?

CKD management centres around prevention of progression. Focus changes as CKD progresses through different stages, utilising the following domains:

- BP and RAS interruption
- AKI management (see Chapter 130 Acute Kidney Injury)
- *Protein intake reduction (controversial)*: 0.8 g/kg/day
- Lipid-lowering therapies
- *Glycaemic control*: target HbA_{1c} 53 mmol/mol (7%)
- *Salt intake reduction*: <90 mmol (2 g) sodium per 24 h (5 g NaCl)
- *Electrolyte management*: calcium, phosphate
- *Anaemia management*: iron, erythropoietin
- *Lifestyle adaptations*: physical activity, weight management, smoking cessation, dietary advice

What are the implications of CKD for the critically unwell patient?

Physiological

- *B*: increased risk of post-operative pulmonary complications
- *C*: increased risk of cardiovascular disease, hypertension, and diabetes
- *D*: autonomic and peripheral neuropathies
- *F*: altered electrolytes and fluid status
- *H*: anaemia, coagulopathies, platelet dysfunction
- *I*: reduced humeral and cell-mediated immunity

Pharmacokinetics

- Increased plasma volume due to renin-angiotensin activation
- Increased volume of distribution
- Increased free drug availability of highly protein-bound drugs and ionised drugs (due to hypoalbuminaemia, acidosis, and thrombocytopaenia)
- Reduced renal excretion of drugs

Unit resources

- Increased requirement for RRT
- Increased nursing dependency

How might you adapt your management in this patient group?

- **Supportive care** as indicated
  - Isotonic solution use

- Consider hyponatraemic effects of free water load from medications prepared in 5% dextrose
- *Meticulous fluid balance assessment*: regular weight monitoring
- **Limitation of nephrotoxins**
- **Adjustment of medication dosing**
- *Vein/artery preservation*: minimise peripheral venepuncture, consider in decision-making
- *Cautious transfusion*: may affect tissue matching if transplantation required in the future

Can you name some drugs that may require dose alterations in patients with reduced GFR?

- Warfarin
- LMWH
- Beta-blockers (50% reduction)
- Opioids
- Antibiotics (e.g. piperacillin/tazobactam, meropenem)
- Local anaesthetics

The renal drug handbook is a useful resource to guide adaptations alongside liaison with pharmacy.

Resources

- Ashley C, Currie A. (Eds.) The Renal Drug Handbook, 3rd ed. Oxford: Radcliffe Publishing Ltd; 2009.
- Nickson C. Life in the Fast Lane: End-Stage Renal Failure. November 2020. Available from: https://litfl.com/end-stage-renal-failure/. (Accessed 09 February 2022.)

---

132. ELECTROLYTE DISORDERS

What do you know about hypokalaemia (/hyperkalaemia)?

An overview of potassium disorders is as follows: (Table 132.1).

What do you know about hypomagnesaemia (/hypermagnesaemia)?

An overview of magnesium disorders is as follows: (Table 132.2).

Can you describe some other therapeutic uses of magnesium?

- *Exacerbation of asthma*: possible role as bronchodilator (3Mg trial)
- *SAH*: prevention of vasospasm (treatment, not prophylaxis) (MASH-2 trial)
- *Pre-eclampsia/eclampsia*: neuronal stabilisation (Magpie trial)
- *Premature labour*: tocolysis
- *Analgesia*: reduction of opioid requirement

(See Chapter 82 Subarachnoid Haemorrhage)

What do you know about hypocalcaemia (/hypercalcaemia)?

An overview of calcium disorders is as follows: (Table 132.3).

When might you also use calcium therapeutically in critical care?

- *Massive transfusion*: counteract calcium chelation by citrate in blood products
- *Calcium channel blocker overdose*: saturate remaining ion channels
- *Hyperkalaemia*: myocardial stabilisation

What do you know about hypophosphataemia (/hyperphosphataemia)?

An overview of phosphate disorders is as follows: (Table 132.4).

Table 132.1 Potassium disorders

K+	Hypokalaemia	Hyperkalaemia
Definition	<3.5 mmol/l: mild <2.5 mmol/l: severe	>5.5 mmol/l: mild >6.5 mmol/l: severe
Causes	Spurious: • Sampling error Reduced intake • Malabsorption Disturbed homeostasis: • Insulin use • Diabetes mellitus • Metabolic alkalosis • Corticosteroid excess • Xanthines • Cirrhosis • B2-agonists • Thyrotoxicosis Increased loss: • Diuretics • Diarrhoea • Vomiting	Spurious: • Haemolysis of sample Increased intake: • Potassium containing solutions (fluids, antibiotics) • Blood transfusion • PN Disturbed homeostasis: • Renal failure • Insulin deficiency • Hypoaldosteronism • Metabolic acidosis • *Drugs*: digoxin, beta-blockers, suxamethonium • Rhabdomyolysis • Tumour lysis syndrome (TLS) Reduced loss • *Drugs*: amiloride, spironolactone, NSAID, ACE-I, ARB, heparin
Features	Skeletal muscle weakness Cardiac arrhythmias	Cardiac arrhythmias (>7 mmol/l, rate of change also significant)
ECG	Ventricular extrasystoles AF ST-segment depression T-wave inversion U-wave elevation	Peaked T-waves Absent P-waves Diminished R-wave amplitude Broad QRS Sinusoidal waveform
Treatment	IV potassium chloride (up to 40 mmol/h via CVC)	Calcium gluconate 10 ml 10% (ECG changes) Insulin and dextrose (10 units short-acting in 50 ml 5% dextrose over 15–30 min) Salbutamol nebulisers
Other	Treat cause Address magnesium also	Treat cause Cardiac monitor if K+ > 6.0 mmol/l RRT if refractory *Potassium binders*: sodium zirconium cyclosilicate (Lokelma®), patiromer Sodium bicarbonate 8.4% 50 ml in cardiac arrest/significant arrhythmia

Table 132.2 Magnesium disorders

Mg²⁺	Hypomagnesaemia	Hypermagnesaemia
Definition	<0.7 mmol/l: mild <0.5 mmol/l: severe	>2.5 mmol/l: mild >7 mmol/l: severe
Causes	Reduced intake: • Dietary Disturbed homeostasis Increased GI loss: • Diarrhoea • Vomiting • Laxative use • Small bowel surgery • IBD	Increased intake: • IV infusions • *Drugs*: magnesium-containing antacids, laxatives, enemas • CKD with exogenous magnesium intake • Pre-eclampsia/eclampsia therapy

(Continued)

Table 132.2 Magnesium disorders (*Continued*)

Mg²⁺	Hypomagnesaemia	Hypermagnesaemia
	Increased renal loss: • Alcohol excess • Diabetes mellitus • Congenital/acquired disease • Diuretics • Proton pump inhibitors	
Features	Cardiovascular: • Hypertension • Angina • Cardiac arrhythmias Neuromuscular hyperexcitability: • Myoclonus • Stridor • Dysphagia • Abdominal pain • Seizures • Reduced level of consciousness	Neuromuscular depression: • Respiratory depression • Apnoea • Loss of deep tendon reflexes
ECG	Prolonged PR, QRS	Prolonged PR, QRS, QT Complete heart block
Treatment	20 mmol in emergency (5 g MgSO₄) Up to 40 mmol per day	IV calcium if life-threatening features Consider forced diuresis ± RRT if this fails
Other	Treat cause Ensure renal function adequate first Correct potassium and calcium (Risk of hypotension, bradycardia, unpleasant flushing with treatment)	Treat cause

Table 132.3 Calcium disorders

Ca²⁺	Hypocalcaemia	Hypercalcaemia
Definition	*<2.1 mmol/l plasma*: mild (*<1.1 mmol/l*: ionised) *<1.8 mmol/l* severe	*>2.6 mmol/l*: mild *>3 mmol/l*: severe
Causes	Spurious: • Hypoalbuminaemia (ionised calcium normal) Disturbed homeostasis: • *Parathyroid related*: hereditary/acquired hypoparathyroidism, hypomagnesaemia • *Vitamin D related*: dietary deficiency, lack of sunlight, anticonvulsant therapy, malabsorption • *Hyperphosphataemia*: TLS, rhabdomyolysis Increased loss • AKI • CKD • Citrate chelation (e.g. massive transfusion)	Increased intake: • Supplement excess Disturbed homeostasis: • *Parathyroid related*: primary hyperparathyroidism, lithium, familial hypocalciuric hypercalcaemia • *Vitamin D related*: intoxication, granulomatous diseases, e.g. sarcoid • *High bone turnover*: hyperthyroidism, immobilisation, thiazides, vitamin A toxicity • *Cancer related*: primary tumour, secondary hyperparathyroidism, paraneoplastic syndromes • PN • Lithium • Hyperthyroidism • Addison's disease
Features	Altered mental state Seizures Tetany Chvostek sign Trousseau sign Laryngospasm Hypotension Cardiac arrhythmias	*Groans*: constipation *Moans*: psychosis *Bones*: bone pain *Stones*: renal stones *Other*: fatigue, depression, confusion, anorexia, nausea, vomiting, peptic ulceration, pancreatitis, muscle weakness (>3.75 mmol/l coma, cardiac arrest)

(*Continued*)

Table 132.3   Calcium disorders (*Continued*)

Ca²⁺	Hypocalcaemia	Hypercalcaemia
ECG	Prolonged QT-interval AV conduction block	Short PR and QT-interval Wide T-wave
Treatment	10 ml 10% calcium chloride/gluconate (0.23/0.68 mmol/ml, respectively)	IV 0.9% NaCl Diuresis Bisphosphonates Calcitonin Calcimimetics if parathyroid surgery-related RRT if above fail
Other	Treat cause Correct magnesium	Treat cause Mobilisation helpful Cancer-related: mithramycin, glucocorticoids

Table 132.4   Phosphate disorders

PO₄³⁻	Hypophosphataemia	Hyperphosphataemia
Definition	*<0.8 mmol/l*: mild *<0.32 mmol/l*: severe	*>1.46 mmol/l*: mild *>4.54 mmol/l*: severe
Causes	Reduced intake: • Malabsorption • Dietary deficiency • Phosphate-binding antacids Disturbed homeostasis: • *Hormonal*: insulin, glucagon, adrenaline, dopamine • *Drugs*: carbohydrate infusion, B2 agonists, steroids, xanthines • Respiratory alkalosis • *Glucose shift*: refeeding, DKA management • *Rapid cell uptake*: hungry bone syndrome, leukaemia • Vitamin D deficiency Increased loss • *Drugs*: acetazolamide, metolazone, tenofovir, imatinib, glucocorticoids, mineralocorticoids, diuretics • Rickets • Osteomalacia RRT	*Spurious*: exogenous • Amphotericin B • Heparin • Tissue plasminogen activator *Spurious*: endogenous • Hyperglobulinaemia • Hyperlipidaemia • Haemolysis • Hyperbilirubinaemia *Increased intake*: exogenous • Laxatives • Fosphenytoin *Increased intake*: endogenous • TLS • Rhabdomyolysis Redistribution: • Metabolic acidosis (e.g. DKA) Reduced loss: • AKI • CKD • *Increased tubular reabsorption*: hypoparathyroidism, bisphosphates, vitamin D toxicity, acromegaly, familial tumoural calcinosis
Features	*B*: respiratory failure, diaphragmatic weakness, failure to wean, left shift of Hb dissociation curve *C*: reduced contractility, arrhythmias *D*: delirium, reduced consciousness, seizures *E*: muscle weakness, myalgia *G*: dysphagia, ileus, insulin resistance *H*: haemolysis, leukocyte dysfunction	Myocardial and vascular calcification Microcirculatory dysfunction in CKD
Treatment	*<0.32 mmol/l*: Phosphate Polyfusor® (50 mmol PO₄³⁻) 500 ml IV over 24 h *<0.64 mmol/l*: Phosphate Sandoz® (16.1 mmol PO₄³⁻) up to 6 per day	Treat cause
Other	Treat cause PN can be adjusted Don't administer phosphate with aluminium, calcium, magnesium salts (bind phosphate and reduce absorption)	Hydration *Insulin/dextrose*: temporising measure RRT in rapid cell turnover or rhabdomyolysis Phosphate binders (e.g. sevelamer) in CKD

(See Chapter 134 Sodium Disorders)

Resources
- Parikh M, Webb ST. Cations: potassium, calcium, and magnesium. CEACCP. 2012;12(4):195–198.
- Wadsworth RL, Siddiqui S. Phosphate homeostasis in critical care. BJA Educ. 2016;16(9):305–309.

133. RHABDOMYOLYSIS

What is rhabdomyolysis?

Rhabdomyolysis is the rupture of skeletal muscle cells. It is a syndrome characterised by the release of muscle cell contents into the systemic circulation with a range of clinical effects. These substances include myoglobin, potassium, phosphate, urate, LDH, ALT, and CK.

Diagnosis is largely clinical, with myoglobinuria and elevated CK providing supporting information. The triad of **weakness**, **myalgia**, and **dark 'coca cola' urine** may be present. The level of CK at which clinical complications will occur is variable, depending on the individual's physiology. Crush syndrome may be a significant contributor to morbidity and mortality in mass casualty incidents.

What are the causes of rhabdomyolysis?

Skeletal muscle cell ischaemia or necrosis may occur by many mechanisms, often in combination:

Traumatic
- *Crush injury, trauma*: entrapment in building collapse, road traffic collisions
- *Compartment syndrome*: long lie, perioperative (e.g. prolonged/dense neuraxial block), tourniquet use
- Electrical injury

Atraumatic
- *Exertional*: seizure, exercise
- *Temperature disruption*: hyper-/hypothermia
- *Genetic*: disorders of glycolysis, gluconeogenesis, mitochondria, G6PD deficiency
- *Drugs/toxins*: cocaine, alcohol, statins, propofol
- *Infection*: influenza, EBV, HIV, *Strep. pyogenes*, *Staph. aureus*
- *Metabolic/electrolyte disorders*: DKA, HHS

What is the pathophysiology of this condition?

Rhabdomyolysis may result in a spiral of further muscle death unless treated. This is followed by a common pathway including ATP depletion and/or cell wall disruption, before the following:

- Na^+/K^+ pump disruption
- Increased intracellular Ca^{2+}
- Altered interaction of actin and myosin
- Prolonged contraction of myocytes
- Mitochondrial dysfunction
- Further muscle necrosis

What are the major complications of rhabdomyolysis?

- AKI
- Compartment syndrome, limb amputation
- Intravascular depletion, third space loss
- Metabolic acidosis
- Multi-organ dysfunction
- DIC

How does rhabdomyolysis lead to AKI?

Multiple mechanisms, including the following:

- Prerenal effects of hypovolaemia with third space fluid shifts or multi-organ dysfunction
- Renal tubule blockage by myoglobin (and urate) crystals in acidic urine
- ROS, haem, and iron causing direct tubular damage
- Sympathetic vasoconstriction of renal vasculature
- Existing poor oxygen saturation in vasa recta
- Haem component of myoglobin implicated in ischaemic tubular injury

What are the priorities in clinical management?

- **Stop precipitant** of rhabdomyolysis
  - High index of suspicion
  - Stop offending agents where possible
  - Antidotes to specific toxins
- **Limit further muscle injury**
  - Organ support to achieve adequate perfusion
  - Fasciotomy in compartment syndrome or high risk (e.g. after vascular surgery)
  - Dantrolene in selected causes (e.g. NMS, MH)
  - Anaesthesia or sedation may be indicated to reduce oxygen demand (e.g. serotonin syndrome).
- **Treat electrolyte disorders**
  - May require insulin, bicarbonate
  - *Caution with calcium (although tricky in severe hyperkalaemia or hyperphosphataemia)*: calcium will be liberated from damaged muscle as injury resolves
  - RRT
- **Prevent AKI**
  - Aggressive volume replacement (may seem counterintuitive if positive balance and third space loss)
  - Debatable role of urinary alkalinisation with sodium bicarbonate (may worsen hypocalcaemia and result in calcium phosphate deposition in the kidney)
  - Aim for polyuria (200 ml/h), debatable role of mannitol
  - May be some role for antioxidants (e.g. desferrioxamine, allopurinol, pentoxifylline)
- **Manage other complications**
  - Appropriate transfusion of red cells and clotting factors in DIC
  - Analgesia

How is limb compartment syndrome diagnosed and managed?

Limb compartment syndrome involves the imbalance of perfusion with tissue requirements in a restricted space. Mechanisms include thrombosis, vascular disruption, prolonged hypotension, and compression by oedema or dressings. (See Chapter 67 Compartment Syndromes)

Diagnosis

- *Clinical examination*: tense, swollen limb compartment, signs of venous congestion, arterial insufficiency (e.g. weak pulses, later signs of tissue ischaemia and necrosis)
- *Pressure measurement*: needle connected to manometer (>30 mmHg significant); tissue perfusion pressure = diastolic BP − compartment pressure

As with any threat to tissue perfusion, early suspicion and optimisation has the potential to limit progression and secondary injury. Existing or inevitable limb compartment syndrome should be managed by fasciotomy. This should take place at the bedside where limb loss is an immediate threat. Longitudinal incisions are performed to divide restrictive tissue and release pressure in affected compartments.

Resources

- Cone J, Inaba K. Lower extremity compartment syndrome. Trauma Surg Acute Care Open. 2017;2:e000094.
- Nathanson MH, Harrop-Griffiths W, Adlington DJ, et al. Regional analgesia for lower leg trauma and the risk of acute compartment syndrome. Anaesthesia. 2021;76(11):1446–1449.
- Williams J, Thorpe C. Rhabdomyolysis. CEACCP. 2013;14(4):163–166.

134. SODIUM DISORDERS

What is severe hyponatraemia?

The severity of hyponatraemia relates to the presence of clinical signs and symptoms rather than the absolute sodium concentration. Severe symptoms may manifest at different degrees of hyponatraemia. Occasionally, patients are well despite profoundly low concentrations.

- $Na^+ < 135\ mmol/l$: hyponatraemia
- $Na^+ < 130\ mmol/l$: clinically significant
- $Na^+ < 125\ mmol/l$: symptoms and signs more prominent

Severe features
- Seizures
- Reduced GCS
- Encephalopathy

How would you approach a patient referred to you with hyponatraemia?

Diagnosis is the key to informing the management direction. In the absence of this, an understanding of the likely pathophysiology can help. A full history, examination, and relevant investigations should be carried out where possible.

Patients with severe symptoms will require a minimum of central venous access and close monitoring in HDU/ICU if appropriate.

History
- Features of hyponatraemia
  - *Severe*: seizures, reduced GCS, encephalopathy
  - *Other*: headache, nausea and vomiting, muscle cramps, confusion, lethargy
- Underlying pathology
  - Known
  - New presentation
- Precipitants
  - *Drugs*: diuretics, SSRIs

Examination – fluid status estimation
- Input/output charting
- Clinical assessment
- Distributive pathology (e.g. capillary leak syndromes)

Investigation
- Often identified on ABG/VBG
- Serum and urine osmolality
- Urinary sodium
- Specific investigations as per suspected cause (e.g. TFT, CXR, urine dip, CT head, echo, US liver)

How would you determine the likely cause of hyponatraemia from this information?

1 Determine serum osmolality (mOsm/kg)
  - *<285*: **hypotonic hyponatraemia** (true hyponatraemia)
  - *285–295*: isotonic hyponatraemia (pseudohyponatraemia)
    - ➢ Hyperproteinaemia
    - ➢ Hyperlipidaemia
  - *>295*: hypertonic hyponatraemia (osmotic diuresis)
    - ➢ Hyperglycaemia
    - ➢ Mannitol
    - ➢ *Glycine irrigation*: TURP syndrome

Table 134.1 Causes of hypotonic hyponatraemia (by urinary sodium, mEq/l)

Hypovolaemic		Euvolaemic		Hypervolaemic	
>20	<20	>20	<20	>20	<20
Renal loss	Extra-renal loss			Renal failure	Other failures
Addison's disease CSWS Osmotic diuresis Salt-losing nephropathy Diuretics	Diarrhoea Vomiting Burns Fistulae Pancreatitis Sweating	SIADH Glucocorticoid insufficiency Diuretics Other drugs	Hypothyroidism Hypotonic fluid Polydipsia	AKI CKD	Nephrotic syndrome Cirrhosis CCF

If true hypotonic hyponatraemia (Table 134.1):

2 Assess volume status
3 Determine urinary sodium (mmol/l)

What is the difference between SIADH and diabetes insipidus?

SIADH and diabetes insipidus are opposing disorders of sodium homeostasis. In SIADH, water retention occurs resulting in **hyponatraemia** and urinary sodium is high. Diabetes insipidus involves polyuric water loss causing **hypernatraemia**.

Causes of SIADH are as follows:

- *Intracranial*: trauma, tumour, infection, SAH, CVA, neurosurgical, epilepsy
- *Pulmonary*: pneumonia, TB, sarcoidosis, abscess
- *Malignancy*: small cell lung cancer, mesothelioma, lymphoma, nasopharyngeal cancer, GI/GU malignancy
- *Drugs*: DDAVP, proton pump inhibitors, SSRI, TCA, haloperidol, carbamazepine, sodium valproate, levetiracetam, cyclophosphamide, oxytocin, MDMA
- *Other*: HIV, acute intermittent porphyria, GBS

Causes of diabetes insipidus are as follows:

- *Central*: brain tumour, head injury, neurosurgical, hypoxic brain injury, CNS infection
- *Nephrogenic*: lithium, hypercalcaemia, hyponatraemia, obstruction, pyelonephritis, congenital, amphotericin B, hypokalaemia

How would you distinguish between SIADH and CSWS?

CSWS and SIADH may appear similar in the following:

- Hypotonic hyponatraemia
- High urinary sodium
- High urine osmolality

However, **patients with CSWS are hypovolaemic** with significant polyuria. SIADH patients tend to be euvolaemic. CSWS is usually self-limiting following an intracranial insult and managed with isotonic saline.

How would you manage hyponatraemia?

If specific aetiology is unconfirmed, management is determined by severity, chronicity, and volume status (acute < 24 h, chronic > 48 h).

All patients

- Ensure no spurious readings, confirm hyponatraemia.
- Treat as chronic hyponatraemia if unclear and no severe symptoms.
- *Review IV/enteral fluid management*: adjust based on volume status.
- Management of haemodynamic instability should be prioritised over risk of sodium increase when 0.9% NaCl used.

Acute severe
- First hour
  - Admit to HDU/ICU
  - Hypertonic saline (3% NaCl) 150 ml IV over 20 min, usually via CVC
  - Check Na^+
  - Repeat until risen by 5 mmol/l
- Switch from 3% to 0.9% NaCl IV slow infusion
- Specific treatment for underlying cause
- Check Na^+ at 6, 12, 24, 48 h

Acute, not severe
- Stop precipitating causes where possible (e.g. diuretics)
- *Hypovolaemic*: restore volume with 0.9% NaCl IV
- Check Na^+ after 4 h
- Treat underlying cause where known

Chronic
- *Hypovolaemic*: restore volume with 0.9% NaCl IV
- *Euvolaemic*: confirm hypotonic hyponatraemia, high urinary sodium
  - TFT, cortisol, short synacthen test if appropriate
  - *Normal*: likely SIADH – fluid restriction
  - *Abnormal*: endocrine disease – treat
- *Hypervolaemic*: treat underlying cause (e.g. fluid restriction to prevent overload)

GUIDELINE RCP 2016 Hyponatraemia

What specific management applies in SIADH?
- *Fürst formula*: **electrolyte free water clearance** = $(Na^+_{urine} + K^+_{urine})/Na^+_{serum}$
  - *<0.5*: fluid restrict to 1.0 l/24 h
  - *0.5–1*: fluid restrict to 0.5 l/24 h
  - *>1.0*: no fluid restriction
- Assess response at 24 and 48 h
- Seek endocrinology review if poor response
  - Demeclocycline 150 mg TDS, or
  - Tolvaptan 15 mg single dose (ADH receptor antagonist)
  - Fluid restriction lifted if these are used

What are the risks of a rapid increase in serum sodium?
Osmotic demyelination syndrome (formerly central pontine myelinolysis) may result from harsh osmotic shifts, resulting in significant morbidity and lasting neurological disability. Brain parenchyma shrinkage may also cause vascular rupture and haemorrhage.

Sodium change should be limited to a maximum of the following:

- 10 mmol/l in the first 24 h
- 8 mmol/l in each subsequent 24 h

What would you use to manage sodium overcorrection?
The use of hypertonic saline confers a risk of over-excretion of water and an undesirably excessive rise in serum sodium; **5% dextrose** may be used to replace free water, but this can be tricky and ineffective.

The '**DDAVP clamp**' is an alternative technique used to prevent overcorrection. Desmopressin, or DDAVP, stimulates V_2 vasopressin receptors in the kidney and subsequent water retention. A typical dose would be 2 µg IV 8 hourly. Prophylactic DDAVP use has been described.

How would you manage a patient with hypernatraemia?
Hypernatraemia is a serum sodium >145 mmol/l. Severe features become more prevalent >160 mmol/l and include altered mental state, hyperreflexia, and seizures.

Establishing the aetiology is again the key to management:

- **Water loss**
  - Diabetes insipidus
  - GI loss
  - Intrinsic renal disease
  - Hypokalaemia
  - Hypercalcaemia
  - Solute diuresis
  - Glucosuria
  - Burns
  - Hyperthermia
- **Reduced water intake**
  - Inappropriate response to thirst
- **Increased solute intake**
  - Salt poisoning
  - Sodium bicarbonate
  - Hypertonic saline
  - Hyperaldosteronism

Management may include the following:

- Treating the cause
- *Water deficit*: rehydration
- *Nephrogenic diabetes insipidus*: thiazide diuretics, sodium restriction, high dose DDAVP, (acetazolamide if lithium-induced)
- *Central diabetes insipidus*: DDAVP, 5% dextrose, strict input/output matching (as prone to adipsia with significant sodium swings)

$$\text{Water deficit} = 0.6 \times \text{premorbid weight} \times \left(1 - 140 / Na^+_{serum}\right)$$

Resources

- Farkas J. PULMCrit. September 2015. Taking Control of Severe Hyponatremia with DDAVP. Available from: https://emcrit.org/pulmcrit/taking-control-of-severe-hyponatremia-with-ddavp/. (Accessed 19 December 2021.)
- Hirst C, Allahabadia A, Cosgrove J. The adult patient with hyponatraemia. CEACCP. 2014;15(5):248–252.
- National Health Service. Diabetes Insipidus: Causes. 2019. Available from: https://www.nhs.uk/conditions/diabetes-insipidus/causes/. (Accessed 09 February 2022.)
- Nickson C. Life in the Fast Lane. Hypernatraemia. November 2020. Available from: https://litfl.com/hypernatraemia/. (Accessed 19 December 2021.)

135. ACUTE LIVER FAILURE

How do you define acute liver failure?

KEY POINT

Acute liver failure (ALF) is the rapid decline in liver function associated with jaundice, coagulopathy, and encephalopathy, with no pre-existing chronic liver disease.

Classification relates to timing from jaundice to encephalopathy. Various systems exist (e.g. O'Grady; Bernuau et al.; Japanese consensus).

O'Grady system for ALF:

- *Hyperacute*: 0–1 week
- *Acute*: 1–4 weeks
- *Subacute*: 4–12 weeks

What are the causes of ALF?

- Paracetamol overdose
- *Drug-induced liver injury*: antibiotics, anti-epileptics, anti-TB drugs, recreational drugs, herbal medicines
- *Viral hepatitis*: hepatitis A/B/E, EBV, CMV, HSV
- Ischaemic hepatitis
- Post-surgical
- Acute fatty liver of pregnancy
- Mushroom poisoning

Patients with acute presentations of chronic autoimmune hepatitis, Wilson disease, or Budd-Chiari syndrome are considered to have ALF if hepatic encephalopathy develops (i.e. despite having pre-existing liver disease).

What is Budd-Chiari syndrome?

Budd-Chiari syndrome is a rare, congestive cause of liver failure caused by obstruction of hepatic veins which usually drain directly into the IVC (i.e. not portal veins). It is characterised by the triad of **abdominal pain**, **ascites**, and **hepatomegaly**. It may be acute or chronic. Causes include hepatic vein thrombus and compression (e.g. from tumour).

US demonstrates loss of hepatic venous signal and reverse flow in the portal vein. Gross ascites should lead to suspicion of this condition, and early imaging is crucial.

What are the manifestations of ALF?

Patients often develop fulminant multi-organ dysfunction.

Loss of metabolic liver function manifests with disorders of the following:

- *Gluconeogenesis*: hypoglycaemia
- *Lactate clearance*: lactic acidosis
- *Ammonia clearance*: hyperammonaemia
- *Synthetic function*: coagulopathy

Other features

- *C*: hypotension, low SVR, high cardiac output, HF, subclinical myocardial injury
- *D*: encephalopathy, cerebral oedema, raised ICP, hypoglycaemia
- *F*: AKI from direct insult (e.g. paracetamol overdose), hypoperfusion, nephrotoxicity
- *G*: pancreatitis, adrenal insufficiency
- *H*: bone marrow suppression
- *I*: sepsis, SIRS

What is the pathophysiology of hepatic encephalopathy?

- Ammonia normally detoxified in liver – this is reduced
- Accumulated ammonia crosses the blood brain barrier
- Ammonia is converted to glutamine in the brain
- Water homeostasis and mitochondrial function disrupted
- Cerebral oedema, neurological dysfunction, raised ICP

Hepatic encephalopathy severity is described by **West Haven grading** as follows:

1 Trivial lack of awareness, euphoria, anxiety, shortened attention span
2 Lethargy/apathy, disorientation, inappropriate behaviour
3 Somnolence, stupor, gross disorientation, confusion
4 Coma

What do you know about paracetamol toxicity?

Paracetamol (or acetaminophen) is a household analgesic medication that is readily available without prescription. Paracetamol toxicity is responsible for significant mortality and thousands of hospital admissions per year in the UK. The metabolite **N-acetyl-p-benzoquinone imine (NAPQI)** is hepatotoxic. **Glutathione** usually metabolises NAPQI, and its deficiency results in greater toxicity. 'Staggered' overdose should also be considered.

Risk factors
- Chronic alcohol excess
- Enzyme inducing medications (e.g. antiepileptics)
- Anti-TB regimes
- *Reduced glutathione stores*: HIV, malnutrition, malignancy

What are the specific management considerations in ALF secondary to paracetamol overdose?

Management involves timely administration of NAC (Parvolex®) as a glutathione donor. The treatment threshold may be determined using the plasma paracetamol concentration and time from ingestion, following a nomogram. However, this has its limitations (e.g. unreliable in mixed or staggered overdose, variable physiology). Administration within 8 h is advocated to reduce mortality.

- Quantify and establish timing of paracetamol overdose
- Assess plasma levels of paracetamol at 4 h (or at presentation if staggered)
- *NAC*: lower mortality if given within 8 h
- *Supportive care*: avoid clotting factor administration unless significant bleeding or advised by transplantation team
- Liver transplantation in severe cases

NAC dosing
- Historic 21-h protocol
  - *First infusion*: 150 mg/kg over 1 h
  - *Second infusion*: 50 mg/kg over 4 h
  - *Third infusion*: 100 mg/kg over 16 h
- More recent 12-h SNAP regimen
  - 100 mg/kg over 2 h
  - 200 mg/kg over 10 h

NAC cessation
- Blood sampled at 1 h before end of 21-h protocol/2 h before end of 12-h protocol
- INR ≤ 1.3
- ALT < 100 U/l
- ALT ≤ 2 × admission value

STUDY

Pettie et al. (2019)

- Paracetamol overdose
- *Intervention*: SNAP regimen vs 21-h NAC protocol
- *Primary*: hepatotoxicity – **no difference (4.3% vs 3.6%)**
- *Secondary*: antihistamine treatment for NAC anaphylactoid reaction – **significantly lower (2.0% vs 11%)**

Table 135.1 King's College criteria for liver transplantation

Paracetamol-induced ALF (any of:)	Non-paracetamol induced ALF (either of:)

• pH < 7.3 (after resuscitation, > 24 h since ingestion)
• Lactate > 3 mmol/l
• All 3 of the following:
  • PT > 100 s (or INR > 6.5)
  • Serum creatinine > 300 µmol/l
  • Grade 3–4 encephalopathy
	• PT > 100 s (INR > 6.5) with any grade encephalopathy
	• Any 3 of the following:
	  • Age < 10 or > 40
	  • *Unfavourable aetiology*: seronegative, drug associated
	  • Jaundice to encephalopathy time > 7 days
	  • PT > 50 s (INR > 3.5)
	  • Serum bilirubin > 300 µmol/l

When should a patient with ALF be discussed with a specialist unit?

The King's College criteria are used for transplantation and form the benchmark for monitoring (Table 135.1).

Suggested tertiary referral criteria are based on the following:

Non-paracetamol aetiology

- pH < 7.30 or HCO_3^- < 18 mmol/l
- INR > 1.8
- Oliguria or Na^+ < 130 mmol/l
- Bilirubin > 300 µmol/l
- Encephalopathy, hypoglycaemia, or metabolic acidosis
- Shrinking liver size

Paracetamol related

- Arterial pH < 7.30 or HCO_3^- < 18 mmol/l
- INR > 3 on day 2, or > 4 thereafter
- Oliguria and/or elevated creatinine
- Altered level of consciousness
- Hypoglycaemia
- Elevated lactate unresponsive to fluid resuscitation

GUIDELINE EASL 2017 Acute liver failure

When is liver transplantation indicated in this setting?

ALF may require treatment with liver transplantation. The European Association for Study of the Liver (EASL) recommend selection based on the King's College or Clichy criteria. Current policy lists several specific indications for super-urgent liver transplantation in the UK. These relate mostly to adaptations of the King's College criteria:

Paracetamol poisoning

- pH < 7.25
- Lactate > 5 mmol/l on admission, > 4 mmol/l at 24 h in presence of encephalopathy
- 2 of 3 'minor' criteria and clinical deterioration (e.g. high ICP, F_iO_2 > 50%, increasing inotrope requirement) in absence of sepsis

Non-paracetamol

- *Favourable aetiologies (e.g. viral, ecstasy, cocaine)*: King's College criteria
- *Other (e.g. seronegative, drug reaction)*: PT > 100 s and:
  - *Encephalopathic*: jaundice to encephalopathy time > 7 days, and bilirubin > 300 µmol/l
  - *Not encephalopathic*: INR > 2 after vitamin K, age < 10 or > 40 years, and PT > 50 s (INR > 3.5)

Other

- *Acute Wilson's disease or Budd-Chiari syndrome*: coagulopathy and encephalopathy
- *Post-liver transplantation*: early hepatic artery thrombosis, early graft dysfunction
- Total absence of liver function (e.g. hepatectomy)

- Live donor developing early severe liver failure
- *Children under 2 years of age*: INR > 4 or grade 3–4 encephalopathy (excludes haematological malignancy, HLH, and DIC)

Outcomes are worse in the acute setting. Absolute contraindications include substance misuse, overwhelming sepsis, refractory shock, AIDS, and uncontrolled intracranial hypertension with suspected permanent neurological damage. Suitability may change with evolving disease.

Criteria in elective transplantation aim to allow selection if anticipated survival without transplantation is less than that obtained with a liver transplant. Projected 5-year survival should be >50% post-transplantation. Disease mortality without transplantation is calculated using the UK model for End-stage Liver Disease (UKELD) score (≥49 predicts >9% mortality at 1 year). Other specific indications exist (e.g. portopulmonary hypertension, hepatopulmonary syndrome).

When is liver transplantation contraindicated in the context of substance misuse?

Management of alcohol-related liver disease is controversial due to the common overlap with alcohol addiction. Transplantation is absolutely contraindicated in the following:

- Alcoholic hepatitis
- >2 episodes in 2 years of non-adherence with medical care (including that of addiction) without satisfactory explanation
- >2 episodes in 2 years of return to drinking following professional advice
- Illicit drug use

Evidence of drinking alcohol whilst on the transplant list will result in permanent removal from the list, and this should be discussed on entry.

Illicit drug use is also a contraindication. Other concerns include poor social support to remain abstinent, lack of motivation to leave drug culture as able, history of cross-dependency, and reluctance to sign a treatment agreement. Stable engagement in substance misuse services is a more relative contraindication.

What is the intensive care management of a patient with ALF?

Candidacy for HDU/ICU admission often more straightforward than in ACLF. Usual considerations apply. The management of ALF and ACLF follows similar principles. (See Chapter 136 Chronic Liver Disease)

- **Specialist input**
  - Determination of aetiology (may affect prognosis)
  - May require early/regular contact with liver unit ± transfer
  - Orthotopic liver transplantation is curative
  - *Hepatic assist devices (e.g. MARS)*: limited evidence but may be used
  - *TIPS*: if major complications of portal hypertension (e.g. refractory ascites, variceal bleeding)
- **Supportive care**
  - *NIV*: HFNO is recommended over NIV
  - *Intubation*: consider in grade 3–4 encephalopathy, or if transfer indicated
  - *Ventilation*: low PEEP (ARDS vs ICP)
  - *Fluid resuscitation with albumin*: especially if serum albumin low
  - *Vasopressors*: noradrenaline first-line + low-dose vasopressin
  - *Nutrition*: may prevent deterioration in encephalopathy
  - *RRT*: CVVH
  - *Antimicrobials*: antibacterial, antifungal cover
  - Avoidance of hepatotoxic and nephrotoxic drugs
  - *NAC*: anti-inflammatory, antioxidant, inotropic, vasodilating effects may be of benefit in non-paracetamol aetiologies
- **Prevention of encephalopathy**
  - *Thiamine (vitamin B1) supplementation*: prevention of Wernicke's
  - Regular lactulose (aiming for several stools per day)
  - *Rifaximin*: reduces GI bacterial overgrowth and ammonia production
  - Maintain CPP (ICP monitoring controversial, particularly with coagulopathy)

- Avoid long-acting sedatives, opioids, medications causing bowel stasis
- *RRT*: removal of ammonia

GUIDELINE   SCCM 2020 Acute liver failure

How are other potential complications addressed?

Coagulopathy
- Assessment with viscoelastic testing in preference to INR, platelet count, or fibrinogen
- Vitamin K routinely
- *Prophylactic proton pump inhibitor cover*: high risk of GI bleeding
- Avoidance of clotting products unless active bleeding (coagulation profile aids prognostication, monitoring, transplant decision-making)
- *VTE prophylaxis*: encouraged, consider infusion over subcutaneous route

Ascites
- Sodium restriction
- Diuresis (e.g. spironolactone)
- Investigation and management of SBP if present (see Chapter 136 Chronic Liver Disease)
- Drainage if SBP or respiratory compromise

Bleeding (see Chapter 139 Gastrointestinal Haemorrhage)

Portopulmonary hypertension (mean PAP > 35 mmHg)
- Riociguat
- Sildenafil
- Prostacyclin analogues (e.g. epoprostenol, treprostinil)
- Endothelin receptor antagonists (e.g. bosentan, ambrisentan)

Other
- *Hepatic hydrothorax*: chest drain only if TIPS not appropriate or palliative intent
- *Budd-Chiari syndrome*: may require surgical/endovascular intervention

(See Chapter 19 Extracorporeal Liver Support)

What is hepatopulmonary syndrome?

Hepatopulmonary syndrome is a state characterised by hypoxaemia and breathlessness secondary to pulmonary vasodilatation and shunting.

It differs from portopulmonary hypertension, which is an elevated mean PAP due to increased PVR.

How is alcoholic hepatitis managed?

Alcoholic hepatitis is a clinical syndrome of jaundice and liver impairment following heavy and prolonged alcohol use.

Care is largely supportive and focuses on prevention of encephalopathy and AKI. Specific treatments are as follows:

- Prednisolone use is controversial due to the demonstration of a non-significant mortality benefit in the **STOPAH** trial. A typical course would involve 40 mg daily for 28 days before abrupt cessation or tapering. Some patients will not respond to steroids and might be identified using the Lille score, facilitating cessation.
- Pentoxifylline has also fallen out of favour with no benefit over placebo and is no longer recommended. Other measures include supportive care as above, especially prevention of AKI.
- *Anti-TNF agents*: not recommended due to risk of death and severe infection.

Maddrey's discriminant function may be calculated to determine which patients will benefit from corticosteroid therapy, with severe hepatitis indicated by a score ≥32 (35% mortality at 28 days). The Glasgow alcoholic hepatitis score is used to predict mortality.

$$\text{Maddrey's discriminant function} = 4.6 \times (\text{patient PT} - \text{normal PT}) + \text{bilirubin in mg/dl}$$

STOPAH (2015)

- Severe alcoholic hepatitis
- *Intervention*: prednisolone vs pentoxifylline vs placebo
- *Primary*: 28-day mortality – **no difference** with prednisolone or pentoxifylline (14% vs 19% vs 17%)

GUIDELINE EASL 2018 Alcohol-related liver disease

Resources

- Bernal W, Wendon J. Acute liver failure. N Engl J Med. 2013;369:2525–2534.
- Kwan LW, Nick M. Management of acute liver failure. CEACCP. 2004;4(2):40–43.
- NHS Blood and Transplant. POL 195/12 – Liver Transplantation: Selection Criteria and Recipient Registration. April 2021. Available from: https://www.odt.nhs.uk/transplantation/tools-policies-and-guidance/policies-and-guidance/. (Accessed 20 March 2022.)

136. CHRONIC LIVER DISEASE

Can you describe some common reasons for patients with chronic liver disease to present to critical care?

- **Decompensation** secondary to:
  - Sepsis
  - AKI
  - UGIB
  - SBP
  - Hepatic encephalopathy
  - Toxins (most commonly, alcohol)
  - Thrombus
  - Tumour
- **Unrelated** medical condition (e.g. MI, pneumonia)
- **Perioperatively**
- **Trauma**

What are the causes of chronic liver disease?

- Infectious
  - *Viral*: hepatitis B/C, EBV, CMV
  - *Bacterial*: Brucellosis
- *Toxins*: alcoholic liver disease, methotrexate, amiodarone
- *Hepatic obstruction*: right HF, Budd-Chiari syndrome
- *Metabolic*: haemochromatosis, Wilson disease, alpha-1-antitrypsin deficiency, non-alcoholic steato-hepatitis (NASH)
- *Autoimmune*: autoimmune hepatitis, primary biliary cholangitis/cirrhosis, primary sclerosing cholangitis
- Secondary sclerosing cholangitis

Chronic liver disease progresses through steatosis (fatty change), to fibrosis, and to cirrhosis. Potential reversibility decreases with progression.

What is decompensated liver disease?

Decompensated cirrhosis (or acute hepatic decompensation) is an acute deterioration of cirrhotic liver disease manifesting with 1 or more of the following:

- **Jaundice**
- **Worsening ascites**
- **Overt encephalopathy**
- **GI haemorrhage**
- **Bacterial infections**
- **Coagulopathy**

Other complications

- *AKI*: hypoperfusion, IAH
- Hepatorenal syndrome (HRS)
- Hepatopulmonary syndrome
- Portopulmonary hypertension
- Cirrhotic cardiomyopathy
- Adrenal insufficiency

What is acute-on-chronic liver failure?

ACLF is a distinct syndrome combining the concept of **SIRS** and **multi-organ dysfunction** with acute decompensation of chronic liver disease. Diagnosis is recommended when organ failure(s) involving high short-term mortality develop.

Short-term mortality of ACLF is higher than in decompensation alone, at around 50%, even in a high-level care environment.

ACLF is **graded by corresponding number of organ failures** (with grade 1a for single renal failure and 1b for single non-kidney organ failure). These are defined by the **CLIF-C ACLF** score, in preference to CLIF SOFA or CLIF Organ Failure scores.

> **GUIDELINE** EASL 2018 Decompensated cirrhosis

What is portal hypertension?

Portal hypertension is the state of relatively elevated pressure in the hepatic portal venous system and sinusoids.

Grading according to **hepatic venous pressure gradient** (HVPG) is as follows:

- *Mild*: 5–10 mmHg
- *Clinically significant*: >10 mmHg

Clinical effects are as follows:

- **Ascites** (serum-ascites albumin gradient [SAAG] >11 g/l implicates portal hypertension)
- **Oesophageal varices**
- **Decompensated cirrhosis**
- At >12 mmHg, varices may bleed
- At >16 mmHg, mortality increases

How is portal hypertension managed?

- Salt restriction
- *Diuresis*: spironolactone, furosemide
- *Non-selective beta blockade*: propranolol, carvedilol
- TIPS

What is involved in the TIPS procedure?

TIPS involves endovascular insertion of a stent to shunt an intrahepatic portal branch into a hepatic vein. Indications include control of variceal bleeding, refractory ascites, and renal hypoperfusion. Complications include hepatic encephalopathy, stent stenosis, thrombosis, bleeding at insertion, and recurrent ascites (i.e. failure). Child C cirrhosis carries a high risk of post-procedure encephalopathy; TIPS is not recommended in this group.

What is HRS?

HRS is a functional renal failure caused by intra-renal vasoconstriction. It occurs in patients with end-stage liver disease, ALF, or alcoholic hepatitis.

HRS was classified originally into type 1 and type 2. Type 1 was more acute, with serum creatinine doubling within 2 weeks; type 2 a stepwise progression of deterioration in creatinine and liver function.

More recently, this has been described as '**HRS-AKI**'. Pathophysiology is thought to involve a multifactorial process as follows:

- Pro-inflammatory cytokines
- Splanchnic vasodilatation, glomerular vasoconstriction, abnormal tubular electrolyte handling (e.g. Na^+)
- Tubular damage results

KEY POINT

HRS-AKI diagnostic criteria are as follows:

- Diagnosis of cirrhosis and ascites
- Diagnosis of AKI
- No response to 2 consecutive days of diuretic withdrawal and plasma volume expansion (HAS 1 g/kg)
- Absence of shock
- No current/recent nephrotoxic drugs
- No macroscopic signs of structural kidney injury (proteinuria, microhaematuria, findings on renal US)

The term 'HRS-NAKI' (non-AKI) has been used for disease not meeting above criteria (equivalent to previous HRS type 2):

- *HRS-AKD*: eGFR < 60 ml/min/1.73 m^2 for < 3 months
- *HRS-CKD*: eGFR < 60 ml/min/1.73 m^2 for ≥3 months

Treatment is with vasoconstrictors (terlipressin or noradrenaline), albumin (20–40 g/day), treatment of any associated infection (e.g. SBP), and supportive care. Liver transplantation is considered as definitive therapy in selected cases.

GUIDELINE ICA 2015 AKI

What is SBP?

SBP is a bacterial infection of ascitic fluid without any intra-abdominal surgically treatable cause of infection. Signs and symptoms may include abdominal pain, distension, erythema, fever, shock, encephalopathy, AKI, and worsening LFTs ± coagulopathy.

It is common in patients with cirrhosis and ascites and is diagnosed by abdominal paracentesis. SBP is confirmed with an **ascitic fluid neutrophil count > 250 cells/mm^3**. This may be accompanied by a positive fluid culture in up to 40% of cases (most commonly, *E. coli*).

Treatment should be initiated upon suspicion with broad-spectrum antibiotics, usually piperacillin/tazobactam or a third-generation cephalosporin for 5–7 days. Treatment efficacy should be confirmed with repeat paracentesis at 48–72 h. Prophylactic antimicrobials will be indicated thereafter.

Albumin is recommended routinely to prevent HRS and improve mortality:

- 1.5 g/kg at diagnosis
- 1 g/kg on day 3

SBP is an indication for ascitic drain insertion for source control. Drainage is reserved for tense ascites causing respiratory impairment otherwise.

Differentials include secondary bacterial peritonitis from other intra-abdominal pathology (e.g. perforation), which should be suspected in the presence of multiple organisms on culture or very high ascitic neutrophil/protein results. Prompt CT imaging should be performed with consideration of surgery where appropriate.

STUDY

Sort et al. (1999)

- Cirrhosis and SBP
- *Intervention*: cefotaxime and albumin vs cefotaxime alone
- *Primary*: renal impairment – **significantly lower (10% vs 33%)**
- *Secondary*: in-hospital mortality – **significantly lower (10% vs 29%)**, 3-month mortality – **significantly lower (22% vs 41%)**

Which scoring systems are used to assess chronic liver disease?

Part of the difficulty in managing critically unwell patients with chronic liver disease is determining candidacy for HDU/ICU admission. The physiological, often multi-organ, disturbance of chronic liver disease causes significant morbidity when coupled with acute disease.

Scoring systems may help in assessing such patients, for example:

- **MELD** (see Chapter 2 Scoring Systems)
- **UKELD**: 12-month mortality, doesn't use RRT criteria
- **Child-Turcotte-Pugh**
  - Ascites, albumin, bilirubin, encephalopathy, INR
  - *12-month survival*: Class A 100%, B 80%, C 45%
  - *Validated for perioperative mortality in abdominal surgery*: Class C 82%
- *CLIF-C ACLF*: 28-day mortality

When is futility considered in ACLF?

The role of transplantation is controversial in ACLF. High complication rates have been observed, and some patients will be too unwell to tolerate the demands of the procedure and ongoing care. Rationing may play a part, particularly due to donor liver availability and existence of other indications with better outcomes.

Futility is difficult to determine. One study found that CLIF-C ACLF score ≥70 after 48 h of intensive care was associated with 100% mortality.

EASL have suggested criteria for withdrawal of intensive care support as follows:

- 7 days after diagnosis and adequate treatment of ACLF-3
- ≥4 organ failures (or CLIF-C ACLF > 64)
- Liver transplantation contraindicated or not available

Resources

- Dimonetto DA, Gines P, Kamath PS. Hepatorenal syndrome: pathophysiology, diagnosis, and management. BMJ. 2020;370:m2687.
- Engelmann C, Thomsen KL, Zakeri N, et al. Validation of CLIF-C ACLF score to define a threshold for futility of intensive care support for patients with chronic liver failure. Crit Care. 2018;22(1):254.
- Passi NN, McPhail MJW. The patient with cirrhosis in the intensive care unit and the management of acute-on-chronic liver failure. J Intensive Care Soc. 2020;23(1):78–86.
- Procopet B, Berzigotti A. Diagnosis of cirrhosis and portal hypertension: imaging, non-invasive markers of fibrosis and liver biopsy. Gastroenterology Rep (Oxf). 2017;5(2):79–89.

137. DIARRHOEA

How would you define diarrhoea?

Diarrhoea is a common symptom in critical care, affecting 14–21% of patients.

Definitions vary but diarrhoea can be defined as follows:

- 3 or more loose/liquid stools per day, with
- Stool weight > 200 g per day, or
- Volume > 250 ml per day

Types 5–7 on the Bristol Stool Chart also constitute diarrhoea.

Why is diarrhoea a problem in critical care?

Diarrhoea is common and can have significant consequences in critical care which might include the following:

- *Infection*: cross-infection or contamination of sterile sites, prevention strategies
- Electrolyte imbalance
- Skin breakdown
- Loss of patient dignity
- High nursing workload
- Increased morbidity and mortality
- Increased LOS

C. difficile infection (CDI) is of particular concern in healthcare systems as a potentially fatal condition that may occur in outbreaks in vulnerable populations. Antimicrobial stewardship and infection prevention and control measures may reduce the impact of this disease. The NHS links CDI outcomes to financial sanctions.

What types of diarrhoea are there?

Diarrhoea may be classified by mechanism, duration, severity, or aetiology.

Mechanism
- Secretory
- Osmotic
- Motoric
- Exudative

Duration
- Acute (<2 weeks)
- Chronic (>4 weeks)

Severity
- *Mild*: self-limiting, no major fluid or electrolyte disturbance
- *Severe*: fluid loss and electrolyte disturbance requiring treatment

Aetiology
- Infectious
  - ➤ *Bacterial*: CDI, E. coli, Salmonella, Shigella, Campylobacter, Staph. aureus, Bacillus cereus, Klebsiella oxytoca, Yersinia enterocolitica, Vibrio cholerae, Vibrio parahaemolyticus/vulnificus, Aeromonas/Plesiomonas
  - ➤ *Viral*: norovirus, rotavirus, adenovirus, CMV, HSV
  - ➤ *Other*: Entamoeba histolytica, Cryptosporidium parvum, Microsporidium spp., Cystisospora belli, Cyclospora cayatanensis, Giardia lamblia
- Non-infectious

or:
- Disease
  - ➤ *Non-specific*: hypoperfusion, hypoalbuminaemia
  - ➤ *Specific*: pancreatitis, IBD, short bowel, specific infections, pancreatic insufficiency, endocrine

- Food/feeding related
  - ➤ Osmotic/motor
  - ➤ Specific intolerance (e.g. lactose)
  - ➤ Bacterial contamination
- Medication related
  - ➤ Laxatives
  - ➤ Prokinetics
  - ➤ Antibiotic associated with/without colitis
  - ➤ Hyperosmolar (e.g. magnesium, sorbitol)
  - ➤ Chemotherapy
  - ➤ Radiotherapy

How do laxative drugs work?

Mechanisms of laxative drugs are as follows:

- Bulk-forming agents (e.g. fibre)
- Emollient (softeners) (e.g. sodium docusate)
- Lubricant (e.g. mineral oil)
- Hyperosmotic (e.g. lactulose, glycerin)
- Saline (e.g. magnesium salts)
- Stimulant (e.g. senna, bisacodyl)

What is the pathophysiology of antibiotic-associated diarrhoea?

Four main mechanisms are as follows:

- *Direct prokinetic effect (motoric)*: erythromycin, azithromycin
- Microbial modification with unmetabolised carbohydrates (osmotic)
- Unmetabolised dihydroxy bile acids due to disturbed microbiota (secretory)
- Colitis from bacterial overgrowth of gut microbiota by *C. difficile* or *K. oxytoca*

How would you manage a patient with diarrhoea in the ICU?

- **Management of infection** if present
  - Stool for *C. difficile* toxin, other specific pathogens (e.g. CMV)
  - Infection prevention measures (e.g. handwashing with soap rather than alcohol gel, visitors to wear apron and gloves, isolation)
- **Treatment of specific causes**
- **Systemic factors**
  - Adequate gut perfusion
  - Optimise nutrition
- **Check medications**
  - Stop laxatives
  - Change preparation where relevant
- **Adjust feed** if appropriate
  - Reduce feed rate
  - Reposition feeding tube
  - Add soluble fibre to prolong transit time
  - Low osmolality feed
- **Symptomatic management**
  - Nursing care
  - Consider bowel management system
  - Antidiarrhoeal medications
- **Manage complications**
  - *Fluid loss*: hydration
  - *Electrolyte disturbance*: replacement
  - *Skin lesions, wound infection*: antimicrobials, nursing care

What is *C. difficile*?

C. difficile is a Gram-positive spore-forming anaerobe that may cause severe colitis, toxic megacolon, and death. Two toxins, A and B, have been identified. Enterotoxin A is associated with increased intestinal permeability, whereas B is responsible for colonic inflammation.

Risk factors
- *Antimicrobials*: quinolones, clindamycin, ampicillin, cephalosporins
- Age > 60 years
- Proton pump inhibitor use
- Exposure to other patients with CDI
- Residence in a chronic care facility
- Severe underlying disease

> **KEY POINT**
>
> CDI is defined as follows:
>
> - Diarrhoea, plus
> - Positive *C. difficile* toxin B (CDT) test, or
> - Results of CDT test pending and clinical suspicion of CDI

How is the severity of CDI graded?

Mild
- WCC normal, and
- <3 episodes of loose stools per day

Moderate
- WCC raised but <15 × 10⁹/l, and
- 3–5 loose stools per day

Severe (any of:)
- WCC > 15 × 10⁹/l
- Serum creatinine > 50% increase above baseline
- Temperature > 38.5°C
- Evidence of severe colitis (abdominal/radiological signs)

Life-threatening (any of:)
- Hypotension
- Ileus (partial/complete)
- Toxic megacolon
- CT evidence of severe disease

What specific treatment is there for *C. difficile*?

- **Enteral antibiotics ideally**
  - *First line*: vancomycin 125 mg 6 hourly for 10 days
  - *Second line/relapse*: fidaxomicin 200 mg 12 hourly for 10 days
  - Third line/life-threatening
    - ➤ Vancomycin 500 mg 6 hourly for 10 days
    - ➤ + IV metronidazole 500 mg 8 hourly for 10 days
    - ➤ Specialist input recommended
- *Surgery*: may be required for life-threatening disease
- **Avoid antimotility agents**
- **Microbiological therapy**
  - *Faecal microbiota transplant*: in recurrent disease >2 episodes
  - *Probiotics/prebiotics*: not recommended as lack of evidence for prevention
  - *Non-toxigenic C. difficile*: under investigation

- **Other**
  - *Rifaximin*: no evidence for preventing recurrence, not recommended
  - *Bezlotoxumab*: may increase time to recurrence, not cost-effective
  - *IVIg*: may be appropriate in severe or recurrent infection, no RCT evidence
  - *Anion exchange resin (e.g. cholestyramine)*: not recommended, may bind antibiotics

GUIDELINE NICE 2021 NG199 Clostridioides difficile

What are probiotics?

- **Probiotics** are live bacteria/yeasts that are promoted as having health benefits by restoration of the natural gut microbiome.
- **Prebiotics** are a food source for usual GI flora – non-digestible food ingredients (e.g. fructo-oligosaccharides). They occur naturally but may also be promoted as supplements.

Resources

- Blaser AR, Deane AM, Fruhwald J. Diarrhoea in the critically ill. Curr Opin Crit Care 2015;21:142–153.
- Department of Health and Health Protection Agency. *Clostridium difficile* infection: How to deal with the problem. December 2008. Available from: https://assets.publishing.service.gov.uk/government/uploads/system/uploads/attachment_data/file/340851/Clostridium_difficile_infection_how_to_deal_with_the_problem.pdf. (Accessed 20 March 2022.)
- Murali M, Ly C, Tirlapur N, et al. Diarrhoea in critical care is rarely infective in origin, associated with increased length of stay and higher mortality. J Intensive Care Soc. 2020;21(1):72–78.
- NHS England. NHS England Patient Safety Domain. *Clostridium difficile* Infection Objectives for NHS Organisations in 2016/17 and Guidance on Sanction Implementation. March 2016. Available from: https://www.england.nhs.uk/patientsafety/wp-content/uploads/sites/32/2016/05/c-diff-objectives-guidance-16-17-v2.pdf. (Accessed 18 December 2021.)
- Wilcox MH. Public Health England: Updated Guidance on the Management and Treatment of *Clostridium difdicile* Infection. May 2013. Available from: https://assets.publishing.service.gov.uk/government/uploads/system/uploads/attachment_data/file/321891/Clostridium_difficile_management_and_treatment.pdf. (Accessed 20 March 2022.)

138.　INFLAMMATORY BOWEL DISEASE

How might patients with inflammatory bowel disease present to critical care?

- **Post-operatively**
  - Elective
    - ➢ Resection if refractory or intolerable side effects of medication
    - ➢ Restorative surgery for intestinal continuity
  - Emergency
    - ➢ Bowel perforation
    - ➢ Toxic megacolon
    - ➢ Life-threatening GI haemorrhage
- **Complications of disease**
  - Acute severe colitis
  - Sepsis
- **Complications of therapy**
  - Medication side effects
  - *Immunosuppression*: sepsis

What challenges might patients with IBD present?

- **Late physiological decompensation** in younger subgroup
- *Immunosuppression*: propensity to sepsis and atypical organisms, side effects
  - *Steroid management*: dependency, supplementation in acute illness
- *Poor nutritional state*: malabsorption syndrome, limited reserve
- **Combined both medical and surgical management**

What are the main forms of chronic IBD?

- **UC** is characterised by mucosal inflammation starting distally, with continuous extension proximally and an abrupt demarcation with non-inflamed mucosa. Local complications are as follows: haemorrhage, adenocarcinoma, toxic megacolon (and subsequent perforation).
- **Crohn's disease** is difficult to define but is a complex chronic inflammatory GI condition with variable onset age, location, and behaviour. It is suggested by skip lesions, ileal involvement, and granulomatous inflammation and can occur along the whole GI tract. Local complications are as follows: strictures, fistulation, perforation.

Despite adequate investigations, 5–15% IBD patients will have unclassifiable disease. Important differentials include other causes of colitis, most notably infective: *C. difficile*, TB, CMV, Shigella, and amoebic dysentery.

> **GUIDELINE** BSG 2019 IBD

What immunosuppressive agents are used in IBD?

Immunosuppressants are used to either induce remission or maintain disease control, with subtle differences in approach between the 2 conditions. In moderate-severe disease, induction of remission is initially achieved using corticosteroids, before consideration of anti-TNF or other medications if refractory (e.g. at 72 h).

- **5-aminosalicylic acid** (5-ASA) (e.g. mesalazine)
- **Thiopurines** (e.g. azathioprine)
- **Corticosteroids** (e.g. prednisolone in UC, budesonide in Crohn's disease)
- **Anti-TNF** (e.g. infliximab, adalimumab, golimumab, certolizumab pegol)
- **Calcineurin inhibitors** (e.g. ciclosporin, tacrolimus)
- **Integrin $\alpha_4\beta_7$ inhibitors** (e.g. vedolizumab)
- **JAK inhibitors** (e.g. tofacitinib)
- **IL-12, IL-23 inhibitors** (e.g. ustekinumab)
- **Anti-metabolite** (e.g. methotrexate)

> **GUIDELINE** ECCO 2020 Crohn's disease

> **GUIDELINE** ECCO 2022 Ulcerative colitis

What are the notable side effects of these drugs (i.e. other than immunosuppression)?

- *5-ASA*: nephrotoxicity
- *Thiopurines*: myelotoxicity, hepatotoxicity, pancreatitis, flu-like symptoms
- *Vedolizumab*: PML
- *Tofacitinib*: Herpes Zoster infection
- *Ciclosporin*: nephrotoxicity, seizures, anaphylaxis, death
- *Methotrexate*: GI and liver toxicity (including fibrosis, cirrhosis), interstitial pneumonitis
- *Ustekinumab*: nasopharyngitis, headache, arthralgia

Infusion reactions are notable with anti-TNF therapies, vedolizumab, and ustekinumab.

Describe the features of acute severe UC.

> **KEY POINT**
>
> Acute severe UC can be defined using the **Truelove and Witts criteria** (in adults) as follows:
>
> - **>6 bloody stools**/day, and
> - **Systemic toxicity**, as ≥1 of the following:
>   - Temperature > 37.8°C
>   - HR > 90
>   - Hb < 105 g/l
>   - CRP > 30 mg/l

How is acute severe UC managed?

- Daily senior gastroenterology review
- Baseline investigations
  - *Bloods (daily)*: FBC, U&E, CRP, albumin
  - *Stool*: MC+S including *C. difficile*
  - Sigmoidoscopy within 24 h including CMV screen
- **Anti-inflammatory treatment**
  - IV hydrocortisone 100 mg 6 hourly/methylprednisolone 60–80 mg daily
  - 5-ASA may need to be withheld
- **Second-line 'rescue' therapy or surgery** if no response in 3 days (see above)
  - Response defined by < 4 stools per day for 2 days and no rectal bleeding
- *VTE prophylaxis*: prothrombotic state
- Management of complications
  - *Surgery in selected cases*: subtotal colectomy and end ileostomy with long rectal stump
  - *Antimicrobials*: broad spectrum
- Avoid bowel static medications and NSAIDs

When would surgical review be indicated?

Acute severe UC carries a 30–40% risk of colectomy, and 10–20% will occur on first admission.

Further imaging is likely to be recommended (CT preferred to X-ray) in addition to surgical review for refractory disease as follows:

- Continued systemic toxicity
- Severe abdominal pain
- Oedema with low serum albumin
- Suspected toxic megacolon or perforation

Colectomy might also be indicated if:

- >8 stools per day, or
- 3–8 stools per day and CRP > 45 mg/l

What is toxic megacolon?

Toxic megacolon is a form of severe colitis which is characterised by non-obstructive colonic dilatation and systemic toxicity. It is defined by the presence of the following 3 criteria:

- Radiographic evidence of **colonic distension ≥6 cm**
- ≥3 of the following:
  - Temperature > 38°C
  - HR > 120
  - Neutrophil leukocytosis > 10.5 × 10⁹/l
  - Anaemia
- ≥1 of the following:
  - Dehydration
  - Altered consciousness

- Electrolyte disturbances
- Hypotension

Resources

- Jain S, Ahuja V, Limdi JK. Optimal management of acute severe ulcerative colitis. Postgrad Med J. 2019;95(1119):32–40.
- Jalan KN, Circus W, Cord WI, et al. An experience with ulcerative colitis: toxic dilatation in 55 cases. Gastroenterology. 1969;57(1):68–82.

---

139.   GASTROINTESTINAL HAEMORRHAGE

What is the difference between upper and lower GI bleeding?

GI bleeding can be classified by the location of its origin in the GI tract. The boundary between the upper and lower tract is the ligament of Treitz, the suspensory ligament of the duodenum.

UGIB is a medical emergency associated with a high mortality. If there is evidence of bleeding once admitted, mortality is as high as 30%. Patients may require intensive care admission due for sequelae of haemorrhagic shock, airway protection, aspiration pneumonitis, or to tamponade bleeding varices when endoscopy has failed.

What are the causes of upper GI haemorrhage?

The most common cause of GI haemorrhage in the UK is peptic ulcer disease, followed by variceal haemorrhage and oesophagitis. Stress ulceration should be considered in critical illness although much better prevented in recent years (see Chapter 18 Stress Ulcer Prophylaxis).

- **Varices**
  - Oesophageal
  - Gastric
- **Ulcers**
  - *Drugs*: NSAIDs, steroids
  - *Infective*: *Helicobacter pylori*
  - Stress ulcer
  - Zollinger-Ellison syndrome
  - Oesophagitis
- *Portal hypertension*: hypertensive gastropathy
- **Vascular**
  - *Dieulafoy lesion*: abnormally prominent arteriole in GI wall
  - Hereditary haemorrhagic telangiectasia
- **Traumatic**
  - Mallory-Weiss tear
  - Post-surgical
  - Aorto-enteric fistula
- **Tumours**
  - Polyps
  - *Malignancy*: adenocarcinoma, lymphoma

How might these patients present?

- Reduced appetite
- Haematemesis
- Melaena
- Haematochezia (or haemochezia)
- Abdominal pain

- Dizziness
- Syncope/collapse
- Cardiac arrest

Which points might you clarify in the history?

- NSAID use
- Anticoagulation or antiplatelet use
- Previous GI bleeding
- History of chronic liver disease
- History of varices
- *Comorbidities*: IHD, HF, renal failure

Are there any risk scores for UGIB?

The Glasgow-Blatchford Score can be used prior to endoscopy to help determine the urgency of intervention and best place of care – specifically, whether or not patients require admission to hospital. The AIM65 score is a better predictor of mortality prior to endoscopy but is less useful in decisions to admit/discharge from hospital. The Rockall Score takes endoscopy findings into consideration in the context of morbidity and mortality prediction.

Glasgow-Blatchford

- Urea, Hb, systolic BP, HR, melaena, syncope, liver disease, cardiac failure
- Factors weighted differently, range 0–23
- *Score 0*: low risk – outpatient management suitable

AIM65

- Albumin < 30 g/l, INR > 1.5, altered mental state, SBP ≤ 90 mmHg, age ≥ 65 years
- 1 point each
- *Score 1*: 1.2% in-hospital mortality (2: 5%, 3: 10%, 4: 17%, 5: 25%)

Rockall

- Age, HR, systolic BP, comorbidities, diagnosis, stigmata of haemorrhage
- *Score ≤2*: good prognosis
- *Score > 7*: 10–30% mortality (up to 25–50% with rebleed)

How do you manage major upper GI haemorrhage?

- Consider intubation if risk of airway compromise due to aspiration or endoscopy
- Management of major haemorrhage (see Chapter 51 Major Haemorrhage)
    - Platelet transfusion threshold 50×10^9/l
    - Reversal of anticoagulants (± haematology input)
    - Restrictive Hb threshold unless unstable or IHD
- *Specific management as per aetiology*: variceal vs non-variceal
- Intervention
    - *Endoscopy*: immediately after resuscitation if unstable; within 24 h if stable
    - *Repeat endoscopy within 24 h*: if rebleeding, high risk of rebleed, or doubt about haemostasis
    - *IR*: if rebleed following endoscopy
    - *Surgery*: if IR not available/successful
- Acid suppression (e.g. proton pump inhibitor) not indicated unless evidence of non-variceal bleeding at endoscopy

STUDY

Villanueva et al. (2013)

- Severe acute UGIB
- *Intervention*: restrictive transfusion (threshold 70 g/l) vs liberal (90 g/l)
- *Primary*: 45-day mortality – **significantly lower (5% vs 9%)**
- *Secondary*: further bleeding, in-hospital complications – **significantly lower**

Would you use TXA when managing GI haemorrhage?

TXA use has not been shown to improve outcomes, and its use has fallen out of favour since the HALT-IT trial, despite it not differentiate between upper and lower GI haemorrhage. The increase in thromboembolic events has not been demonstrated in other TXA trials, but the patient population differs significantly. Most clinicians would not use TXA in their management of GI haemorrhage, and it is not mentioned in the relevant guidelines.

STUDY

HALT-IT (2020)

- GI bleeding
- *Intervention*: TXA 1 g then infusion 3 g/24 h vs placebo
- *Primary*: death due to bleeding within 5 days – **no difference**
- *Secondary*: 24-h/28-day mortality, rebleeding, interventions, transfusion – no difference; VTE – **significantly higher**

GUIDELINE   NICE 2016 CG141 UGIB

GUIDELINE   BSG 2020 UGIB Care Bundle

What is the specific management of variceal haemorrhage?

- **Vasoconstrictors**
  - Terlipressin 2 mg 6° until haemostasis (max 5 days)
  - Somatostatin alternatively, octreotide third line
- *Prophylactic antibiotics*: significant mortality related to pneumonia in patients with cirrhosis
- *Endoscopy*: variceal band ligation or injection with N-butyl-2-cyanoacrylate

If failed endoscopy:

- **Temporising measures**
  - Balloon tamponade recommended
  - Possible role for oesophageal stenting but not yet recommended
- **TIPS**
  - Selected patients
  - <72 h of index bleed

STUDY

Escorsell et al. (2016)

- Cirrhosis and oesophageal variceal bleeding refractory to medical and endoscopic treatment
- *Intervention*: oesophageal covered metal stent vs balloon tamponade
- *Primary*: composite of survival at day 15, control of bleeding, absence of serious adverse events – **significantly higher (66% vs 20%)**

GUIDELINE   BSG 2015 Variceal haemorrhage

What is the specific management of non-variceal haemorrhage?

- **Endoscopy**
  - *Mechanical treatment*: clips
  - Thermal coagulation with adrenaline
  - Fibrin or thrombin with adrenaline
  - (Adrenaline monotherapy not recommended)

- *As above*: **repeat endoscopy** if rebleed ± IR ± surgery
- **High-dose proton pump inhibitor** after endoscopy if stigmata of recent bleed seen
- *H. pylori* **eradication therapy** if identified

GUIDELINE BSG 2002 Non-variceal haemorrhage

How is balloon tamponade achieved?

- Appropriate airway management established
- Specific orogastric tube with additional channels inserted (e.g. Sengstaken-Blakemore, Minnesota)
    - Gastric balloon, oesophageal balloon, gastric aspiration port, oesophageal aspiration port
- Gastric balloon inflated with 500 ml air (± oesophageal balloon up to 30–45 mmHg)
    - Confirmed on CXR
    - Occludes oesophageal varices more proximally at gastro-oesophageal junction
    - Also tamponades gastric varices
    - Oesophageal balloon used if this fails
- Traction may be applied using weight of approximately 0.5–1 kg
    - Release regularly to prevent necrosis
    - Remove after 24 h
- Other possible complications include oesophageal rupture and aspiration

What is the significance of lower GI haemorrhage?

Lower GI haemorrhage usually presents with fresh PR bleeding, and patients are less likely to be unstable. Common causes include diverticular disease (most common), IBD, and neoplasia. Resuscitation will need to be balanced with urgency of investigation as with upper GI haemorrhage.

Risk stratification
- Stable vs unstable (shock index > 1)
- *If stable*: major vs minor – determined by risk assessment tool (e.g. Oakland score)

Initial investigation
- *Minor*: urgent outpatient investigation or equivalent if admitted for other reason.
- *Major*: next available inpatient colonoscopy.
- Unstable
    - **CT angiography** is recommended initially.
    - **Upper GI endoscopy** is indicated if no source is identified on CT.
        - ➢ To rule out brisk UGIB causing lower GI presentation
        - ➢ If patient stabilises with resuscitation, this may be first line prior to CT.
    - **Catheter angiography and embolisation within 60 min** if CT positive
    - *Colonoscopy may be indicated*: only used in around 2% cases regardless of stability
    - *Laparotomy*: last resort unless exceptional circumstances

KEY POINT

- Shock index = heart rate/systolic BP
- Also studied in context of trauma mortality, transfusion requirement, peri-intubation cardiac arrest, and sepsis

GUIDELINE BSG 2019 Lower GI bleeding

Resources
- Elsayed IAS, Battu PK, Irving S. Management of acute upper GI bleeding. BJA Educ. 2017;17(4):117–123.
- Saltzman JR, Tabak YP, Hyett BH, et al. A simple risk score accurately predicts in-hospital mortality, length of stay, and cost in acute upper GI bleeding. Gastroint Endosc. 2011;74(6):1215–1224.

What is refeeding syndrome?

There is no consensus definition of refeeding syndrome. It can be described as a potentially life-threatening syndrome of metabolic disturbance characterised by electrolyte and fluid shift upon reintroduction of feeding after a period of starvation.

Metabolic abnormalities include the following:

- Glucose metabolism imbalance
- Hypophosphataemia
- Hypokalaemia
- Hypomagnesaemia
- Thiamine deficiency

The reported incidence in critical care varies largely due to the unclear definition. Malnourished patients have a 60 times greater risk of hypophosphataemia, which has an all-cause mortality of 18%.

What is the pathophysiology of refeeding syndrome?

The pathophysiology of refeeding syndrome encompasses 2 phases: starvation/malnutrition and refeeding. The severity of features is related to increasing caloric load and is unrelated to route of feeding.

Starvation
- Glycogenolysis, gluconeogenesis, protein catabolism occur
- Depletion of protein, fat, minerals, electrolytes, vitamins
- Salt and water intolerance

Refeeding
- Switch to catabolism
- Fluid, salt, nutrient intake
- Shift from using free fatty acids and ketones to carbohydrate metabolism
- Increased insulin secretion
- Increased protein, fat, and glycogen synthesis
- Increase in uptake of glucose, K^+, Mg^{2+}, PO_4^{3-}, increased thiamine utilisation
- Pre-existing intracellular compartment depletion causes wide concentration gradient
- Rapid depletion of extracellular ions
- Sodium retention to maintain neutral osmotic gradient, followed by water

Pathophysiology of metabolic disturbances
- *Hypokalaemia*: rapid cellular uptake of K^+ as glycogen and protein synthesised
- *Hypophosphataemia*: increased phosphorylation of glucose
- *Hypomagnesaemia*: cellular uptake of Mg^{2+}
- *Thiamine depletion*: used as cofactor in glycolysis

Who is at risk of refeeding syndrome in critical care?

Risk factors for refeeding syndrome are described by NICE (Table 140.1). Patients admitted to critical care often have several risk factors.

Table 140.1   Risk factors for refeeding syndrome

≥1 of:	≥2 of:
• BMI < 16 kg/m² • Unintentional weight loss >15% in last 3–6 months • Little or no nutritional intake >10 days • Low K^+/PO_4^{3-}/Mg^{2+} prior to feeding	• BMI < 18 kg/m² • Unintentional weight loss >10% in last 3–6 months • Little or no nutritional intake >5 days • History of alcohol abuse or drugs including insulin, chemotherapy, antacids, diuretics

Which patient groups are at risk of malnutrition?

Low intake
- *Starvation*: iatrogenic, hunger strikes
- Chronic swallowing problems
- Anorexia nervosa
- Alcoholism
- Depression
- Malignancy
- Chronic infectious diseases
- Catabolic illness
- Post-operative patients
- Morbid obesity with profound weight loss
- Homelessness, social deprivation
- Idiosyncratic/eccentric diets

Excess losses/decreased absorption
- Vomiting
- Diarrhoea
- GI tract inflammation
- Chronic pancreatitis
- Chronic antacid use
- Chronic high-dose diuretic use
- After bariatric surgery

What are the complications of refeeding syndrome?

Refeeding syndrome encompasses a spectrum of disorders ranging from patients who are asymptomatic with risk factors to those with life-threatening features. These may include the following:

- *A/B*: pulmonary oedema, failure to wean
- *C*: oedema, CCF, cardiomyopathy, arrhythmias
- *D*: Wernicke's encephalopathy, seizures, altered mental state, hyperglycaemia
- *G*: severe diarrhoea if gut atrophy

What measures can be taken to prevent and treat refeeding syndrome in high-risk patients?

- **Dietitian/nutrition team involvement**
  - Appropriate screening
  - Refer if at risk
  - Adjust feed components as required
- **Manage underlying condition**
- **Cardiovascular support**
  - Monitor for arrhythmias
  - Restore circulating volume
- **Vitamin supplementation**
  - Immediately (30 min) before and for first 10 days of feeding
  - Thiamine 200–300 mg daily, vitamin B co-strong 1–2 tablets 8 hourly, or
  - Daily IV vitamin B preparation (e.g. Pabrinex®)
- **Slow introduction of feed**
  - 10 kcal/kg/day initially
  - 5 kcal/kg/day in extreme cases (BMI < 14 kg/m^2, starvation > 15 days)
  - Increase to meet full needs by 4–7 days

- **Baseline electrolyte supplementation**
  - Increased requirement, omit only if plasma levels high pre-feeding
  - Potassium (2–4 mmol/kg/day)
  - Magnesium (0.2 or 0.4 mmol/kg/day, IV vs PO)
- Monitoring
  - *Daily bloods*: U&E, Mg^{2+}, PO_4^{3-}, Ca^{2+}
  - Glucose several times per day
  - Adjust feed as required
  - Treat significant electrolyte disturbance
- Cautious fluid balance
  - Minimise input as long as renal function maintained
  - Restrict sodium intake

(See Chapter 17 Nutrition and Chapter 132 Electrolyte Disorders)

Resources

- McKnight CL, Newberry C, Sarav M, et al. Refeeding syndrome in the critically ill: a literature review and clinician's guide. Curr Gastroenterol Rep. 2019;21(11):58.
- Stanga Z, Brunner A, Leuenberger M, et al. Nutrition in clinical practice – the refeeding syndrome: illustrative cases and guidelines for prevention and treatment. Eur J Clin Nutr. 2008;62(6):687–694.

141. BLEEDING AND CLOTTING DISORDERS

What are the causes of bleeding in critically unwell patients?

Reduced haemostasis
- Coagulation factor deficiency
  - *Consumptive*: sepsis, DIC, cardiac surgery
  - *Loss*: major haemorrhage
  - *Production*: vitamin K deficiency/antagonists
- Platelet deficiency/function
  - *Consumptive*: sepsis, DIC, extracorporeal support, splenomegaly
  - *Loss*: major haemorrhage
  - *Production*: myelosuppression, bone marrow failure

Hyperfibrinolysis
- *Inherited*: haemophilia, factor XIII deficiency, dysfibrinogenaemias
- Acquired
  - *Primary*: cirrhosis, acute promyelocytic leukaemia (APML)
  - *Secondary*: trauma, thrombolysis, CPB, amyloid, placental disease

Secondary disruption of haemostasis
- Hypothermia (temperature < 34°C)
- Acidosis (pH < 7.25)
- *Hypocalcaemia*: notable in massive blood transfusion

Outline the key features of the inherited bleeding disorders.
- *Haemophilia A*: factor VIII deficiency
- *Haemophilia B*: factor IX deficiency
- *Haemophilia C*: factor XI deficiency
- *von Willebrand's disease*: vWF quality/quantity defect
- *Rare*: factor II, V, VII, X, XIII deficiencies; dysfibrinogenaemia

Haemophilia A and B are X-linked recessive disorders, therefore affecting males. Severity is proportional to magnitude of factor deficiency. Features include spontaneous bleeding, significant bleeding after trauma, haemarthrosis in weight-bearing joints, muscle haematomas, and GU bleeding. ICH is the commonest cause of death.

Von Willebrand's disease is the commonest inherited bleeding disorder at 1:100 prevalence, but it is only significant in 1:10000 of those affected. vWF is required in platelet adhesion/aggregation and carriage of factor VIII. It is characterised by easy bruising from trivial trauma (including mucosal – nose, gums, bowel).

What are the causes of clotting catastrophes in critically unwell patients?

'Thrombotic storm' can occur in several conditions characterised by the following:

- Underlying procoagulant state
- Trigger to initiate clotting process
- Rapid development of new thromboembolic events

In these states, prompt antithrombotic therapy will improve outcome and good long-term prognosis can be achieved if the thrombotic cycle is interrupted early.

Catastrophic thrombotic syndromes

- Catastrophic antiphospholipid syndrome
- DIC
- TTP
- HIT
- Trousseau's syndrome
- Pregnancy
- COVID-19 infection
- VITT

(See Chapter 86 Cerebral Venous Sinus Thrombosis, Chapter 124 COVID-19, Chapter 145 Heparin-Induced Thrombocytopaenia, Chapter 147 Thrombotic Thrombocytopaenic Purpura, and Chapter 154 Rheumatology)

What do you know about DIC?

DIC is a syndrome resulting from inappropriate thrombin activation, resulting in fibrin formation, platelet/endothelial activation, and fibrinolysis. It may present with bleeding, thrombosis, or purpura fulminans. Diagnosis is based on the presence of a causative condition with a typical coagulation test profile. Mortality is approximately 40–80%.

Laboratory testing reveals the following:

- Prolonged PT
- Prolonged APTT
- Thrombocytopaenia
- Low fibrinogen
- Elevated fibrin degradation products (e.g. D-dimer)
- Microangiopathic haemolytic anaemia (MAHA) may be present.

Management centres around treating the underlying cause and providing supportive care. Thrombosis is rare but may present with peripheral gangrene and require heparinisation.

Transfusion in DIC is as follows:

- Stable, non-bleeding patients do not usually require platelet or clotting factor transfusion.
- *Platelets < 10–20 × 10⁹/l*: bleeding or planned intervention may trigger transfusion.
- No benefit of antithrombin transfusion in bleeding
- *Antifibrinolytics (e.g. TXA) contraindicated* (may increase thrombosis)

Purpura fulminans is a rare condition associated with extensive tissue thrombosis and haemorrhagic skin necrosis. It usually follows infection, particularly of viral or meningococcal origin. Protein C deficiency may be contributory, and protein C concentrate may be of benefit.

When might you suspect heritable thrombophilia?

Heritable thrombophilias include the following:

- Loss of function
  - Protein C deficiency
  - Protein S deficiency
  - Antithrombin deficiency
- Gain of function
  - Factor V Leiden
  - Antiphospholipid syndrome

Significant heritable thrombophilia should be suspected with the following:

- **Venous thrombosis at early age** (<40 years)
- **Apparent thrombosis-prone family** (>2 others symptomatic)
- **Children with purpura fulminans**
- **Pregnant women at risk of venous thrombosis**
- **Skin necrosis with oral vitamin K antagonists**

Testing is not usually indicated in unselected patients with CVC-related venous or arterial thrombosis.

> **GUIDELINE** BSH 2010 Thrombophilia

(See Chapter 51 Major Haemorrhage)

Resources

- Loo J, Spittle DA, Newnham M. COVID-19, immunothrombosis and venous thromboembolism: biological mechanisms. Thorax. 2021;76(4):412–420.
- Ridley S, Taylor B, Gunning K. Medical management of bleeding in critically ill patients. CEACCP. 2007;7(4):116–121.
- Shah UH, Narayanan M, Smith JG. Anaesthetic considerations in patients with inherited disorders of coagulation. CEACCP. 2015;15(1):26–31.
- Singh MY. Approach to the coagulopathic patient in the intensive care unit. Indian J Crit Care Med. 2019;23(Suppl3):S215–S220.
- Sinha S, Todi SK. Clotting catastrophies in the intensive care unit. Indian J Crit Care Med. 2019;23(Suppl3):S197–S201.

142.   HAEMATOLOGICAL MALIGNANCY

Which haematological malignancies are you aware of?

There are many types of haematological malignancy, often classified by cell origin and chronicity (Figure 142.1). These may present as new diagnoses, complications of intensive treatments, or relapsed disease. In the context of critical care:

Commonly admitted

- **Acute myeloid leukaemia** (AML) (e.g. APML presenting with DIC)
- **Acute lymphoblastic leukaemia** (ALL)
- **High-grade NHL** (e.g. diffuse large B-cell lymphoma [DLBCL], Burkitt's, mantle cell, T cell)

Less commonly involved

- Hodgkin lymphoma (majority curable)
- Myeloma

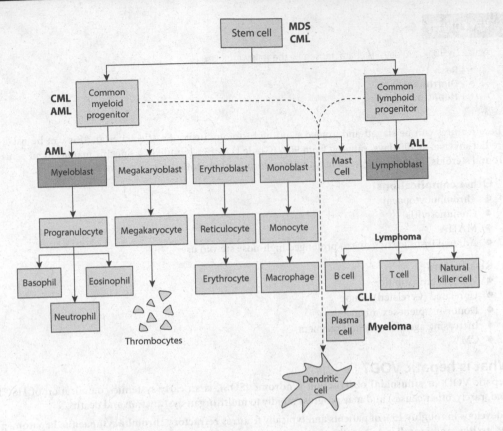

Figure 142.1   Cell origins of haematological malignancies.

MDS, myelodysplastic syndromes; AML, acute myeloid leukaemia; ALL, acute lymphoblastic leukaemia; CLL, chronic lymphocytic leukaemia.

- Chronic myeloid leukaemia
- Chronic lymphocytic leukaemia (CLL)
- Low-grade NHL (e.g. follicular, marginal zone)

What is haematopoietic stem cell transplantation (HSCT)?

HSCT involves transplantation of stem cells derived from bone marrow, peripheral blood, or umbilical cord blood. This can be from the patient's own bone marrow (**autologous**) or a donor (**allogenic**). HSCT is used in some haematological malignancies with curative intent. Allogenic transplantation requires long-term immunosuppressive therapy. Other indications include other malignancies and non-malignant conditions such as MS and mucopolysaccharidosis.

There is great variability in technique – cell origin, cell donor (HLA matching), and intensity of conditioning (destruction of bone marrow with radiotherapy or drugs prior to transplantation). Both short-term toxicity and long-term toxicity are significantly higher with allogenic than autologous HSCT (10–30% vs 3% mortality).

Engraftment is the incorporation of stem cells into the marrow, resulting in reconstitution of haematopoiesis. It typically takes up to 4 weeks to occur and signifies a functioning transplant.

Complications of HSCT include acute/chronic GvHD, graft failure, infection, haemorrhage, veno-occlusive disease (VOD), autoimmune disorders, and secondary malignancies. Patients will require irradiated blood products.

(See Chapter 70 The Post-Transplant Patient)

What is acute GvHD?

GvHD is a reaction in which a graft mounts an immune response against the recipient's body.

Acute GvHD (<100 days) is characterised by the following:

- **Rash**
- **Diarrhoea**
- **Hepatitis**

These features can be staged and graded pending histology (using Seattle criteria). This can be used to predict survival at 100 days, ranging from 90% (Grade I) to 23% (Grade IV). Specific management centres around steroids, immunosuppressants, and extracorporeal phototherapy.

Other complications
- Thrombocytopaenia
- Conjunctivitis
- MAHA
- Adrenal insufficiency due to prolonged high-dose steroid use

Risk factors
- HLA incompatibility
- Unrelated (vs related) donor
- Donor-recipient sex mismatch
- Increasing age of donor and recipient
- CMV

What is hepatic VOD?

Hepatic VOD, or **sinusoidal obstruction syndrome (SOS)**, is an early systemic complication of HSCT (and, rarely, other causes) and may progress rapidly to multi-organ dysfunction and death.

It develops in roughly 15% of patients and typically features **refractory thrombocytopaenia, hepatomegaly, ascites**, and **jaundice** 1–2 weeks post-transplantation. Diagnosis is often clinical due to the risks of liver biopsy and poor sensitivity of US. Seattle or Baltimore criteria can be used, taking into account the significance of jaundice/hyperbilirubinaemia, ascites/weight gain, and painful hepatomegaly.

The pathophysiology involves damage to sinusoidal epithelial cells and hepatocytes in zone 3 of liver acini following cytokine release and haemostatic activation. Hepatocellular necrosis and fibrosis result in vascular occlusion.

VOD resolves over 2–3 weeks and may require organ support in the meantime. Renal perfusion, whilst avoiding fluid overload, is a management priority. Specific agents and TIPS are under evaluation.

Mortality ranges from 20 to 50% and might be caused by hepatic failure, HRS, pulmonary VOD, interstitial pneumonitis, pulmonary haemorrhage, GI bleeding, or CCF.

What is tumour lysis syndrome (TLS)?

TLS may be spontaneous or the result of chemotherapy or steroid use for certain malignancies. It is more commonly associated with acute leukaemias and high-grade lymphomas (particularly Burkitt's). Diagnosis involves clinical and laboratory criteria.

Laboratory TLS: Cairo-Bishop criteria (absolute values below or 25% increase from baseline) are as follows:

- Uric acid ≥ 476 µmol/l
- $K^+ ≥ 6$ mmol/l
- $PO_4^- ≥ 1.45$ mmol/l
- $Ca^{2+} ≤ 1.75$ mmol/l

Clinical TLS: laboratory TLS and any of the following:

- Seizure
- Cardiac arrhythmia
- Increase in serum creatinine ≥1.5 × upper limit of normal

Management priorities
- Hydration
- Management of hyperkalaemia (may involve RRT)
- Rasburicase (recombinant urate oxidase, under specialist direction)
- Monitoring of electrolytes, early detection where possible
- Avoid correction of hypocalcaemia unless symptomatic or ECG changes present (exacerbates AKI)
- *Prophylaxis*: rasburicase/allopurinol, euvolaemia

(See Chapter 155 Oncology)

Resources
- Beed M, Levitt M, Bokhari SW. Intensive care management of patients with haematological malignancy. CEACCP. 2010;10(6):167–171.
- Kumar S, Delve LD, Kamath PS, et al. Hepatic veno-occlusive disease (sinusoidal obstruction syndrome) after hematopoietic stem cell transplantation. Mayo Clin Proc. 2003;78(5):589–598.

143. HAEMOGLOBINOPATHIES

Why are haemoglobinopathies significant to critical care?

Haemoglobinopathies are disorders affecting Hb. They are usually inherited conditions caused by mutations in genes coding for the components of Hb, affecting its structure, quality, and quantity:

- *Quality/structure*: Hb variants (e.g. HbS, HbO, HbE, HbC, HbD)
- *Quantity*: β thalassaemia, α thalassaemia, δβ thalassaemia

Hb is a fundamental requirement for organ perfusion and respiration due to its role in transporting oxygen. Reduction in its function by the above conditions will have significant multisystem effects.

What is the pathophysiology of sickle cell disease?

- Mutation on chromosome 11
- Amino acid substitution on β-globin subunit of HbA, forming HbS
- HbS unstable, precipitates if deoxygenated, forms curved, sickle-shaped cells
- Higher HbS proportion related to propensity of cell to sickle
- *Sickle cell trait (heterozygous)*: benign, sickling under significant stress only
- *Sickle cell disease (homozygous)*: haemolytic anaemia, vaso-occlusion, pain, organ damage, reduced life expectancy

What are the clinical effects of sickle cell disease?

Acute crises
- *Vaso-occlusive*: acute chest syndrome, abdominal, bone (cause severe pain)
- *Aplastic/hypoplastic*: marrow suppression/failure
- **Haemolytic**
- **Sequestration** (splenic)

Other features
- *A*: prominent maxilla, lymphoid hypertrophy, OSA
- *B*: pulmonary infarcts, chronic respiratory failure, pain, dyspnoea, haemoptysis
- *C*: cardiomegaly, CCF, PAH
- *D*: CVA, ICH

- *E*: aseptic necrosis, leg ulcers
- *F*: CKD, priapism
- *G*: gallstones, hepatomegaly
- *H*: splenic infarction, splenomegaly
- *I*: functional asplenism

What are the specific priorities in the acute management of patients with sickle cell disease?

- May require rapid screening in emergency setting (e.g. SICKLEDEX® test)
- *Supportive care*: particularly **analgesia**, **rehydration**
- Transfusion if indicated
  - *Thorough transfusion history*: patient may carry an information card
  - Specialist input prior to transfusion
  - Viral screening if regularly transfused
  - *Specialised blood products*: HbS negative, <10 days old (<7 if exchange), extended antibody screening
- Prevention/management of crisis
  - Appropriate HbS fraction and Hb concentration
  - Adequate oxygenation, perfusion pressure, hydration, temperature, analgesia
  - Prevention of venous stasis
  - Early treatment of precipitants (e.g. infection)

When might transfusion be indicated in sickle cell disease?

Acute anaemia in the context of aplastic/sequestration crises is defined as a decrease in Hb ≥20 g/dl below baseline. Transfusion may be performed by simple 'top up' or exchange transfusion. Exchange transfusion uses a similar set-up to plasma exchange via a femoral venous line, wide-bore peripheral IV access in each antecubital fossa, or a portacath.

Indications include the following:

- **Top up**
  - Aplastic crisis
  - *Sequestration*: hepatic/splenic
  - Severe anaemia in pregnancy
  - Delayed haemolytic transfusion reaction
- **Exchange**
  - CVA
  - Acute multi-organ dysfunction
  - Severe sepsis
  - Elective low-/medium-risk surgery

Other indications managed with **either method**: ACS, stroke prevention, sickle complications in pregnancy, high maternal/fetal/obstetric risk, recurrent ACS, or recurrent painful crises.

Transfusion is not recommended in uncomplicated vaso-occlusive crises, and there is no evidence to support shortening in the duration of painful crises.

GUIDELINE BSH 2017 Sickle transfusion

What therapeutic targets are recommended in sickle cell disease?

- *HbS < 30%*: stroke prevention, acute ischaemic stroke (and Hb > 100)
- *Hb > 90 g/dl*: pre-operative
- *Hb > 100 g/dl*: emergency surgery, some elective surgery with Hb <90 g/dl and SS
- Avoid transfusing to above Hb 80 g/dl in sequestration crisis
- Avoid transfusing to above Hb 100 g/dl if Hb <90 g/dl and not regularly transfused

What is the significance of the thalassaemias to critical care?

An awareness of the thalassaemias will aid management of affected patients. These hereditary conditions are characterised by defective synthesis of the alpha or beta chains in Hb.

Alpha thalassaemias
- Reduced erythrocyte life span due to increased splenic uptake.
- Combined with sickle cell genes, HbS-thalassaemia may result in severe disease with microcytic haemolytic anaemia and vaso-occlusive crises.

Beta thalassaemias
- Thalassaemia minor
  - Heterozygous
  - Mild hypochromic microcytic anaemia
  - Hb 20–30 g/dl lower than expected
- Thalassaemia major
  - Homozygous
  - Profound anaemia
  - Repeated blood transfusions required

Important considerations
- Similar airway considerations to sickle cell disease from marrow hyperplasia
- Appropriate Hct
- Assessment of cardiac function if haemosiderosis present
- May have undergone splenectomy, associated immunocompromise, OPSI risk

(See Chapter 61 Splenic Injury)

Resource
- Wilson M, Forsyth P, Whiteside J. Haemoglobinopathy and sickle cell disease. CEACCP. 2010;10(1):24–28.

---

144. HAEMOPHAGOCYTIC LYMPHOHISTIOCYTOSIS

What is haemophagocytic lymphohistiocytosis?

HLH is a syndrome of dysregulated immune function, characterised by **severe inflammation, fever, cytopaenias**, and **organ dysfunction**.

It is similar and/or related to other inflammatory states including MAS, sepsis-induced hyperinflammation, and PIMS-TS. Other terminology for HLH includes hyperferritinaemic syndrome, MAS-like syndrome, sepsis-HLH overlap syndrome, and viral-associated haemophagocytic syndrome.

HLH can be familial (fHLH) or secondary/acquired (sHLH). An increased awareness of this condition has followed the COVID-19 pandemic, after some patients were found to have an HLH-like syndrome.

(See Chapter 110 PIMS-TS)

What is MAS?

MAS is a historical term, synonymous with HLH in the context of autoimmune disease. Associations are as follows:

- Systemic juvenile idiopathic arthritis (10%)
- Adult-onset Still's disease
- SLE

- Rheumatoid arthritis
- Systemic vasculitis
- IBD

What other causes of sHLH have been recognised?

Infection is the most common cause, with **EBV** most commonly implicated.

- **Infection**
  - *Viral*: EBV, CMV, HSV, VZV, HHV, hepatitis, HIV, parvovirus, influenza
  - *Bacterial*: *Mycobacteria, Rickettsia, Legionella, Staph.* spp.
  - *Parasitic*: Leishmaniasis, *Plasmodium falciparum, Toxoplasma* spp.
  - *Fungal*: Histoplasmosis, *Pneumocystis jirovecii, Candida* spp., *Aspergillus* spp.
- **Malignancy**
  - *Direct*: lymphomas, some solid tumours
  - *Treatment*: chemotherapy, stem cell transplant, novel immune therapies

What is the pathogenesis?

This is not fully understood and is thought to involve failure of negative feedback controlling inflammation:

- May involve individual susceptibility and/or background inflammation
- HLH triggered by failure to clear antigen from infected tumour/autoimmune cells and antigen-presenting dendritic cells
- *Uncontrolled immune stimulation*: activation and proliferation of macrophages and cytotoxic T lymphocytes
- Cytokine storm
- Hyperinflammation, end-organ damage, haemophagocytosis (phagocytosis of haematopoietic cells)

How is HLH diagnosed?

A high index of suspicion should follow any presentation of an unwell patient with unexplained fever, cytopaenias, and organ dysfunction.

Other clinical features include hepatosplenomegaly, lymphadenopathy, and skin features (erythroderma, petechiae, purpura). Organ dysfunction may include ARDS, shock, cardiomyopathy, AKI, and neurological impairment including seizures.

Workup might include the following approach in critical care:

- *Serum ferritin*: significant elevation
- If ferritin elevated, investigate further
  - *Serial bloods*: FBC, ferritin, triglycerides, fibrinogen, LFTs, LDH
  - Calculate HScore
- Consider alternative diagnoses
- Involve other specialties ± HLH expert
- Bone marrow aspiration may be indicated

Diagnosis may then be made based on clinical probability.

What do you know about HLH scoring systems?

There are 2 main scoring systems: HLH-2004 and HScore.

HLH-2004 is a diagnostic framework involving 8 parameters. A score of ≥5 results in a diagnosis of HLH. It has only been validated in children and requires specialised tests.

The **HScore** is a bedside probability scoring tool which allocates points for severity of features. A total score >169 has 93% sensitivity and 86% specificity for HLH. Parameters included the following:

- Temperature
- Organomegaly
- Number of cytopaenias
- Triglycerides
- Fibrinogen
- Haemophagocytosis on bone marrow aspirate

- Ferritin
- Serum ALT
- *Known immunosuppression*: HIV or long-term immunosuppressive therapy

What specific therapy can be used to manage HLH?

Immunosuppression is the mainstay of specific treatment and should be guided by a specialist. Strategies include the following:

- **Steroids** (e.g. hydrocortisone, methylprednisolone, dexamethasone if CNS involvement)
- **Anakinra** (IL-1 receptor antagonist, alternative to steroids if trigger unclear)
- **IVIg**
- *Second line*: etoposide (particularly for malignancy)
- *Maintenance*: ciclosporin

Parallel therapies might include antimicrobials, rituximab (EBV), antiretroviral therapy (HIV), or targeted cancer chemotherapy or biological therapy. Treatment of any underlying cause is crucial where identified.

What is the prognosis of HLH?

- 40% acute mortality
- 80% acute mortality in malignancy-associated HLH, 5-year survival < 5%
- *ICU patients*: 52–68% hospital mortality
- Mortality worse with shock or severe thrombocytopaenia
- Maximum serum ferritin directly correlates with mortality risk
- Rapid fall in serum ferritin with treatment associated with favourable short-term outcome

Resource

- Bauchmuller K, Manson JJ, Tattersall R. Haemophagocytic lymphohistiocytosis in adult critical care. J Intensive Care Soc. 2020;21(3):256–268.

---

145. HEPARIN-INDUCED THROMBOCYTOPAENIA

What is heparin-induced thrombocytopaenia?

HIT is a prothrombotic syndrome that may result from administration of exogenous heparin compounds. It has also been called heparin-induced thrombocytopaenia thrombosis (HITT).

Two types of HIT have been described, with different pathogenesis and clinical features (Table 145.1). UFH usage carries a 1–5% incidence of HIT, compared with <1% with LMWH. It is more common in females and post-operative patients on the ICU. It is rare in medical and obstetric patients.

Clinical HIT manifests in 5% patients undergoing orthopaedic surgery receiving UFH and 2.4% patients undergoing cardiac surgery. The incidence in ICU is <2%. Reported incidence in pregnant women on LMWH is 0%.

Table 145.1 Comparison of HIT subtypes

	Type I	Type II
Significance	Less common	More common
Thrombocytopaenia	Mild (usually ≥100 × 10⁹/l)	Significant
Mechanism	Non-immune	Immune
Features	Usually benign	Thrombotic sequelae common
Scenarios	Sepsis, burns, vascular disease	Trauma, surgery, neoplasm, inflammation
Approach	Heparin can be continued	Heparin cessation/replacement

What is the pathophysiology of HIT?

HIT occurs after exposure to heparin. Heparin usually causes mild platelet aggregation.

Both processes involve PF4. PF4 is made by megakaryocytes and stored in platelet α-granules. When platelet activation occurs, PF4 is released and binds to compounds on cell surfaces. PF4 then inhibits megakaryocyte formation and angiogenesis and modulates the immune response. Certain conditions will cause significant PF4 release. Anti-PF4 is also produced in VITT. (See Chapter 86 Cerebral Venous Sinus Thrombosis)

Type I (non-immune)
- Heparin binds to PF4
- Inhibition of adenyl cyclase
- Decrease in intracellular cAMP
- Lower platelet activation threshold
- Mild platelet aggregation and thrombocytopaenia

Type II (immune)
- Heparin displaces PF4
- PF4 undergoes structural change, and a **PF4/heparin complex** is formed
- PF4/heparin acts as an antigen, triggering an immune response
- IgG antibodies (anti-PF4) are released and bind to these complexes
- Platelet Fc receptor clustering results in platelet activation
- Arterial thrombosis occurs
- Other contributors to thrombosis
  - Platelet fragmentation into prothrombotic microparticles, causing venous thrombosis
  - Antibodies may bind to monocyte Fc receptors, resulting in tissue factor release
  - HIT antibodies causing platelet adhesion to vessel walls, forming platelet-leukocyte aggregates
  - Elevated vWF and thrombomodulin

What is the differential diagnosis for thrombocytopaenia in ICU?

- **Decreased production**
  - Sepsis
  - *Drugs*: vancomycin, chemotherapy
  - Alcohol excess
  - Bone marrow failure
- **Consumption**
  - PE
  - VITT
  - Major trauma
  - HELLP syndrome
  - TTP
- **Dilutional**
  - Fluid resuscitation
  - Massive transfusion
- **Distributive**
  - Hypersplenism
  - Hypothermia
- **Destruction**
  - *Immune*: immune thrombocytopaenic purpura (ITP), SLE, antiphospholipid syndrome, HIT
  - *Other*: DIC, intravascular devices (ECMO, IABP, LVAD, PAC)
- **Spurious**: EDTA-induced pseudothrombocytopaenia

Can you name some other manifestations of HIT?

Common
- VTE
- PE
- *Arterial thrombus*: stroke, ACS, peripheral arterial thrombosis

Rare

- Skin lesions
- Adrenal haemorrhage
- Venous limb gangrene
- Total global amnesia
- Acute systemic reaction
- Sudden collapse and death
- Warfarin-induced skin necrosis

What is your diagnostic approach to HIT in critical care?

The issues surrounding HIT diagnosis relate to the immediate need to manage patients' coagulation whilst waiting for a specialist test result and the broad differential diagnosis of thrombocytopaenia. In addition, the pathogenic process may occur without clinically significant HIT.

HIT will often present with thrombocytopaenia in the first instance. Baseline platelet count is important in any patient about to receive any form of heparin. Post-op patients and those who have had cardiopulmonary bypass should also have this repeated at 24 h after heparin starting. Suspicion should be triggered by a platelet count fall of ≥30% and/or new thrombosis or other manifestation of HIT.

Half of those with the condition will have thrombosis. A thorough investigation of heparin administration timing, thrombotic features, and other causes should be carried out.

Specific investigation should start in the form of pretest probability scoring. The **4Ts score** was described by Warkentin in 2003 with the following parameters (highest scoring criteria given):

- *Thrombocytopaenia*: > 50% fall, platelet nadir ≥20 × 10^9/l
- *Timing*: onset day 5–10, or ≤1 day if exposure within last 30 days
- *Thrombosis*: new thrombosis, skin necrosis, acute systemic reaction post bolus
- *oTher cause*: no other evident cause of thrombocytopaenia

A score of 6–8 indicates high, 4–5 indicates intermediate, and 0–3 indicates low probability.

How would you manage a case of suspected HIT?

If the pretest probability of HIT is low, HIT can be excluded without further laboratory investigation.

Intermediate and high pretest probability is as follows:

- **Stop heparin** (including flush solutions and regional heparin for dialysis)
- **Use alternative anticoagulant** at full dosage
  - *Direct thrombin inhibitors*: argatroban, lepirudin, bivalirudin
  - *Factor Xa inhibitors*: danaparoid (suitable in pregnancy)
  - Fondaparinux or DOAC may be suitable in stable patients
  - Anticoagulation for 3 months if thrombotic complication (4 weeks if not)
- *Vitamin K (IV)*: if on vitamin K antagonist at time of suspicion/diagnosis
- **Avoid platelet transfusion** unless significant bleeding
- **Await laboratory tests**
- **Haematologist involvement**

> **GUIDELINE** BCSH 2012 HIT

What specific tests are available for HIT?

- **Platelet activation (functional) assays**
  - Multiplate® platelet aggregometer (90% sensitivity)
  - Standard light transmission platelet aggregometry
  - Heparin-induced platelet activation assay (HIPA)
  - Serotonin release assay (SRA)
- **Antigen assays**
  - *ELISA*: detect IgG/A/M to PF4/heparin
  - Particle gel immunoassay
  - Particle immunofiltration assay

Type of assay is important alongside pretest probability. HIPA and SRA have high sensitivities, and a negative test can rule out HIT. However, most clinicians will only have access to antigen assays making clinical judgement essential.

What implications does HIT have on future management?

Heparin should be avoided until antibody negative. Until then, **bivalirudin** is recommended in the context of urgent surgery and coronary intervention.

Patients with a history of HIT may receive heparin for short periods (e.g. for cardiopulmonary bypass). This should still ideally occur > 100 days after previous exposure to avoid rapid-onset HIT with anti-HIT antibodies excluded.

Vitamin K antagonists (e.g. warfarin) are contraindicated until platelet count has normalised and should be reintroduced slowly.

Resources

- Cuker A, Arepally GM, Chong BH, et al. American Society of Hematology 2018 guidelines for management of venous thromboembolism: heparin-induced thrombocytopenia. Blood Adv. 2018;27:3360–3392.
- Sakr Y. Heparin-induced thrombocytopenia in the ICU: an overview. Crit Care. 2011;15(2):211.

146. PORPHYRIA

What are the porphyrias?

The porphyrias mostly encompass uncommon conditions involving disorders of haem synthesis. They are mostly inherited and involve deficiencies in enzyme activity and are characterised by acute neurovisceral attacks and/or skin photosensitivity:

Acute porphyrias

- *Acute intermittent porphyria*: hydroxymethylbilane synthase (affected enzyme)
- *Hereditary coproporphyria*: coproporphyrinogen oxidase
- *Variegate porphyria*: protoporphyrinogen oxidase
- *5-aminolaevulinic acid (ALA) dehydratase deficiency porphyria*

Non-acute porphyrias (not susceptible to neurovisceral attacks)

- *Erythropoietic protoporphyria*: ferrochelatase
- *Porphyria cutanea tarda*: uroporphyrinogen decarboxylase
- *Congenital erythropoietic porphyria*: uroporphyrinogen synthase
- *X-linked erythropoietic protoporphyria*: ALA synthase 1 and 2 (increased activity)

Critical care interventions may be required to support those suffering from acute attacks. Prevention is the key, where possible, and an awareness of these conditions and precipitants is also invaluable in stable porphyria patients admitted to critical care for other reasons.

What is the pathophysiology involved in acute neurovisceral attacks?

- Haem supply to cells is dependent on a multistage synthetic pathway.
- Enzymes along this pathway may be affected in different porphyria disorders (Table 146.1).
- Enzyme activity change usually leads to accumulation of substrate (porphyrins).
- Porphyrin release into the circulation results in a spectrum of clinical features.
- Acute attacks manifest when hepatic haem requirements are increased.

Table 146.1   Haem synthesis pathway and the porphyrias

	Compound	Enzyme	Porphyria
1	Succinyl CoA + glycine	ALA synthase	X-linked erythropoietic porphyria
2	ALA	ALA dehydrogenase	**5-ALA dehydratase deficiency porphyria**
3	Porphobilinogen	Porphobilinogen deaminase	**Acute intermittent porphyria**
4	Hydroxymethylbilane	Uroporphyrinogen synthase	Congenital erythropoietic porphyria
5	Uroporphyrinogen III	Uroporphyrinogen decarboxylase	Porphyria cutanea tarda
6	Coproporphyrinogen III	Coproporphyrinogen oxidase	**Hereditary coproporphyria**
7	Protoporphyrinogen IX	Protoporphyrinogen oxidase	**Variegate porphyria**
8	Protoporphyrin IX	Ferrochelatase	Protoporphyria
9	Haem		

Note: Acute porphyrias are listed in **bold**.

What might precipitate an acute attack?

- *Medications*: cytochrome P450 induction/inhibition
- *Calorie deficiency*: fasting, absorption disorders
- *Hormonal variation*: menstrual cycle
- Pregnancy
- Alcohol
- *Other physiological stress*: infection, pain, surgery

What are the clinical features of acute neurovisceral attacks?

- **CNS**
  - *Seizures (5–30%)*: compounded by hyponatraemia (30%)
  - *Psychiatric symptoms (20–30%)*: depression, anxiety, hallucinations, paranoia, insomnia
  - *Altered mental state*: agitation, confusion
  - Encephalopathy
- **ANS**
  - Diffuse abdominal pain (90%)
  - Hypertension
  - Tachycardia
  - Cardiac arrest
  - Nausea, vomiting, constipation
  - Urinary retention
- **Peripheral nervous system**
  - *Motor neuropathy in distal muscles (20–68%)*: weakness, paralysis, bulbar dysfunction
  - *Pain*: legs, back
  - *Sensory symptoms*: paraesthesia

How would you diagnose an acute neurovisceral attack?

- High index of suspicion with clinical features
- Random urine sample for urinary porphobilinogen (always elevated acutely)
  - Protect from light
  - Qualitative results should be confirmed by quantitative testing

Following this, the underlying disorder should be confirmed with further light-protected samples:

- *Plasma porphyrins*: fluorescence emission wavelength
- *Faecal porphyrins*: excretion patterns

How would you manage the patient with an acute neurovisceral attack?

- *Specific treatment*: **haem arginate**
- **Supportive care** as required
  - *Respiratory weakness*: ventilatory support as indicated

- *Cardiovascular instability*: atenolol, propranolol, labetalol, nifedipine, vasopressors/inotropes
- *Progressive neuropathy*: likely to need HDU/ICU, specialist involvement
- *Seizures*: lorazepam, diazepam, levetiracetam
- *Psychiatric symptoms*: olanzapine, risperidone
- *Hyponatraemia*: avoid glucose only solutions, may require hypertonic saline
- *Malnutrition*: dietetic support (high carbohydrate, IV glucose if no enteral route)
- *Management of symptoms*: analgesia (e.g. PCA), antiemetics, urethral catheterisation
- *Management of precipitant*: analgesia, fluid replacement, medication adjustment
- **Exclude other causes** of abdominal pain
- *Confirmation of diagnosis*: send random urine for porphobilinogen
- *Advice from porphyria specialist*: 24/7 National Acute Porphyria Service (NAPS) in UK
- **Follow up** with porphyria specialist (likely to involve clinical geneticist)

What do you know about haem arginate?

Human haemin is available as haem arginate for use in acute attacks. It is available through NAPS.

Indications
- **Progressive neuropathy** (prevents further damage but does not reverse it)
- **Hyponatraemia**
- **Seizures**
- **Refractory pain or vomiting**

Dosing
- 3 mg/kg (maximum 250 mg) once daily for 4 days
- Concentrated haem solution is diluted in saline and given over 30–40 min

Adverse effects include local irritation and thrombophlebitis – consider using large cannula or CVC and flushing with 250 ml 0.9% saline after use. CVC obstruction with haem deposits is possible.

Which critical care medications should be avoided in those with porphyria?

- *Anaesthetic agents*: ketamine, thiopental, etomidate, halothane
- *Analgesia*: dexmedetomidine
- *Cardiovascular*: amiodarone, diltiazem, hydralazine, indapamide, methyldopa, metolazone, spironolactone, verapamil
- *CNS*: nitrazepam, valproate, phenytoin, phenobarbital
- *Antimicrobials*: clarithromycin, clindamycin, erythromycin, fluconazole, itraconazole, rifampicin, sulphamethoxazole, trimethoprim
- *Other*: ergometrine, mifepristone

Online drug databases are a valuable source of information if any doubt clinically.

Resources
- Ruthirago D, Julayanont P, Rassameehiran S. Presentations associated with porphyrias in intensive care units. SWRCCC. 2016;4(16):45–50.
- Wilson-Baig N, Badminton M, Schulenburg-Brand D. Acute hepatic porphyria and anaesthesia: a practical approach to the prevention and management of acute neurovisceral attacks. BJA Educ. 2021;21(2):66–74.

147.   THROMBOTIC THROMBOCYTOPAENIC PURPURA

What are the thrombotic microangiopathies?

TMAs are a group of diseases with microvascular or macrovascular occlusion characterised by intraluminal thrombus formation, alongside microangiopathic haemolytic anaemia and thrombocytopaenia (MAHAT).

TMAs include the following:

- TTP
- HUS
- Other conditions presenting with MAHAT (e.g. transplant-associated microangiopathy)

GUIDELINE BCSH 2012 TTP

What is TTP?

KEY POINT

TTP is a rare, life-threatening disorder within the TMA group defined by the following:

- MAHA
- Moderate-to-severe thrombocytopaenia
- Absence of other identifiable cause

TTP was originally described as a pentad of MAHA, thrombocytopaenia, neurological signs, AKI, and fever. However, all features are not always present. Presentation is usually with **neurological sequelae**, **bleeding tendency** (bruising, haematuria), or **multi-organ failure**.

- *Neurological features*: seizures, altered mental state, paresis, aphasia, visual disturbance
- AKI requiring RRT is usually a late feature except in congenital cases. Early severe renal impairment is more typical of HUS.
- Cardiac and GI dysfunction may also manifest.
- Untreated mortality is 90%, with most occurring within 24 h and in women.

What causes TTP?

TTP results from **reduced activity of the ADAMTS-13 enzyme** (<10%). ADAMTS-13 is a protease which acts to cleave vWF into a functional form. Its expansion is 'a disintegrin and metalloprotease with a thrombospondin type 1 motif, member 13'.

Cleaving of vWF is required on release from the endothelium. If this is reduced, large multimers of vWF will cause platelet aggregates, typically in the brain, heart, and kidney microvasculature resulting in organ failure. Haemolysis occurs as red blood cells are sheared at these sites.

This may arise in the following situations:

Primary (most common)
- ADAMTS-13 activity impaired by autoimmune process

Secondary (also immune-mediated)
- *Infection*: HIV
- *Drugs*: quinine, simvastatin, trimethoprim, interferon
- Pregnancy
- *Autoimmune*: SLE, Sjogren's syndrome, rheumatoid arthritis

Congenital
- Mutational defect in ADAMTS-13 gene causing enzyme deficiency

How would you investigate suspected TTP?

TTP should be suspected in any patient with MAHAT in the absence of another identifiable cause. Some investigations should be taken before time-critical treatment is started.

- **Urgent**
  - *ADAMTS-13 enzyme assay and antibody screen*: do not wait for result before treating
  - *FBC, blood film*: high reticulocytes, low platelets, low Hb, fragments

- *Haptoglobin*: reduced
- *U&E*: AKI
- Pregnancy test if appropriate
- *Troponin*: cardiac involvement
- *LDH*: raised in haemolysis
- TFT, amylase, HIV, HAV, HBV, HCV
- *Autoantibodies*: ANA, rheumatoid factor, La, anti-cardiolipin, lupus anticoagulant
- *Blood group and antibody screen*: for transfusion if required
- *Coagulation screen, LFT, direct antiglobulin (Coombs') test*: usually normal

- **After treatment started**
  - *Urinalysis*: proteinuria
  - *Stool culture*: if diarrhoea
  - Echocardiogram
  - *CT head*: if neurological signs
  - *CT thorax/abdomen/pelvis ± tumour markers*: if considering malignancy

How would you manage suspected TTP in critical care?

TTP is likely to require critical care involvement ± airway, cardiovascular, renal, and GI support. Specific priorities include the following:

Definitive therapy

- *Haematologist involvement*: may require transfer to specialist centre
- *Plasma exchange*: within 4–8 h 24/7 (significant mortality reduction)
  - Request solvent/detergent-treated FFP ideally
  - 1.5 plasma volumes × 3, then 1 plasma volume per day
  - Consider stopping when platelets > 150×10^9/l for 2 days
- *FFP infusion*: if delayed plasma exchange
- *Steroids*: after plasma exchange started
  - Methylprednisolone 1 g IV (or prednisolone enterally 1 mg/kg) for 3 days
  - Proton pump inhibitor
  - Folic acid 5 mg OD
- *Caplacizumab (anti-vWF Ig fragment)*: reduces long-term complications in acquired TTP (i.e. not congenital), recommended from 2020 as an option in combination with plasma exchange and immunosuppression

Transfusion

- Packed red cells for anaemia (target 70 g/l in most)
- Avoid platelets unless life-threatening bleeding
- HBV vaccination may be considered once platelets >50×10^9/l

Specific cases

- *Antiretroviral therapy*: immediately if HIV causative (liaise with HIV physician)
- Treatment of underlying cancer may be indicated.
- *Rituximab*: if neurological/cardiac involvement or refractory/relapsing TTP
- Ciclosporin may be considered as second-line therapy in relapsing acquired TTP.
- Splenectomy in the non-acute phase has been carried out to reduce relapse rate.

VTE prophylaxis

- LMWH when platelets >50×10^9/l
- Aspirin 75 mg daily

What is HUS?

HUS is characterised by **MAHAT with AKI**. It lies on the same spectrum as TTP with a more indolent presentation following a trigger event:

- *Typical/epidemic (diarrhoea-positive, 'D +')*: E. coli 0157 or Shigella infection, causing bloody diarrhoea
- *Atypical ('D –')*: infection (S. pneumoniae, HIV), drugs (quinine, bleomycin), malignancy, pregnancy, autoimmune (SLE, antiphospholipid syndrome)

Mortality is much lower than in TTP, particularly in typical HUS, which is managed more supportively.

Atypical HUS (complement-mediated TMA) is more concerning. Blood should be sent for C3, C4, factor H, factor I concentrations, and antibodies against complement components before initiating urgent PLEX. There may be a role for the complement inhibitor, eculizumab, in atypical HUS. Renal ± liver transplantation may be required.

GUIDELINE BCSH & British Transplantation Society Atypical HUS

Resources

- National Institute for Health and Care Excellence. Caplacizumab with Plasma Exchange and Immunosuppression for Treating Acute Acquired Thrombotic Thrombocytopenic Purpura: Technology Appraisal Guidance [TA667]. December 2020. Available from: https://www.nice.org.uk/guidance/ta667. (Accessed 04 March 2022.)
- Scully M, Cataland S, Coppo P, et al. Consensus on the standardization of terminology in thrombotic thrombocytopenic purpura and related thrombotic microangiopathies. J Thromb Haemost. 2016;15(2):312–322.

148. ADRENOCORTICAL DISORDERS

What disorders of adrenocortical function are you aware of?

Hyperaldosteronism (hypertension, low K⁺, alkalosis)

- *Primary*: adrenal adenoma (Conn's syndrome), bilateral adrenal hyperplasia
- *Secondary*: any condition with low effective arterial blood volume → increased renin secretion (e.g. low cardiac output state, cirrhosis, nephrotic syndrome)

Cushing's syndrome (hypertension, diabetes mellitus, low K⁺, bruising, muscle wasting, altered habitus)

- *ACTH dependent*: pituitary adenoma (Cushing's disease), ectopic ACTH
- *ACTH independent*: adrenal tumour, exogenous steroids

Adrenocortical insufficiency

- *Primary = Addison's disease (adrenal pathology)*: autoimmune, TB, metastasis, adrenalectomy, haemorrhage, drugs (e.g. etomidate), critical illness-related corticosteroid insufficiency (CIRCI)
- *Secondary (ACTH deficiency)*: hypopituitarism, prolonged corticosteroid therapy
- *Tertiary (hypothalamic)*: infarct, malignancy

What are the features of acute adrenocortical insufficiency (Addisonian crisis)?

- *C*: vasoplegia, distributive shock, high cardiac output, postural hypotension
- *D*: altered consciousness, dizziness, lethargy, fatigue, weakness
- *E*: abdominal pain, vomiting
- *F*: dehydration
- *Chronic features*: skin crease/buccal pigmentation (if primary disease), anorexia
- *Associated autoimmune disease*: hyper-/hypothyroidism, pernicious anaemia, type 1 diabetes mellitus, vitiligo
- *Initial blood results*: hypoglycaemia, hyponatraemia, hyperkalaemia, uraemia, eosinophilia

Which investigations are indicated?

- *Initial*: glucose, U&E, random cortisol, ACTH, FBC, CRP, pregnancy test
- *Delayed*: short synacthen test, adrenal antibodies, imaging (brain, adrenal)
- *Imaging is only indicated in selected cases*: primary disease with negative antibodies; or secondary disease without history of exogenous steroids

What are the management priorities in this condition?

- **Glucocorticoid**
  - *Known adrenal insufficiency*: IV hydrocortisone 200 mg loading, 100 mg 6° maintenance
  - *Undiagnosed*: IV dexamethasone 4–6 mg – will not influence subsequent short synacthen test but not used routinely in the UK in place of hydrocortisone
- **Mineralocorticoid**
  - Sodium replaced by IV fluid so rarely required
  - May be indicated in primary insufficiency if steroid chosen has weak mineralocorticoid activity – usually added later (e.g. fludrocortisone 50–100 µg daily)
- **Fluid resuscitation**
- **Correction of hypoglycaemia**: may require glucose in addition to steroid
- **Management of underlying cause**

What is 'CIRCI'?

KEY POINT

CIRCI is a state of hypothalamic impairment during critical illness, characterised by dysregulated systemic inflammation. It manifests as a relative corticosteroid deficiency.

Suggestive features

- *A/B*: persistent hypoxia
- *C*: refractory hypotension, reduced sensitivity to catecholamines, high cardiac index
- *D*: delirium, coma, asthenia
- *E*: nausea, vomiting, feed intolerance, fever

Investigations may reveal hypoglycaemia, hyponatraemia, hyperkalaemia, metabolic acidosis, and hypereosinophilia. There is no single test that can diagnose CIRCI reliably. Total plasma cortisol and stimulation tests may be of use.

GUIDELINE SCCM 2017 CIRCI

What are the equivalent doses of commonly used steroids?

- Hydrocortisone 100 mg
- Prednisolone 25 mg
- Methylprednisolone 20 mg
- Dexamethasone 3.75 mg

When are steroids indicated in the management of critically ill patients?

Many conditions throughout medicine have been managed with steroids (Table 148.1).

STUDY

CORTICUS (2008)

- Septic shock
- *Intervention*: hydrocortisone 50 mg 6° 6 days then tapered to day 12 vs placebo
- *Primary*: 28-day mortality in short corticotropin non-responders – **no difference**
- Secondary: 28-day mortality – no difference, time to reversal of shock – **significantly lower (3.3 vs 5.8 days)**

Table 148.1   Use of steroids in specific conditions requiring critical care

	Benefit	Dose	No benefit
A	*Anaphylaxis*: second-line therapy	200 mg hydrocortisone	
	Airway oedema: prevention of post-extubation stridor	40 mg methylprednisolone (4 h prior)	
B	*COPD*: acute exacerbation	30 mg prednisolone	CAP
	Asthma: acute exacerbation	40–50 mg prednisolone	
	PJP: HIV patients	40 mg prednisolone/60 mg methylprednisolone	
	COVID-19 pneumonitis: oxygen requirement	6 mg dexamethasone	
	Possible role in ARDS		
C	Septic shock (controversial)	200 mg hydrocortisone per 24 h	Cardiac surgery
D	*Bacterial meningitis*: especially *S. pneumoniae*	10 mg dexamethasone (6°)	• TBI (harm) • Spinal cord injury (harm) • GBS
	Intracerebral tumour/abscess: oedema, high ICP	16 mg dexamethasone (PO)	
E	Chronic steroid use (stress dose supplementation)	Specific to risk	
	Adrenal crisis	100 mg hydrocortisone (200/24 h)	
	Myxoedema coma	100 mg hydrocortisone	
Misc.	*Immune modulation*: autoimmune/inflammatory disease, transplant rejection		
	Organ donation: brain stem death inflammatory response	15 mg/kg methylprednisolone	

STUDY

Marik et al. (2017)

- Severe sepsis or septic shock
- *Intervention*: addition of vitamin C + hydrocortisone + thiamine vs standard care (single-centre retrospective study, not RCT)
- *Primary*: hospital mortality – **significantly lower (8.5% vs 40.4%)**
- *Secondary*: duration of vasopressors, requirement for RRT – **significantly lower**; ICU LOS – no difference
- Allegations of research fraud were submitted in 2022

STUDY

ADRENAL (2018)

- Septic shock
- *Intervention*: hydrocortisone 200 mg/24 h IV infusion 7 days or until ICU discharge vs placebo
- *Primary*: 90-day mortality – **no difference**
- *Secondary*: 28-day mortality, shock recurrence, time to hospital discharge, organ support, infection) – no difference; days to resolution of shock, time to cessation of MV, time to discharge from ICU, blood transfusion – **significantly lower**

APROCCHSS (2018)

- Septic shock
- *Intervention*: hydrocortisone 50 mg 6 hourly + fludrocortisone 50 µg daily 7 days vs placebo
- *Primary*: 90-day mortality – **significantly lower (43% vs 49.1%)**, NNT 17
- *Secondary*: mortality at ICU/hospital discharge – **significantly lower**; days free from vasopressors, organ-failure free days – **significantly higher**; 28-day mortality – no difference

(See individual chapters associated with other conditions in Table 148.1 for relevant trials: **Meduri et al., DEXA-ARDS, RECOVERY, REMAP-CAP, CRASH, NASCIS 2.**)

When is the use of steroids not supported by the evidence?

Trials have demonstrated no benefit, or even harm, from corticosteroid use in the following:

- CAP
- Cardiac surgery
- TBI
- Spinal cord injury
- GBS

Resources

- Davies M, Hardman J. Anaesthesia and adrenocortical disease. CEACCP. 2005;5(4):122–126.
- Owen K, Turner H, Wass J. (Eds.) Oxford Handbook of Endocrinology & Diabetes, 4th ed. New York: Oxford University Press; 2022.
- Sheldrick K. Evidence of Fabricated Data in a Vitamin C Trial by Paul E Marik et al in CHEST. March 2022. Available from: http://kylesheldrick.blogspot.com/2022/03/evidence-of-fabricated-data-in-vitamin.html. (Accessed 14 April 2022.)
- Young A, Marsh S. Steroid use in critical care. BJA Educ. 2018;18(5):129–134.

149. DIABETES EMERGENCIES

What is diabetic ketoacidosis?

Diabetic ketoacidosis (DKA) is a disordered metabolic state characterised by hyperglycaemia, ketonaemia, and acidosis.

It is a complication of diabetes mellitus with a reported incidence ranging from 8 to 51: 1000 patient years in patients with type 1 diabetes and maximal in 18–24 year olds. Mortality is <1% in the UK with cerebral oedema the leading cause of death. Others include severe hyperkalaemia, ARDS, and precipitants (e.g. pneumonia, MI, sepsis).

KEY POINT

DKA diagnostic criteria (all 3 of the following):

- *Diabetes*: capillary blood glucose > **11** mmol/l (or known to have diabetes mellitus)
- *Ketones*: capillary sample > **3** mmol/l (or urine ketones ≥++)
- *Acidaemia*: **pH < 7.3** (and/or **HCO_3^-** < **15** mmol/l)

What causes DKA?

DKA is precipitated by an event on top of underlying diabetes mellitus resulting in absolute or relative insulin deficiency. Most cases arise in those with type 1 but up to a third occur in type 2 (termed 'ketosis-prone type 2 diabetes'). DKA may be the first presentation of type 1 diabetes mellitus, with or without a precipitant.

Precipitants
- **Stress response**
  - Infection
  - Non-compliance with or adjustment to usual therapy
  - MI
  - CVA
  - Trauma/surgery
- **Altered carbohydrate metabolism**
  - *Drugs*: corticosteroids, thiazines, sympathomimetics (e.g. terbutaline)
  - Alcohol excess
  - Pancreatitis
  - Eating disorders

Pathophysiology
- Insulin deficiency.
- Accompanying rise in glucagon, cortisol, growth hormone, catecholamine secretion.
- Increased hepatic gluconeogenesis and glycogenolysis.
- Hyperglycaemia.
- *Enhanced lipolysis increases serum free fatty acids*: metabolised to ketone bodies.
- *Ketone bodies cause significant acidosis*: 3-beta-hydroxybutyrate (BHB, predominant blood ketone), acetone, acetoacetate.
- *Fluid depletion*: osmotic diuresis in hyperglycaemia, vomiting, reduced intake when obtunded.

In which settings does DKA present to critical care?
- Organ dysfunction requiring support
- Severe abnormality in biochemistry
- Peripartum complication
- Perioperative complication
- Secondary issue in patient with another critical illness (e.g. cardiogenic shock, sepsis)

Multiple pathologies often coexist, and management of haemodynamics may be complicated by the potentially multifactorial aetiology of shock.

In which differentials is the presence of ketones prominent?
Alcoholic ketoacidosis usually involves euglycaemia, and history taking is the key. BHB should be measured instead of urine ketones (acetoacetate production can be suppressed).

Starvation acidosis is usually slower in onset and better compensated than DKA, despite ketone levels sometimes > 6 mmol/l. Insulin secretion is reduced, increasing lipolysis and ketosis.

When would you admit a patient with DKA to critical care?
A minimum of level 2 (HDU) care is recommended if:

- Age 18–25/elderly/pregnant
- Cardiac/renal failure
- Serious comorbidity
- Severe DKA

Severe DKA is indicated by the following:

- *B*: S_pO_2 < 92% on air
- *C*: systolic BP < 90 mmHg, HR > 100 or < 60 min⁻¹
- *D*: GCS < 12
- *F*:
  - Blood ketones > 6 mmol/l
  - pH < 7.1
  - HCO_3^- < 5 mmol/l
  - K⁺ < 3.5 mmol/l on admission to hospital
  - Anion gap > 16 mmol/l

What are the specific priorities in management of severe DKA?

Current guidance is subdivided into management priorities at different time points:

- *0–1 h*: immediate assessment and **resuscitation**
- 1–6 h: clearance of **ketones** and suppression of ketogenesis
- 6–12 h: continued biochemical improvement and avoidance of **complications**
- 12–24 h: **normalisation** of parameters and resolution of DKA

Restoration of circulating volume

- Crystalloid bolus × 500 ml until systolic BP > 90 mmHg
- *Maintenance*: next litre over 1 h (1000 ml/h)
- Further 3 × litre bags over next 8 h at 2, 2, 4 hourly (500, 500, 250 ml/h)
- *Caution in specific groups*: younger, elderly, cardiac/renal failure
- NaCl 0.9% recommended over balanced crystalloid
  - Allows premixed potassium chloride solutions to be used (National Patient Safety Agency [NPSA] recommendation)
  - No RCT evidence of faster DKA resolution on ward with Hartmann's

Potassium replacement

- Add KCl 40 mmol/h to maintenance fluid unless K⁺ > 5.5 mmol/l

Reduce ketonaemia

- Fixed rate insulin infusion (FRII) 0.1 unit/kg/h (no priming bolus dose)
- Use 50 ml 0.9% NaCl with 50 units human soluble insulin
- Continue usual long acting insulin analogue if usually taken
- If blood glucose < 14 mmol/l
  - Add 10% glucose 125 ml/h
  - Consider FRII reduction to 0.05 unit/kg/h
- Refractory DKA should prompt an increase in FRII by 1 unit/h until targets achieved

Targets in DKA:

- Ketones 0.5 mmol/l/h fall or
- HCO_3^- 3 mmol/l/h rise
- Glucose 3 mmol/h fall
- K⁺ in normal range

Avoidance of complications

- *Admission to HDU/ICU if indicated*: consideration of central venous access
- Thromboprophylaxis
- Maintain UO > 0.5 ml/kg/h (catheterise if no urine at 60 min or obtunded)
- Monitoring
  - Hourly glucose, ketones, potassium, pH, HCO_3^- initially

- 4° U&E
- Step down frequency as stability allows

Other
- Manage underlying precipitant (e.g. antimicrobials, management of ACS/CVA)
- Management of symptoms
  - *Vomiting*: antiemetics, NG decompression
- Supportive care
  - Sodium bicarbonate may be indicated in myocardial dysfunction with low pH
- *Specialist input*: diabetes team referral

(See Chapter 105 Diabetic Ketoacidosis in Children)

How would you manage the patient recovering from DKA?
DKA resolution can be defined as **ketones < 0.6 mmol/l** and **venous pH > 7.3.**

Hyperchloraemic acidosis secondary to 0.9% NaCl may delay normalisation of pH and bicarbonate despite resolution of ketonaemia.

When DKA has resolved (i.e. the patient is biochemically stable as defined above), subcutaneous insulin can be reinstituted. In addition, venous HCO_3^- should be > 18 mmol/l. The patient must have a reliable nutritional intake (e.g. return to baseline of usually eating and drinking). If not, a variable rate insulin infusion should be used.

- Involve specialist diabetes team and use local guidelines.
- Restart subcutaneous insulin.
- Discontinue IV insulin infusion at least 30 min after subcutaneous short-acting insulin has been given.
- Arrange follow-up with specialist team (review prior to discharge if newly diagnosed).

What is HHS?
HHS is a complication of type 2 diabetes mellitus characterised by **hyperglycaemia**, **hypovolaemia**, and **increased serum osmolality** (often without significant acid-base disturbance).

It has a more insidious onset and carries a higher mortality with complications including MI, stroke, peripheral arterial occlusion, seizures, cerebral oedema, and central pontine myelinolysis. Terminology was updated from hyperosmotic non-ketotic (HONK) coma due to better reflection of the biochemical and clinical picture. A mixed picture of HHS and DKA is possible. The prevalence is increasing in children with the rise of type 2 diabetes in this population.

KEY POINT

HHS:

- Hyperglycaemia (≥**30** mmol/l)
  - Absence of hyperketonaemia (≤3 mmol/l)
  - Absence of acidosis (pH ≥ 7.3, HCO_3^- ≥ 15 mmol/l)
- Hypovolaemia
- Serum osmolality ≥ **320** mOsm/kg ($2Na^+$ + glucose + urea)

GUIDELINE   JBDS-IP 2022 HHS

How would you manage the critically unwell HHS patient?
The immediate priority is to restore circulating volume. Subsequent management aims to achieve gradual normalisation in osmolality. The underlying cause should be treated whilst preventing complications (e.g. thomboembolism, electrolyte derangement, osmotic demyelination syndrome, cerebral oedema, fluid overload).

Normalise osmolality
- **Replace fluid and electrolyte losses**
  - 0.9% sodium chloride (initial rise in sodium expected)

➢ 0.45% sodium chloride if osmolality not falling and positive fluid balance
➢ Oral water as soon as tolerated
- **Normalise blood glucose**
  ➢ *Fluids*: 0.9% NaCl 1 litre over 1 h, more rapidly if hypotensive
  ➢ *FRII*: indicated at low dose (0.05 units/kg/h) in **ketonaemia** (BHB > 1 mmol/l or urine > 2+), DKA dosing (0.1 units/kg/h) in mixed DKA and HHS, or refractory disease once euvolaemic

Indications for admission to critical care
- B: S_pO_2 < 92% on air
- C: systolic BP < 90 mmHg, HR > 100 or < 60 min^{-1}, macrovascular event
- D: GCS < 12
- F
  ➢ Osm > 350 mOsm/kg
  ➢ Na^+ > 160
  ➢ pH < 7.1
  ➢ K^+ < 3.5 or > 6 mmol/l on admission
  ➢ UO < 0.5 ml/kg/h
  ➢ Creatinine > 200 μmol/l
  ➢ Hypothermia
- Serious comorbidity

Targets
- Gradual decline in osmolality 3–8 mOsm/kg/h
- Positive fluid balance 2–3 l in 6 h
- Sodium fall ≤10 mmol/l per 24 h
- Glucose fall ≥5 mmol/l/h

Resolution (usually > 24 h, longer than DKA)
- Measured/calculated serum osmolality < 300 mOsm/kg
- Hypovolaemia corrected (UO ≥0.5 ml/kg/h)
- Cognitive status back to premorbid state
- Blood glucose < 15 mmol/l

What do you know about euglycaemic ketoacidosis?

Euglycaemic DKA is that occurring in patients known to have diabetes but with a normal or not significantly elevated raise in serum glucose. It is managed as per hyperglycaemic DKA with the inclusion of measures taken when glucose <14 mmol/l. pH and ketones are the more significant biochemical measurements in diagnosis and management.

There is a risk of developing euglycaemic DKA in patients taking SGLT2 inhibitors (e.g. dapagliflozin, canagliflozin), particularly if they have a concomitant stress response such as infection or surgery. Morning dosage should be adjusted when fasting on the day of, surgery and presentation may be up to several weeks later during the recovery period.

What is meant by a target of 'normoglycaemia' in critical care?

Hyperglycaemia has been associated with worse outcomes in several conditions. However, tight control might increase the risk of hypoglycaemic episodes, particularly with lower targets. 'Normoglycaemia' involves a balance of these 2 factors. In the majority of patients, a serum glucose target of 6–10 mmol/l is appropriate.

STUDY

NICE-SUGAR (2009)

- Critically unwell adults
- *Intervention*: intensive (target 4.5–6 mmol/l) vs conventional (<10 mmol/l) glucose control
- *Primary*: 90-day mortality – **significantly higher**
- *Secondary*: 28-day mortality, LOS, organ support – no difference; severe hypoglycaemia – **significantly higher (6.8% vs 0.5%)**

How would you manage a severely hypoglycaemic patient on the critical care unit?

Hypoglycaemia is a lower-than-normal blood glucose. It is classified as 'mild' if self-treated or 'severe' if third-party assistance is required.

Features can be described as autonomic (e.g. sweating, palpitations), neuroglycopaenic (e.g. confusion, incoordination), or general malaise (e.g. headache, nausea). Hypoglycaemia can progress to coma, hemiparesis, and seizures, with potential for long-term neurological deficits.

Prevention is ideal. Inpatients with blood glucose <4.0 mmol/l should be treated. Enteral carbohydrate is preferred where possible.

Initial therapy
- *Enteral route, cooperative*: 15–20 g quick-acting carbohydrate (e.g. glucose tablet, 200 ml fruit juice)
- *Enteral route, uncooperative*: 1.5–2 tubes 40% glucose gel between teeth and gums (or IM glucagon)
- *No enteral route, agitated, or seizures*: 75–100 ml 20% glucose or 150–200 ml 10% glucose over 15 min (or IM glucagon)
- Further glucose check 15 min later, repeat as required if <4 mmol/l

Glucagon 1 mg IM can be used when IV access is not available but can take up to 15 min to work. It may also cause significant vomiting or be ineffective (e.g. in liver disease, alcohol intoxication, or malnourished states). It is licenced in insulin overdose but may also be used in sulphonylurea-induced hypoglycaemia.

IV 50% glucose solution is significantly hyperosmolar and carries an increased risk of extravasation injury as well as higher post-treatment glucose levels. It can be difficult to administer due to its high viscosity.

Further management
- *Poor enteral absorption*: maintenance glucose infusion (e.g. 10% at 100 ml/h)
- *Refractory cases*: hydrocortisone, octreotide
- *Manage underlying cause*: investigations as indicated (e.g. insulin, C-peptide, ketones, cortisol, LFT)

Causes
- Liver failure
- Adrenal insufficiency
- Self-administration of insulin
- Sepsis
- *Drugs*: sulphonylureas, fluoroquinolones, phenytoin, haloperidol, propranolol, ACEI, NSAIDs
- *Other*: hypothyroidism, post-gastric bypass (delayed dumping syndrome), insulinoma, starvation/exercise, pregnancy, alcohol, renal failure
- *Monitoring error*: occult presentation with spuriously 'normal' ABG (unintentional use of glucose-containing flush solution)

GUIDELINE JBDS-IP 2018 Hypoglycaemia

Resources
- Association of Anaesthetists of Great Britain and Ireland. Peri-operative management of the surgical patient with diabetes 2015. Anaesthesia. 2015;70(12):1427–1440.
- Farkas J. The Internet Book of Critical Care: Hypoglycaemia. September 2021. Available from: https://emcrit.org/ibcc/hypoglycemia. (Accessed 10 February 2022.)

150. PHAEOCHROMOCYTOMA

What is a phaeochromocytoma?
A phaeochromocytoma is a rare catecholamine-secreting tumour of the adrenal medullary chromaffin cells.

It was thought that 10% are extra-adrenal, 10% malignant, 10% bilateral, 10% normotensive, and 10% familial. More recent data suggest approximately 30% are malignant and around 30–40% are familial. Hormones secreted include noradrenaline, adrenaline, and dopamine. Secretion can be constant or episodic.

Paragangliomas are related tumours of extra-adrenal paraganglia that may also secrete catecholamines.

Outline the synthesis and metabolism of catecholamines.
The **synthetic pathway** is as follows:

- Phenylalanine
- Tyrosine
- DOPA
- Dopamine
- Noradrenaline
- Adrenaline

Metabolism
- Dopamine is metabolised by MAO to products including homovanillic acid.
- NA and adrenaline are metabolised by MAO and **catechol-O-methyltransferase** (COMT).
  - NA metabolites include normetanephrine.
  - Adrenaline metabolites include metanephrine.
  - Both are precursors of the metabolite vanillylmandelic acid.

How do phaeochromocytomas present to critical care?

General features
- Classical presentation is a triad of headache, palpitations, and sweating
- 90% hypertensive
- *Other*: anxiety, lethargy, nausea, weight loss, hyperglycaemia, tremor, abdominal pain
- Frequently an incidental finding on imaging

Acute crisis
- MODS
- *B*: pulmonary oedema (multifactorial)
- *C*: Takotsubo cardiomyopathy, catecholamine-induced myocarditis, hypertensive crisis (precipitants: exertion, some foods, emotion, drugs), arrhythmias, MI, refractory hypertension in critical care
- *D*: stroke, ICH, seizures
- *E*: GI ischaemia/ileus
- *F*: AKI
- *H*: DIC
- *Other*: hyperthermia, gangrene

Diagnosis is by measuring **plasma/urine metanephrines**. Other investigations include 24-h urinary catecholamines, vanillylmandelic acid, and homovanillic acid. Diagnosis in the critically unwell patient may be confounded by false-positive tests due to the influence of renal impairment and medications including SNRIs, alpha/beta-blockers, MAOI, stimulant drugs of abuse, and sympathomimetics.

Imaging is indicated to localise the disorder, initially with **adrenal CT**. Functional imaging with MIBG is used pre-operatively to detect multiple tumours or metastases.

How is a phaeochromocytoma crisis managed?
Emergency management follows similar principles to those in stable patients:

- Supportive care as indicated
- Cardiovascular
  - *BP control*: initially **alpha blockade** (phentolamine, phenoxybenzamine), followed by **beta blockade**
  - *Reversal of circulating volume depletion*: fluids, sodium
  - *Arrhythmia/rate control*: selective beta blockade after alpha (e.g. atenolol)
  - *Myocardial optimisation*: echo, ECG
- Management of glucose and electrolyte disturbance
- Investigation of differential diagnoses

Surgery is planned once stable – BP controlled, infrequent ectopics, no ST changes, effective alpha blockade (e.g. postural hypotension).

(See Chapter 73 Hypertension)

What are the intraoperative priorities during resection of a phaeochromocytoma?

- Appropriate timing of surgery with cardiovascular stability
- *Avoidance of catecholamine release*: procedural, drug related
- Haemodynamic stability during tumour handling
- Manage hypotension after tumour devascularised

Patients often require several infusions to manipulate haemodynamics and attenuate the stress response. Options include magnesium sulphate, remifentanil, dexmedetomidine, phentolamine, sodium nitroprusside, GTN, nicardipine, esmolol. Noradrenaline and vasopressin may be required for hypotension after fluid balance has been optimised.

How might a patient be managed post-operatively?

- Arterial BP monitoring > 24 h
  - *Persistent hypertension*: incomplete resection, metastasis, unintentional ligation of renal artery
  - *Hypotension*: drugs, tumour devascularisation (abrupt catecholamine deficiency and chronic receptor downregulation), residual alpha blockade, myocardial dysfunction, bleeding
- *Analgesia*: pain may contribute to hypertension and confound clinical picture
- Corticosteroid replacement if bilateral adrenalectomy
- Blood glucose monitoring for rebound hyperinsulinism

What is carcinoid crisis?

Carcinoid syndrome classically arises due to liver or 'post-hepatic' (distal to portal venous system) metastasis of neuroendocrine tumours, facilitating the release of hormones into the systemic circulation. These include serotonin, catecholamines, and brady/tachykinins. Clinical effects of high circulating hormone levels include wheeze, breathlessness, flushing, palpitations, diarrhoea, and abdominal pain.

Carcinoid crisis is an exacerbation of carcinoid syndrome which may be precipitated by physiological stress including surgery, anaesthesia, and chemotherapy. It may present with severe bronchospasm, labile BP, arrhythmias, altered mental state, and diarrhoea. Octreotide can be used prophylactically and therapeutically.

Resources

- Clement D, Ramage D, Srirajaskanthan R. Review article update on pathophysiology, treatment, and complications of carcinoid syndrome. J Oncol. 2020;8341426.
- Connor D, Boumphrey S. Perioperative care of phaeochromocytoma. BJA Educ. 2016;16(5):153–158.
- Nickson C. Life in the Fast Lane: Pheochromocytoma. November 2020. Available from: https://litfl.com/pheochromocytoma/. (Accessed 10 February 2022.)
- Owen K, Turner H, Wass J. (Eds.) Oxford Handbook of Endocrinology & Diabetes, 4th ed. New York: Oxford University Press; 2022.

151. PITUITARY DISEASE

How might pituitary disease present?

- Incidental finding
- Lesion mass effect (macroadenoma > 10 mm)
  - Headache

- *Visual field defect*: compression of optic nerves
- *Large tumours*: hypopituitarism, cranial nerve palsies, hydrocephalus
- Hypersecretion
  - *ACTH*: Cushing's disease
  - *GH*: acromegaly
  - *Prolactin*: irregular menstruation, galactorrhoea, breast growth, sexual dysfunction
  - *ADH*: SIADH
  - *TSH*: hyperthyroidism (rare, due to TSHoma/thyrotropinoma)
  - *FSH*: ovarian hyperstimulation syndrome (rare)
- Hyposecretion
  - Panhypopituitarism
  - *ACTH*: adrenocortical insufficiency
  - *GH*: short stature, developmental delay
  - *Prolactin*: ovarian dysfunction, sexual dysfunction
  - *ADH*: diabetes insipidus
  - *TSH*: hypothyroidism
  - *FSH, LH*: hypogonadotrophic hypogonadism

Hormone secretion

- *Anterior pituitary*: ACTH, GH, prolactin, FSH, LH, TSH, endorphins, encephalins, MSH
- *Posterior pituitary*: ADH, oxytocin
- (*Hypothalamus*: TRH, CRH, GHRH, GnRH, somatostatin, dopamine)

What are the priorities in management of the post-op patient who has undergone transsphenoidal pituitary surgery?

- Admission to high dependency area
- *Surgical review*: neurosurgery/ENT
- Supportive care
  - **Optimise perfusion**
  - **Avoid nasal CPAP** (sleep apnoea prevalent)
  - **Prevent post-operative nausea and vomiting**
  - **Analgesia**
  - **Nasal hygiene** (e.g. sinus spray, removal of packs after 24 h)
- Hormone replacement
  - **Glucocorticoids**
    - ➢ 100 mg pre-op, 8 hourly post-op, reduce around day 3
    - ➢ May not be required in Cushing's patients
  - Others as per post-op hormonal function
    - ➢ *Acromegaly*: growth hormone test and oral glucose tolerance test 1–2 weeks post-op
    - ➢ *Cushing's*: monitor morning cortisol, start hydrocortisone if low
    - ➢ Specialist endocrinology review of new basal pituitary function
- Detection and management of complications
  - *DI (usually within 24 h, resolution after 1 week)*: monitor UO, U&E
  - *Hyponatraemia*: SIADH/CSWS (see Chapter 134 Sodium Disorders)
  - *Local damage/bleeding*: monitor neurology including eye movements, visual fields, acuity
  - *CSF rhinorrhoea*: dip for glucose, send fluid for Tau protein
  - Meningitis

What is pituitary apoplexy?

Pituitary apoplexy is a rare syndrome of hypoperfusion of the pituitary gland leading to infarction. It is life- and sight-threatening and requires a high index of suspicion. Characteristic features relate to hormone deficiencies and mass effect.

It is usually caused by bleeding into a pre-existing tumour combined with a precipitant:

- Hypertension
- Surgery

- Anticoagulants
- Radiotherapy
- Trauma
- Episode of severe hypoperfusion
- Sickle crisis

Sheehan's syndrome is hypopituitarism secondary to pituitary hypoperfusion in the puerperium (usually due to haemorrhage).

Patients may present with sudden onset headache, vomiting, visual disturbances, cranial nerve signs, altered consciousness, and occasionally meningism. Life-threatening features may include **cardiovascular collapse** (adrenal insufficiency) and **seizures** (hyponatraemia).

Specific acute management will involve the following:

- *Investigations*: U&E, LFT, FBC, coagulation screen, hormone levels, visual field assessment
- *Glucocorticoid replacement first*: bolus, then continuous infusion
- Surgery may be indicated for decompression
- Specialist input
- Other hormone replacement as indicated

Resources

- Alexandraki KI, Grossman AB. Management of hypopituitarism. J Clin Med. 2019;8(12):2153.
- Kerr DE, Wenham T, Newell-Price J. Endocrine problems in the critically ill 2: endocrine emergencies. BJA Educ. 2017;17(11):377–382.
- Menon R, Murphy PG, Lindley AM. Anaesthesia and pituitary disease. CEACCP. 2011;11(4):133–137.
- Owen K, Turner H, Wass J. (Eds.) Oxford Handbook of Endocrinology & Diabetes, 4th ed. New York: Oxford University Press; 2022.

---

152. THYROID CRISES

What is thyroid storm and what causes it?

Thyroid storm is a rare thyrotoxic crisis characterised by an extreme hypermetabolic state. Mortality is up to 75%.

It typically presents with chronic progression of thyrotoxicosis with crises precipitated by stressors such as pregnancy, trauma, surgery, MI, GI bleeding, and DKA.

Causes of thyrotoxicosis include Grave's disease, toxic multinodular goitre, adenoma, and levothyroxine intoxication.

What are the clinical features?

Thyroid storm is a continuation of the clinical spectrum of thyrotoxicosis with end-organ dysfunction. Diagnosis is clinical. The **Burch-Wartofsky Point Scale** may help in systemic decompensation. A score of 25–44 is suggestive and ≥45 highly suggestive of thyroid storm.

It includes the following criteria with variable weighting depending on severity of features:

- Thermoregulatory dysfunction (pyrexia)
- *Cardiovascular*: heart rate (tachycardia), AF, CCF
- *GI-hepatic dysfunction*: diarrhoea, abdominal pain, nausea/vomiting, jaundice
- *CNS disturbance*: agitation, delirium psychosis, extreme lethargy, seizures, coma
- Precipitant history

Serum thyroid hormone levels do not correlate with severity of disease in this condition. Features of underlying disease might be present (e.g. goitre, exophthalmos, other autoimmune signs). Complications may also include rhabdomyolysis and progression to multi-organ dysfunction.

GUIDELINE American Thyroid Association 2011 Hyperthyroidism

What are the specific management priorities in thyroid storm?

- **Management of underlying disease trigger**
- **Inhibition of thyroid hormone synthesis**, release, and conversion to T3
  - Propylthiouracil first line (e.g. enteral 500–1000 mg loading then 250 mg 4 hourly)
    - ➤ Carbimazole second line (or IV methimazole – not available in the UK)
  - Iodine ≥1 h after antithyroid drugs (e.g. potassium iodide, Lugol's iodine)
- **Corticosteroid prophylaxis against relative adrenal insufficiency** (e.g. IV hydrocortisone 300 mg loading then 100 mg 8 hourly, or dexamethasone)
- **Inhibition of peripheral effects**
  - Beta blockade (e.g. propranolol 60–80 mg 4 hourly first line, esmolol infusion, diltiazem)
  - *Management of arrhythmias*: amiodarone
  - Cardiac output monitoring
  - Fluid resuscitation
  - *Thermoregulation*: may require active cooling, avoid salicylates
  - *Refractory disease*: PD, plasma exchange, thyroidectomy (around day 10)

What is thyrotoxic periodic paralysis?

Thyrotoxic (or hypokalaemic) periodic paralysis is a rare complication of thyrotoxicosis which is characterised by elevated T3/T4 and hypokalaemia. A profound attack of muscle weakness/paralysis may develop and last several days, occasionally requiring critical care support. Management of thyrotoxicosis and hypokalaemia are the key. There is a risk of overshoot hyperkalaemia.

What is myxoedema coma and what are the possible causes?

Myxoedema coma is a life-threatening complication of hypothyroidism. Mortality is 20–60%.

Most cases occur in patients with primary hypothyroidism. Precipitants include MI, HF, stroke, drugs (e.g. amiodarone), and cessation of levothyroxine therapy. Advanced age and frailty are important risk factors.

What are the clinical features?

Myxoedema coma is more common in females over 60 years old. TSH will be elevated and T4 reduced. Features are as follows:

- *B*: respiratory failure (altered response to hypoxia/hypercarbia), pleural effusions
- *C*: bradycardia, LV hypertrophy, BBB, torsade de pointes, cardiac failure
- *D*: reduced consciousness, sluggish reflexes
- *E*: hypothermia, high LDH, hypoglycaemia
- *F*: rhabdomyolysis, hyponatraemia
- *H*: anaemia, acquired von Willebrand's disease
- *Other*: dry skin, hair loss, macroglossia, obesity

What are the specific management priorities?

- Management of underlying precipitating disease
- **Corticosteroid replacement** prior to thyroid hormones (most have adrenal impairment)
- **Thyroid hormone replacement**
  - *Enteral T4*: levothyroxine sodium
  - *IV T3*: liothyronine sodium (second line)
- *Supportive care as indicated*: ventilation, electrolyte/fluid management, warming

What is non-thyroidal illness syndrome (NTIS)?

NTIS is a syndrome of hypothalamic-pituitary-thyroid axis disruption found in critically ill patients. The degree of dysfunction is proportional to underlying disease severity.

Features

- Low T3 (triiodothyronine)
- Low/normal TSH
- Low T4 in severe illness (predictive of mortality, particularly with raised cortisol)

Pathophysiology is poorly understood, and there is no evidence for thyroid hormone replacement in critical care. Existing therapy should be continued.

Resources

- Fliers E, Bianco AC, Langouche L, et al. Thyroid function in critically ill patients. Lancet Diabetes Endocrinol. 2015;3(10):816–825.
- Kerr DE, Wenham T, Newell-Price J. Endocrine problems in the critically ill 2: endocrine emergencies. BJA Educ. 2017;17(11):377–382.

153. DERMATOLOGY

Why is skin important in critical care?

Skin provides several important functions. It acts as a physical barrier and has roles in moisture and temperature regulation, sensation, and immunity.

The environment of critical care, combined with acute illness, may threaten skin integrity and result in significant morbidity including sepsis and multi-organ dysfunction. A number of primary and secondary skin conditions may also require critical care support.

What common skin conditions might arise during a critical care stay?

- Intertrigo
- Miliaria (heat rash)
- Pressure ulcers
- Peripheral gangrene (shock, vasoconstrictor use)
- Extravasation injury

What is acute skin failure and what might cause it?

Acute skin failure may be defined as total dysfunction of the skin. The skin and underlying tissue may die as a result of hypoperfusion.

Primary skin conditions which may present to critical care are as follows:

- *Infection*: necrotising fasciitis, cellulitis, erysipelas
- *TSS*
- *Drugs*: SJS, TEN, drug reaction with eosinophilia and systemic symptoms (DRESS) syndrome
- *Immunological*: erythema multiforme, pemphigus vulgaris, immunotherapy-related dermatitis
- *Inflammatory*: acute generalised pustular psoriasis, erythroderma

Burns are another important cause of acute skin failure, and management of the above will follow similar principles to burns management. Examples of other conditions with significant skin involvement include anaphylaxis/anaphylactoid involvement (e.g. vancomycin flushing syndrome) and meningococcal septicaemia. (See Chapter 54 Burns)

Erythroderma is an inflammatory condition in which widespread erythema and oedema affects > 90% of the skin surface and is associated with exfoliation.

A **severe cutaneous adverse reaction (SCAR)** is the terminology for certain drug reactions including SJS, TEN, DRESS, and acute generalised exanthematous pustulosis (AGEP).

What is DRESS syndrome?

DRESS syndrome is a rare but potentially life-threatening adverse drug reaction.

Causative agents include the following:

- *Antiepileptics*: carbamazepine, lamotrigine, phenytoin, valproate
- *Antimicrobials*: ampicillin, cefotaxime, dapsone, anti-TB drugs, linezolid, metronidazole, vancomycin, trimethoprim-sulphamethoxazole, quinine, sulphasalazine, streptomycin
- *Antivirals*: abacabir, nevirapine
- *Antidepressant*: fluoxetine
- *Biologic*: imatinib, efalizumab
- *NSAID*: celecoxib, ibuprofen
- *Other*: allopurinol, ranitidine

Clinical features
- 'Lag phase' 2–6 weeks from trigger
- Prodromal fever and malaise
- Skin changes
    - Erythematous morbilliform rash
    - Facial involvement first, spread to trunk and upper limbs before lower limbs
    - Diffuse, pruritic, may become confluent
    - May have pustulation and target lesions
    - Commonly painful
    - Usually > 50% BSA
    - 20–30% progress to exfoliative dermatitis
- *Lymphatic*: lymphadenopathy
- *Haematological*: eosinophilia, leukocytosis/leukopaenia, MAS
- *Hepatic*: transaminitis, fulminant hepatic failure
- *Renal*: AKI
- *Respiratory*: mild involvement to ARDS
- *Cardiovascular*: myocarditis (hypersensitivity vs necrotising)
- *Other*: meningoencephalitis, gastroenteritis, endocrine dysfunction

Diagnosis may be difficult and involves scoring systems (RegiSCAR, J-SCAR) alongside specialist input and biopsy where practical. Management will involve removal of the causative agent and systemic steroids.

What do you know about SJS and TEN?

SJS and TEN are life-threatening dermatological emergencies. They lie on a spectrum of skin reactions characterised by severe mucocutaneous involvement, epidermal loss, and systemic upset. Definitions relate to percentage of BSA with skin detachment:

- *<10%*: SJS
- *10–30%*: TEN/SJS overlap
- *>30%*: **TEN**

Drugs are responsible for 85% cases. Common causative agents include sulphonamides, beta lactams, allopurinol, anticonvulsants, and NSAIDs. Infective causes include CMV and mycoplasma. Acute GvHD may cause a similar clinical picture to SJS/TEN but is managed differently. (see Chapter 142 Haematological Malignancy)

Features
- *Prodromal illness*: fever, sore throat, malaise
- Painful erythematous skin over trunk/face/limbs
- Macules > targetoid lesions > blisters > sheet-like skin loss
- *Nikolsky's sign*: dislodgement of epidermis with direct pressure
- Extensive mucosal and cutaneous necrosis in 2–3 days

What is the mortality of TEN?

The mortality of TEN is about 30%. The SCORe of TEN (SCORTEN) and ABCD-10 criteria can be used to predict mortality at time of admission to hospital based on specific risk factors.

ABCD-10 uses 5 criteria (points in brackets) as follows:

- Age ≥ 50 (1)
- Bicarbonate serum level < 20 mmol/l (1)
- Cancer (active) (2)
- Dialysis prior to admission (3)
- Epidermal detachment > **10%** (1)

Mortality by ABCD-10 score is as follows:

0   2.3%
1   5.4%
2   12.3%
3   25.2%
4   45.7%
5   67.4%
6   83.6%

SCORTEN also utilises heart rate (≥120 min⁻¹) and serum glucose (>14 mmol/l) and age criteria ≥40 years.

Mortality by SCORTEN is as follows:

0–1   3.2%
2   12.1%
3   35.3%
4   58.3%
≥5   90%

How would you manage the critical care patient with acute skin failure?

Similar principles are followed to those in burns management (See Chapter 54 Burns):

- *Resuscitation and supportive care as indicated*: including analgesia/sedation
- Consideration of referral/transfer to tertiary burns centre
- *Multidisciplinary approach*: dermatologist input, regular ophthalmological review
- Barrier nursing
- Insertion of lines through non-lesional skin
- Careful handling of skin to prevent further damage
- Regular surveillance cultures for infection
- *Avoidance of soiling affected skin*: bowel management system
- *Surgical input*: debridement, washout, skin grafts

Resources

- Bastuji-Garin S, Fouchard N, Bertocchi M, et al. SCORTEN: A severity-of-illness score for toxic epidermal necrolysis. J Invest Dermatol. 2000;115(2):149–153.
- Bromley M, Marsh S, Layton A. Dermatological complications of critical care. BJA Educ. 2021;21(22): 408–413.
- Bromley M, Marsh S, Layton A. Life-threatening skin conditions presenting to critical care. BJA Educ. 2021;21(10):376–383.
- Noe MH, Rosenbach M, Hubbard RA, et al. Development and validation of a risk prediction model for in-hospital mortality among patients with Stevens-Johnson syndrome/toxic epidermal necrolysis – ABCD-10. JAMA Dermatol. 2019;155(4):448–454.
- Scrace B, Fityan A, Bigham C. Drug reactions with eosinophilia and systemic symptoms. BJA Educ. 2020;20(10):65–71.

Why are rheumatological diseases important in critical care?

Rheumatological disorders encompass those involving the musculoskeletal system and systemic autoimmune diseases:

- *Rheumatoid arthritis and variants*: Sjogren's, Felty syndrome
- *Seronegative arthropathies*: ankylosing spondylitis, psoriatic, reactive arthritis, IBD
- *Connective tissue diseases*: SLE, systemic sclerosis, polymyositis, dermatomyositis, mixed connective tissue disease, Marfan syndrome
- *Vasculitides*
- *Degenerative*: OA, spondylolisthesis
- *Other*: gout, pseudogout

Many have systemic effects, and patients may present to critical care due to the following:

- Progression or complications of underlying condition
- *Complications of therapy*: side effects, infection
- *Unrelated condition (e.g. trauma)*: may be exacerbated by underlying condition

Why might management of patients with rheumatological diseases in critical care be complex?

- Multisystem involvement
- May result in multi-organ dysfunction
- High mortality in critical care
- Complicated pharmacotherapy with significant side effects (e.g. immunocompromise)
- Differential diagnosis broad/overlapping (e.g. infection vs disease flare up)
- Unusual life-threatening complications (e.g. MAS, scleroderma renal crisis)

Which vasculitides are you aware of?

ANCA-associated vasculitidies (AAV) are conditions involving autoimmune disease of blood vessels, characterised by the presence of ANCA in the blood.

- **Microscopic polyangiitis (MPA)**
- **Granulomatosis with polyangiitis (GPA)** (formerly 'Wegener's granulomatosis')
- **Eosinophilic granulomatosis with polyangiitis (EGPA)** (formerly 'Churg-Strauss syndrome')
- **Single-organ ANCA-associated vasculitidies (AAV)**
- **Behçet's syndrome**

Notable systemic effects
- *MPA*: glomerulonephritis, CKD to ESRF
- *GPA*: subglottic stenosis, diffuse alveolar haemorrhage, glomerulonephritis (may be rapidly progressive)
- *EGPA*: nasal polyps, asthma, conduction block, myocarditis, pericarditis, MI

Can you describe some systemic effects of rheumatological diseases that are relevant to critical care?

- *A*: kyphoscoliosis, risk of atlanto-occipital subluxation, sinusitis, cricoarytenoid dysfunction, laryngeal amyloidosis/nodules, temporomandibular joint involvement
- *B*: restrictive lung disease, PTX, emphysema, haemorrhage, effusion, costochondral disease
- *C*: aortic root disease, valve prolapse/incompetence, hypertension, pulmonary hypertension, CCF, vasculitis, effusion, tamponade, myocarditis, endocarditis
- *D*: peripheral neuropathy, autonomic dysfunction, kerato-conjunctivitis

- *E*: thin skin, joint hyper/hypomobility, arthritis, challenging positioning, vulnerability to pressure sores
- *F*: glomerulonephritis
- *G*: GI bleeding, weight loss, dysmotility, hepatosplenomegaly
- *H*: anaemia
- *I*: pyrexia, HLH/MAS

(See Chapter 144 Haemophagocytic Lymphohistiocytosis.

Outline the specific pharmacotherapies that you might encounter in these patients.

Reduction of inflammatory burden is a priority, and aggressive immunosuppression is often started early with disease-modifying anti-rheumatic drugs (DMARDs) first line.

- *DMARDs*: methotrexate, sulphasalazine, leflunomide, hydroxychloroquine
- **New-generation biologics**
  - *Anti-TNF*: infliximab, etanercept, adalimumab
  - *Anti-CD20 (B-cell depletion)*: rituximab
  - *IL-6 antagonists*: tocilizumab
  - *T-cell co-stimulators*: abatacept
- *Alkylating agents*: cyclophosphamide
- *NSAIDs*: ibuprofen, naproxen, celecoxib
- *Steroids*: methylprednisolone, prednisolone

Can you name some significant side effects of these therapies?

- *DMARDs*: marrow suppression (neutropaenic sepsis), liver/renal toxicity, rash, GI upset
- *Methotrexate*: pneumonitis, bone marrow toxicity
- *Biologics*: immunosuppression (atypical infection – TB, PJP, fungal, CMV), antibody depletion (JC virus reaction, PML), marrow suppression, exacerbation of demyelination, infusion reaction
- *Cyclophosphamide*: marrow suppression, pancreatitis, SIADH, AKI, hepatotoxicity

Methotrexate pneumonitis is potentially reversible with its cessation and sufficient physiological reserve for recovery. Improvement may be seen within days.

What is catastrophic antiphospholipid syndrome?

Antiphospholipid syndrome is a disorder characterised by recurrent venous and arterial thrombosis, pregnancy disorders, and the presence of antiphospholipid antibodies. It is often found in patients with other inflammatory autoimmune diseases.

Catastrophic antiphospholipid syndrome is a rarer, accelerated disease which leads to multi-organ failure with 50% mortality despite treatment. TMA of small vessels is thought to be responsible following a precipitating event (e.g. infection, surgery, trauma).

Management involves specialist input, heparinisation, IVIg/plasma exchange, and immunomodulation.

What is scleroderma renal crisis?

Systemic sclerosis is an autoimmune condition involving inflammation and fibrosis of multiple organs including the skin.

Scleroderma renal crisis is a syndrome of rapidly progressive hypertension with **AKI**. It occurs in 5–10% of patients with systemic sclerosis.

Reduced renal perfusion and excessive renin release after thickening of inter-lobar/arcuate arteries are thought to be responsible. Patients may present with headache, visual disturbance, and encephalopathy and seizures. Cardiovascular complications include LV dysfunction, pulmonary oedema, dysrhythmias, and myocarditis/pericarditis. MAHA may be seen.

Management involves use of ACEI, which may seem counterintuitive in AKI. Other therapies include calcium channel blockers, labetalol, nitrates, and plasma exchange. RRT is required in 25% – only 40–60% of these patients will recover independent renal function, which may take up to 3 years.

Resources

- Bell A, Tattersall R, Wenham T. Rheumatological conditions in critical care. BJA Educ. 2016;16(12):427–433.
- Chetcuti S, Jones RB, Varley J. Heritable connective tissue diseases, vasculitides, and the anaesthetist. BJA Educ. 2016;16(9):316–322.
- Fombon F, Thompson JP. Anaesthesia for the adult patient with rheumatoid arthritis. CEACCP. 2006;6(6): 235–239.

---

155. ONCOLOGY

Why might oncology patients be referred to critical care?

- **Related to cancer**
  - New presentation (e.g. airway compression by lymphoma)
  - Local spread (e.g. massive haemoptysis)
  - Other complication (e.g. PE, spontaneous TLS)
- **Related to treatment**
  - *Surgery*: curative, debulking, palliative (e.g. defunctioning stoma for bowel obstruction, biliary drainage)
  - *Chemotherapy*: neutropaenic sepsis, pneumonitis, TLS, mucositis
  - *HSCT*: sepsis, GvHD
  - *Immunotherapy*: immune-related reactions in most systems
  - *Chimeric antigen receptor T cell (CAR-T)*: CRS, immune effector cell-associated neurotoxicity syndrome (ICANS)
- **Unrelated condition** (e.g. trauma)

Can you name some common complications of chemotherapeutic agents?

- *Bleomycin*: pulmonary fibrosis (oxygen-sensitive)
- *Cisplatin*: renal toxicity, electrolyte disturbance
- *Cyclophosphamide*: idiopathic interstitial pneumonitis, haemorrhagic cystitis
- *Ciclosporin* hypertension, TTP
- *Doxorubicin*: cardiomyopathy
- *Methotrexate*: renal toxicity, pneumonitis
- *5-fluorouracil*: coronary/cerebral vasospasm (ACS/CVA-like presentation)

What is febrile neutropaenia?

Febrile neutropaenia is an oncological emergency which may develop in any patient receiving cytotoxic chemotherapy (up to 50% patients or 80% in haematology patients). Mortality is approximately 10%.

KEY POINT

Febrile neutropaenia is defined as follows:

- Oral temperature >38.3°C, or
- Two consecutive readings >38.0°C for 2 h, in the presence of
- Absolute neutrophil count (or expected to fall) <**0.5** × 109/l

---

Neutropaenic sepsis is defined in keeping with the Sepsis 3 definition. Neutropaenic patients without fever but with other features consistent with sepsis should be managed similarly.

Bacteraemia may result from translocation from non-sterile sources (mouth, skin, GI tract), colonisation of indwelling devices, or de novo (e.g. pneumonia, UTI). A minimum of 2 sets of blood cultures should be taken on presentation: peripheral, CVC if present (e.g. Hickman line).

Common organisms
- *P. aeruginosa*
- *Staph. aureus*
- *Streptococcus* spp.

Other considerations
- *Pneumocystis jirovecii*: if respiratory symptoms and prolonged lymphopaenia or steroid use
- *Fungal causes*: poor response to broad-spectrum antibiotics and history of prolonged neutropaenia

GUIDELINE ESMO 2016 Febrile neutropaenia

How is febrile neutropaenia managed?

Pharmacological
- Empirical broad-spectrum antibiotics within 60 min of presentation
- *G-CSF*: consider if colitis/mucositis or prolonged neutropaenia likely (reduces duration of neutropaenia but no evidence of improved clinical outcomes if started after symptoms develop)
- Antimicrobial prophylaxis alongside high-risk chemotherapy regimes (e.g. antifungal, antiviral, PJP)

Non-pharmacological
- Appropriate investigation of source including detailed history where possible – often not identified
- Specific source control as required (e.g. abscess drainage)
- Judicious use and replacement of indwelling devices
  - Early removal associated with improved survival if haemodynamically unstable
- Consideration of high flow oxygen over NIV
- Involvement of microbiologist
- Reverse barrier nursing
- *Neutropaenic colitis (typhlitis)*: early surgical review, CT, bowel rest (high risk of deterioration, perforation, bowel necrosis)

(See Chapter 142 Haematological Malignancy)

What is immunotherapy?

- *Immune checkpoint inhibitors (ICI)*: monoclonal antibodies, relatively new class used in some malignancies – 43.6% of US cancer patients received ICIs in 2018
- *CAR-T therapy*: intent of long-term disease control, that is 'cure' (ALL, lymphoma)
- Non-specific immunotherapies
  - *Cytokines*: IL-2, interferons (renal cell carcinoma) – largely replaced by ICIs
  - BCG (bladder cancer)
- Cancer vaccines (prostate cancer)

What is the mode of action behind CAR-T therapy?

- T cells are removed from the patient
- These are genetically modified with chimeric antigen receptors
- Chimeric cells are cloned and returned to patient
- This triggers an immune response against malignant cells

What are the significant side effects of immunotherapies?
Infusion reactions, CRS, and secondary HLH may result from most immunotherapies. Specific syndromes are more common with different types

Monoclonal antibodies
- *Respiratory*: pneumonitis, PE
- *Cardiovascular*: cardiomyopathy, dysrhythmias, ACS

- *Neurotoxicity*: PRES, ischaemic stroke, ICH, aseptic meningitis, encephalopathy
- *Renal*: interstitial nephritis, TMA, TLS

CAR-T

- **CRS** is "a supraphysiological response following any immune therapy that results in the activation or engagement of endogenous/infused T-cells and/or other immune effector cells".
  - Most common toxicity with CAR-T (occurs in 60–95%).
  - May cause ARDS.
  - Up to 20% require high-dose vasopressors.
  - Severe cases managed with anti-IL-6 therapy (e.g. tocilizumab) and steroids.
- *ICANS*: updated terminology for cytokine-release encephalopathy syndrome and encephalopathy/neurotoxicity related to CAR-T.
  - Tremor, headache, confusion, seizures, coma, paresis, cerebral oedema.
  - Managed with anakinra (crosses blood-brain-barrier unlike anti-IL-6).

ICI can cause immune-related adverse events (15–90%). These occur any time during/after treatment and are managed with immunosuppression:

- Pneumonitis (2–4%)
- *Cardiovascular (<1%)*: myocarditis, pericarditis, arrhythmias, cardiomyopathy, ventricular dysfunction
- *Neurological toxicity (1%)*: polyneuropathy, facial nerve palsy, demyelination, myaesthenia gravis, GBS, PRES, transverse myelitis, enteric neuropathy, encephalitis, aseptic meningitis
- *Renal (<1%)*: nephritis, nephrotic syndrome, TLS
- *GI*: hepatitis (5–10%), diarrhoea (27–54%)
- *Other*: thyroid dysfunction (21%), hypophysitis (1–16%), type 1 diabetes mellitus (<1%), skin toxicity (34–45%), arthralgia (2012%), ocular toxicity

GUIDELINE ESMO 2017 Toxicities from immunotherapy

What is HIPEC?

Hyperthermic intraperitoneal chemotherapy (HIPEC) is a form of chemotherapy that is applied directly during cytoreductive surgery to optimise delivery of cytotoxic agents. It is heated to >40°C and works over 60–90 min. Complications include pancreatitis, bleeding, and inflammatory reactions.

How would you assess a patient referred to critical care with underlying malignancy?

- **Physiology**
  - *Patient wishes*: informal, advanced directives, discussions about resuscitation
  - Comorbidities
  - Frailty
  - *Reserve*: may be disproportionate to age, etc. (e.g. due to therapies used)
  - *Functional status*: change over time
- **Pathology**
  - *Expected malignant disease course prior to acute episode*: ideally seek specialist input
  - *Nature of acute process*: reversibility in isolation vs with cancer
  - *Likely effects of treatment*: side effects, iatrogenesis, deconditioning

What are the challenges of admitting patients with malignancy to critical care?

The decision whether to admit a patient with cancer to the critical care unit is often challenging. The decision-making process will revolve around the balance of perceived benefit to the patient and the potential burdens of admission, as with any referral.

More specific to patients with malignancy, the perceived benefit may incorporate a judgement on life expectancy with or without critical care involvement. This will be with a view to not prolonging the dying process. There may be a fine line between this and depriving those who may benefit from critical care.

Challenges

- Extensive range of malignant diseases and stages in disease process at presentation to critical care
- Limited evidence available to inform decision-making (selection bias with observational studies)
- Many scoring systems don't perform well in those with malignancy.
- Physician judgement has been found to be unreliable in predicting outcome in some studies.
- Details about tertiary management and investigations may not be accessible within the required time frame. On-call oncology services should be available to advise.
- Difference in experience at tertiary cancer centre unit vs others
- Evolving range of therapies available with need for ongoing learning
- Prognosis may be uncertain in an acute presentation with new diagnosis without histology or complete staging information.
- Acceptable benefits or burdens of treatment will vary between individuals. Combined with reduced capacity, this is difficult to assess.
- *Improved outcomes over recent decades*: a growing number of patients are admitted to critical care with decrease in mortality. Many stage 4 'metastatic' cancers have >50% 5-year survival (e.g. stage 4 melanoma may be 'cured' – alive and disease free for several years following treatment).

Careful patient selection is crucial, and it may be extremely difficult to tell who will benefit from admission and specific support. There is a need for decision-making to be individualised with multidisciplinary collaboration.

(See Chapter 156 Prognostication)

Resources

- Beed M, Levitt M, Bokhari SW. Intensive care management of patients with haematological malignancy. CEACCP. 2010;10(6):167–171.
- Gutierrez C, McEvoy C, Munshi L, et al. Critical care management of toxicities associated with targeted agents and immunotherapies for cancer. Crit Care Med. 2020;48(1):10–21.
- Haslam A, Prasad V. Estimation of the Percentage of US patients with cancer who are eligible for and respond to checkpoint inhibitor immunotherapy drugs. JAMA Netw Open, 2019;2(5):e192535.
- Koutsoukou A. Admission of critically ill patients with cancer to the ICU: many uncertainties remain. ESMO Open. 2016;2(4):e000105.
- Lewis A, Chaft J, Girotra M, et al. Immune checkpoint inhibitors: a narrative review of considerations for the anaesthesiologist. Br J Anaesth. 2020;124(3):251–260.
- Stephens RS. Neutropenic fever in the intensive care unit. Oncologic Critical Care. 2019:1297–1311.

PALLIATIVE CARE

156. PROGNOSTICATION

What is prognostication?

Prognostication can be defined as the process of prophesying future events.

In medical scenarios, prognostication is the process by which a clinician attempts to predict a patient's outcome, usually to inform treatment decisions.

How is prognostication carried out in critical care?

Prognostication is inherently difficult and is often based on the combination of clinical experience and evidence-based medicine. It features in several decision-making processes in critical care as follows:

- Admission
- Treatment limitations
  - Mechanical ventilation
  - Renal replacement therapy
  - Extracorporeal life support
- Appropriateness of tracheostomy (potentially facilitating long-term airway/respiratory support)
- Withdrawal of life-sustaining treatment
- Decision to operate (e.g. emergency laparotomy in a comorbid or irreversibly unwell patient)

A patient's acute pathology and premorbid physiology should be considered in making a judgement. This may need to be done to the best ability with the information available before a full history can be ascertained. This judgement can be considered alongside the burdens of the decision, and what may be deemed an acceptable quality of life for the patient.

Multi-disciplinary assessment is often ideal but may be limited in time-critical situations.

(See Chapter 60 Emergency Laparotomy, Chapter 155 Oncology, and Chapter 157 Withdrawal of Life-Sustaining Treatment)

How might prognosis be assessed after a cardiac arrest?

In the unconscious post-arrest population:

- Two thirds will die before hospital discharge.
- Two thirds of those deaths will be due to neurological injury.

The ERC has released guidance on prognostication which has been adopted widely. Basic principles include the following:

- Exclusion of reversible causes of poor neurological state
- Multi-modal assessment
- Evidence-based prediction of poor neurological outcome

Supportive care should be facilitated for 72 h (if stable) before judgement can be made. This period goes hand in hand with temperature control recommendations. Prognostication can include some signs available earlier than this retrospectively (as detailed below). (See Chapter 27 Out-of-Hospital Cardiac Arrest)

KEY POINT

Poor outcome likely if at 72 h if all 3 of the following:

- Unconscious
- GCS motor score ≤3
- ≥2 of:
  - Pupillary (light) and corneal reflexes absent bilaterally
  - CT/MR shows diffuse and extensive anoxic injury
  - EEG highly malignant (>24 h)
  - Status myoclonus (≤72 h)
  - SSEP N20 wave absent bilaterally
  - NSE > 60 µg/l (at 48 h +/ 72 h)

Notes
- *Status myoclonus*: continuous and generalised, ≥30 min
- *Highly malignant EEG*: burst suppression or suppressed background ± periodic discharges
- Caution should be exercised if discordant signs are present (indicating a potentially good outcome).

GUIDELINE ERC ESICM 2021 Post-resuscitation care

The FOUR (Full Outline of UnResponsiveness) score can be used in the assessment of comatose patients after cardiac arrest, and is thought to be more useful than GCS in this context as more detail is provided within lower GCS scores. Four domains are each scored 0–4, with a lower score indicating higher severity (Table 156.1).

Table 156.1   The FOUR score with comparison to GCS criteria

	Eye response	Motor response in upper limbs	Brain stem reflexes (absence of)	Respiratory pattern
0	E1	M1	Pupillary, corneal, cough	Breathing at ventilator rate or apnoea
1	E2	M2	Pupillary, corneal	Breathing above ventilator rate
2	E3	Flexion to pain	Pupillary or corneal	Not intubated, irregular
3	Open, not tracking	M5	One pupil wide and fixed	Not intubated, Cheyne-Stokes
4	Tracking or blinking to command	Thumbs up, fist, or peace sign	Not absent	Not intubated, regular

What is considered a good neurological outcome after brain injury?

- CPC 1–2
- mRS 0–3

Neurological outcome is usually assessed from 6 to 12 months post-injury onwards.

CPC

1. Good cerebral performance (conscious, able to work, mild deficit)
2. Moderate cerebral disability (conscious, independent ADLs, sheltered work)
3. Severe cerebral disability (conscious, dependent due to brain function)*
4. Coma or vegetative state (any degree of impaired consciousness without brain death)
5. Brain death

* CPC 3 can range from an ambulant state to severe dementia or paralysis.

mRS

0	No symptoms
1	Symptoms, no significant disability (all ADLs)
2	Slight disability (not all ADLs, can look after own affairs)
3	Moderate disability (requires help, walks without assistance)
4	Moderately severe disability (assistance to walk and for bodily needs)
5	Severe disability (bedbound, incontinent, constant nursing care)
6	Dead

Do you know any predictors of good neurological outcome?

EEG
- Continuous or nearly continuous activity within 12 h of ROSC
- Presence of early reactivity
- Improvement of auditory discrimination

MR
- Absence of diffusion weighted imaging abnormalities within 1 week of ROSC

What is frailty?

Frailty is difficult to define but can be described as a multidimensional phenotype of vulnerability predisposing to adverse outcomes.

There is a paucity of evidence surrounding frailty in critical care, with potential for bias. However, it can be suggested that increased frailty is less likely to be compatible with the physiological reserve necessary to survive various aspects of a critical care stay with an acceptable outcome.

Physical phenotype of frailty
- Reduced walking speed
- Reduced physical activity
- Reduced grip strength
- Weight loss (4.5 kg in 1 year)
- Exhaustion

It may be graded using various models. The Rockwood Clinical Frailty Scale (CFS) is used most widely in critical care in which a score of 5–8 is considered frail, and 9 is a separate concept for terminal illness:

> **KEY POINT**
>
> CFS
>
> 1. *Very fit*: robust, active, energetic, motivated
> 2. *Fit*: no active disease symptoms, active occasionally
> 3. *Managing well*: well controlled medical problems, not regularly active
> 4. *Very mild frailty*: symptoms limit activities
> 5. *Mild frailty*: more evident slowing, help with high order activities (e.g. finances)
> 6. *Moderate frailty*: help with housework and all outside activities
> 7. *Severe frailty*: completely dependent for personal care
> 8. *Very severe frailty*: approaching end of life, could not recover from mild illness
> 9. *Terminally ill*: life expectancy <6 months, not otherwise living with severe frailty

What is 'performance status'?

The World Health Organization refers to 'performance status' in the form of the Eastern Cooperative Oncology Group (ECOG) Performance Status Scale (or Zubrod Score). It was originally used to estimate a patient's ability to perform ADL in the context of malignancy. It is used to guide prognosis and treatment options. (See Chapter 155 Oncology)

Performance status can be used as an approximation of premorbid functional capacity and has been applied to critical care, with impairment associated with several adverse outcomes (e.g. increased ICU and hospital mortality).

> **KEY POINT**
>
> ECOG Performance Status Scale
>
> 0   Fully active
> 1   Restricted in strenuous activity, able to carry out light work
> 2   Ambulatory, self-caring, unable to carry out work activities
> 3   Limited self-care, confined to bed/chair > 50% waking h
> 4   Completely disabled, dependent for care, confined to bed/chair
> 5   Dead

Resources

- De Biasio JC, Mittel AM, Mueller AL, et al. Frailty in critical care medicine: a review. Anesth Analg. 2020;130(6):1462–1473.
- Oken MM, Creech RH, Tormey DC, et al. Toxicity and response criteria of the Eastern Cooperative Oncology Group. Am J Clin Oncol. 1982;5(6):649–655.
- Wijdicks FM, Bamlet WR, Maramattom BV, et al. Validation of a new coma scale: The FOUR score. Ann Neurol. 2005;58(4):585–593.
- Zampieri FG, Bozza FA, Moralez GM, et al. The effects of performance status one week before hospital admission on the outcomes of critically ill patients. Intensive Care Med. 2017;43(1):39–47.

157. WITHDRAWAL OF LIFE-SUSTAINING TREATMENT

What is palliative care?

Palliative care is the **holistic care** of patients with **advanced, progressive, incurable illness** with the aim to support patients to live well until they die, and to die with dignity.

Palliative care focuses on the management of symptoms and provision of psychological, social, and spiritual support.

What is meant by the term 'end-of-life'?

A patient may be approaching the 'end of their life' when it is likely that they will die within the next 12 months. This includes many patients in the population admitted to critical care.

'End stage' describes the final period or phase of a progressive disease leading to death.

What is futility?

Futility is a subjective term used to describe the perceived non-benefit of treatment and covers several interpretations as follows:

- *Physiological*: unable to maintain acceptable physiology
- *Quantitative*: low chance of succeeding
- *Qualitative*: cannot achieve an acceptable quality
- *Imminent demise*: will not change the fact that the patient is imminently dying
- *Lethal conditions*: underlying condition will not be affected and will lead to death soon

This terminology is avoided in GMC guidance in favour of determining the potential 'overall benefit' to the patient. This involves weighing proposed benefits, burdens, and risks of treatments. These may include non-clinical considerations. Sufficient information should be provided on the options available.

> **GUIDELINE**   GMC 2010 Treatment and care towards the end of life

Which principles apply to decision-making in end-of-life care?

- Equalities and human rights
- Presumption in favour of prolonging life
- Presumption of capacity
- Maximising capacity to make decisions
- Overall benefit

The Ethicus-2 (2021) study described variations in practice worldwide as follows.

> **STUDY**
>
> Ethicus-2 (2021)
>
> - Adult ICU patients who died or had limitations of life-sustaining treatment
> - Prospective observational study including 14.6% of ICU admissions
> - *11.8% admissions involved limitations*: Commonly withholding life-sustaining treatment (44.1%) and its withdrawal (36.4%), and 1 in 5 with limitations survived to hospital discharge
> - Shortening of the dying process was uncommon (0.5%)
> - 14% died due to failure of CPR (range from 3.7% in Northern Europe to 65.4% in Africa)

How would you approach decision-making for the adult who lacks capacity to decide?

GMC guidance outlines a stepwise approach as follows:

- Be clear what **decisions** must be made.
- Check for potentially **legally binding** advance decision/directive refusing treatment.
- Enquire as to whether someone holds legal **authority** to decide (and scope of authority).
- Take **responsibility** for deciding which treatment will provide overall benefit to the patient where no legal proxy exists, consulting those close to the patient and members of the healthcare team.

Special circumstances

- *Patients lacking capacity with no known advocates*: **independent mental capacity advocate (IMCA)** may be appointed for certain decisions (non-instructed advocacy).
- *Children*: may be made '**wards of court**' after petition to the High Court, which will then take over responsibility for decision-making on their behalf.

What is the role of relatives or others close to the patient in this context?

Persons close to the patient can help to ensure that the patient receives good care at the end of life through the provision of information. They may provide information about the patient's wishes, preferences, feelings, beliefs, and values but do not make decisions.

If they do not have legal authority to make decisions on behalf of the patient who lacks capacity, their role is only to advise the team. Decisions should take the information provided into account.

How would you approach a disagreement about decisions surrounding end-of-life care?

Efforts should be made to reach an agreement on the best course of action. However, disagreements do occur. These may be between team members (e.g. opinions of intensivist and surgeon) or between the team and persons close to the patient.

Strategies to resolve disagreements may include the following:

- Seeking advice from a more experienced colleague
- Involving an independent advocate
- Holding a case conference or ethics consultation
- Using mediation services

Legal advice may need to be sought if these fail and an independent court ruling may be sought to provide a thorough exploration of the issues and reassurance.

What would you tell a family member about withdrawal of life-sustaining treatment?

An explanation of what is going to happen should take place if appropriate and communication is often split between the medical and nursing teams. Subjects that might be covered include the following:

- The aim not to prolong death, but to relieve symptoms and maintain dignity
- Likely procedures involved (e.g. extubation)
- Likely physiological changes
- Uncertainty about duration of dying process, or more information when this is more apparent
- Support provided should they wish to be present
- What they might see or hear
- How perceived symptoms will be managed
- What happens when death occurs, confirmation, care after death, certification

How might organ support be withdrawn in critical care?

- Individualised assessment of the nature of life-sustaining treatment being provided
- Non-comfort medications stopped
  - It may be reasonable to continue antiepileptics
- *Monitoring*: silencing alarms ± partial/complete removal of monitoring
- Assessment for relevant signs/symptoms and appropriate treatment, for example:
  - Opioids for pain/discomfort
  - Haloperidol/midazolam for agitation
  - Infusions may be required/continued
  - Supplemental oxygen may be required for symptomatic relief
- Sequential reduction in support (with ongoing symptomatic relief)
  - Vasoactive medications stopped
  - Reduction in ventilatory support
  - Extubation to air

Do you know of any adaptations in special circumstances?

- **Ongoing requirement for sedation (e.g. refractory status epilepticus)**
  - This is subject to differing opinions regarding the doctrine of double effect.
  - It may be reasonable to continue sedation – more so in certain conditions (e.g. status epilepticus).
- **NIV**
  - CPAP withdrawal became a more prominent concern during the COVID-19 pandemic.
  - Weaning F_IO_2 (to 0.21) and pressure support may be appropriate if patient appears comfortable.
  - The machine may then be turned off and the mask removed.
- **Mechanical circulatory support and ECMO**
  - *Patient may be awake/aware*: communication and symptom control are crucial.
  - Decannulation or clamping may not be practical and cause distress.
  - Reduction in pump/gas flow may be appropriate.
- **ICD**
  - Device deactivation should have been discussed before implantation.
  - Repeated shocks can cause significant distress.
  - Deactivation can be achieved by technicians.
  - In an emergency, a doughnut magnet can be taped over the device (closing an internal switch).
- **Organ donation after circulatory death**
  - Intubation of the body may be required, potentially causing ethical unease.
  - Check the staff member present is prepared to do this.

Resources
- Beattie J. British Heart Foundation. ICD Deactivation at the End of Life: Principles and Practice: A Discussion Document for Healthcare Professionals [M106]. 2013. Available from: https://www.bhf.org.uk/informationsupport/publications/living-with-a-heart-condition/icd-deactivation-at-the-end-life. (Accessed 4 January 2022.)
- Braganza MA, Glossop AJ, Vora VA. Treatment withdrawal and end-of-life care in the intensive care unit. BJA Educ. 2017;17(12):396–400.
- Webber N, Avari M, Harridge G, et al. Implementing a novel protocol for withdrawal of CPAP support in COVID-19 patients: a case series. Clin Med (Lond). 2021;21(4):e392–e394.
- Winston E. Dying on ECMO – How Do We Care for the dying patient on mechanical support? 2020. Available from: https://intensiveblog.com/dying-on-ecmo-how-do-we-care-for-the-Dying-Patient-on-Mechanical-Support/. (Accessed 4 January 2022.)

---

158. DEATH

What is the definition of death?

> **KEY POINT**
>
> Death is the irreversible loss of the **capacity for consciousness**, combined with irreversible loss of the **capacity to breathe**.

- This implies the irreversible loss of those essential characteristics which are necessary to the existence of a living human person.
- Both criteria are required. Conditions exist in which either may be present (e.g. patient in a vegetative state has, by definition, lost the capacity for consciousness).
- Notably a person has not died due to the absence of mechanical cardiac function.
- Diagnosis does not require the cessation of all neurological activity in the brain, but these criteria imply an absence of activity pertaining to human life (i.e. ability to feel, be aware of, or do anything).

What are some of the consequences of death for an individual?

- Cessation of requirements to continue resuscitation
- Loss of personhood and individual rights
- Formal registration of the death and certification
- Execution of a will, estate transfer, payment of life insurance
- Religious or social ceremonies
- Possible post-mortem examination
- Opportunity for organ donation
- Disposition of the body

How might death be diagnosed?

An appropriately trained clinician may perform verification of life extinct (VLE) using somatic, cardiore-spiratory, or neurological criteria.

Can you describe somatic criteria in more detail?

Somatic criteria relate to the general recognition of death by another person. They are more commonly used in the community, for example by paramedics. Certain conditions indicate reliably that an irreversible loss of functions has occurred. These are often used where there has been a significant delay between death and discovery, or in catastrophic trauma.

These conditions are known as 'recognition of life extinct' (ROLE) criteria:

- Decapitation
- Massive cranial and cerebral disruption
- Hemicorporectomy or similar massive injury
- Massive truncal injury incompatible with life
- Incineration (>95% full thickness burns)
- Decomposition or putrefaction
- *Rigor mortis and hypostasis*: beware similar situations (e.g. drug ingestion causing abnormal rigidity immediately after cardiac arrest)
- Neonatal maceration

How is death diagnosed by cardiorespiratory criteria?

Cardiorespiratory criteria require both:

- **Continuous apnoeic asystole**
- **Loss of consciousness**

Practically, this should involve the following examination:

1 **Cessation of circulatory system**
   - No central pulses on palpation
   - No heart sounds on auscultation
   - (*Supplementary*: asystole on continuous ECG display; absence of pulsatile flow using direct intra-arterial pressure monitoring; absence of contractile activity on echocardiography)
2 **Cessation of respiratory system**
   - No respiratory effort seen
   - No breath sounds on auscultation

Cardiorespiratory arrest must have occurred for a minimum of **5 min** before proceeding.

3 **Cessation of cerebral function**
   - Pupils dilated and not reactive to light
   - No corneal reflexes
   - No motor response to painful central stimulus

Who can verify life extinct?

It is not mandated for this to be done by a doctor, but one should be informed after any VLE. Certain experienced nursing staff and other clinicians may do this, subject to appropriate governance.

A doctor is more likely to be required in some circumstances:

- Sudden death
- Uncertain cause
- Suspected suspicious circumstances
- Result of an untoward event (e.g. fall)
- Coroner's referral or consented hospital post-mortem examination indicated
- Patient is under 18 years old
- Organ donation proceeding

> **GUIDELINE**   DOH Northern Ireland (2019) Verifying life extinct

When is the time of death?

This is the time at which **VLE is completed**. In hospital settings, there is often somatic recognition by nursing staff before informing a doctor. VLE should be performed as soon as possible after death becomes obvious (or is first considered) and should be on the same calendar day where possible. This time is important in determining the start of consequences given above (e.g. execution of a legal will).

If using neurological criteria, it is the time at which the **first set of tests is completed**. (See Chapter 159 Diagnosis of Death by Neurological Criteria)

How does diagnosis of death differ in children?

VLE does not apply to the fetus or preterm neonate (<37 weeks corrected gestational age). Neurological criteria should not be used in the preterm neonate. From **37 weeks**, any of the 3 sets of criteria may be used.

Cardiorespiratory criteria still mandate a minimum of 5 min of observation. Subtle differences relate to the difficulty of examining very young children. Adult criteria can be used from **2 months** corrected gestational age.

37 weeks to 2 months corrected gestational age:

- *Cessation of circulatory system*: no heart sounds (auscultation or asystole on ECG)
- *Cessation of respiratory system*: no respiratory effort observed, no breath sounds
- *Cessation of cerebral function*: no spontaneous movement or response to stimulation

In this age range, neurological criteria also differ slightly and it is rarely possible to diagnose brain stem death. A further 24-h observation period is an additional precondition. Drug level measurements are advocated. Ancillary tests are under evaluation.

What are the roles of the coroner and medical examiner in relation to critical care?

The medical examiner system has been introduced in the UK to provide greater scrutiny of all deaths, including those not referred to the coroner. It also aims to provide a better service for the bereaved and improve the quality of death certification and mortality data. A senior medical doctor will carry out this role in each geographical region.

A coroner is an independent judicial officer responsible for investigating a patient's cause of death in certain circumstances (in England and Wales in the UK; Scotland involves the Procurator Fiscal). They aim to ascertain who the deceased was and how, when, and where death occurred. This may involve a post-mortem examination, imaging, and/or inquest (legal inquiry).

The clinical team is responsible for referring appropriate cases and they may require to write statements or attend relevant inquests.

Indications for referral include the following:

- *Mechanism*: unnatural, trauma, self-harm, neglect, poisoning, notifiable accidents/diseases, anaesthesia, post-operative
- Unknown identity or cause
- Custody or other state detention

Potential conclusions

- Natural causes
- Accident/misadventure
- Industrial disease
- Dependence on drugs/non-dependent abuse of drugs
- Attempted/self-induced abortion
- Disasters subject to public inquiry
- Unlawful killing
- Lawful killing
- Suicide
- *Open*: insufficient evidence to determine cause
- *Narrative*: describes circumstances in more detail, not bound by above categories

The coroner may also write a Prevention of Future Deaths Report under Regulation 28 if it appears that other deaths may occur in similar circumstances. The receiving organisation must reply within 56 days detailing planned actions as a result of the report.

> **GUIDELINE**   UK Legislation 2013 The Coroners (Investigations) Regulations 2013

What should be done if a death is suspicious?

The body and the area around it should be secured and not disturbed and the police and coroner have been contacted.

What is meant by the term 'last offices'?

'Last offices' is a historical term used to describe care after death, specifically the physical preparation of the body.

Care after death involves the following:

- Honouring spiritual/cultural wishes
- Preparing the body for transfer to the mortuary
- Offering relatives the opportunity to participate, support to do so
- Maintaining privacy and dignity
- Protection of health and safety of those coming into contact with the body
- Honouring wishes for organ/tissue donation
- Returning the deceased person's possessions to their relatives

Preparation of the body depends on the requirement for coronial involvement.

- With coronial involvement
  - Leave all lines in situ if forensic investigation is required, including catheter bag contents
  - Keep infusions attached but clamped if circumstances are suspicious
  - Do not wash or begin mouth care
  - Leave tracheal tubes in situ
- Without coronial involvement
  - Position, close eyes, support jaw
  - Mouth care, replace dentures
  - Tidy the hair, clean, dress, remove jewellery as specified
  - Remove mechanical devices, contain leakages, spigot remaining tubes
  - Keep dressings, sutures, clips, cannulae, fresh stoma bag

Resources

- National End of Life Care Programme and National Nurse Consultant Group (Palliative Care). Guidance for Staff Responsible for Care after Death (Last Offices). June 2011. Available from: https://www.england.nhs.uk/improvement-hub/wp-content/uploads/sites/44/2017/10/Guidance-for-Staff-Responsible-for-Care-after-Death.pdf. (Accessed 04 January 2022.)
- National Health Service. The National Medical Examiner System. 2022. Available from: https://www.england.nhs.uk/establishing-medical-examiner-system-nhs/. (Accessed 20 April 2022.)

---

159. DIAGNOSIS OF DEATH BY NEUROLOGICAL CRITERIA

What are the preconditions to diagnose death by neurological criteria?

- GCS 3 requiring mechanical ventilation
- Irreversible brain damage of known aetiology

GUIDELINE AoMRC 2008 Diagnosis and confirmation of death

What are the likely causes of brain stem death?

- *Intra-cranial*: traumatic brain injury, spontaneous intra-cranial haemorrhage, and ischaemic stroke
- *Extra-cranial*: profound hypoxia

Which conditions would need to be excluded to proceed with this diagnostic pathway?

All reversible pharmacological, metabolic, or endocrinological causes of coma and apnoea should be excluded:

- Metabolic and endocrine criteria
- Residual effect of drugs that can contribute to unconsciousness (e.g. sedatives, narcotics, hypnotics, tranquilisers)
- Residual effects of neuromuscular blocking agents

If any doubt, specific drug levels and antagonists can be used. Presence of residual block can be measured using peripheral nerve stimulators, if necessary (Table 159.1).

In which red flag conditions is caution advised?

- <6 h after loss of the last brain stem reflex
- <24 h after loss of the last brain stem reflex when aetiology is primarily anoxic damage
- <24 h of re-warming following hypothermia
- Neuromuscular disorders
- Steroids given in space occupying lesions such as abscesses
- Prolonged fentanyl infusions
- Aetiology primarily located to the brain stem or posterior fossa
- Therapeutic decompressive craniectomy

If possible, a period of cardiorespiratory stability should be achieved prior to testing:

- MAP > 60 mmHg consistently
- $P_aCO_2 < 6.0$ kPa
- $P_aO_2 > 10$ kPa
- pH 7.35–7.45

Table 159.1   Metabolic criteria for diagnosis of death by neurological criteria

Criterion	Minimum	Maximum
Core temperature (°C)	34	
Serum Na⁺ (mmol/l)	115	160
Serum K⁺ (mmol/l)	2	
Serum PO₄³⁻ (mmol/l)	0.5	3
Serum Mg²⁺ (mmol/l)	0.5	3
Blood glucose (mmol/l)	3	20

How is brain stem death testing performed?

Testing is divided into 2 sections:

- Brain stem reflexes (cranial nerve tests)
- Apnoea testing

For the diagnosis of death, there must be absence of specified brain stem reflexes and apnoea despite hypercarbia (Table 159.2). Apnoea testing is only performed if brain stem reflexes are found to be absent first.

Testing must be performed by at least 2 doctors who have been registered with the GMC (or equivalent) for at least 5 years and are competent in performing brain stem death testing. They should not have any conflict of interest in testing, particularly in organ donation.

The full set of tests is performed twice, typically with the 2 doctors swapping roles of tester and observer for each set.

How is the apnoea test performed?

KEY POINT

Apnoea test:

- Take baseline ABG (1)
- Pre-oxygenate patient and obtain cardiovascular stability, if possible
- Reduce minute ventilation to allow P_aCO_2 to rise to >6 kPa (consider 6.5 if known chronic CO_2 retainer) and pH < 7.4
- Confirm with ABG (2)
- Disconnect from mechanical ventilation and provide oxygen using CPAP circuit
- Observe for evidence of spontaneous respiration for 5 min
- Repeat ABG (3) post-apnoea test to ensure P_aCO_2 has increased by at least 0.5 kPa

When is the time of death?

Death is confirmed on completion of the second set of tests. However, the legal time of death is when the first set of tests is complete.

Table 159.2   Cranial nerve testing for diagnosis of death

Test	Afferent	Efferent
Pupillary response to light	II	III
Corneal reflex	V	VII
Supra-orbital pressure	V	VII
Vestibulo-ocular reflex	VIII	III, VI
Gag reflex	IX	X
Cough reflex	IX	X

In which situations might diagnosing death by neurological criteria be challenging?

- Extensive maxillo-facial injuries (cranial nerve testing impossible)
- High cervical spine injuries (aetiology of apnoea unreliable)

Ancillary testing can be used in conjunction with clinical examination:

- *Neurophysiological*: loss of **brain activity** (e.g. EEG, evoked potentials)
- *Radiological*: absence of **cerebral blood flow** (e.g. CT angiography, transcranial Doppler)

How does ECMO affect this process?

- Altered pharmacokinetics of palliative care medications
- Apnoea test affected by clearance of CO_2

With VV-ECMO, sweep gas can be manipulated as cerebral and peripheral P_aCO_2 should be identical. In VA- or hybrid ECMO, cerebral circulation may differ and multiple sites must be sampled – the highest pH and lowest P_aCO_2 should be used. Specialist input is recommended (e.g. neurology, neurointensive care) and ancillary tests may be helpful.

> **GUIDELINE**   FICM ICS 2018 Neurological criteria on ECMO

Resource

- Faculty of Intensive Care Medicine. Form for the Diagnosis of Death Using Neurological Criteria – Long Version. 2021. Available from: https://www.ficm.ac.uk/sites/ficm/files/documents/2021-10/Form_for_the_ Diagnosis_of_Death_using_Neurological_Criteria-long_version.pdf. (Accessed 04 January 2022.)

160.   DONATION AFTER BRAIN STEM DEATH

Why is the critical care management of the brain stem dead organ donor important?

Standardised protocols for management of heart beating donors have demonstrated improved organ retrieval. On average a donation after brain stem death (DBD) donor donates 3.3 organs.

What challenges might managing the DBD donor present?

- Cardiovascular instability including hypotension (81%) and arrhythmias (25%)
- Diabetes insipidus (65%)
- Neurogenic pulmonary oedema (18%)
- *Electrolyte disturbance*: in particular metabolic acidosis (11%), hypernatraemia, hypokalaemia, and hyperglycaemia
- DIC (28%)
- Hypothermia

What are the immediate objectives?

- Methylprednisolone for all donors
- Recruitment manoeuvres to correct atelectasis caused by apnoea test
- Correction of hypovolaemia
- Introduction of vasopressin (weaning noradrenaline/adrenaline)
- Glycaemic control
- Identification and correction of diabetes insipidus

Which systems-based optimisation would you carry out?

> **KEY POINT**
>
> Physiological targets in the organ donor:
>
> - $P_aO_2 > 10$ kPa
> - pH > 7.25
> - MAP 60–80 mmHg
> - UO 0.5–2 ml/kg/h
> - $Na^+ < 150$ mmol/l
> - Glucose 4–10 mmol/l
> - Normothermia

Respiratory
- Lung recruitment manoeuvres
- Lung protective ventilation
- Regular chest physio and suctioning
- 30–45° head up
- Appropriate cuff pressure
- Appropriate patient positioning and turns
- Consider bronchoscopy and bronchial lavage (therapeutic, lung donation)

Cardiovascular
- Review fluid status, correct hypovolaemia
- Commence cardiac output/flow monitoring
- *If vasopressors required*: vasopressin at 0.5–4 units/h (reduce/stop other support as able)
- *Preferred inotrope*: dopamine (dobutamine second line)

Fluids and metabolic
- Methylprednisolone 15 mg/kg (max 1 g)
- IV crystalloids or NG water if hypernatraemic
- If UO > 4 ml/kg/h consider diabetes insipidus, treat with vasopressin ± DDAVP
- Continue NG feed

Thrombo-embolic prevention
- Thrombo-embolic stockings ± compression devices as applicable
- Continue or prescribe low molecular weight heparin

What further investigation or monitoring might be indicated?
- Arterial line (left radial/brachial)
- Central line (right IJV/SCV)
- May require active warming to normothermia
- 12 lead ECG
- Troponin in all cardiac arrest cases
- Echo
- CXR post-recruitment manoeuvres
- Review and stop unnecessary medications

How does organ donation proceed after brain stem death?
The donation process is more predictable than with circulatory death. An anaesthetist may be involved in managing the donor and should be contacted early. Once assent has been given and the retrieval team

is present on site, the patient can be transferred to theatre. A laparotomy and sternotomy are performed. After inspection, vessels may be ligated or cross-clamped depending on organ donated.

Intra-operative anaesthetic management includes the following:

- Warming
- *Monitoring*: F_iO_2, E_tCO_2, BP, intracardiac pressures
- Managing haemodynamic disturbance
- Moderation of spinal reflexes and autonomic responses
- Administration of antibiotics, fluids
- Lung recruitment manoeuvres

Resource
- Corbett S, Trainor, Gaffney A. Perioperative management of the organ donor after diagnosis of death using neurological criteria. BJA Educ. 2021;21(5):194–200.

---

161. DONATION AFTER CIRCULATORY DEATH

When can organ donation occur after circulatory death?

Donation after circulatory death (DCD) can take place after controlled or unexpected cardiac arrest if donors are eligible. The main limitation of DCD, other than eligibility, is susceptibility of organs to warm ischaemia, translated from timings surrounding withdrawal of life-sustaining treatment and retrieval.

DCD is increasing. Demand for organs is rising with the ageing population and accompanying increasing prevalence of organ failures. In addition, DBD has not increased, with the donor group largely coming from those with traumatic injuries and advances in traffic safety over recent decades. Organ support technology has improved, with some DCD organs (e.g. kidneys) now achieving similar long-term outcomes to those from DBD.

How are donors described in the donation pathway?

Both DCD and DBD donors can be classified as follows by the WHO:

- *Possible deceased organ donor*: medical suitability suspected in patient with devastating injury or disease
- *Potential donor*: death anticipated or confirmed
- *Eligible donor*: dead and organ(s) medically suitable
- *Actual donor*: assent given, eligible donor in whom operative incision made or from whom at least 1 organ was recovered for this purpose
- *Utilised donor*: actual donor from whom at least 1 organ was transplanted

Can you name some clinical contraindications to organ donation?

Absolute contraindications are as follows:

- Age ≥ 85 years
- CJD
- History of Ebola virus infection
- WNV infection
- *TB*: active/untreated

Most potential donors with the following will be ineligible:

- Active cancer (excluding some primary brain tumours)
- HIV (rarely donation occurs to other HIV-positive patients if infection present, but not disease)

Organ-specific contraindications also exist.

What legislation exists surrounding 'consent' for donation in the UK?

Organ donation law varies across the UK. Above the age of 18:

Wales
- Deemed consent (2015)
- Considered to have no objection to become a donor unless previously opted out

England
- Opt out system (2020)
- Considered to agree to become a donor unless previously opted out

Scotland
- Deemed authorisation (2021)
- Considered to be willing to become a donor unless previously opted out

Northern Ireland
- Currently opt in, ongoing consultation
- May change in 2023 to opt out system

Practically speaking, the wishes of persons close to the patient will be considered and it is very unlikely that donation will proceed if there is objection despite the presence of opt out systems.

What is the difference between controlled and uncontrolled donation?

Controlled donation describes organ retrieval after expected death (e.g. withdrawal of life-sustaining treatment). Uncontrolled donation occurs after unexpected and irreversible cardiac arrest.

Maastricht classes **III and IV are controlled**. Classes I, II, and V are uncontrolled.

KEY POINT

The Modified Maastricht Classification is as follows:

I. Dead on arrival
II. Unsuccessful resuscitation
III. **Anticipated cardiac arrest**
IV. **Cardiac arrest in brain-dead donor**
V. Unexpected arrest in ICU patient

What are the practical stages involved in controlled DCD in the intensive care unit?

- Decision to withdraw life-sustaining treatment
- Assessment of suitability for organ donation
- Consent/authorisation (involving discussion with relatives and coroner)
- Maintenance of stability
- Withdrawal of life-sustaining treatment (when retrieval team present, often near theatre)
- Palliative care
- Diagnosis of death using circulatory criteria (5 min)
- Brief period for family, if required (5 min)
- Organ retrieval in theatre
- Care after death ('last offices'), family viewing of body, if required
- Team debriefing

Importantly, the transplant team should not be involved in the decision-making or care for the donor patient before death has been confirmed.

What do you know about organ ischaemic time?

Ischaemic time will result in ischaemic organ injury and influence the outcome of the graft in the recipient.

Donor functional warm ischaemia time
- Starts when systolic BP < 50 mmHg, S_aO_2 < 70%, or both (i.e. not the onset of asystole)
- Ends when cold perfusion takes place (cold organ preservation)

Graft cold ischaemia time
- Starts at cold perfusion
- Ends at removal of graft from cold storage

Graft warm ischaemia time
- Starts at removal from cold storage
- Ends at reperfusion (i.e. removal of arterial clamp)

Can you give some examples of how ischaemic time might affect organ suitability for transplantation?
Maximum functional warm ischaemic time (minutes):

- *Liver*: 30 (20 in suboptimal donors)
- *Pancreas*: 30
- *Lung*: 60 (to reinflation rather than cold perfusion)
- *Kidney*: 120 (+ further 120 min in selected donors)

Is it ethically justifiable to perform heart transplantation from a DCD donor?
Heart transplantation has been performed after DCD. There is an apparent contradiction in diagnosing death on circulatory or 'cardiac' grounds, whilst considering the heart viable for transplantation.

From an ethical standpoint, the diagnosis of death applies to the person as a whole, rather than individual organs. In such circumstances it is likely that systemic features have caused the irreversible loss of the capacity to breathe or be conscious, rather than end-stage cardiac disease. The heart may therefore be restarted and transplanted into a recipient.

What ex vivo perfusion techniques are there?
Machine perfusion is often used to improve viability of organs during the time required for transfer to a recipient. This is frequently the case with DCD kidney transplantation.

Lung transplantation will require protection from aspiration and hypoxia. Additional optimisation of organs for transplantation includes the following:

- Tracheal intubation after confirmation of death
- A single recruitment manoeuvre should be performed at least 10 min after mechanical asystole.
- This is followed by CPAP to oxygenate the alveolar epithelium (e.g. 5 cmH_2O).

A donor heart may be perfused ex vivo using the direct procurement and machine perfusion (DPP) technique.

It is also possible to achieve perfusion in vivo using the thoraco-abdominal normothermic regional perfusion (TA-NRP) technique. Thoracic and abdominal organs are perfused in situ after the cerebral circulation is isolated. A period of stability should follow before in-situ assessment of function. Cardioplegia solution is given before explanation to an external system.

Resources
- Flood S, Tordoff C. A new heart for organ donation after circulatory death. BJA Educ. 2020;20(4):126–132.
- Manara AR, Murphy PG, O'Callaghan G. Donation after circulatory death. Br J Anaesth. 2012;108(Suppl 1):i108–121.
- NHS Blood and Transplant. Organ Donation Laws. 2022. Available from: https://www.organdonation.nhs.uk/uk-laws/. (Accessed 29 August 2022.)
- Zalewska K. POLICY POL 188/5.2 Clinical Contraindications to Approaching Families for Possible Organ Donation. December 2015. Available from: http://odt.nhs.uk/pdf/contraindications_to_organ_donation.pdf. (Accessed 14 April 2022.)

SECTION 2: ORGAN SUPPORT

OSCILLATE (2013)	Ferguson ND, Cook DJ, Guyatt GH, et al. High-frequency oscillation in early acute respiratory distress syndrome. N Engl J Med. 2013;368(9):795–805.
OSCAR (2013)	Young D, Lamb SW, Shah S, et al. High-frequency oscillation for acute respiratory distress syndrome. N Engl J Med. 2013;368(9):806–813.
CESAR (2009)	Peek GJ, Mugford M, Tiruvoipati R, et al. Efficacy and economic assessment of conventional ventilatory support versus extracorporeal membrane oxygenation for severe adult respiratory failure (CESAR): a multicentre randomised controlled trial. Lancet. 2009;374(9698):1351–1363.
EOLIA (2018)	Combes A, Hajage D, Capellier G, et al. Extracorporeal membrane oxygenation for severe acute respiratory distress syndrome. N Engl J Med. 2018;378(21):1965–1975.
PROSEVA (2014)	Guérin C, Reignier J, Richard JC, et al. Prone positioning in severe acute respiratory distress syndrome. N Engl J Med. 2013;368(23):2159–2168.
SUPERNOVA (2019)	Combes A, Fanelli V, Pham T, et al. Feasibility and safety of extracorporeal CO_2 removal to enhance protective ventilation in acute respiratory distress syndrome: the SUPERNOVA study. Intensive Care Med. 2019;45(5):592–600.
REST (2021)	McNamee JJ, Gillies MA, Barrett NA, et al. Effect of lower tidal volume ventilation facilitated by extracorporeal carbon dioxide removal vs standard care ventilation on 90-day mortality in patients with acute hypoxemic respiratory failure: The REST randomized clinical trial. JAMA. 2021;326(11):1013–1023.
Subirà et al. (2019)	Subirà C, Hernández G, Vásquez A, et al. Effect of pressure support vs T-piece ventilation strategies during spontaneous breathing trials on successful extubation among patients receiving mechanical ventilation: a randomized clinical trial. JAMA. 2019;321(22):2175–2182.
TracMan (2013)	Young D, Harrison DA, Cuthbertson BH, et al. Effect of early vs late tracheostomy placement on survival in patients receiving mechanical ventilation. JAMA. 2013;309(20):2121–2129.
SPLIT (2015)	Young P, Bailey M, Beasley R, et al. Effect of a buffered crystalloid solution vs saline on acute kidney injury among patients in the intensive care unit. JAMA. 2015;314(16):1701–1710.
SMART (2018)	Semler MW, Self WH, Wanderer JP, et al. Balanced crystalloids versus saline in critically ill adults. N Engl J Med. 2018;378(9):829–839.
PLUS (2022)	Finfer S, Micallef S, Hammond N, et al. Balanced multielectrolyte solution versus saline in critically ill adults. N Engl J Med. 2022;386(9):815–826.
FEAST (2011)	Maitland K, Kiguli S, Opoka RO, et al. Mortality after fluid bolus in African children with severe infection. N Engl J Med. 2011;364(26):2483–2495.
SAFE (2004)	The SAFE Study Investigators. A comparison of albumin and saline for fluid resuscitation in the intensive care unit. N Engl J Med. 2004;350(22):2247–2256.
ALBIOS (2014)	Caironi P, Tognoni G, Masson S, et al. Albumin replacement in patients with severe sepsis or septic shock. N Engl J Med. 2014;370(15):1412–1421.
CHEST (2012)	Myburgh JA, Finfer S, Bellomo R, et al. Hydroxyethyl starch or saline for fluid resuscitation in intensive care. N Engl J Med. 2012;367(20):1901–1911.
6S (2012)	Perner A, Haase N, Guttormsen AB, et al. Hydroxyethyl starch 130/0.42 versus ringer's acetate in severe sepsis. N Engl J Med. 2012;367(2):124–134.

ABC (2008)	Girard TD, Kress JP, Fuchs BD, et al. Efficacy and safety of a paired sedation and ventilator weaning protocol for mechanically ventilated patients in intensive care (Awakening and Breathing Controlled trial): a randomised controlled trial. Lancet. 2008;371(9607):126–134.
SLEAP (2012)	Mehta S, Burry L, Cook D, et al. Daily sedation interruption in mechanically ventilated critically ill patients cared for with a sedation protocol: a randomized controlled trial. JAMA. 2012;308(19):1985–1992.
TTM (2013)	Nielsen N, Wetterslev J, Cronberg T, et al. Targeted temperature management at 33 °C versus 36 °C after cardiac arrest. N Engl J Med. 2013;369(23):2197–2206.
TTM 48 (2017)	Kirkegaard H, Søreide E, de Haas I, et al. Targeted temperature management for 48 vs 24 hours and neurologic outcome after out-of-hospital cardiac arrest: a randomized clinical trial. JAMA. 2017;318(4):341–350.
TTM2 (2021)	Dankiewicz J, Cronberg T, Lilja G, et al. Hypothermia versus normothermia after out-of-hospital cardiac arrest. N Engl J Med. 2021;384(24):2283–2294.
TICACOS (2011)	Singer P, Anbar R, Cohen J, et al. The tight calorie control study (TICACOS): a prospective, randomized, controlled pilot study of nutritional support in critically ill patients. Intensive Care Med. 2011;37(4):601–609.
CALORIES (2014)	Harvey SE, Parrott F, Harrison DA, et al. Trial of the route of early nutritional support in critically ill adults. N Engl J Med. 2014;371(18):1673–1684.
PermiT (2005)	Arabi YM, Aldawood AS, Haddad SH, et al. Permissive underfeeding or standard enteral feeding in critically ill adults. N Engl J Med. 2015; 372(25):2398–2408.
EPaNIC (2011)	Casaer MP, Mesotten D, Hermans G, et al. Early versus late parenteral nutrition in critically ill adults. N Engl J Med. 2011;365(6):506–517.
SUP-ICU (2018)	Krag M, Marker S, Perner A, et al. Pantoprazole in patients at risk for gastrointestinal bleeding in the ICU. N Engl J Med. 2018;379(23):2199-2208.
ATN (2008)	VA/NIH Acute Renal Failure Trial Network. Intensity of renal support in critically ill patients with acute kidney injury. N Engl J Med. 2008;359(1):7–20.
RENAL (2009)	The RENAL Replacement Therapy Study Investigators. Intensity of continuous renal-replacement therapy in critically ill patients. N Engl J Med. 2009;361(17):1627–1638.
IVOIRE (2013)	Joannes-Boyau O, Honoré PM, Perez P, et al. High-volume versus standard-volume haemofiltration for septic shock patients with acute kidney injury (IVOIRE study): a multicentre randomized controlled trial. Intensive Care Med. 2013;39(9):1535–1546.
Zarbock et al. (2020)	Zarbock A, Küllmar M, Kindgen-Milles D, et al. Effect of regional citrate anticoagulation vs systemic heparin anticoagulation during continuous kidney replacement therapy on dialysis filter life span and mortality among critical care patients with acute kidney injury: a randomized clinical trial. JAMA. 2020;324(16):1629–1639.

SECTION 3: ON THE ICU

ARDSNet (2000)	The Acute Respiratory Distress Syndrome Network. Ventilation with lower tidal volumes as compared with traditional tidal volumes for acute lung injury and the acute respiratory distress syndrome. N Engl J Med. 2000;342(18):1301–1308.
ALVEOLI (2004)	The National Heart, Lung, and Blood Institute ARDS Clinical Trials Network. Higher versus lower positive end-expiratory pressures in patients with the acute respiratory distress syndrome. N Engl J Med. 2004;351(4):327–336.
ROSE (2019)	The National Heart, Lung, and Blood Institute PETAL Clinical Trials Network. Early neuromuscular blockade in the acute respiratory distress syndrome. N Engl J Med. 2019;380(21):1997–2008.
ACURASYS (2010)	Papazian L, Forel J-M, Gacouin A, et al. Neuromuscular blockers in early acute respiratory distress syndrome. N Engl J Med. 2010;363(12):1107–1116.
Meduri et al. (2007)	Meduri GU, Golden E, Freire AX, et al. Methylprednisolone infusion in early severe ARDS: results of a randomized controlled trial. Chest. 2007;131(4):954–963.

DEXA-ARDS (2020)	Villar J, Ferrando C, Martínez C, et al. Dexamethasone treatment for the acute respiratory distress syndrome: a multicentre, randomised controlled trial. Lancet Respir Med. 2020;8(3):267–276.
SOAP II (2010)	De Backer D, Biston P, Devriendt J, et al. Comparison of dopamine and norepinephrine in the treatment of shock. N Engl J Med. 2010;362(9):779–789.
ANDROMEDA-SHOCK (2019)	Hernández G, Ospina-Tascón GA, Damani LP, et al. Effect of a resuscitation strategy targeting peripheral perfusion status vs serum lactate levels on 28-day mortality among patients with septic shock: the ANDROMEDA-SHOCK randomized clinical trial. JAMA. 2019;321(7):654–664.
Rivers et al. (2001)	River E, Nguyen B, Havstad S, et al. Early goal-directed therapy in the treatment of severe sepsis and septic shock. N Engl J Med. 2001;345(19):1368–1377.
ICU-ROX (2019)	The ICU-ROX Investigators and the Australian and New Zealand Intensive Care Society Clinical Trials Group. Conservative oxygen therapy during mechanical ventilation in the ICU. N Engl J Med. 2020;382(11):989–998.
HOT-ICU (2021)	Schjørring OL, Klitgaard TL, Perner A, et al. Lower or higher oxygenation targets for acute hypoxemic respiratory failure. N Engl J Med. 2021;384(14):1301–1311.
ARISE (2014)	The ARISE Investigators and the ANZICS Clinical Trials Group. Goal-directed resuscitation for patients with early septic shock. N Engl J Med. 2014;371(16):1496–1506.
ProCESS (2014)	The ProCESS Investigators. A randomized trial of protocol-based care for early septic shock. N Engl J Med. 2014;370(18):1683–1693.
ProMISe (2015)	Mouncey PR, Osborn TM, Power S, et al. Trial of Early, goal-directed resuscitation for septic shock. N Engl J Med. 2015;372(14):1301–1311.
SEPSISPAM (2014)	Asfar P, Meziani F, Hamel J. High versus low blood-pressure target in patients with septic shock. N Engl J Med. 2014;370(17):1583–1593.
65 (2020)	Lamontagne F, Richards-Belle A, Thomas K, et al. Effect of reduced exposure to vasopressors on 90-day mortality in older critically ill patients with vasodilatory hypotension: a randomized clinical trial. JAMA. 2020;323(10):938–949.
VASST (2008)	Russell JA, Walley KR, Singer J, et al. Vasopressin versus norepinephrine infusion in patients with septic shock. N Engl J Med. 2008;358(9):877–887.
PROWESS (2001)	Bernard GR, Vincent J, Laterre P, et al. Efficacy and safety of recombinant human activated protein C for severe sepsis. N Engl J Med. 2001;344(10):699–709.
PROWESS-SHOCK (2012)	Ranieri VM, Thompson BT, Barie PS, et al. Drotrecogin alfa (activated) in adults with septic shock. N Engl J Med. 2012;366(22):2055–2064.
CITRIS-ALI (2019)	Fowler AA, Truwit JD, Hite RD, et al. Effect of vitamin c infusion on organ failure and biomarkers of inflammation and vascular injury in patients with sepsis and severe acute respiratory failure: the CITRIS-ALI randomized clinical trial. JAMA 2019;322(13):1261–1270.
LOVIT (2022)	Lamontagne F, Masse MH, Menard J, et al. Intravenous vitamin C in adults with sepsis in the intensive care unit. N Engl J Med. 2022;386(25):2387–2398.
PARAMEDIC2 (2018)	Perkins GD, Ji C, Deakin CD, et al. A randomized trial of epinephrine in out-of-hospital cardiac arrest. N Engl J Med. 2018;379(8):711–721.
TOMAHAWK (2021)	Desch S, Freund A, Akin I, et al. Angiography after out-of-hospital cardiac arrest without ST-segment elevation. N Engl J Med. 2021;385(27):2544–2553.
ARREST (2020)	Yannopoulos D, Bartos J, Raveendran G, et al. Advanced reperfusion strategies for patients with out-of-hospital cardiac arrest and refractory ventricular fibrillation (ARREST): a phase 2, single centre, open-label, randomised controlled trial. Lancet. 2020;396(10265):1807–1186.
DahLIA (2016)	Reade MC, Eastwood GM, Bellomo R, et al. Effect of dexmedetomidine added to standard care on ventilator-free time in patients with agitated delirium. JAMA. 2016;315(14);1460–1468.
Hope-ICU (2013)	Page VJ, Ely EW, Gates S, et al. Effect of intravenous haloperidol on the duration of delirium and coma in critically ill patients (Hope-ICU): a randomised, double-blind, placebo-controlled trial. Lancet Respir Med. 2013;1(7):515–523.

SECTION 6: RESUSCITATION

ITACTIC (2020)	Baksaas-Aasen K, Gall LS, Stensballe J, et al. Viscoelastic haemostatic assay augmented protocols for major trauma haemorrhage (ITACTIC): a randomized, controlled trial. Intensive Care Med. 2021;47(1):49–59.
CRASH-2 (2010)	CRASH-2 trial collaborators. Effects of tranexamic acid on death, vascular occlusive events, and blood transfusion in trauma patients with significant haemorrhage (CRASH-2): a randomised, placebo-controlled trial. Lancet. 2010;376(9734):23–32.
CRASH-3 (2019)	The CRASH-3 trial collaborators. Effects of tranexamic acid on death, disability, vascular occlusive events and other morbidities in patients with acute traumatic brain injury (CRASH-3): a randomised, placebo-controlled trial. Lancet. 2019;394(10210):1713–1723.
PROPPR (2015)	Holcomb JB, Tilley BC, Baraniuk S. Transfusion of plasma, platelets, and red blood cells in a 1:1:1 vs a 1:1:2 ratio and mortality in patients with severe trauma: the PROPPR randomized clinical trial. JAMA. 2015;313(5):471–482.
CRYOSTAT-1 (2015)	Curry N, Rourke C, Davenport R, et al. Early cryoprecipitate for major haemorrhage in trauma: a randomised controlled feasibility trial. Br J Anaesth. 2015;115(1):76–83.
TRICC (1999)	Hébert PC, Wells G, Blajchman MA, et al. A multicenter, randomized, controlled clinical trial of transfusion requirements in critical care. N Engl J Med. 1999;340(6):409–417.
TRISS (2014)	Holst LB, Haase N, Wetterslev J, et al. Lower versus higher hemoglobin threshold for transfusion in septic shock. N Engl J Med. 2014;371(15):1381–1391.
TRICS-III (2017)	Mazer CD, Whitlock RP, Fergusson DA, et al. Restrictive or liberal red-cell transfusion for cardiac surgery. N Engl J Med. 2017;377(22):2133–2144.

SECTION 7: SURGERY

IMPROVE (2014)	IMPROVE trial investigators. Observations from the IMPROVE trial concerning the clinical care of patients with ruptured abdominal aortic aneurysm. Br J Surg. 2014;101(3):216–224.

SECTION 8: CARDIOTHORACICS

ISIS-2 (1988)	ISIS-2 (Second International Study of Infarct Survival) Collaborative Group. Randomised trial of intravenous streptokinase, oral aspirin, both, or neither among 17,187 cases of suspected acute myocardial infarction: ISIS-2. Lancet. 1988;2(8607):349–360.
NORDISTEMI (2010)	Bøhmer E, Hoffmann P, Abdelnoor M, et al. Efficacy and safety of immediate angioplasty versus ischaemia-guided management after thrombolysis in acute myocardial infarction in areas with very long transfer distances results of the NORDISTEMI (NORwegian study on DIstinct treatment of ST-elevation myocardial infarction). J Am Coll Cardiol. 2010;55(2):102–110.
POISE (2008)	POISE Study Group. Effects of extended-release metoprolol succinate in patients undergoing non-cardiac surgery (POISE trial): a randomised controlled trial. Lancet. 2008;371(9627):1839–1847.
REMATCH (2001)	Rose EA, Gelijns AC, Moskowitz AJ, et al. Long-term use of a left ventricular assist device for end-stage heart failure. N Engl J Med. 2001;345(20):1435–1443.
SHOCK (1999)	Hochman JS, Sleeper LA, Webb JG, et al. Early revascularization in acute myocardial infarction complicated by cardiogenic shock. N Engl J Med. 1999;341(9):625–634.
IABP-SHOCK II (2012)	Thiele H, Zeymer U, Neumann FJ, et al. Intraaortic balloon support for myocardial infarction with cardiogenic shock. N Engl J Med. 2012;367(14):1287–1296.
CARRESS-HF (2012)	Bart BA, Goldsmith SR, Lee KL, et al. Ultrafiltration in decompensated heart failure with cardiorenal syndrome. N Engl J Med. 2012;367(24):2296–2304.
PAC-Man (2005)	Harvey S, Harrison DA, Singer M, et al. Assessment of the clinical effectiveness of pulmonary artery catheters in management of patients in intensive care (PAC-Man): a randomised controlled trial. Lancet. 2005;366(9484):472–477.

SECTION 9: NEUROSCIENCES

MASH-2 (2012)	Mees SMD, Algra A, Vandertop WP, et al. Magnesium for aneurysmal subarachnoid haemorrhage (MASH-2): a randomised placebo-controlled trial. Lancet. 2012;380(9836):44–49.
ULTRA (2021)	Post R, Germans MR, Tjerkstra MA, et al. Ultra-early tranexamic acid after subarachnoid haemorrhage (ULTRA): a randomised controlled trial. Lancet. 2020;397(10269):112–118.
STASH (2014)	Kirkpatrick PJ, Turner CL, Smith C, et al. Simvastatin in aneurysmal subarachnoid haemorrhage (STASH): a multicentre randomised phase 3 trial. Lancet Neurol. 2014;13(7):666–675.
ISAT (2005)	Molyneux AJ, Kerr RSC, Clarke M, et al. International subarachnoid aneurysm trial (ISAT) or neurosurgical clipping versus endovascular coiling in 2143 patients with ruptured intracranial aneurysms: a randomised comparison of effects on survival, dependency, seizures, rebleeding, subgroups, and aneurysm occlusion. Lancet. 2005;366(9488):809–817.
DECRA (2011)	Cooper DJ, Rosenfeld JV, Murray L, et al. Decompressive craniectomy in diffuse traumatic brain injury. N Engl J Med. 2011;364(16):1493–1502.
RESCUEicp (2016)	Hutchinson PJ, Kolias AG, Timfeev IS, et al. Trial of decompressive craniectomy for traumatic intracranial hypertension. N Engl J Med. 2016;375(12):1119–1130.
CRASH (2004)	CRASH trial collaborators. Effect of intravenous corticosteroids on death within 14 days in 10008 adults with clinically significant head injury (MRC CRASH trial): randomised placebo-controlled trial. Lancet. 2004;364(9442):1321–1328.
Eurotherm3235 (2015)	Andrews PJD, Sinclair HL, Rodriguez A, et al. Hypothermia for Intracranial hypertension after traumatic brain injury. N Engl J Med. 2015;373(25):2403–2412.
POLAR (2018)	Cooper DJ, Nichol AD, Bailey M, et al. Effect of early sustained prophylactic hypothermia on neurologic outcomes among patients with severe traumatic brain injury. JAMA. 2018;320(21):2211–2220.
INTERACT2 (2013)	Anderson CS, Heeley E, Huang Y, et al. Rapid blood-pressure lowering in patients with acute intracerebral hemorrhage. N Engl J Med. 2013;368(25):2355–2365.
ATACH-2 (2016)	Qureshi AI, Palesch YY, Barsan WG, et al. Intensive blood-pressure lowering in patients with acute cerebral haemorrhage. N Engl J Med. 2016;375(11):1033–1043.
TICH-2 (2018)	Sprigg N, Flaherty K, Appleton JP, et al. Tranexamic acid for hyperacute primary IntraCerebral Haemorrhage (TICH-2): an international randomised, placebo-controlled, phase 3 superiority trial. Lancet. 2018;391(10135):2107–2115.
STICH (1998)	Morgenstern LB, Frankowski RF, Shedden P, et al. Surgical treatment for intracerebral haemorrhage (STICH): a single-center, randomized clinical trial. Neurology. 1998;51(5):1359–1363.
STICH II (2013)	Mendelow AD, Gregson BA, Rowan EN, et al. Early surgery versus initial conservative treatment in patients with spontaneous supratentorial intracerebral haematomas (STICH II): a randomised trial. Lancet. 2013;382(9890):397–408.
STITCH[Trauma] (2015)	Mendelov AD, Gregson BA, Rowan EN, et al. Early surgery versus initial conservative treatment in patients with traumatic intracerebral hemorrhage (STITCH [Trauma]): the first randomized trial. J Neurotrauma. 2015;32(17):1312–1323.
NINDS (1995)	The National Institute of Neurological Disorders and Stroke rt-PA Stroke Study Group. Tissue plasminogen activator for acute ischemic stroke. N Engl J Med. 1995;333(24):1581–1587.
IST-3 (2012)	The IST-3 collaborative group. The benefits and harms of intravenous thrombolysis with recombinant tissue plasminogen activator within 6 h of acute ischaemic stroke (the third international stroke trial [IST-3]): a randomised controlled trial. Lancet. 2012;379(9834):2352–2363.
EuroHYP-1 (2018)	Schwab S. EuroHYP-1 Final Report: Publishable Summary. November 2018. Available from: https://cordis.europa.eu/docs/results/278/278709/final1-final-report-publishable-summary-30nov2018-vf1-0.pdf. (Accessed 5 January 2023.)

DAWN (2018)	Nogueira RG, Jadhav AP, Haussen DC, et al. Thrombectomy 6 to 24 hours after stroke with a mismatch between deficit and infarct. N Engl J Med. 2018;378(1):11–21.
DEFUSE 3 (2018)	Albers GW, Marks MP, Kemp S, et al. Thrombectomy for stroke at 6 to 16 hours with selection by perfusion imaging. N Engl J Med. 2018;378(8):708–718.
DESTINY (2007)	Jüttler E, Schwab S, Schmiedek P, et al. Decompressive surgery for the treatment of malignant infarction of the middle cerebral artery (DESTINY): a randomized, controlled trial. Stroke. 2007;38(9):2518–2525.
DECIMAL (2007)	Vahedi K, Vicaut E, Mateo J, et al. Sequential-design, multicenter, randomized, controlled trial of early decompressive craniectomy in malignant middle cerebral artery infarction (DECIMAL Trial). Stroke. 2007;38(9):2506–2517.
HAMLET (2009)	Hofmeijer J, Kappelle LJ, Algra A, et al. Surgical decompression for space-occupying cerebral infarction (the hemicraniectomy after middle cerebral artery infarction with life-threatening edema trial [HAMLET]): a multicentre, open, randomised trial. Lancet Neurol. 2009;8(4):326–333.
DESTINY II (2011)	Jüttler E, Bösel J, Amiri H, et al. DESTINY II: DEcompressive Surgery for the Treatment of malignant INfarction of the middle cerebral arterY II. Int J Stroke. 2011;6(1):79–86.
HYBERNATUS (2016)	Legriel S, Lemiale V, Schenck M, et al. Hypothermia for neuroprotection in convulsive status epilepticus. N Engl J Med. 2016;375(25):2457–2467.
Brouwer et al. (2015)	Brouwer MC, McIntyre P, Prasad K, et al. Corticosteroids for acute bacterial meningitis. Cochrane Database Syst Rev. 2015;2015(9):CD004405.
NASCIS 2 (1990)	Bracken MB, Shepard MJ, Collins WF, et al. A randomized, controlled trial of methylprednisolone or naloxone in the treatment of acute spinal-cord injury. Results of the Second National Acute Spinal Cord Injury Study. N Engl J Med. 1990;322(20):1405–1411.

SECTION 10: OBSTETRICS

INTERCOVID (2021)	Villar J, Ariff S, Gunier RB, et al. Maternal and neonatal morbidity and mortality among pregnant women with and without COVID-19 infection: the INTERCOVID multinational cohort study. JAMA Pediatr. 2021;175(8):817–826.
Magpie (2002)	The Magpie Trial Collaborative Group. Do women with pre-eclampsia, and their babies, benefit from magnesium sulphate? The Magpie Trial: a randomised placebo-controlled trial. Lancet. 2002;359(9321):1877–1890.
WOMAN (2017)	WOMAN Trial Collaborators. Effect of early tranexamic acid administration on mortality, hysterectomy, and other morbidities in women with post-partum haemorrhage (WOMAN): an international, randomised, double-blind, placebo-controlled trial. Lancet. 2017;389(10084):2105–2116.

SECTION 13: MEDICINE

3Mg (2013)	Goodacre S, Cohen J, Bradburn M, et al. Intravenous or nebulised magnesium sulphate versus standard therapy for severe acute asthma (3Mg trial): a double-blind, randomised controlled trial. Lancet Respir Med. 2013;1(4):293–300.
Middleton et al. (2019)	Middleton PG, Mall MA, Dřevínek P, et al. Elexacaftor–Tezacaftor–Ivacaftor for cystic fibrosis with a single Phe508del allele. N Engl J Med. 2019;381(19):1809–1819.
Delclaux et al. (2000)	Delclaux C, L'Her E, Alberti C, et al. Treatment of acute hypoxemic nonhypercapnic respiratory insufficiency with continuous positive airway pressure delivered by a face mask: a randomized controlled trial. JAMA. 2000;284(18):2352–2360.
FLORALI (2015)	Frat JP, Whille AW, Mercat A, et al. High-flow oxygen through nasal cannula in acute hypoxemic respiratory failure. N Engl J Med. 2015;372(23):2185–2196.
DIABOLO (2016)	Faisy C, Meziani F, Planquette B, et al. Effect of acetazolamide vs placebo on duration of invasive mechanical ventilation among patients with chronic obstructive pulmonary disease: a randomized clinical trial. JAMA. 2016;315(5):480–488.

REMAP-CAP (2020) Corticosteroid	The Writing Committee for the REMAP-CAP Investigators. Effect of hydrocortisone on mortality and organ support in patients with severe COVID-19: the REMAP-CAP COVID-19 corticosteroid domain randomized clinical trial. JAMA. 2020;324(13):1317–1329.
RECOVERY (2021) Dexamethasone	The RECOVERY Collaborative Group. Dexamethasone in hospitalized patients with Covid-19. N Engl J Med. 2021;384(8):693–704.
REMAP-CAP (2021) IL-6	The REMAP-CAP Investigators. Interleukin-6 receptor antagonists in critically ill patients with Covid-19. N Engl J Med. 2021;384(16):1491–1502.
RECOVERY (2022) Casirivimab/imdevimab	RECOVERY Collaborative Group. Casirivimab and imdevimab in patients admitted to hospital with COVID-19 (RECOVERY): a randomised, controlled, open-label, platform trial. Lancet. 2022;399(10325):665–676.
RECOVERY (2022) Baricitinib	RECOVERY Collaborative Group. Baricitinib in patients admitted to hospital with COVID-19 (RECOVERY): a randomised, controlled, open-label, platform trial and updated meta-analysis. Lancet. 2022;400(10349):359–368.
MOPETT (2013)	Sharifi M, Bay C, Skrocki L, et al. Moderate pulmonary embolism treated with thrombolysis (from the "MOPETT" Trial). Am J Cardiol. 2013;111(2):273–277.
PEITHO (2014)	Meyer G, Vicaut E, Danays T, et al. Fibrinolysis for patients with intermediate-risk pulmonary embolism. N Engl J Med. 2014;370(15):1402–1411.
STARRT-AKI (2020)	The STARRT-AKI Investigators for the Canadian Critical Care Trials Group, the Australian and New Zealand Intensive Care Society Clinical Trials Group, the United Kingdom Critical Care Research Group, the Canadian Nephrology Trials Network, and the Irish Critical Care Trials Group. Timing of initiation of renal-replacement therapy in acute kidney injury. N Engl J Med. 2020;383(3):240–251.
AKIKI (2016)	Gaudry S, Hajage D, Schortgen F, et al. Initiation strategies for renal-replacement therapy in the intensive care unit. N Engl J Med. 2016;375(2):122–133.
ELAIN (2016)	Zarbock A, Kellum JA, Schmidt C, et al. Effect of early vs delayed initiation of renal replacement therapy on mortality in critically ill patients with acute kidney injury: the ELAIN randomized clinical trial. JAMA. 2016;315(20):2190–2199.
BICAR-ICU (2018)	Jaber S, Paugam C, Futier E, et al. Sodium bicarbonate therapy for patients with severe metabolic acidaemia in the intensive care unit (BICAR-ICU): a multicentre, open-label, randomised controlled, phase 3 trial. Lancet. 2018;392(10141):31–40.
Sort et al. (1999)	Sort P, Navasa M, Arroyo V, et al. Effect of intravenous albumin on renal impairment and mortality in patients with cirrhosis and spontaneous bacterial peritonitis. N Engl J Med. 1999;341(6):403–409.
Villanueva et al. (2013)	Villanueva C, Colomo A, Bosch A, et al. Transfusion strategies for acute upper gastrointestinal bleeding. N Engl J Med. 2013;368(1):11–21.
HALT-IT (2020)	The HALT-IT Trial Collaborators. Effects of a high-dose 24h infusion of tranexamic acid on death and thromboembolic events in patients with acute gastrointestinal bleeding (HALT-IT): an international randomised, double-blind, placebo-controlled trial. Lancet. 2020;395(10241):1927–1936.
Escorsell et al. (2016)	Escorsell À, Pavel O, Cárdenas A, et al. Esophageal balloon tamponade versus esophageal stent in controlling acute refractory variceal bleeding: A multicenter randomized, controlled trial. Hepatology. 2016;63(6):1957–1967.
Pettie et al. (2019)	Pettie JM, Caparrotta TM, Hunter RW, et al. Safety and efficacy of the snap 12-hour acetylcysteine regimen for the treatment of paracetamol overdose. EClinicalMedicine. 2019;11:11–17.
STOPAH (2015)	Thursz MR, Richardson P, Allison M, et al. Prednisolone or pentoxifylline for alcoholic hepatitis. N Engl J Med. 2015;372(17):1619–1628.
CORTICUS (2008)	Sprung CL, Annane D, Keh D, et al. Hydrocortisone therapy for patients with septic shock. N Engl J Med. 2008;358(2):111–124.
Marik et al. (2017)	Marik PE, Khangoora V, Rivera R, et al. Hydrocortisone, vitamin c, and thiamine for the treatment of severe sepsis and septic shock: a retrospective before-after study. Chest. 2017;151(6):1229–1238.
ADRENAL (2018)	Venkatesh B, Finfer S, Cohen J, et al. Adjunctive glucocorticoid therapy in patients with septic shock. N Engl J Med. 2018;378(9):797–808.

| APROCCHSS (2018) | Annane D, Renault A, Brun-Buisson C, et al. Hydrocortisone plus fludrocortisone for adults with septic shock. N Engl J Med. 2018;378(9):809–818. |
| NICE-SUGAR (2009) | The NICE-SUGAR Study Investigators. Intensive versus conventional glucose control in critically ill patients. N Engl J Med. 2009;360(13):1283–1297. |

SECTION 14: PALLIATIVE CARE

| Ethicus-2 (2021) | Avidan A, Sprung CL, Schefold JC, et al. Variations in end-of-life practices in intensive care units worldwide (Ethicus-2): a prospective observational study. Lancet. Respir Med. 2021;9(10):1101–1110. |

SECTION 1: ORGANISATIONAL ISSUES

FICM ICS 2022 GPICS 2.1	The Faculty of Intensive Care Medicine, Intensive Care Society. Guidelines for the Provision of Intensive Care Services, version 2.1. July 2022. Available from: https://www.ics.ac.uk/Society/Guidelines/GPICS/Society/Guidance/GPICS_Version_2.1.aspx?hkey=5dda1ac0-eec7-4b9c-881f-e72f4882d639. (Accessed 1 September 2022.)
ICS FICM 2019 Transfer	Intensive Care Society, The Faculty of Intensive Care Medicine. Guidance On: The Transfer of The Critically Ill Adult. May 2019. Available from: https://www.ics.ac.uk/ICU/Guidance/PDFs/Patient_Transfer_Guidance. (Accessed 16 January 2022.)
NHS 2018 Never Events	NHS Improvement. Never Events list 2018: First published January 2018 (last updated February 2021). Available from: https://www.england.nhs.uk/wp-content/uploads/2020/11/2018-Never-Events-List-updated-February-2021.pdf. (Accessed 14 November 2021.)
NHS 2020 Major Incidents	NHS England. Clinical Guidelines for Major Incidents and Mass Casualty Events. September 2020. Available from: https://www.england.nhs.uk/wp-content/uploads/2018/12/B0128-clinical-guidelines-for-use-in-a-major-incident-v2-2020.pdf. (Accessed 21 February 2022.)
ICS AoA 2021 Fire	Kelly FE, Bailey CR, Aldridge P, et al. Fire safety and emergency evacuation guidelines for intensive care units and operating theatres: for use in the event of fire, flood, power cut, oxygen supply failure, noxious gas, structural collapse or other critical incidents. Anaesthesia. 2021;76(10):1377–1391.

SECTION 2: ORGAN SUPPORT

FICM ICS 2018 ARDS	The Faculty of Intensive Care Medicine, Intensive Care Society. Guidelines on the Management of Acute Respiratory Distress Syndrome. July 2018. Available from: https://www.ics.ac.uk/ICU/Guidance/PDFs/Management_of_ARDS. (Accessed 18 January 2022.)
FICM ICS 2019 Proning	The Faculty of Intensive Care Medicine, Intensive Care Society. Guidance For: Prone Positioning in Adult Critical Care. November 2019. Available from: https://static1.squarespace.com/static/5e6613a1dc75b87df82b78e1/t/5e72187c06c2956228316545/1584535679039/FICM-ICS-Prone-Position-Adult-Full.pdf. (Accessed 18 January 2022.)
Resuscitation Council UK NSGBI SBNS 2014 Neurosurgery	Working group of the Resuscitation Council (UK), Neuroanaesthesia Society of Great Britain and Ireland, Society of British Neurological Surgeons 2014. Management of cardiac arrest during neurosurgery in adults: Guidelines for healthcare providers. August 2014. Available from: https://www.resus.org.uk/sites/default/files/2020-05/CPR_in_neurosurgical_patients.pdf. (Accessed 18 January 2022.)
ICS 2020 Conscious Proning	Bamford P, Bentley A, Dean J, et al. ICS Guidance for Prone Positioning of the Conscious COVID Patient 2020. 2020. Available from: https://static1.squarespace.com/static/5e6613a1dc75b87df82b78e1/t/5e99e7f60755047b87934d6e/1587144697447/2020-04-12+Guidance+for+conscious+proning.pdf. (Accessed 18 January 2022.)
ELSO 2017 ECLS	ELSO Guidelines for Cardiopulmonary Extracorporeal Life Support. Extracorporeal Life Support Organization, Version 1.4. August 2017. Ann Arbor, MI, USA. Available from: https://www.elso.org/ecmo-resources/elso-ecmo-guidelines.aspx. (Accessed 20 March 2022.)
ELSO 2021 VV ECMO	Tonna JE, Abrams D, Brodie D, et al. Management of Adult Patients Supported with Venovenous Extracorporeal Membrane Oxygenation (VV ECMO): Guideline from the Extracorporeal Life Support Organization (ELSO). ASAIO J. 2021;67(6):601–610.

NTSP ICS 2020 Tracheostomy	The Short-life Standards and Guidelines Working Party of the UK National Tracheostomy Safety Project. Guidance for: Tracheostomy Care. August 2020. Available from: https://www.ficm.ac.uk/sites/ficm/files/documents/2021-11/2020-08%20Tracheostomy_care_guidance_Final.pdf. (Accessed 18 January 2022.)
ESC 2021 Cardiac pacing	Glikson M, Nielsen JC, Kronborg MB, et al. 2021 ESC Guidelines on cardiac pacing and cardiac resynchronization therapy: Developed by the Task Force on cardiac pacing and cardiac resynchronization therapy of the European Society of Cardiology (ESC) With the special contribution of the European Heart Rhythm Association (EHRA). Eur Heart J. 2021;42(35):3247–3520.
NCS ESICM 2014 Multimodal monitoring	Le Roux P, Menon DK, Citerio G, et al. The International Multidisciplinary Consensus conference on multimodality monitoring In neurocritical care: a list of recommendations and additional conclusions: a statement for healthcare professionals from the Neurocritical Care Society and the European Society of Intensive Care Medicine. Neurocrit Care. 2014;21(Suppl 2):S282–S296.
ERC 2021 Post-resuscitation care	Nolan JP, Sandroni C, Böttiger BW, et al. European Resuscitation Council and European Society of Intensive Care Medicine guidelines 2021: post-resuscitation care. Intensive Care Med. 2021;47:369–421.
ERC-ESICM 2022 Temperature management	Sandroni C, Nolan JP, Andersen LW, et al. ERC-ESICM guidelines on temperature control after cardiac arrest in adults. Intensive Care Med. 2022;48(3):261–269.
NICE 2017 CG32 Nutrition	National Institute for Health and Care Excellence. Nutrition support for adults: oral nutrition support, enteral tube feeding and parenteral nutrition: Clinical guideline [CG32]. February 2006 (Updated August 2017). Available from: https://www.nice.org.uk/guidance/cg32/chapter/1-Guidance. (Accessed 19 January 2022.)
ESPEN 2019 Nutrition	Singer P, Blaser AR, Berger MM, et al. ESPEN guideline on clinical nutrition in the intensive care unit. Clin Nutr. 2019;38(1):48–79.
KDIGO 2012 AKI	Kidney Disease: Improving Global Outcomes (KDIGO) Acute Kidney Injury Work Group. KDIGO clinical practice guideline for acute kidney injury. Kidney Inter Suppl. 2012;2(1):1–138.
American Society for Apheresis 2019 Therapeutic apheresis	Padmanabhan A, Connelly-Smith L, Aqui N, et al. Guidelines on the use of therapeutic apheresis in clinical practice – evidence-based approach from the writing committee of the American Society for Apheresis: The Eighth Special Issue. J Clin Apher. 2019;34(3);171–354.
BCSH 2015 Apheresis	Howell C, Douglas K, Cho G, et al. Guideline on the clinical use of apheresis procedures for the treatment of patients and collection of cellular therapy products. Transfus Med. 2015;25(2):57–78.
NICE 2009 CG83 Rehabilitation	National Institute for Health and Care Excellence. Rehabilitation after critical illness in adults: Clinical guideline [CG83]. March 2009. Available from: https://www.nice.org.uk/guidance/cg83. (Accessed 10 February 2022.)
NICE 2017 QS158 Rehabilitation	National Institute for Health and Care Excellence. Rehabilitation after critical illness in adults: Quality standard [QS158]. September 2017. Available from: https://www.nice.org.uk/guidance/qs158. (Accessed 10 February 2022.)

SECTION 3: ON THE ICU

FICM ICS 2018 ARDS	The Faculty of Intensive Care Medicine, Intensive Care Society. Guidelines on the management of Acute Respiratory Distress Syndrome. July 2018. Available from: https://www.ficm.ac.uk/sites/ficm/files/documents/2021-10/Guidelines_on_the_Management_of_Acute_Respiratory_Distress_Syndrome.pdf. (Accessed 30 March 2022.)
BTS 2017 Oxygen	O'Driscoll BR, Howard LS, Earis J, et al. BTS guideline for oxygen use in adults in healthcare and emergency settings. Thorax. 2017;72(Suppl 1):ii1–ii90.
ELSO 2021 E-CPR	Richardson AC, Tonna JE, Nanjayya V, et al. Extracorporeal cardiopulmonary resuscitation in adults. Interim Guideline Consensus Statement from the Extracorporeal Life Support Organization. ASAIO J. 2021;67(3):221–228.
SSC 2021 Sepsis	Evans L, Rhodes A, Waleed A, et al. Surviving sepsis campaign: International Guidelines for Management of Sepsis and Septic Shock 2021. Crit Care Med. 2021;49(11):e1063–e1143.

Resuscitation Council UK 2021 Adult advanced life support	Soar J, Deakin CD, Nolan JP, et al. Resuscitation Council UK: Adult advanced life support Guidelines. May 2021. Available from: https://www.resus.org.uk/library/2021-resuscitation-guidelines/adult-advanced-life-support-guidelines. (Accessed 20 January 2022.)
ERC ESICM 2021 Post-resuscitation care	Nolan JP, Sandroni C, Böttiger BW, et al. European Resuscitation Council and European Society of Intensive Care Medicine Guidelines 2021: Post-resuscitation care. Resuscitation. 2021;161:220–269.
ICS 2017 Eye care	Lightman S, Montgomery H. Ophthalmic Services Guideline: Eye Care in the Intensive Care Unit (ICU). June 2017. Available from: https://www.rcophth.ac.uk/wp-content/uploads/2021/01/Intensive-Care-Unit.pdf. (Accessed 20 January 2022.)
NICE 2019 CG103 Delirium	National Institute for Health and Care Excellence. Delirium: prevention, diagnosis and management: Clinical guideline [CG103]. July 2010 (Updated March 2019). Available from: https://www.nice.org.uk/guidance/cg103. (Accessed 07 March 2022.)
ICS 2014 Analgesia & Sedation	Whitehouse T, Snelson C, Grounds M. (Eds.) Intensive Care Society Review of Best Practice for Analgesia and Sedation in the Critical Care. June 2014. Available from: https://www.wyccn.org/uploads/6/5/1/9/65199375/sedation_for_patients_in_icu_2014.pdf. (Accessed 27 April 2022.)
PADIS 2018	Devlin JW, Skrobik Y, Gélinas C, et al. Clinical Practice Guidelines for the Prevention and Management of Pain, Agitation/Sedation, Delirium, Immobility, and Sleep Disruption in Adult Patients in the ICU. Crit Care Med. 2018;46(9):e825–e873. Available from: https://www.nice.org.uk/guidance/cg103/. (Accessed 20 January 2022.)

SECTION 4: TOXICOLOGY

UK Legislation 1983 Mental Health Act 1983	Legislation.gov.uk. 1983. Mental Health Act 1983. Chapter 20. Available from: https://www.legislation.gov.uk/ukpga/1983/20/contents. (Accessed 15 January 2022.)
UK Legislation 2005 Mental Capacity Act 2005	Legislation.gov.uk. 2005. Mental Capacity Act 2005. Available from: https://www.legislation.gov.uk/ukpga/2005/9/contents. (Accessed 15 January 2022.)
BMA 2020 DOLS	British Medical Association. Deprivation of Liberty Safeguards - guidance for doctors. September 2020. Available from: https://www.bma.org.uk/media/3087/bma-deprivation-of-liberty-safeguards-guidance-september-2020.pdf. (Accessed 15 January 2022.)
FICM 2021 Midnight Laws	The Faculty of Intensive Care Medicine. Midnight Laws. Available from: https://www.ficm.ac.uk/midnightlaws. (Accessed 15 January 2022.) • Deprivation of Liberty in Intensive Care (July 2021) • Approaching Plans for the Person with a Disability (England & Wales) (November 2020) • Approaching Plans for the Person with a Disability (Scotland) (November 2020) • Disclosure of Genetic Information to a Relative without a Patient's Consent (November 2020) • Child Protection and Safeguarding (May 2020) • Relatives Recording Conversations (October 2019) • Disagreement on Best Interests (England and NI) (August 2019) • Disagreement regarding the treatment of patients who lack capacity (Scotland) (August 2019) • Police Access to Critical Care Patients (August 2019)
RCEM 2022 Acute Behavioural Disturbance	The Royal College of Emergency Medicine. Best Practice Guideline: Acute Behavioural Disturbance in Emergency Departments. February 2022. Available from: https://rcem.ac.uk/wp-content/uploads/2022/01/Acute_Behavioural_Disturbance_Final.pdf. (Accessed 15 April 2022.)
AoA 2010 Severe Local Anaesthetic Toxicity	Association of Anaesthetists. AAGBI Safety Guideline: Management of Severe Local Anaesthetic Toxicity. 2010. Available from: https://anaesthetists.org/Portals/0/PDFs/Guidelines%20PDFs/Guideline_management_severe_local_anaesthetic_toxicity_v2_2010_final.pdf?ver=2018-07-11-163755-240&ver=2018-07-11-163755-240. (Accessed 15 January 2022.)

SECTION 5: AIRWAY

WAO 2020 Anaphylaxis	Cardona V, Ansotegui I, Ebisawa M, et al. World Allergy Organization Anaphylaxis Guidance 2020. World Allergy Organ J. 2020;13(10):100472.
Resuscitation Council UK 2021 Anaphylaxis	Working Group of Resuscitation Council UK. Emergency treatment of anaphylaxis: Guidelines for healthcare providers. May 2021. Available from: https://www.resus.org.uk/sites/default/files/2021-05/Emergency%20Treatment%20of%20Anaphylaxis%20May%202021_0.pdf. (Accessed 17 January 2022.)
Resuscitation Council UK 2021 Adult BLS	Perkins G, Colquhoun M, Deakin CD, et al. Resuscitation Council UK: Adult basic life support Guidelines. May 2021. Available from: https://www.resus.org.uk/library/2021-resuscitation-guidelines/adult-basic-life-support-guidelines. (Accessed 17 January 2022.)
Resuscitation Council UK 2021 Paediatric BLS	Skellett S, Maconochie I, Bingham B, et al. Resuscitation Council UK: Paediatric basic life support Guidelines. May 2021. Available from: https://www.resus.org.uk/library/2021-resuscitation-guidelines/paediatric-basic-life-support-guidelines. (Accessed 17 January 2022.)
DAS 2017 Critically ill	Higgs A, McGrath BA, Goddard C, et al. Guidelines for the management of tracheal intubation in critically ill adults. Br J Anaesth. 2017;120:323–352.
NTSP 2012 Tracheostomy emergencies	McGrath B, Bates L, Atkinson D, Moore J. Multidisciplinary guidelines for the management of tracheostomy and laryngectomy airway emergencies. Anaesthesia. 2012;67(9):1025–1041.

SECTION 6: RESUSCITATION

NICE 2016 NG39 Major trauma	National Institute for Health and Care Excellence. Major trauma: assessment and initial management. February 2016. Available from: https://www.nice.org.uk/guidance/ng39/resources/major-trauma-assessment-and-initial-management-pdf-1837400761285. (Accessed 17 January 2022.)
RCEM 2019 Traumatic cardiac arrest	The Royal College of Emergency Medicine. Best Practice Guideline: Traumatic Cardiac Arrest in Adults. September 2019. Available from: https://rcem.ac.uk/wp-content/uploads/2021/10/RCEM_Traumatic_Cardiac_Arrest_Sept2019_FINAL.pdf. (Accessed 19 April 2022.)
EAST 2015 Emergency department thoracotomy	Mark S, Haut ER, Van Arendonk K, et al. An evidence-based approach to patient selection for emergency department thoracotomy: A practice management guideline from the Eastern Association for the Surgery of Trauma. J Trauma Acute Care Surg. 2015;79(1):159–173.
ERC 2015 Special circumstances	Truhlář A, Deakin CD, Soar J, et al. European Resuscitation Council Guidelines for Resuscitation 2015 Section 4. Cardiac arrest in special circumstances. Resuscitation. 2015;95:148–201.
European Guideline 2019 Major bleeding and coagulopathy following trauma	Spahn DR, Bouillon B, Cerny V, et al. The European guideline on management of major bleeding and coagulopathy following trauma: fifth edition. Crit Care. 2019;23(1):98.
BSH 2015 Major haemorrhage	Hunt BJ, Allard S, Keeling D, et al. A practical guideline for the haematological management of major haemorrhage. Br J Haematology. 2015;170(6):788–803.
ESICM 2020 Transfusion	Vlaar AP, Oczkowski S, de Bruin S, et al. Transfusion strategies in non-bleeding critically ill adults: a clinical practice guideline from the European Society of Intensive Care Medicine. Intensive Care Med. 2020;46(4):673–696.
BSH 2012 Transfusion reactions	Tinegate H, Birchall J, Gray A, et al. Guideline on the investigation and management of acute transfusion reactions: Prepared by the BCSH Blood Transfusion Task Force. Br J Haematol. 2012;159(2):143–153.
ESPEN 2013 Major burns	Rousseau AF, Losser MR, Ichai C, et al. ESPEN endorsed recommendations: Nutritional therapy in major burns. Clin Nutr. 2013;32(4):497–502.
ICS 2019 Gas embolism	The Intensive Care Society. Management of Patients with Gas Embolism: Guidance For Intensive Care and Resuscitation Teams. August 2019. Available from: https://www.ics.ac.uk/ICU/Guidance/PDFs/Gas_Embolism_guidance. (Accessed 17 January 2022.)

AoA 2020 Malignant hyperthermia	Hopkins PM, Girard T, Dalay S, et al. Malignant hyperthermia 2020: Guideline from the Association of Anaesthetists. October 2020. Available from: https://anaesthetists.org/Portals/0/PDFs/Guidelines%20PDFs/Guideline%20Malignant%20hyperthermia%202020.pdf?ver=2021-01-13-144236-793. (Accessed 17 January 2022.)

SECTION 7: SURGERY

ERAS 2018 Colorectal surgery	Gustafsson UO, Scott MJ, Hubner M, et al. Guidelines for perioperative care in elective colorectal surgery: Enhanced Recovery After Surgery (ERAS®) Society Recommendations 2018. World J Surg. 2019;43(3):659–695.
Gut 2005 Acute pancreatitis	UK Working Party on Acute Pancreatitis. UK guidelines for the management of acute pancreatitis. Gut. 2005;54(Suppl 3):iii1–iii9.
WSES 2019 Severe pancreatitis	Leppäniemi A, Tolonen M, Tarasconi A, et al. 2019 WSES guidelines for the management of severe acute pancreatitis. World J Emerg Surg. 2019;14:27.
ESVS 2019 AAA	Wanhainen A, Verzini F, Van Herzeele I, et al. European Society for Vascular Surgery (ESVS) 2019 Clinical Practice Guidelines on the Management of Abdominal Aorto-iliac Artery Aneurysms. Eur J Endovasc Surg. 2019;57(1):8–93.
NICE 2020 NG156 AAA	National Institute for Health and Care Excellence. Abdominal aortic aneurysm: diagnosis and management: NICE guideline [NG156]. March 2020. Available from: https://www.nice.org.uk/guidance/ng156/. (Accessed 30 March 2022.)
WSACS 2013 Abdominal compartment syndrome	Kirkpatrick AW, Roberts DJ, De Waele J, et al. Intra-abdominal hypertension and the abdominal compartment syndrome: updated consensus definitions and clinical practice guidelines from the World Society of the Abdominal Compartment Syndrome. Intensive Care Med. 2013;39(7):1190–1206.
Small Bowel and Nutrition Committee 2006 Short bowel	Nightingale J, Woodward JM. Guidelines for management of patients with a short bowel. Gut. 2006;55(Suppl 4):iv1–iv12.

SECTION 8: CARDIOTHORACICS

ESC ESH 2018 Hypertension	Williams B, Mancia G, Spiering W, et al. 2018 ESC/ESH Guidelines for the management of arterial hypertension. Eur Heart J. 2018;39(33):3021–3104.
ESC 2015 Infective endocarditis	Habib G, Lancellotti P, Antunes M, et al. 2015 ESC Guidelines for the management of infective endocarditis: The Task Force for the Management of Infective Endocarditis of the European Society of Cardiology (ESC). Eur Heart J. 2015;36(44):3075–3128.
ESC 2017 STEMI	Ibanez B, James S, Agewall S, et al. 2017 ESC Guidelines for the management of acute myocardial infarction in patients presenting with ST-segment elevation: The Task Force for the management of acute myocardial infarction in patients presenting with ST-segment elevation of the European Society of Cardiology (ESC). Eur Heart J. 2018;39(2):119–177.
ESC 2020 NSTE-ACS	Collet JP, Thiele H, Barbato E, et al. 2020 ESC Guidelines for the management of acute coronary syndromes in patients presenting without persistent ST-segment elevation: The Task Force for the management of acute coronary syndromes in patients presenting without persistent ST-segment elevation of the European Society of Cardiology (ESC). Eur Heart J. 2021;42(14):1289–1367.
NICE 2020 NG185 ACS	National Institute for Health and Care Excellence. Acute coronary syndromes: NICE guideline [NG185]. November 2020. Available from: https://www.nice.org.uk/guidance/ng185. (Accessed 24 January 2022.)
ESC 2015 Ventricular arrhythmias	Priori SG, Blomström-Lundqvist C, Mazzanti A, et al. 2015 ESC Guidelines for the management of patients with ventricular arrhythmias and the prevention of sudden cardiac death: The Task Force for the Management of Patients with Ventricular Arrhythmias and the Prevention of Sudden Cardiac Death of the European Society of Cardiology (ESC). Eur Heart J. 2015;36(41):2793–2867.

ESC 2021 Heart failure	McDonagh TA, Metra M, Adamo M, et al. 2021 ESC Guidelines for the diagnosis and treatment of acute and chronic heart failure: Developed by the Task Force for the diagnosis and treatment of acute and chronic heart failure of the European Society of Cardiology (ESC) with the special contribution of the Heart Failure Association (HFA) of the ESC. Eur Heart J. 2021;42(36):3599–3726.
ESC ERS 2015 Pulmonary hypertension	Galiè N, Humbert M, Vachiery JL, et al. 2015 ESC/ERS Guidelines for the diagnosis and treatment of pulmonary hypertension: The Joint Task Force for the Diagnosis and Treatment of Pulmonary Hypertension of the European Society of Cardiology (ESC) and the European Respiratory Society (ERS). Eur Heart J. 2016;37:67–119.

SECTION 9: NEUROSCIENCES

NICE 2021 SAH (Draft)	National Institute for Health and Care Excellence. Guideline: Subarachnoid haemorrhage caused by a ruptured aneurysm: diagnosis and management: Draft for consultation, February 2021. 2021. Available from: https://www.nice.org.uk/guidance/GID-NG10097/documents/draft-guideline. (Accessed 25 January 2022.)
Brommeland et al. 2018 BCVI	Brommeland T, Helseth E, Aarhus M, et al. Best practice guidelines for blunt cerebrovascular injury (BCVI). Scandinavian Journal of Trauma, Resuscitation and Emergency Medicine 2018;26:90.
NICE 2019 CG176 Head injury	National Institute for Health and Care Excellence. Head injury: assessment and early management: Clinical guideline [CG176]. January 2014 (Updated September 2019). Available from: https://www.nice.org.uk/guidance/cg176. (Accessed 04 March 2022.)
BTF 2016 TBI	Carney N, Totten AM, O'Reilly C, et al. Brain Trauma Foundation: Guidelines for the Management of Severe Traumatic Brain Injury 4th Ed. September 2016. Available from: https://braintrauma.org/uploads/13/06/Guidelines_for_Management_of_Severe_TBI_4th_Edition.pdf. (Accessed 28 January 2022.)
SIBICC 2019 TBI	Hawryluk GWJ, Aguilera S, Buki A, et al. A management algorithm for patients with intracranial pressure monitoring: the Seattle International Severe Traumatic Brain Injury Consensus Conference (SIBICC). Intensive Care Med. 2019;45(12):1783–1794.
ESO 2014 Spontaneous ICH	Steiner T, Salman RA, Beer R, et al. European Stroke Organisation (ESO) guidelines for the management of spontaneous intracerebral haemorrhage. Int J Stroke. 2014;9(7):840–855.
NICE 2019 NG128 Stroke and TIA	National Institute for Health and Care Excellence. Stroke and transient ischaemic attack in over 16s: diagnosis and initial management: NICE guideline (NG128). May 2019. Available from: https://www.nice.org.uk/guidance/ng128/. (Accessed 01 February 2022.)
AHA ASA 2019 Early management of stroke	Powers WJ, Rabinstein AA, Ackerson T, et al. Guidelines for the Early Management of Patients With Acute Ischemic Stroke: 2019 Update to the 2018 Guidelines for the Early Management of Acute Ischemic Stroke: A Guideline for Healthcare Professionals From the American Heart Association/American Stroke Association. Stroke. 2019;50(12):e344–e418.
ICS 2021 VITT	Intensive Care Society. *Intensive Care guidance for the management of vaccine induced immune-thrombocytopenia and thrombosis (VITT).* May 2021. Available from: https://www.ics.ac.uk/Society/COVID-19/COVID-19_Knowledge_Sharing_Summaries. (Accessed 02 February 2022.)
RCP 2020 PDOC	Royal College of Physicians. Prolonged disorders of consciousness following sudden onset brain injury: National clinical guidelines. London: Royal College of Physicians; 2020.
BMA & RCP 2018 CANH	British Medical Association and Royal College of Physicians. Clinically assisted nutrition and hydration (CANH) and adults who lack the capacity to consent: Guidance for decision-making in England and Wales. London: British Medical Association and Royal College of Physicians; 2018.
NICE 2021 CG137 Epilepsies	National Institute for Health and Care Excellence. Epilepsies: diagnosis and management. January 2012 (Updated May 2021). Available from: https://www.nice.org.uk/guidance/cg137. (Accessed 03 February 2022.)

NCS 2012 Status epilepticus	Brophy GM, Bell R, Claassen J, et al. Guidelines for the Evaluation and Management of Status Epilepticus. Neurocritical Care. April 2012. Available from: http://wfccn.org/wp-content/uploads/2018/02/Guidelines-for-the-Evaluation-and-Management-of-Status-Epilepticus.pdf. (Accessed 03 February 2022.)
JSS 2016 Meningitis	McGill F, Heyderman RS, Michael BD, et al. The UK joint specialist societies guideline on the diagnosis and management of acute meningitis and meningococcal sepsis in immunocompetent adults. J Infect. 2016;72(4):405–438.
NICE 2015 CG102 Paediatric meningitis	National Institute for Health and Care Excellence. Meningitis (bacterial) and meningococcal septicaemia in under 16s: recognition, diagnosis and management: Clinical guideline [CG201]. June 2010 (Updated February 2015). Available from: https://www.nice.org.uk/guidance/cg102. (Accessed 04 February 2022.)
IEC 2013 Encephalitis	Venkatesan A, Tunkel AR, Bloch KC, et al. Case definitions, diagnostic algorithms, and priorities in encephalitis: consensus statement of the international encephalitis consortium. Clin Infect Dis. 2013;57(8):1114–1128.
Neurology 2020 Myaesthenia gravis	Narayanaswami P, Sanders DB, Wolfe G, et al. International Consensus Guidance for Management of Myasthenia Gravis: 2020 Update. Neurology. 2021;96(3):114–122.
NICE 2016 NG41 Spinal injury	National Institute for Health and Care Excellence. Spinal injury: assessment and initial management. NICE Guideline [NG41]. February 2016. Available from: https://www.nice.org.uk/guidance/ng41. (Accessed 05 February 2022.)

SECTION 10: OBSTETRICS

RCoA 2018 Enhanced maternal care	Royal College of Anaesthetists. Care of the critically ill woman in childbirth; enhanced maternal care. August 2018. Available from: https://www.rcoa.ac.uk/sites/default/files/documents/2020-06/EMC-Guidelines2018.pdf. (Accessed 23 January 2022.)
OAA DAS 2015 Airway	Mushambi MC, Kinsella SM, Popat M, at al. Obstetric Anaesthetists' Association and Difficult Airway Society guidelines for the management of difficult and failed tracheal intubation in obstetrics.Anaesthesia. 2015;70(11):1286–1306.
NICE 2019 NG133 Hypertension in pregnancy	National Institute for Health and Clinical Excellence. Hypertension in pregnancy: diagnosis and management: NICE Guideline [NG133]. June 2019. Available from: https://www.nice.org.uk/guidance/ng133/. (Accessed 23 January 2022.)
RCOG 2016 PPH	Royal College of Obstetricians & Gynaecologists. Prevention and Management of Postpartum Haemorrhage: Green-top Guideline No. 52. BJOG. 2017;124(5):e106–149.
NICE 2019 NG121 Existing conditions or complications	National Institute for Health and Clinical Excellence. Intrapartum care for women with existing medical complications or obstetric complications: NICE Guideline [NG121]. March 2019 (Updated April 2019). Available from: https://www.nice.org.uk/guidance/ng121. (Accessed 23 January 2022.)
RCOG 2012 Bacterial sepsis	Royal College of Obstetricians & Gynaecologists. Bacterial Sepsis following Pregnancy: Green-top Guideline No. 64b. April 2012. Available from: https://www.rcog.org.uk/globalassets/documents/guidelines/gtg_64b.pdf. (Accessed 23 January 2022.)
RCOG 2019 Maternal Collapse	Chu J, Johnston TA, Geoghegan J, on behalf of the Royal College of Obstetricians and Gynaecologists. Maternal collapse in pregnancy and the puerperium. BJOG. 2020;127:e14–e52.

SECTION 11: PAEDIATRICS

NICE 2021 NG9 Bronchiolitis	National Institute for Health and Care Excellence. Bronchiolitis in children: diagnosis and management: NICE guideline. June 2015 (Updated August 2021). Available from: https://www.nice.org.uk/guidance/nh9. (Accessed 04 March 2022.)

ACC AHA 2008 ACHD	Warnes CA, Williams RG, Bashore TM, et al. ACC/AHA 2008 Guidelines for the Management of Adults with Congenital Heart Disease: A Report of the American College of Cardiology/American Heart Association Task Force on practice Guidelines (writing committee to develop guidelines on the management of adults with congenital heart disease). Circulation. 2008;118(23):e714–e833.
BSPED 2021 Children and young people with DKA	British Society for Paediatric Endocrinology and Diabetes. BSPED Interim Guideline for the Management of Children and Young People under the age of 18 years with Diabetic Ketoacidosis. 2021. Available from: https://www.bsped.org.uk/media/1943/bsped-guideline-for-the-management-of-children-and-young-people-under-the-age-of-18-years-with-diabetic-ketoacidosis-2021.pdf. (Accessed 05 January 2022.)
Resuscitation Council UK 2021 Newborn resuscitation	Fawke J, Wyllie J, Madar J, et al. Newborn resuscitation and support of transition of infants at birth Guidelines. May 2021. Available from: https://www.resus.org.uk/library/2021-resuscitation-guidelines/newborn-resuscitation-and-support-transition-infants-birth. (Accessed 05 January 2022.)
Resuscitation Council UK 2021 PALS	Skellett S, Maconochie I, Bingham B, et al. Paediatric advanced life support Guidelines. May 2021. Available from: https://www.resus.org.uk/library/2021-resuscitation-guidelines/paediatric-advanced-life-support-guidelines. (Accessed 05 January 2022.)
SSC 2020 Sepsis in children	Weiss SL, Peters MJ, Alhazzani W, et al. Surviving Sepsis Campaign International Guidelines for the Management of Septic Shock and Sepsis-Associated Organ Dysfunction in Children. Pediatr Crit Care Med. 2020;21(2):e52–e106.
RCPCH 2020 PIMS-TS	Royal College of Paediatrics and Child Health. Guidance: Paediatric multisystem inflammatory syndrome temporally associated with COVID-19. September 2020. Available from: https://www.rcpch.ac.uk/resources/paediatric-multisystem-inflammatory-syndrome-temporally-associated-covid-19-pims-guidance. (Accessed 6 January 2022.)

SECTION 12: MICROBIOLOGY

NHS 2022 Infection prevention and control	NHS England and NHS Improvement. National infection prevention and control manual for England. June 2022. Available from: https://www.england.nhs.uk/wp-content/uploads/2022/04/C1676_National-Infection-Prevention-and-Control-IPC-Manual-for-England-version-21_July-2022.pdf. (Accessed 29 August 2022.)
PHE 2022 HCID	Public Health England Oct 2018 (Updated May 2021). Guidance: High consequence infectious diseases (HCID). October 2018 (Updated August 2022). Available from: https://www.gov.uk/guidance/high-consequence-infectious-diseases-hcid. (Accessed 31 August 2022.)
BHIVA 2020 HIV Testing	Palfreeman A, Peto T, Buckley A, et al. British HIV Association/British Association for Sexual Health and HIV/British Infection Association Adult HIV Testing Guidelines 2020. 2020. Available from: https://www.bhiva.org/file/5f68c0dd7aefb/HIV-testing-guidelines-2020.pdf. (Accessed 24 January 2022.)
WHO 2021 Malaria	World Health Organization. WHO Guidelines for malaria. July 2021. Available from: https://www.who.int/publications/i/item/guidelines-for-malaria. (Accessed 24 January 2022.)

SECTION 13: MEDICINE

BTS SIGN 2019 Asthma	Scottish Intercollegiate Guidelines Network and British Thoracic Society. British guideline on the management of asthma: A national clinical guideline. July 2019. Available from: https://www.brit-thoracic.org.uk/quality-improvement/guidelines/asthma/. (Accessed 06 February 2022.)
BTS 2019 Bronchiectasis	Hill AT, Sullivan AL, Chalmers JD, et al. British Thoracic Society Guideline for bronchiectasis in adults. Thorax. 2019;74(Suppl 1):1–69.
NICE 2019 NG138 CAP	National Institute for Health and Care Excellence. Pneumonia (community-acquired): antimicrobial prescribing: NICE guideline [NG138]. September 2019. Available from: https://www.nice.org.uk/guidance/ng138. (Accessed 06 February 2022.)

PHE 2019 Influenza	Dunning J, Dabrera G, Pebody R, et al. Public Health England: Seasonal influenza: Guidance for adult critical care units. November 2019. Available from: https://assets.publishing.service.gov.uk/government/uploads/system/uploads/attachment_data/file/846879/Adult_Seasonal_Influenza_Critical_Care_Guidance.pdf. (Accessed 07 February 2022.)
BTS 2009 CAP	Lim WS, Baudouin SV, George RC, et al. BTS guidelines for the management of community acquired pneumonia in adults: update 2009. Thorax. 2009;64(Suppl 3):iii1–iii55.
GOLD 2017 COPD	Global Initiative for Chronic Obstructive Lung Disease, Inc. Pocket Guide to COPD Diagnosis, Management, and Prevention: A Guide for Health Care Professionals. 2017. Available from: https://goldcopd.org/wp-content/uploads/2016/12/wms-GOLD-2017-Pocket-Guide.pdf. (Accessed 02 March 2022.)
NICE 2019 NG115 COPD	National Institute for Health and Care Excellence. Chronic obstructive pulmonary disease in over 16s: diagnosis and management: NICE guideline [NG115]. December 2018 (Updated July 2019). Available from: https://www.nice.org.uk/guidance/ng115. (Accessed 07 February 2022.)
BTS ICS 2016 Acute hypercapnic respiratory failure	Davidson AC, Banham S, Elliott M, et al. BTS/ICS guideline for the ventilatory management of acute hypercapnic respiratory failure in adults. Thorax. 2016;71(Suppl 2):ii1–ii35.
NICE 2022 NG191 COVID-19	National Institute for Health and Care Excellence. COVID-19 rapid guideline: Managing COVID-19. Version 27.2. March 2021 (Updated July 2022). Available from: https://www.nice.org.uk/guidance/ng191. (Accessed 31 August 2022.)
NICE 2020 NG187 COVID-19 Vitamin D	National Institute for Health and Care Excellence. COVID-19 rapid guideline: vitamin D: NICE guideline [NG187]. December 2020. Available from: https://www.nice.org.uk/guidance/ng187. (Accessed 31 August 2022.)
ICS 2020 COVID-19 Airway	Intensive Care Society. COVID-19 Airway management principles. March 2020. Available from: https://www.ics.ac.uk/Society/COVID-19/PDFs/Airway_Management. (Accessed 31 August 2022.)
NTSP 2020 COVID-19 Tracheostomy	National Tracheostomy Safety Project. NTSP considerations for tracheostomy in the Covid-19 outbreak. March 2020. Available from: https://www.ics.ac.uk/Society/COVID-19/PDFs/Tracheostomy_and_COVID-19. (Accessed 31 August 2022.)
RCP 2021 Ethical dimensions of COVID-19	Royal College of Physicians. Ethical dimensions of COVID-19 for frontline staff. February 2021. Available from: https://www.rcplondon.ac.uk/news/ethical-guidance-published-frontline-staff-dealing-pandemic. (Accessed 07 February 2022.)
BTS 2010 Pleural disease	British Thoracic Society Pleural Disease Guideline Group. BTS Pleural Disease Guideline 2010. Thorax. 2010;65(Suppl 2):ii18–ii31.
ESC/ERS 2019 PE	Konstantinides SV, Meyer G, Becattini C, et al. 2019 ESC Guidelines for the diagnosis and management of acute pulmonary embolism developed in collaboration with the European Respiratory Society (ERS). Eur Heart J. 2020;41(4):543–603.
BTS 2008 ILD	Wells AU, Hirani N. Interstitial lung disease guideline: the British Thoracic Society in collaboration with the Thoracic Society of Australia and New Zealand and the Irish Thoracic Society. Thorax. 2008;63(Suppl 5):v1–v58.
KDIGO 2012 CKD	Kidney Disease: Improving Global Outcomes (KDIGO) CKD Work Group. KDIGO 2012 clinical practice guideline for the evaluation and management of chronic kidney disease. Kidney Inter Suppl. 2013;3(1):1–150.
RCP 2016 Hyponatraemia	Argentesi G, Jackson S, Clayton J, et al. 2016 Hyponatraemia: NUH guideline for initial assessment and management. 2016. Available from: https://www.rcplondon.ac.uk/file/4721/download. (Accessed 19 December 2021.)
SCCM 2020 Acute liver failure	Nanchal R, Subramanian R, Karvellas CJ, et al. Guidelines for the management of adult acute and acute-on-chronic liver failure in the ICU: cardiovascular, endocrine, hematologic, pulmonary, and renal considerations. Crit Care Med. 2020;48(3):e173–e191.
EASL 2017 Acute liver failure	European Association for the Study of the Liver. EASL Clinical Practical Guidelines on the management of acute (fulminant) liver failure. J Hepatol. 2017;66(5):1047–1081.

EASL 2018 Decompensated cirrhosis	European Association for the Study of the Liver. EASL Clinical Practice Guidelines for the management of patients with decompensated cirrhosis. J Hepatol. 2018;69(2):406–460.
EASL 2018 Alcohol-related liver disease	European Association for the Study of the Liver. EASL Clinical Practice Guidelines: Management of alcohol-related liver disease. J Hepatol. 2018;69(1):154–181.
ICA 2015 AKI	Angeli P, Ginès P, Wong F, et al. Diagnosis and management of acute kidney injury in patients with cirrhosis: Revised consensus recommendations of the International Club of Ascites. J Hepatol. 2015;62(4):968–974.
NICE 2021 NG199 Cloistridioides difficile	National Institute for Health and Care Excellence. Clostridioides difficile infection: antimicrobial prescribing: NICE guideline [NG199]. July 2021. Available from: https://www.nice.org.uk/guidance/ng199. (Accessed 09 February 2022.)
BSG 2019 IBD	Lamb CA, Kennedy NA, Raine T, et al. British Society of Gastroenterology consensus guidelines on the management of inflammatory bowel disease in adults. Gut. 2019;68(Suppl 3):s1–s106.
ECCO 2020 Crohn's Disease	Torres J, Bonovas S, Doherty G, et al. ECCO Guidelines on Therapeutics in Crohn's Disease: Medical Treatment. J Crohns Colitis. 2020;14(1):4–22.
ECCO 2022 Ulcerative Colitis	Raine T, Bonovas S, Burisch J, et al. ECCO Guidelines on Therapeutics in Ulcerative Colitis: Medical Treatment. J Crohns Colitis. 2022;16(1):2–17.
NICE 2016 CG141 UGIB	National Institute for Health and Care Excellence. Acute upper gastrointestinal bleeding in over 16s: management: Clinical guideline [CG141]. June 2012 (Updated August 2016). Available from: https://www.nice.org.uk/guidance/cg141. (Accessed 09 February 2022.)
BSG 2020 UGIB Care bundle	Siau K, Hearnshaw S, Stanley A, et al. British Society of Gastroenterology (BSG)-led multisociety consensus care bundle for the early clinical management of acute upper gastrointestinal bleeding. Frontline Gastroenterol. 2020;11(4):311–323.
BSG 2015 Variceal haemorrhage	Tripathi D, Stanley AJ, Hayes PC, et al. UK guidelines on the management of variceal haemorrhage in cirrhotic patients. Gut. 2015;64(11):1680–1704.
BSG 2002 Non-variceal haemorrhage	British Society of Gastroenterology Endoscopy Committee. Non-variceal upper gastrointestinal haemorrhage: guidelines. Gut. 2002;51(Suppl 4):iv1–iv6.
BSG 2019 Lower GI bleeding	Oakland K, Chadwick G, East JE, et al. Diagnosis and management of acute lower gastrointestinal bleeding: guidelines from the British Society of Gastroenterology. Gut. 2019;68(5):776–789.
BSH 2010 Thrombophilia	Baglin T, Gray E, Greaves M, et al. Clinical guidelines for testing for heritable thrombophilia. Br J Haematol. 2010;149(2):209–220.
BSH 2017 Sickle transfusion	Davis BA, Allard S, Qureshi, et al. Guidelines on red cell transfusion in sickle cell disease. Part II: indications for transfusion. Br J Haematol. 2017;176(2):192–209.
BCSH 2012 HIT	Watson H, Davidson S, Keeling D. Guidelines on the diagnosis and management of heparin-induced thrombocytopenia: second edition. Br J Haematol. 2012;159(5):528–540.
BCSH 2012 TTP	Scully M, Hunt BJ, Benjamin S, et al. Guidelines on the diagnosis and management of thrombotic thrombocytopenic purpura and other thrombotic microangiopathies. Br J Haematol. 2012;158(3):323–335.
BCSH British Transplantation Society 2010 Atypical HUS	Taylor CM, Machin S, Wigmore SJ, et al. Clinical practice guidelines for the management of atypical haemolytic uraemic syndrome in the United Kingdom. Br J Haematol. 2010;148(1):37–47.
SCCM 2017 CIRCI	Annane D, Pastores SM, Rochwerg B, et al. Guidelines for the diagnosis and management of critical illness-related corticosteroid insufficiency (CIRCI) in critically ill patients (Part I): Society of Critical Care Medicine (SCCM) and European Society of Intensive Care Medicine (ESICM) 2017. Intensive Care Med. 2017;45(12):1751–1763.
JBDS-IP 2021 DKA	Joint British Diabetes Societies for inpatient care. The Management of Diabetic Ketoacidosis in Adults. June 2021. Available from: https://abcd.care/sites/abcd.care/files/site_uploads/JBDS_02%20_DKA_Guideline_amended_v2_June_2021.pdf. (Accessed 10 February 2022.)

JBDS-IP 2022 HHS	Joint British Diabetes Societies Inpatient Care Group. The Management of Hyperosmolar Hyperglycaemic State (HHS) in Adults. February 2022. Available from: https://abcd.care/sites/abcd.care/files/site_uploads/JBDS_Guidelines_Current/JBDS_06_The_Management_of_Hyperosmolar_Hyperglycaemic_State_HHS_%20in_Adults_FINAL_0.pdf. (Accessed 14 April 2022.)
JBDS-IP 2018 Hypoglycaemia	Joint British Diabetes Societies for inpatient Care. The Hospital Management of Hypoglycaemia in Adults with Diabetes Mellitus. 3rd ed. February 2018. Available from: http://www.diabetologists-abcd.org.uk/JBDS/JBDS_HypoGuideline_FINAL_280218.pdf. (Accessed 14 April 2022.)
ATA AACE 2011 Hyperthyroidism	Bahn RS, Burch HB, Cooper DS, et al. Hyperthyroidism and Other Causes of Thyrotoxicosis: Management Guidelines of the American Thyroid Association and American Association of Clinical Endocrinologists. Endocr Pract. 2011;17(3):456–520.
ESMO 2016 Febrile neutropaenia	Klastersky J, de Naurois K, Rolston K, et al. Management of febrile neutropaenia: ESMO Clinical Practice Guidelines. Ann Oncol. 2016;27(Suppl 5):v111–v118.
ESMO 2017 Toxicities from immunotherapy	Haanen JBAG, Carbonnel F, Robert C, et al. Management of toxicities from immunotherapy: ESMO Clinical Practice Guidelines for diagnosis, treatment and follow-up. Ann Oncol. 2017;28(Suppl 4):iv119–iv142.

SECTION 14: PALLIATIVE CARE

ERC ESICM 2021 Post-resuscitation care	Nolan JP, Sandroni C, Böttiger BW, et al. European Resuscitation Council and European Society of Intensive Care Medicine Guidelines 2021: Post-resuscitation care. Resuscitation. 2021;161:220–269.
GMC 2010 Treatment and care towards the end of life	General Medical Council. Treatment and care towards the end of life: good practice in decision making. May 2010. Available from: https://www.gmc-uk.org/-/media/documents/Treatment_and_care_towards_the_end_of_life___English_1015.pdf_48902105.pdf. (Accessed 04 January 2022.)
UK Legislation 2013 The Coroners (Investigations) Regulations 2013	Legislation.gov.uk. The Coroners (Investigations) Regulations 2013. Chapter 28. 2013. Available from: https://www.legislation.gov.uk/uksi/2013/1629/part/7/made. (Accessed 20 April 2022.)
AoMRC 2008 Diagnosis and confirmation of death	Academy of Medical Royal Colleges. A code of practice for the diagnosis and confirmation of death. 2008. Available from: https://aomrc.org.uk/wp-content/uploads/2016/04/Code_Practice_Confirmation_Diagnosis_Death_1008-4.pdf. (Accessed 04 January 2022.)
DOH Northern Ireland (2019) Verifying life extinct	Department of Health (Northern Ireland). Guidelines for Verifying Life Extinct. Version 0.15. 2019. Available from: https://www.health-ni.gov.uk/sites/default/files/publications/health/Guidelines%20for%20Verifying%20Life%20Extinct.pdf. (Accessed 4 January 2022.)
FICM ICS 2018 Neurological criteria on ECMO	Meadows CIS, Toolan M, Slack A, et al. Supplementary Guidance for the Diagnosis of Death using Neurological Criteria when the patient is supported with extracorporeal membrane oxygenation (ECMO). 2018. Available from: https://www.ficm.ac.uk/sites/ficm/files/documents/2021-10/supplementary_guidance_for_the_diagnosis_of_death.pdf. (Accessed 31 March 2022.)
NHSBT 2012 Donor optimisation	NHS Blood and Transplant. Donation after Brain stem Death (DBD) Donor Optimisation Extended Care Bundle. Available from: https://nhsbtdbe.blob.core.windows.net/umbraco-assets-corp/4522/donor-optimisation-extended-care-bundle.pdf. (Accessed 04 January 2022.)

INDEX

Printed in the United States
by Baker & Taylor Publisher Services